SEEKING VALUE

Balancing Cost and Quality in Psychiatric Care

**Group for the Advancement of Psychiatry
Mental Health Services Committee**

Andres Barkil-Oteo, M.D.
Joseph Battaglia, M.D.
Colleen Bell, M.D.
Glen Davis, M.D.
Bruce Fage, M.D.
Joanna Fried, M.D.
Elizabeth Janopaul-Naylor, M.D.
Michelle Joy, M.D.
Nubia Lluberes, M.D.
Hunter McQuistion, M.D.
Jules M. Ranz, M.D.
Manish Sapra, M.D., M.M.M.
Deepika Sastry, M.D.
Sosunmolu O. Shoyinka, M.D.
Mardoche Sidor, M.D.
Anna Skiandos, D.O.
Wesley E. Sowers, M.D.
Michael J. Vergare, M.D.
Donovan Wong, M.D.

SEEKING VALUE

Balancing Cost and Quality in Psychiatric Care

Edited by

Wesley E. Sowers, M.D.
Jules M. Ranz, M.D.

AMERICAN
PSYCHIATRIC
ASSOCIATION
PUBLISHING

First Edition

Manufactured in the United States of America on acid-free paper
24 23 22 21 20 5 4 3 2 1

American Psychiatric Association Publishing
800 Maine Avenue SW
Suite 900
Washington, DC 20024-2812
www.appi.org

Library of Congress Cataloging-in-Publication Data

Names: Sowers, Wesley E., editor. | Ranz, Jules M., editor. | Group for the Advancement of Psychiatry. Committee on Mental Health Services, issuing body. | American Psychiatric Association Publishing, publisher.

Title: Seeking value : balancing cost and quality in psychiatric care / edited by Wesley E. Sowers, Jules M. Ranz.

Description: First edition. | Washington, DC : American Psychiatric Association Publishing, [2021] | Includes bibliographical references and index.

Identifiers: LCCN 2020037121 (print) | LCCN 2020037122 (ebook) | ISBN 9780873182256 (paperback) (alk. paper) | ISBN 9780873182263 (ebook)

Subjects: MESH: Mental Health Services—economics | Health Care Reform | Quality Assurance, Health Care | Social Values | United States

Classification: LCC RC440.8 (print) | LCC RC440.8 (ebook) | NLM WM 30 AA1 | DDC 362.196890068—dc23

LC record available at https://lccn.loc.gov/2020037121

LC ebook record available at https://lccn.loc.gov/2020037122

British Library Cataloguing in Publication Data

A CIP record is available from the British Library.

Contents

Part II

Where We Want to Go

Systems Interventions

Part III

Where We Want to Go

Professional Interventions

Part IV

Special Value Opportunities

Part V

Conclusions

Contributors

George Alvarado, M.D.
Medical Director, Behavioral Health, Northwell Health Solutions, Manhasset, New York

Elie G. Aoun, M.D.
General, Addictions and Forensic Psychiatrist

Ali Abbas Asghar-Ali, M.D.
Associate Director for Education, South Central MIRECC; Director, Geriatric Psychiatry Fellowship; Associate Professor, Baylor College of Medicine, Michael E. DeBakey VA Medical Center, Houston, Texas

Margaret E. Balfour, M.D., Ph.D.
Chief of Quality and Clinical Innovation, Connections Health Solutions; Associate Professor of Psychiatry, University of Arizona, Tucson, Arizona

Joseph Battaglia, M.D.
Assistant Professor of Psychiatry, Albert Einstein College of Medicine, Bronx, New York

Colleen Bell, M.D., FACHE, FAPA
Medical Director of Behavioral Health, Sulzbacher Center, Jacksonville, Florida

Victor J. A. Buwalda, M.D., Ph.D.
Chief Psychiatrist and Medical Director, Novadic-Kentron, Centre for Addiction Treatment, Vught, The Netherlands; Affiliated Researcher, Department of Psychiatry, Amsterdam University Medical Centers, Amsterdam, The Netherlands

Peter L. Chien, M.D., M.A.
Medical Director, Acute Recovery Center, Edward Hines, Jr. VA Hospital, Hines, Illinois; Affiliate Associate Professor, Department of Psychiatry and Behavioral Neurosciences, Loyola University Chicago, Maywood, Illinois

Allen S. Daniels, Ed.D.
Behavioral Health Consultant, Cincinnati, Ohio

Bruce Fage, M.D., FRCPC
Psychiatrist, Centre for Addiction and Mental Health, Toronto, Ontario, Canada

Mark Graham, LCSW
Vice President, Program Services, Coordinated Behavioral Care, New York, New York

Elizabeth Haase, M.D.
Associate Professor, Department of Psychiatry, University of Nevada School of Medicine, Reno, Nevada; Medical Director of Behavioral Health, Carson Tahoe Regional Medical Center, Carson City, Nevada; Chair, Climate Committee, Group for the Advancement of Psychiatry, Dallas, Texas

Ben W. Hunter, M.D.
Medical Director of Outpatient Services, Skyland Trail; Adjunct Assistant Professor, Emory University School of Medicine, Atlanta, Georgia

Kenneth G. Hunter
President, FTF Consulting LLC, Bluffton, South Carolina

Elizabeth Janopaul-Naylor, M.D.
Child and Adolescent Psychiatry Fellow, Clinical Instructor, New York University School of Medicine, New York, New York

Michelle Joy, M.D.
Attending Psychiatrist, Corporal Michael J. Crescenz VA Medical Center; Clinical Assistant Professor of Psychiatry, Perelman School of Medicine, Philadelphia, Pennsylvania

Gary J. Kennedy, M.D.
Vice Chair for Education, Professor of Psychiatry and Behavioral Science, and Director, Division of Geriatric Psychiatry and Training Program, Montefiore Medical Center, Albert Einstein College of Medicine; Department of Psychiatry and Behavioral Science, Montefiore Medical Center, Bronx, New York

Zev Labins, M.D.
Clinical Assistant Professor, Mt Sinai School of Medicine, New York, New York

Frances R. Levin, M.D.
Kennedy-Leavy Professor of Psychiatry, Department of Psychiatry, Columbia University, New York, New York

Collins Lewis, M.D.
Associate Professor of Psychiatry, Emeritus, Washington University Medical School, St. Louis, Missouri

Madeleine Lipshie-Williams, M.D.
Resident Physician, UCLA-Olive View Psychiatry Training Program, Sylmar, California

Nubia Lluberes, M.D., CCHP-MH, FAPA
Clinical Assistant Professor of Psychiatry, University of Texas Medical Branch, (UTMB), Richmond, Texas; Clinical Director, Jester-IV Unit, UTMB-Correctional Manage Care (UTMB-CMC)

Gabrielle Marzani, M.D.
Associate Professor, Department of Psychiatry and Neurobehavioral Sciences, University of Virginia, Charlottesville, Virginia

Brian G. Mitchell, Pharm.D., BCPS, BCPP
Residency Program Director, PGY2 Psychiatric Pharmacy Residency Program; Clinical Pharmacy Specialist—Psychiatry, Michael E. DeBakey VA Medical Center; Assistant Professor, Baylor College of Medicine, Department of Psychiatry and Behavioral Sciences, Houston, Texas

Keris Jän Myrick, M.B.A., M.S.
Chief, Peer and Allied Health Professions, Los Angeles County Department of Mental Health, Los Angeles, California

Ashwin A. Patkar, M.D.
Chief, Avance Psychiatry and Adjunct Professor of Psychiatry, Rush University Medical Center, Raleigh, North Carolina

Jorge R. Petit, M.D.
President/CEO, Coordinated Behavioral Care, New York, New York

Jules M. Ranz, M.D.
Clinical Professor of Psychiatry, Department of Psychiatry, Columbia University Medical Center, New York, New York; Senior Advisor to Community Psychiatric Nurse Practitioner Fellowship, Community Healthcare Network

Kyle E. Rodenbach, M.D.
Clinical Assistant Professor, Department of Psychiatry, University of Wisconsin School of Medicine and Public Health, Madison, Wisconsin

Patrick Runnels, M.D., M.B.A.
Chief Medical Officer, Population Health–Behavioral Health and Director, Population Health Education, University Hospitals; Director, Public and Community Psychiatry Fellowship, Case Western Reserve School of Medicine, Cleveland, Ohio

Sy Atezaz Saeed, M.D., M.S.
Professor and Chair, Department of Psychiatry and Behavioral Medicine, Brody School of Medicine; Director, Center for Telepsychiatry and e-Behavioral Health, East Carolina University; Executive Director, North Carolina Statewide Telepsychiatry Program, Greenville, North Carolina

Manish Sapra, M.D., M.M.M.
Executive Director, Behavioral Health Service Line, Northwell Health, Manhasset, New York; Clinical Assistant Professor of Psychiatry, Hofstra University, New York

Deepika Sastry, M.D., M.B.A., FAPA
Staff Psychiatrist, Louis Stokes Cleveland VA Medical Center; Assistant Professor, University Hospitals Cleveland Medical Center, Cleveland, Ohio

Alessandra Scalmati, M.D., Ph.D.
Associate Professor of Psychiatry and Behavioral Science and Associate Director, Geriatric Psychiatry Training Program, Montefiore Medical Center, Albert Einstein College of Medicine; Department of Psychiatry and Behavioral Science, Montefiore Medical Center, Bronx, New York

Amanda Semidey, LCSW
Vice President, Care Coordination Services, Coordinated Behavioral Care, New York, New York

Steven S. Sharfstein, M.D.
Clinical Professor of Psychiatry, University of Maryland; Past President, Group for the Advancement of Psychiatry; Past President, American Psychiatric Association; President Emeritus, Sheppard Pratt Health System, Baltimore, Maryland

Sosunmolu O. Shoyinka, M.D., M.B.A.
Chief Medical Officer, Philadelphia Department of Behavioral Health and Intellectual disAbility Services, Philadelphia, Pennsylvania

Wesley E. Sowers, M.D.
Clinical Professor of Psychiatry, University of Pittsburgh Medical Center; Director, Center for Public Service Psychiatry, Western Psychiatric Hospital, Pittsburgh, Pennsylvania

David A. Stern, M.D.
Director, Student Mental Health and Wellness; Assistant Professor, New York Medical College, Hawthorne, New York

Maria A. Sullivan, M.D., Ph.D.
Executive Medical Director, Medical Affairs, Alkermes LLC, Waltham, Massachusetts; Associate Professor of Clinical Psychiatry, Columbia University, New York, New York

Arthur Robin Williams, M.D., M.B.E.
Assistant Professor, Department of Psychiatry, Columbia University, New York, New York

Donovan Wong, M.D.
Medical Director, Didi Hirsch Mental Health Services, Culver City, California

Disclosure of Competing Interests

The following contributors to this book have indicated a financial interest in or other affiliation with a commercial supporter, a manufacturer of a commercial product, a provider of a commercial service, a nongovernmental organization, and/or a government agency, as listed below:

Ashwin A. Patkar, M.D.—Dr. Patkar is on the speakers bureau for Otsuka and Janssen Pharmaceuticals. He is a consultant to Allergan and U.S. World Meds. He has received grant support from Allergan, Sunovion, and Envivo Pharmaceuticals. He is a shareholder in Generys Biopharma and Synapse. His spouse is a shareholder in Centers of Psychiatric Excellence.

Ali Abbas Asghar-Ali, M.D.—Dr. Asghar-Ali receives research support from U.S. Department Veterans Affairs Merit Award and the Patient-Centered Outcomes Research Institute for research on ketamine for treatment-resistant depression.

Wesley E. Sowers, M.D.—Dr. Sowers is a consultant to Deerfield Behavioral Health Inc.

Maria A. Sullivan, M.D., Ph.D.—Dr. Sullivan is an employee and shareholder of Alkermes Inc.

Donovan Wong, M.D.—Dr. Wong is a shareholder of Doctor on Demand, a telemedicine company.

The following contributors have indicated that they have no financial interests or other affiliations that represent or could appear to represent a competing interest with the contributions to this book:

Elie G. Aoun, M.D.
Colleen Bell, M.D., FACHE, FAPA
Peter L. Chien, M.D., M.A.
Allen S. Daniels, Ed.D.
Bruce Fage, M.D., FRCPC
Mark Graham, LCSW
Elizabeth Janopaul-Naylor, M.D.
Collins Lewis, M.D.
Nubia Lluberes, M.D., CCHP-MH, FAPA
Gabrielle Marzani, M.D.
Jorge R. Petit, M.D.
Jules M. Ranz, M.D.
Sy Atezaz Saeed, M.D., M.S.
Manish Sapra, M.D., M.M.M.
Deepika Sastry, M.D., M.B.A., FAPA
Amanda Semidey, LCSW
Sosunmolu O. Shoyinka, M.D., M.B.A.
David A. Stern, M.D.
Arthur Robin Williams, M.D., M.B.E.

Preface

Health care in the United States costs too much and is of very uneven quality, and many individuals cannot access the care they need. The crisis of health care in the United States is a chronic problem that has persisted for decades, and because of vested economic interests and the polarizing politics of the twenty-first century, solutions, even the simplest ones, allude us. For psychiatric care, as well as more broadly conceptualized behavioral health care, the situation is more ambiguous and in some ways more critical. The investment and costs of behavioral health care, in contrast to general health care, are much more modest and in many sectors significantly lower than what is necessary. The low investment in behavioral health care contributes to the overall poor value of our health care system, because many of the high costs and poor outcomes in general health care are a direct result of lack of access to psychiatric treatment. Furthermore, we do not fund basic preventive actions that focus on mental health, such as regular exercise, nutrition, violence reduction, and education. These deficits are indicative of the stigma associated with mental illness and the devaluation of mental health care. Payers often resist paying for this care by questioning the "necessity" of treatment. Employers often discount the legitimacy of mental disability and often terminate employees with decreased productivity due to mental illness.

Both patients and doctors suffer in the U.S. scenario. Patients and their families have had to take on a greater share of the burden of expensive treatment due to high deductibles, large copays, and limited coverage. Clinicians are harassed with multiple regulatory requirements, burdening them with extra paperwork and time-consuming electronic health records, and high expectations for productivity in our fee-for-service environment.

The U.S. health system compares poorly with the rest of the world on every metric of health as well as cost. Our outcomes are significantly worse. Compared with other developed Western democracies, our costs are two to three times higher. Prices are extraordinarily high in the United States for virtually every health care "product." An outside observer is struck by the fact that health care is not considered a right or a public service in the United

States. As former CEO of Sheppard Pratt, the largest not-for-profit behavioral health system in the country, I marveled at our difficulties in collecting payments for essential behavioral health services at the same time that our special education services were reimbursed well. Education is considered a right in the United States. Health care is not.

In the United States, we have a mixed system of both public and private financing. The profit motive has placed additional burdens on the effectiveness and efficiency of health care. Extraordinary waste abounds in the U.S. health care system, ranging from two to four times that of other developed nations. To collect the bills at Sheppard Pratt, we had to employ several dozen individuals to interact with hundreds of insurance companies with complex copayments and rules for coordination of benefits. On top of that, our clinicians had to contend with managed care reviews, which often took many hours to avoid denial of payment.

This volume, superbly edited by Wesley Sowers and Jules Ranz, emphasizes that the value of psychiatric treatment and mental health care goes beyond the individual patient. The impact of limited access to mental health treatment on family, community, and the population at large has never been quantified adequately to justify to policy makers the major public and private investments in care and prevention. The value of mental health treatment for medical well-being and reduced medical costs, as well as quality of life, has a growing research base. This work is quite enticing as we think about value. Increased productivity of the nation's workforce is also an area of much promise in establishing the value of mental health treatment. Improving the interface between corrections and mental health is yet another way to enhance the value equation.

With its focus on value, this volume makes an excellent diagnosis of our ailing health care system. With a special focus on psychiatry and behavioral health care, it also suggests actions that can change our dysfunctional health care system for the better. Each chapter is written by leaders from the Group for the Advancement of Psychiatry, referred to as "America's think tank for mental health," and others who are deeply concerned about the experience of clinicians, individuals, and families as they endeavor to access quality health care and pay for these services. In addition to making a diagnosis, this volume provides a menu of reforms, both large and small, that would improve the experience of patients, improve outcomes, lower costs, and make the practice of psychiatry more fulfilling. Psychiatrists can provide transformational leadership in the current environment for care, and even more so in the future. However, psychiatrists cannot do this alone. They must work closely with other medical colleagues as well as nonmedical leaders in systems of care that have a close relationship to the process of recovery in the community. Employment, income support, and housing address the social determinants of illness and health that are strategic for individuals with mental illness and addiction. Working with peers and self-help are other key components for the change that is necessary to improve the value equation. Our advocacy is needed more than ever.

We know we can do better. A lot better. Read this book and see how.

Steven S. Sharfstein, M.D.

Introduction

This book is the product of the Mental Health Services Committee (MHSC) of the Group for the Advancement of Psychiatry (GAP). GAP is an organization of thought leaders in many branches of psychiatry, and the MHSC is one of 32 standing committees focused on a wide array of topics. As its name implies, MHSC has a broad mandate, and over the years it has directed its attention primarily toward issues related to systems of education and service provision. In the past 15 years, the committee has carried out several projects, and its findings or positions have often been published in one form or another.

One of the projects that occupied the committee from 2006 to 2014 was an attempt to define the role of psychiatrists in mental health systems. An article published in 2006 (Ranz et al. 2006) used American Psychiatric Association data to demonstrate that psychiatric practice has increasingly been taking place in publicly funded settings, as opposed to private practice. The article suggested that this trend demanded an examination of how psychiatric residents are being prepared to work in organizational settings.

In 2012, the MHSC described the extent to which psychiatric residents at 12 sites across the country were being trained in systems-based practices (Ranz et al. 2012). The study suggested that systems-based practices could be described by four factors, which the committee converted into four roles named 1) patient care advocate, 2) team member, 3) information integrator, and 4) resource manager. In 2014, the committee published a qualitative analysis of the residents' experience with the training they were receiving in systems-based practices and found that it was usually quite limited. The committee continued to examine the implications of these findings, with emphasis on the role of resource manager. It concluded that training to perform in this role was being seriously neglected (Arbuckle et al. 2014; Fried et al. 2014).

In addition to working on this long-term project, the committee developed several other interests between 2008 and 2016. One subgroup began to put together a pamphlet on career development stemming from a concern over the lack of satisfaction experienced by many psychiatrists who found themselves in jobs that did not coincide with their values and career expectations. A related topic taken up by the committee was the reduction in the scope of psychiatric training and practice, at the expense of developing skills in clinical activities such as individual, group, and family therapies. Another subgroup explored the ways and circumstances in which psychiatrists should provide primary care to the patients they serve (Sowers et al. 2016). The committee also explored ethical issues related to the misuse of diagnoses to access entitlements, and by extension, the meaning and usefulness of the current diagnostic system. A consideration of prescribing practices included the relevance of cost in the process, as well as pharmaceutical industry influence in clinical decision making (Barkil-Oteo et al. 2014).

In the early part of 2017, the MHSC began to consider future directions and ways to link the projects that had been explored in the preceding years. In doing so, a common theme began to emerge. All of these activities were related to improving the quality and/or the cost of the care that our systems deliver. They also fit well with our exploration of the role of psychiatrists as resource managers. Discussions took place in the context of growing recognition of the Triple Aim, introduced by Berwick and colleagues (2008) at the Institute for Healthcare Improvement. Triple Aim initiatives are designed to 1) improve the experience of care, 2) improve the health of populations, and 3) reduce the per capita costs of care for populations. Improving the experience of health care providers was later added as a fourth aim (Berwick et al. 2008; Institute for Healthcare Improvement 2017).

These concepts coalesced and led the committee to consider the need to elaborate them more clearly for issues related to emotional health. As it further researched the topic, the MHSC became aware that very little had been written on this topic or the role of psychiatrists in promoting value-based care. As a result, the decision was made to undertake the writing of this book.

In the first chapter of this book, we attempt to define *value*. The word *value* is commonly defined as outcomes divided by costs. This quotient can be calculated through the collection of data on specific measurements. However, a less tangible aspect of value also exists but is not so easily measured. It is sometimes described as "social value" or the well-being of society. Measurements of social goods are not always coherent or easily agreed upon and will often shift when considered by various stakeholder groups. We have attempted to include both aspects of value determinations in our writing and to consider them from various viewpoints. Throughout the book you will see this interplay between these two concepts of value and the clash between the interests of various constituents of the health care system.

The other concept that emerged during the writing of this book was the interdependent relationship between emotional health and physical health. These two aspects of health have an inseparable impact, and attempting to consider mental health independently would have been counterproductive. As a result, in many cases our research led us to consider value in the context of the health care system in general, and think about how its structure impeded the achievement of value throughout.

Part I of the book, titled "Where We Have Been," provides a historical overview of the forces that convinced us that this book would be a useful addition to the ongoing discussion of seeking value in U.S. behavioral health care. The chapter authors consider the origins of the disjoint systems of care that currently exist and provide some comparative information about the U.S. system relative to those of other developed nations. The impacts of social and political determinants of health in this country are also considered in this section, along with some of the initiatives that have actually improved the value of services in behavioral health to date.

Part II, "Where We Want to Go: Systems Interventions," focuses on correcting the flaws in our current fragmented systems. Important aspects of a solution include rethinking the way we finance health care, considering the role of market forces, and creating the right balance of financial incentives, along with changing the priorities and structures of our systems that have led to the poor health outcomes this country has experienced. Additional elements of needed change that are discussed are integration of services, prevention and health promotion, development of a peer workforce, applications of technology, and elimination of administrative waste.

Part III, "Where We Want to Go: Professional Interventions," turns attention to many of the enhancements that can be achieved without radical change in the systems in which services are provided. It pays particular attention to what the psychiatric profession and individual psychiatrists can do to improve value in these systems. Expansion of consultative roles, provision of the skills needed, alliance with other professionals and teamwork, reform of our diagnostic systems, cost consciousness in prescribing, advocacy, and leadership initiatives are all considered as interventions that can improve the value we seek.

Part IV, "Special Value Opportunities," discusses a variety of opportunities to improve population health and social well-being in areas of policy and practice that go beyond the typical role of clinicians and health care administrators, and in many cases beyond what we normally think of as health care. Harm reduction to address addictions, interventions to mitigate the impact of climate change, elimination of counterproductive incarceration practices, incorporation of healthy practices in the workplace, and reconsideration of care at the end of life all have ramifications for the reduction of social costs and population health that extend beyond their immediate, tangible health advantages.

The final chapter, in Part V ("Conclusions"), serves as an attempt to integrate the recommendations made throughout the book into a coherent framework or "vision" for health care reform. We recognize that the ideal is not always attainable in the short term, and that compromises may be needed to achieve an incremental reform that can eventually lead to the "best balance." The chapter presents some strategies and structures to help guide future reform efforts.

We recognize that a book of this type is rarely read straight through, from cover to cover. Each chapter is designed to stand on its own and to provide a coherent perspective on the topic it tackles. As a result, there is a small amount of unavoidable redundancy in some of the chapters. For example, while there is no chapter specifically dealing with depression, it is referred to in many of the chapters in this book. In many cases, when overlap occurs, readers will be referred to other chapters that contain a more complete treatment of the issue. Although we have attempted to provide a comprehensive view of problems and possibilities related to high-value systems of care, it is likely that we have missed some opportunities. It is our hope that psychiatrists, and other behavioral health practitioners, who read this book will participate in the search for value, which is arguably the most difficult challenge we face, and fill any gaps we have left. We hope that all readers will be inspired to delve further into processes that create value and that these pages will be useful to those who advocate for the changes that are so badly needed in the U.S. health care systems.

Wesley E. Sowers, M.D.
Jules M. Ranz, M.D.

Group for the Advancement of Psychiatry Mental Health Services Committee Members

Andres Barkil-Oteo, M.D., Joseph Battaglia, M.D., Colleen Bell, M.D., Glen Davis, M.D., Bruce Fage, M.D., Joanna Fried, M.D., Elizabeth Janopaul-Naylor, M.D., Michelle Joy, M.D., Nubia Lluberes, M.D., Hunter McQuistion, M.D., Jules M. Ranz, M.D., Manish Sapra, M.D., M.M.M., Deepika Sastry, M.D., Sunmolu Shoyinka, M.D., Mardoche Sidor, M.D., Anna Skiandos, D.O., Wesley E. Sowers, M.D., Michael J. Vergare, M.D., Donovan Wong, M.D.

Special thanks to Sara Hamel for her editorial assistance.

References

Arbuckle MR, Weinberg M, Barkil-Oteo A, et al: The neglected role of resource manager in residency training. Acad Psychiatry 38(4):481–484, 2014

Barkil-Oteo A, Stern DA, Arbuckle MR: Addressing the cost of health care from the front lines of psychiatry. JAMA Psychiatry 71(6):619–620, 2014

Berwick DM, Nolan TW, Whittington J: The triple aim: care, health, and cost. Health Aff (Millwood) 27(3):759–769, 2008

Fried JL, Arbuckle MR, Weinberg M, et al: Psychiatry residents' experiences with systems-based practice: a qualitative survey. Acad Psychiatry 38(4):414–419, 2014

Institute for Healthcare Improvement: The Triple Aim or the Quadruple Aim? Four points to help set your strategy. November 28, 2017. Available at: www.ihi.org/communities/blogs/the-triple-aim-or-the-quadruple-aim-four-points-to-help-set-your-strategy. Accessed February 2, 2020.

Ranz JM, Vergare MJ, Wilk JE, et al: The tipping point from private practice to publicly funded settings for early and mid-career psychiatrists. Psychiatr Serv 57(11):1640–1643, 2006

Ranz JM, Weinberg M, Arbuckle M, et al: A four-factor model of systems-based practices in psychiatry. Acad Psychiatry 36(6):473–478, 2012

Sowers W, Arbuckle M, Shoyinka S: Recommendation for primary care provided by psychiatrists. Community Ment Health J 52(1):379–386, 2016

Part I

Where We Have Been

1

Defining and Measuring Value

Bruce Fage, M.D., FRCPC
Manish Sapra, M.D., M.M.M.
Margaret E. Balfour, M.D., Ph.D.

This book is intended to help an array of behavioral health stakeholders to better understand and improve the value of psychiatric care and, more broadly, health services in general. As will become clear in subsequent chapters of this book, emotional health and physical health are tightly intertwined, and the systems and interventions that address health issues in the population will affect both of these conditions. In seeking value from our systems of care, we will explore in this book a wide variety of complex topics, such as health care financing, prevention, clinical practice, and workplace wellness. But first, we must begin with a fundamental question: What is *value?* How is it defined? Who should define it? How can it be measured?

Although there are multiple formal approaches to defining and measuring value in health systems, they can all be distilled to the simple core definition of outcomes divided by cost (V=outcomes/cost; Porter 2012). *Value* is sometimes referred to as cost-effectiveness or colloquially as getting the "biggest bang for the buck." In a broad definition of value, cost may include time, money, social impact, and other resources that may be direct (monetary) or indirect (social disruption) in nature. This determination is often complicated when there is disagreement about what the best outcomes are. Key stakeholders—providers, purchasers, suppliers, payers, and patients/consumers—may deem different outcomes important. Disagreement about value is primarily a disagreement about which outcomes are most important and whether or not the resources necessary to achieve them can be justified. Therefore, whoever has the power to decide which outcomes will define success holds a significant amount of influence.

Another, less tangible but no less important, concept of value has more philosophical and soul-searching implications. All individuals have personal "values" related to beliefs and customs (i.e., kindness, power, security). Communities or organizations may have shared values (i.e., individualism, conservation, acquisition), which may extend to entire states or nations. These "values" will influence what outcomes a particular stakeholder group will choose or prioritize. For example, many of those who go into health care have a desire to make meaningful contributions to society. If recovery-oriented (person-centered, collaborative) care is selected to improve the lives of the people in the population, those involved will want to ensure that the care is being delivered consistently and comprehensively. They will choose outcomes that reflect well-being, such as client satisfaction, independent living, or employment. Another stakeholder, such as an insurer or other payer, may be motivated by profit. The outcome they choose might be reduced use of expensive services or products, such as inpatient care or expensive medications.

In many cases there are "social values" that almost all constituents of the community agree upon, such as reduced violence, incarceration or homelessness, or increased employment, nutrition, or education level. Even though these outcomes are agreed upon, the means for achieving them, as well as the acceptable level of cost (both direct and indirect) associated with any proposed solutions, may be controversial. An example of these conflicts might be the outcome of reduced gun-related violence. For some members of the community, an inexpensive solution might be restricting or banning the sale or private ownership of guns. To other members, that solution is unacceptably costly in terms of personal rights and self-protection; they might propose better gun safety education and further arming responsible members of society, which will be an unacceptably ineffective solution to the first group. These controversies are the meat of political discord and often stand in the way of progress toward these common interests.

Although stakeholders will have different motivations, regardless of their personal values, they will want to set goals and to know to what extent they are achieving them and at what cost. Ideal solutions to an identified opportunity to increase value will allow all stakeholders to improve their conditions. Any useful discussion of enhancing value must define *quality* through a consensus of stakeholders. Finding indicators of quality and cost parameters that everyone can agree upon can be very challenging, but when they are discovered, they enable an objective assessment of the value everyone is seeking. In health care, creating accountability by measuring adherence to the indicators of quality that are selected, and establishing acceptable expenses for the methods used to achieve them, will allow systems to move toward greater value in the services and interventions they provide. This will benefit both the health of the organizations and the individuals providing care, giving meaning to the hard work put in day after day, and the populations they serve.

In this chapter, we provide an overview of current approaches to defining and paying for value in health care and describe methods for measuring and improving behavioral health outcomes. We conclude with a discussion of the challenges and potential for future advancements in the measurement of quality, cost, and person-centered outcomes. Subsequent chapters delve into the details of creating, financing, and maximizing value. We hope this opening chapter will provide a foundation to help the reader keep sight of the ultimate goal, which is to build sustainable models of care that improve the health and well-being of populations and communities.

Cost of Mental Illness and Substance Use

In 2010, the World Health Organization (WHO) estimated that mental health and substance use disorders accounted for a loss of 183.9 million disability-adjusted life years (DALYs), or 7.4% of all DALYs worldwide (Whiteford et al. 2013). Despite a relatively low contribution to overall years of life lost, mental health and substance use disorders are the leading cause of years lost to disability worldwide, with over 75% stemming from depression, anxiety, and illicit drug and alcohol use. Notably, the burden of mental health and substance use disorders increased by 37.6% between 1990 and 2010, an increase that was largely attributable to population growth and aging (Whiteford et al. 2013). These estimates are likely conservative; because of a variety of factors (including the exclusion of personality disorders from disease burden calculations), the burden of mental illness may be underestimated by almost one-third (Vigo et al. 2016).

In the United States, health spending is expected to grow at an average rate of 5.5% per year between 2017 and 2026, approximately 1% faster than the average expected growth in the gross domestic product (GDP). As a result, health spending as a percentage of GDP is expected to rise from 17.9% in 2016 to 19.7% in 2026, reaching $5.7 trillion annually (Centers for Medicare and Medicaid Services 2018b). The United States spends the most on health care from a per capita basis than any other nation in the Organisation for Economic Co-operation and Development (OECD), at almost 2.5 times the average among the 35 member countries, and 25% higher than the next highest spending country, Switzerland (Organisation for Economic Co-operation and Development 2017). Despite the higher level of spending, the people of the United States, on average, do not appear to enjoy improved access or quality on several metrics. For instance, the United States has the second highest rate of patients skipping physician consultation because of cost (22.3%) and by far the highest rate of patients forgoing prescription medication because of cost (18%), although wait times are less of a concern compared with some other OECD countries. From a quality metric perspective, the performance for the United States is mixed, with some metrics, such as 30-day mortality after acute myocardial infarction, being middle of the pack, and others, such as number of admissions to hospital for an exacerbation of congestive heart failure, trending toward the higher end. Even with high rates of spending, the United States does not have the best outcomes. Despite the prevalence and growing availability of evidence-based psychiatric treatments for mental illnesses, stigma at the individual and system levels plays a complex role in creating barriers to care at multiple levels (Corrigan et al. 2014). In addition to the direct costs of care provision, it is likely that many costs associated with mental disorders are indirect, including costs incurred from reduced labor supply and earnings, public income support payments, and consequences such as homelessness and incarceration (Insel 2008). With an emerging focus on mental health and concerted efforts to destigmatize mental illness, it is time for patients and providers to develop quality frameworks and demand value in mental health care.

The health care industry is facing many challenges in the United States. With increasing expenditures as compared with other high-income nations, there is no bigger challenge than reducing costs of services (Anderson et al. 2003). One way to reduce costs is to provide accountable or value-based care. As mental health providers adapt to these challenges, they have to face the daunting task of coming up with ways to measure quality, cost, and benefits, and thus defining value in mental health care provided to consumers.

Health care costs in the United States are driven in large part by the high costs of services in acute care facilities, expensive pharmaceuticals, and administrative costs, primarily in medical settings (Papanicolas et al. 2018). A 2015 report on utilization of Medicaid recipients noted that about 20% of the members have a behavioral health diagnosis but that this cohort accounted for 50% of total Medicaid expenditures (Medicaid and CHIP Payment and Access Commission 2015). Thus, when defining the value of mental health services, providers and policy makers need to assess the value of services in the interface between physical health and mental health. Mental health can cause significant effects on recovery from somatic illnesses; this has been widely studied in relation to access to care, compliance with treatment, and response to treatment. Patients with moderate to severe mental illness have a higher prevalence of physical comorbidities (Parks et al. 2006). Mental illness and substance use comorbidities are also related to higher total cost of care. These findings are not unique to the United States. In the United Kingdom, the National Health Services has studied and confirmed high costs related to mental health comorbidities in patients with chronic medical illnesses (Naylor et al. 2016). A landmark U.S. report commissioned by the American Psychiatric Association (Melek et al. 2018) highlights an opportunity for significant savings if comorbid psychiatric conditions are effectively treated in individuals suffering from chronic medical conditions. Using data from insurance claims, the authors reported on total health care costs of individuals suffering from chronic conditions in cohorts with and without comorbid mental health and substance use conditions. Individuals identified as having comorbid conditions were noted to have significantly higher costs. Furthermore, it was noted that the increased costs were related to expenditures for treating physical illnesses.

There is growing acknowledgment of social determinants of health and their effect on health care outcomes and costs. WHO's Commission on Social Determinants of Health has defined social determinants of health as "the conditions in which people are born, grow, live, work and age" (www.who.int/social_determinants/en). According to a national study on the modifiable factors that can affect health outcomes, such as life expectancy and quality of life, clinical care accounted for only 16% of the outcomes (Anderson et al. 2003). Other factors, such as socioeconomic status and health behaviors, are deemed much more influential in affecting the health of communities (Hood et al. 2016). As the awareness of social determinants of health grows, multiple stakeholders are starting to address them and at times are coming together to improve conditions in our communities to promote healthy behaviors and quality of life.

As part of New York State's Delivery System Reform Incentive Payment program, large health systems and community-based organizations collaborated to develop programs to address unstable housing and food insecurity (Feliciano and Romanelli 2017). Medicaid plans have introduced initiatives to screen for social determinants and reimburse for some social interventions (Bachrach et al. 2018). With regard to seeking value in these efforts, an emerging theme is to how to leverage improvements in social determinants of health and align them in value purchasing arrangements. This can be both a welcome change and a challenge for mental health delivery service organizations. Although the increasing focus on social determinants of health is relatively new to both payers and large health systems, many mental health service delivery organizations have been contributing to this work for decades. The challenge lies in measuring work and effort in nontraditional sectors and quantifying its value; this will require investment in a robust infrastructure around use of data analytics to capture and properly attribute the benefits of the work done outside the traditional health care delivery model. Social determinants of health are considered in greater detail in Chapter 4, "Social Determinants of Health."

The broad trend of consolidation in the health care industry has increased our ability to invest in large-scale programs. Growth of technology has been another catalyst in bringing change to traditional ways of providing mental health care. Some of the new initiatives in this regard have been in areas of integration of mental health services with primary care, as well as wider implementation of electronic health records, digital therapy tools, and telepsychiatry. These new offerings bring with them challenges of developing models for reimbursement in the existing fee-for-service payment methodology. Hopefully, the move toward value-based payments will align incentives with models for innovative solutions that promote accessible and high-quality mental health care.

Current Approaches to Maximizing Value

There are multiple established value-based strategies that seek to maximize outcomes and reduce associated costs. To better understand these varied approaches, one needs first to consider the stakeholders within the health system who have an interest in these outcomes and associated costs (Allen et al. 2017):

- *Providers*, such as physicians, hospitals, and health systems, facilitate the delivery of health care services.
- *Purchasers* include employers and government.
- *Suppliers* include pharmaceutical corporations and medical equipment or specialty vendors.
- *Payers* are the commercial and publicly available insurance plans.
- *Patients/consumers* are the intended recipients of health care services.

Although the interests and desired outcomes for each stakeholder group may overlap, at times they might stand in opposition to one another. Established value strategies attempt, in various ways, to address the needs of each stakeholder. We explore some formal value strategies—value-based insurance design (V-BID), cost-effective analysis (CEA), value-driven population health (VDPH), and the Triple (or Quadruple) Aim—to broaden the understanding of value in mental health services.

Value-Based Insurance Design

V-BID is an approach to cost sharing between payer and service users that attempts to balance costs associated with a specific intervention with the expected outcome (Chernew et al. 2014). Because almost all health-related interventions have associated risks in addition to potential benefits, clinicians and patients typically weigh these factors when making a decision about whether to proceed. Additionally, the risks and benefits will vary according to each patient's individual clinical situation. In traditional insurance reimbursement systems, when accessing a service, patients may need to make a copayment, the amount of which is generally constant per service and does not take patient variables into account. V-BID attempts to factor the clinical outcomes of the intervention or service into the copayment, such that services that provide the greatest overall benefit for the health of a population (i.e., preventive or primary care services) would require a lower copayment from patients who receive them, whereas services that have limited benefit for the health of a client or overall population (i.e., cosmetic surgery or life-sustaining interventions at the end of life) would have higher copayments attached. V-BID insurance plans attempt to recognize clinical nuances of specific situations and to take into account that the benefit of an intervention depends on both patient and provider factors, including where and when the service is delivered in the course of the disease process (Fendrick and Chernew 2017).

High-deductible health plans are another way that payers attempt to share costs with patients and discourage the overuse of unnecessary services. These plans, however, may also discourage the use of necessary services, thereby increasing the rate of cost-related nonadherence to evidence-based services. For example, a study reviewing the effect of these plans on diabetes mellitus management found that low-income patients experienced statistically significant increases in the number of visits to the emergency department for preventable acute complications of diabetes mellitus (Wharam et al. 2017). High-value health plans, predicated on V-BID, make use of low deductibles and copayments for the proactive management of chronic diseases while requiring higher deductibles for services that are perceived as lower value. This approach attempts to control costs and improve outcomes through better disease management, requiring less high-expense tertiary care. Insurance can be tailored to encourage specific behaviors in persons with chronic diseases. For example, patients with diabetes mellitus would have a low or no deductible for routine eye examinations, given the relatively higher risk of developing diabetic retinopathy. Patients who do not have diabetes mellitus would have a higher copayment or deductible for a similar eye exam, because it is less likely to have a significant benefit. Clearly, the use of variable cost sharing based on evidence of which practices are most likely to be beneficial to a particular person would encourage prevention and reduce the usage of expensive acute care resources for patients further along the disease continuum.

Several barriers exist to the implementation of V-BID (Chernew et al. 2014). From a payer or purchaser perspective, the reduction in copayments for higher-value and preventive services may result in increased access to these services, and thereby costs. Although in theory this could result in lower costs over the long term, it may result in increased costs in the short term. In addition, the selection of high-value services is predicated on two key factors: medical evidence to identify high-value interventions, and methods of determining which patients would receive the most benefit from them. Although there are certainly evidence-based treatments within mental health services, there is insufficient research to effectively identify or distinguish high- and low-value services. Data on patient characteristics and systems to manage these data are necessary to determine which patients would qualify for which services. Personal health information on risk factors and past medical history would be necessary to understand which patients would benefit from which services, and data infrastructure would be needed to store and meaningfully interpret this information.

Cost-Effective Analysis

CEA is an analytic tool that attempts to compare the costs and effects of alternative services for the same health concerns. It acknowledges the limited availability of resources and seeks to prioritize the achievement of the best health possible within those limitations (Neumann and Sanders 2017). CEA uses a ratio of incremental cost to incremental effect, and is differentiated from other cost analyses by the use of health outcomes as a measure—such as the use of DALYs or quality-adjusted life years (QALYs), cases of disease prevented, or years of life gained—as opposed to monetary measures (Sanders et al. 2016). CEA is applied by payers, suppliers, and providers as part of a focused inquiry into potential alternatives to determine which option would deliver the best health outcomes at the lowest cost.

QALYs represent a way of measuring quality and quantity of life and are calculated by multiplying a quality-of-life score (commonly referred to as the utility value) by length of time (Prieto and Sacristan 2003). Perfect health is assigned a utility value of 1, death is 0, and the full range of human health experience lies in between. For example, a year of life lived in perfect health is equivalent to 1 QALY, and a year lived in less than perfect health would be worth less than 1. By combining gains from improved quality and quantity of life into a single measure, QALYs can then be calculated for different treatments and can be used to compare cost-effectiveness. For example, suppose treatment A and treatment B are both used to manage condition X. Treatment A provides 3 years of perfect health (3 QALYs) and costs $50 per treatment, and treatment B provides 2 years of perfect health (2 QALYs) and costs $100 per treatment. Treatment A has a cost per QALY of $16.70, whereas treatment B has a cost per QALY of $50, making treatment A more cost-effective in this oversimplified illustration.

Several techniques have been established for measuring QALYs and determining the quality-of-life score for various conditions, including the visual analogue scale, the standard gamble, and the time trade-off (Knapp and Mangalore 2007). In the visual analogue scale, participants rate a state of ill health between 0 (worst health or death) and 100 (perfect health). The standard gamble is rooted in the von Neumann and Morgenstern (1944) theory of preference measurement. In the standard gamble method, individuals are given a choice: they can either remain in a state of poor health for a defined time period or choose a medical intervention that has a certain probability of either restoring them to perfect health or ruining their health. The probability is varied until the individual has equal preference for both options, and the utility value is determined from this metric (Bleichrodt and Johannesson 1997). In the time trade-off method, respondents are asked to decide between staying in a state of ill health (reduced utility) for a period of time, or returning to perfect health with a shorter life expectancy. The time is varied until there is no preference, and the utility value is calculated from this measure. In addition, established tools are available in the literature that can be used to generate QALY measures based on multiple health attributes (Knapp and Mangalore 2007).

The concept of a QALY is not without controversy. In studies involving mental health, QALYs have been used as an outcome measure with mixed success; it is suspected that some of the aforementioned methods of measuring QALYs and utility scores may be more effective for physical rather than mental health and that standard QALY-generating tools are not sensitive for the symptoms, functional issues, and quality-of-life concerns relevant to people experiencing mental illness (Knapp and Mangalore 2007). Even when QALYs are appropriately measured, health systems must address "willingness to pay." In health care, this amounts to determining how much is appropriate to spend per QALY gained by a particular treatment. In the United States, many cost-effective analyses use a benchmark of $50,000 per QALY in the assessment of cost-effectiveness for medical interventions. The roots of the establishment of this number are unclear and thought to stem from a decision in the 1970s to mandate Medicare coverage for patients with end-stage renal disease, because the cost-effectiveness of dialysis was approximately $50,000 per QALY at the time (Grosse 2008). However, determining a reasonable cost-effectiveness threshold for the QALY is a controversial and challenging process that necessitates an open discussion of the monetary value of human existence.

Part of the disagreement over the usefulness and validity of the $50,000 threshold derives from its adoption in the 1990s and the fact that inflation has not been taken into consideration since then. Some organizations, including WHO, have suggested that a threshold of two to three times the average per capita annual income may be more realistic; in the United States, this figure would be approximately $120,000–$180,000 based on a per capita average income of $60,000. The United States has legislated, through the Patient Protection and Affordable Care Act of 2010, against the explicit use of cost-per-QALY thresholds, but the usage persists (Neumann et al. 2014). Although a general threshold may be helpful as guidance for policy and decision makers, decisions about health care spending are complex and contextual. WHO has outlined limitations to the use of an explicit threshold, including the need to consider the spending in the context of other health system needs (Marseille et al. 2015). Being below the cost-effectiveness threshold alone does not necessarily make a particular treatment option the best one for the overall health of the population. Other factors, such as the health care budget and other pressing health system needs, must be considered. Funding is not infinite, and decisions will still need to be made regarding which interventions to implement, even if multiple interventions are below the threshold. In addition, these thresholds are largely untested. Although social willingness to pay may be a conceptually appropriate way to define *social value*, basing a cost-effectiveness threshold on a country's per capita GDP blatantly discriminates against those who are poor and is an arbitrary threshold that is not usually grounded in evidence of overall social benefit.

Value-Driven Population Health

VDPH is a relatively new approach that combines a theoretical underpinning with management frameworks in an effort to maximize the value of every dollar spent on population health (Allen et al. 2017). It aims to tackle the concurrent problems of high health care costs and mediocre aggregate health outcomes. It recognizes that contributions from five key stakeholder groups—providers, purchasers, suppliers, payers, and patients/consumers—play a role in the current problems facing health systems, and each group needs to manage outcomes and costs in combination to foster alignment. From a managerial perspective, VDPH provides a system of objectives, measures, and tools designed to improve stakeholder role performance.

Triple (or Quadruple) Aim

The Triple Aim is an approach that defines three key aims that are essential for the improvement of a health system: improving the experience of care, improving the health of populations, and reducing per capita costs of care (Berwick et al. 2008). The approach recognizes that each aim is critical to sustainable health system success and that the three do not function independently of one another. Making change in one may affect the others positively or negatively. For example, reducing the misuse or overuse of a diagnostic test may reduce per capita costs of care and have a negligible effect on population health. Increasing access to publicly funded psychotherapy may improve the experience of care and the health of the population but potentially increase per capita costs. Recently, there has been an increased focus on a fourth aim—improved provider experience—as a missing component of the Triple Aim and something that is essential for sustained health improvement. Over 46% of U.S. physicians report symptoms of burnout, and a principal driver of provider satisfaction is the ability to provide quality care (Bodenheimer and Sinsky 2014) (Table 1–1). Care providers and their supporting teams are human. Patients want quality care, and their care teams want to provide it. Physician and staff turnover can lead to disruptions in care and cumbersome searches to find replacements. Provider job satisfaction is critical to the long-term sustainability of health system and care delivery.

Measuring and Improving Quality Outcomes

The scientific approach to quality improvement (QI) in medicine can be traced as far back as Florence Nightingale's groundbreaking statistical analysis of the relationship between hygiene and mortality among soldiers wounded in the Crimean War in the 1850s (Kudzma 2006). However, the importance of QI did not come to the full attention of the U.S. health care industry until a series of landmark reports published in 2000–2001 by the Institute of Medicine (IOM), since renamed the National Academy of Medicine. *To Err Is*

TABLE 1–1. Health care's Quadruple Aim

Improving the patient's experience of care (including both patient satisfaction and clinical quality)
Improving the health of populations
Improving the per capita costs of health care
Improving the work life of clinicians and staff (including joy and meaning in work)

Human: Building a Safer Health System (Institute of Medicine 2000) exposed the troubling state of American health care, specifically the 45,000–100,000 annual deaths linked to preventable medical errors. A follow-up report, *Crossing the Quality Chasm: A New Health System for the 21st Century* (Institute of Medicine 2001), concluded that health care lagged other industries in terms of quality and safety by at least a decade and called for a fundamental redesign of the entire health system rather than incremental or piecemeal attempts at addressing the problem. Together, these works heralded a national call to action and laid out a framework for health care to systematically approach quality and safety as a priority.

The Institute of Medicine (1990) has defined quality as "the degree to which health services for individuals and populations increase the likelihood of desired health outcomes and are consistent with current professional knowledge" (p. 21), and defined safety as "freedom from accidental injury" when interacting in any way with the health care system (Institute of Medicine 2000, p. 4). It identified six aims to guide health care organizations in their improvement efforts (Table 1–2).

Building on this work, the Institute for Healthcare Improvement (IHI) introduced the concept of the Triple Aim in 2008 (Berwick et al. 2008), and a fourth aim, focused on improving the work life of clinicians and staff, was added in 2014 (Bodenheimer and Sinsky 2014) (see Table 1–1). Subsequent work by the IOM, IHI, and other key organizations, such as the Centers for Medicare and Medicaid Services (CMS), the Joint Commission, and CARF International, has further advanced the field of QI in health care. All have recognized a need to learn from and adapt advances in QI from other high-reliability fields such as manufacturing and aviation. A detailed discussion of applied QI methods (e.g., Plan-Do-Study-Act, Lean Six Sigma) is beyond the scope of this chapter, but these methods are considered further in Chapter 2, "Evolution of Funding and Quality Control in Health Care." For the purposes of this discussion, suffice it to say that a fundamental first step for any QI endeavor is the development of measures that reflect the quality of care being delivered. As Sir William Thomson, better known as Lord Kelvin, famously said, "If you cannot measure it, you cannot improve it."

TABLE 1–2. Aims to guide health care organizations in their improvement efforts

Safe: avoiding injuries to patients from the care that is intended to help them.
Effective: providing services based on scientific knowledge to all who could benefit and refraining from providing services to those not likely to benefit.
Patient-centered: providing care that is respectful of and responsive to individual patient preferences, needs, and values, and ensuring that patient values guide all clinical decisions.
Timely: reducing waits and sometimes harmful delays for both those who receive and those who give care.
Efficient: avoiding waste, in particular waste of equipment, supplies, ideas, and energy.
Equitable: providing care that does not vary in quality because of personal characteristics such as gender, ethnicity, geographic location, and socioeconomic status.

Source. Institute of Medicine 2001, pp. 39–40.

The Value of Quality Measurement

Quality measurement is often considered a necessary evil that one must undertake to meet regulatory requirements (and to get paid, as value-based contracting gains popularity). When designed and used effectively, however, quality measures reflect something more fundamental: they are the incarnation of value. *Value* in this context refers to both cost-effectiveness and the personal/social definitions of value discussed in the introduction to this chapter. This multifaceted definition of value is intertwined with the Quadruple Aim. Outcome measurement helps us determine how effectively we are using our resources to provide high-quality care that improves population health. Measuring adherence to personal and social values ascribes meaning and purpose for our work.

Aligning Metrics With Values

One technique to align quality measures with values is via the adoption of a Critical-to-Quality (CTQ) tree. This tool is designed to help an organization translate what the customer values into discrete measures (Lighter 2013). This tool has been used in the development of a core measure set for behavioral health crisis services (Balfour et al. 2016). A CTQ tree begins with a broad customer need. In the example shown in Figure 1–1, the customers are key stakeholders (providers, purchasers, suppliers, payers, and patients/consumers) and the need is "excellence in crisis services." This broad goal is broken down into quality drivers that the customer uses to determine whether or not the broader goal is met. In this example, the drivers representing the customer's values were defined as timely, safe, accessible, least restrictive, effective, consumer and family centered, and collaborative ("partnership"). These are consistent with the IOM's six aims for quality health care—that it be safe, effective, patient-centered, timely, efficient, and equitable (Institute of Medicine 2001; see Table 1–1)—while also focusing attention on goals unique to the behavioral health crisis setting. The final step is to define measurable performance standards for each driver. For example, measuring the percentage of patients discharged to the community (instead of a higher level of care) reflects performance for the driver "least restrictive."

Types of Metrics

It is important to understand various types of measures and at what point their application is most effective to support improvement efforts. Dr. Avedis Donabedian—an early pioneer of quality measurement in health care—developed the commonly used Structure-Process-Outcome model (Donabedian 2002):

1. *Structure:* the environment in which care is delivered. Metrics may describe organizational structure, resources, or staffing (e.g., staff-to-patient ratios, presence or absence of on-site psychiatrist).
2. *Process:* the techniques and processes used to deliver care. Metrics may describe the use of screening tools (e.g., percentage of patients screened for suicide risk) or the speed with which a specific intervention is completed (e.g., door-to-doctor time).
3. *Outcome:* the result of the patient's interaction with the health care system (e.g., injury, death, quality of life, change in symptom rating scales, readmissions).

Different types of measures are appropriate for different settings and purposes. Outcome measures are the most desirable. However, sometimes it is not feasible to collect outcome data, or it is not within the scope of an organization to change an outcome on its own. In these situations, a process or structure metric is more appropriate.

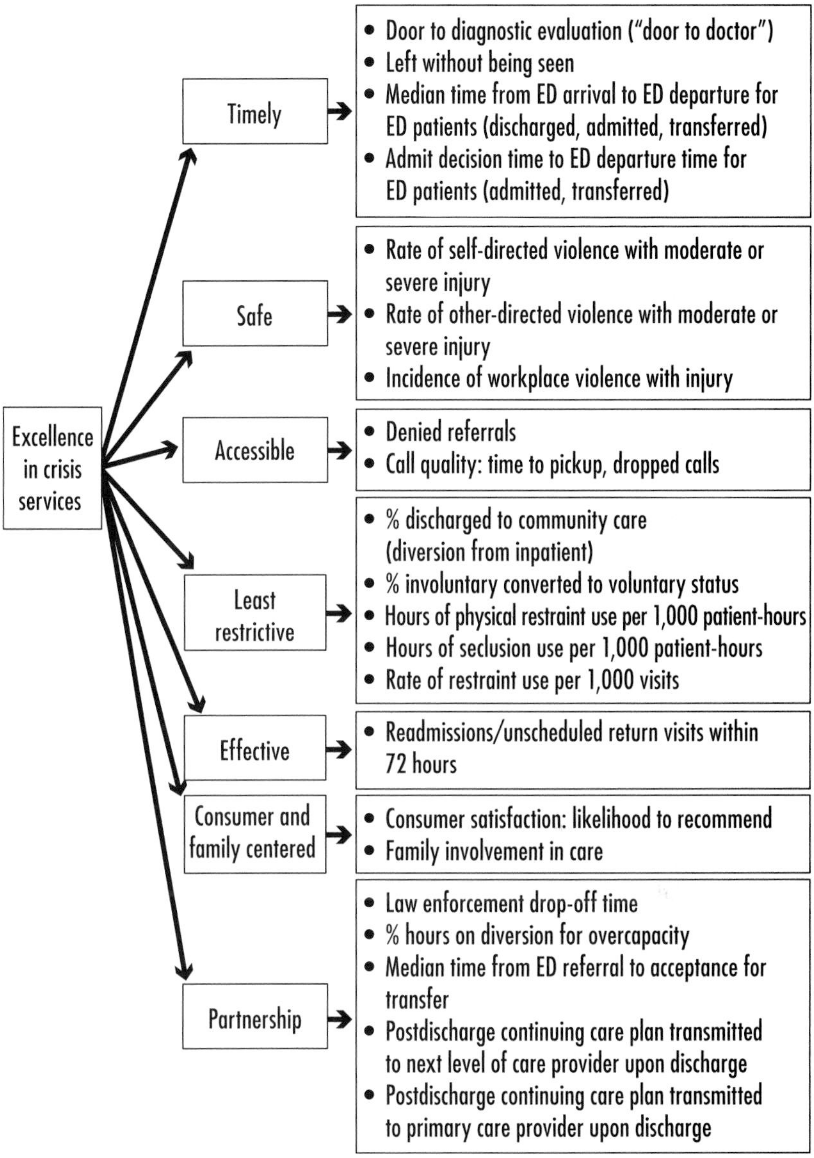

FIGURE 1–1. Critical-to-quality (CTQ) tree.

Example illustrating how a CTQ tree can be adapted to translate values into discrete metrics.

Source. Reprinted from Balfour ME, Tanner K, Jurica JS, et al.: "Crisis Reliability Indicators Supporting Emergency Services (CRISES): A Framework for Developing Performance Measures for Behavioral Health Crisis and Psychiatric Emergency Programs." *Community Mental Health Journal* 52(1):1–9, 2016. Copyright © 2016 Springer Nature. Used with permission under the terms of the Creative Commons Attribution 4.0 International License (http://creativecommons.org/licenses/by/4.0/).

Considerations for Implementation

Many frameworks exist to inform the selection and implementation of individual quality measures. A simple and straightforward approach, described by Hermann and Palmer (2003), requires that measures are meaningful, feasible, and actionable. The following list provides some key considerations regarding each of these requirements.

- *Meaningfulness:* Does the measure reflect a process that is clinically important? Is there evidence supporting the measure? Compared with other fields, there is a less robust evidence base for behavioral health measures, so we must often rely on face validity or adapt measures for which there is evidence in other settings. When possible, measures should be selected or adapted from items that have been endorsed by organizations that set standards for quality measurement, such as the National Quality Forum, the Centers for Medicare and Medicaid Services, the Joint Commission on Accreditation of Healthcare Organizations, and the Agency for Healthcare Research and Quality. Most of these organizations maintain online databases of measures available for use or adaptation.
- *Feasibility:* Is it possible to collect the data needed to provide the measure? If so, can this be done accurately, quickly, and easily? Data must be produced within a short time frame in order to be actionable. An organization's quality department staff should be able to spend most of its time addressing identified problems rather than performing time-consuming manual chart audits. With the advent of electronic health records, it is now possible to design processes that support automated reporting, making it feasible to quickly obtain data that were previously too complex or labor intensive to collect via chart abstraction.
- *Actionability:* Do the measures provide direction for future quality improvement activities? Are there established benchmarks toward which to strive? Are the factors leading to suboptimal performance within the span of control of the organization to address? For example, a stand-alone behavioral health crisis program is in a position to identify many problems in the community-wide system of care (e.g., lack of housing, ineffective outpatient follow-up after discharge) and can be instrumental in collaborating with system partners to help fix these larger issues (Balfour et al. 2018). However, the organization's own core measures must be within its sphere of influence to improve, or else there is the tendency to blame problems on external factors rather than focus on the problems it can address.

Quality Measurement in Behavioral Health

Behavioral health has lagged behind the rest of the medical field in terms of quality measurement. Behavioral health systems have long existed in a silo apart from the rest of the house of medicine, partly due to financing structures. Many behavioral health services are financed by Medicaid and various locally administered funds and are thus beholden to local regulation as much as nationwide federal standards. In both public and private sectors, managed care organizations often "carve out" behavioral health services into a separate managing entity, further leading to fragmentation and silos. Even federally funded behavioral health systems such as Medicare often exclude behavioral health when developing their measurement systems. For example, the Hospital Consumer Assessment of Healthcare Providers and Systems (HCAHPS), a patient satisfaction survey required by CMS for all hospital inpatients, excludes psychiatric inpatients (Centers for Medicare and Medicaid Services 2018a). Similarly, the Health Information Technology for Economic and Clinical Health (HITECH) Act provided financial incentives for health care organizations to demonstrate "meaningful use" of electronic health records to improve quality outcomes but did not include psychiatric facilities (Cohen 2015).

Currently, the most widely used behavioral health measures focus on inpatient psychiatric services, substance use screening, and outpatient depression care. The Hospital Based Inpatient Psychiatric Services core measure set was developed by the Joint Commission on Accreditation of Healthcare Organizations and adopted by CMS for its Inpatient Psychiatric Facility Quality Reporting program (Joint Commission 2019). The measure set includes metrics related to seclusion and restraint use, substance use screening, antipsychotic polypharmacy, and care coordination. The CMS Merit-based Incentive Payment System for physicians includes several measures related to depression screening, metabolic monitoring for patients taking antipsychotics, and coordination of follow-up care (Centers for Medicare and Medicaid Services 2019).

Fortunately, there is increasing momentum to develop additional standards and measures for behavioral health. The Interdepartmental Serious Mental Illness Coordinating Committee, an advisory committee created by the 21st Century Cures Act, recommended that federal quality and measurement initiatives include behavioral health in its initial report (Interdepartmental Serious Mental Illness Coordinating Committee 2017). The American Psychiatric Association is supporting measure development via the PsychPRO registry (American Psychiatric Association 2020) and has recently received grant funding from CMS to develop additional behavioral health measures for the Quality Payment Program (American Psychiatric Association 2018).

The opportunity to guide our own measure development is a pivotal moment for psychiatry. Via the selection and endorsement of measures, professional organizations and regulatory agencies can incentivize improvement in strategic areas of behavioral health care delivery. For example, the increasing focus on the 25-year mortality gap (Parks et al. 2006) between individuals with serious mental illness and the general population has increased emphasis on the value of whole-person health. This has led to the adoption of measures related to physical health and behavioral health integration. Physical health screening and disease management measures have become increasingly employed in behavioral health settings, and the Certified Community Behavioral Health Clinics demonstration program includes multiple measures related to preventive care and screening for diabetes and smoking cessation (Substance Abuse and Mental Health Services Administration 2010). Conversely, measures related to depression and substance use screening are increasingly common in primary care settings, which support the adoption of integrated/collaborative care models and measurement-based care.

An important challenge will be to develop measures supporting the delivery of recovery-oriented care. The Substance Abuse and Mental Health Services Administration (2012) defines *recovery* as "a process of change through which individuals improve their health and wellness, live a self-directed life, and strive to reach their full potential." Thus, recovery is both a process *and* an outcome, a fact that does not fit neatly into the frameworks described earlier in this chapter. However, application of the Critical-to-Quality approach (see earlier subsection "Aligning Metrics With Values") would focus on the key attributes included in the above definition of *recovery* to inform the development of more specific metrics. Improved health, wellness, and reaching one's full potential can be captured in quality-of-life measures. Self-direction is more complex, but a promising place to start is with measures of consumer satisfaction and shared decision making, both of which have been correlated with better treatment engagement and outcomes (Joosten et al. 2009; Lanfredi et al. 2014). Measuring recovery in this way reflects a more holistic concept of value that includes not only *what* care we as psychiatrists deliver, but also *how* we do so.

Conclusion

As the personal and economic burden of mental illness increases, there is a clear need to understand value in the context of mental health services. As a profession, psychiatry must participate in discussions and decision making surrounding the question of value. *Value* can be broadly defined as outcomes divided by costs, but the negotiations surrounding which outcomes are most important and how much should be spent are complex and challenging to navigate. There are multiple facets to value in mental health beyond the quality over cost equation in delivery of services. Mental health conditions are often unrecognized and undertreated in our communities (Kessler et al. 2005). Improving access—and beyond that, focusing on preventive care—is a new frontier for demonstrating the value of mental health services in our communities.

As noted earlier in this chapter (see "The Cost of Mental Illness and Substance Use"), costs for care are high for patients with mental health conditions because of the high prevalence of physical comorbidities. Thus, as new payment models develop that focus on shared savings programs, we see a great opportunity for increasing value by expanding access and improving the mental health care delivery models. Another area of value that needs further exploration is the interface of social services and health care delivery. Mental health service providers are well suited to guide this work because they have the most experience in working with the biopsychosocial model and have been working collaboratively with social service agencies for decades.

No discussion on improving value is complete without addressing the waste and inefficiencies that exist in the current system. It is estimated that in the United States, about 30% of health care costs are attributed to waste in the system (Berwick and Hackbarth 2012). Our field needs to analyze the true costs of our practices and invest in the comparative research of effectiveness of various treatment modalities. Among the various areas of waste that have been identified in health care, improving preventive care, enhancing care coordination, and reducing fragmented care are significant areas of opportunity in mental health services.

As experts in mental health, psychiatrists can play a unique role in defining value by working to bridge differences in perspectives between the various stakeholders involved in mental health care. Psychiatrists are often poised at the interface of the major stakeholder groups—providers, purchasers, suppliers, payers, and patients/consumers—and can link the evidence and clinical perspectives to the broader systems organization. The various stakeholder groups may have differing opinions on the outcomes that are most important and what they are worth. Psychiatrists have an opportunity to lead educational initiatives and foster a shared understanding of the biopsychosocial approach to managing patients appropriately. It is critical that psychiatrists remain engaged in administrative processes and focused on leading system change. One must be involved in order to influence, and we psychiatrists can use our collective voice to advocate for systems that deliver high-value care for all.

References

Allen H, Burton W, Fabius R: Value-driven population health: an emerging focus for improving stakeholder role performance. Popul Health Manag 20(6):465–474, 2017

American Psychiatric Association: APA awarded CMS funding to develop quality measures. September 21, 2018. Available at: www.psychiatry.org/newsroom/news-releases/apa-awarded-cms-funding-to-develop-quality-measures. Accessed February 4, 2020.

American Psychiatric Association: PsychPRO: APA's Mental Health Registry. 2020. Available at: www.psychiatry.org/psychiatrists/registry. Accessed February 4, 2020.

Anderson GF, Hussey P, Petrosyan V: It's still the prices, stupid: why the U.S. spends so much on health care, and a tribute to Uwe Reinhardt. Health Aff (Milwood) 22(3):89–105, 2003

Bachrach D, Guyer J, Meier S, et al: Enabling sustainable investment in social interventions: a review of Medicaid managed care rate-setting tools. The Commonwealth Fund, January 31, 2018. Available at: www.commonwealthfund.org/publications/fund-reports/2018/jan/enabling-sustainable-investment-social-interventions-review. Accessed February 4, 2020.

Balfour ME, Tanner K, Jurica JS, et al: Crisis Reliability Indicators Supporting Emergency Services (CRISES): a framework for developing performance measures for behavioral health crisis and psychiatric emergency programs. Community Ment Health J 52(1):1–9, 2016

Balfour ME, Zinn T, Cason K, et al: Provider-payer partnerships as an engine for continuous quality improvement. Psychiatr Serv 69(6):623–625, 2018

Berwick DM, Hackbarth AD: Eliminating waste in U.S. health care. JAMA 307(14):1513–1516, 2012

Berwick DM, Hackbarth AD, Whittington J: The Triple Aim: care, health, and cost. Health Aff (Milwood) 27(3):759–769, 2008

Bleichrodt H, Johannesson M: Standard gamble, time trade-off and rating scale: experimental results on the ranking properties of QALYs. J Health Econ 16(2):155–175, 1997

Bodenheimer T, Sinsky C: From Triple to Quadruple Aim: care of the patient requires care of the provider. Ann Fam Med 12(6):573–576, 2014

Centers for Medicare and Medicaid Services: HCAHPS Quality Assurance Guidelines V13.0. March 2018a. Available at: https://hcahpsonline.org/globalassets/hcahps/quality-assurance/2018_qag_v13.0.pdf. Accessed June 11, 2020.

Centers for Medicare and Medicaid Services: National health expenditures projections: 2017–2026. February 14, 2018b. Available at: www.cms.gov/Research-Statistics-Data-and-Systems/Statistics-Trends-and-Reports/NationalHealthExpendData/Downloads/NHEProjSlides.pdf. Accessed February 4, 2020.

Centers for Medicare and Medicaid Services: Explore measures and activities. 2019. Available at: https://qpp.cms.gov/mips/explore-measures/quality-measures?py=2019#measures. Accessed February 4, 2020.

Chernew M, Fendrick A, Kachniarz B: Value-based insurance design, in Encyclopedia of Health Economics. Edited by Culyer AJ. New York, Elsevier, 2014, pp 446–453

Cohen D: Effect of the exclusion of behavioral health from health information technology (HIT) legislation on the future of integrated health care. J Behav Health Serv Res 42(4):534–539, 2015

Corrigan P, Druss B, Perlick D: The impact of mental illness stigma on seeking and participating in mental health care. Psychol Sci Public Interest 15(2):37–70, 2014

Donabedian A: An Introduction to Quality Assurance in Health Care. New York, Oxford University Press, 2002

Feliciano A, Romanelli D: A brief report on the experiences of the community-based organizations in DSRIP 2016. New York Commission on the Public's Health System, 2017. Available at: www.cphsnyc.org/cphs/reports/a-brief-report-on-the-experience. Accessed February 4, 2020.

Fendrick A, Chernew M: Precision benefit design—using "smarter" deductibles to better engage consumers and mitigate cost-related nonadherence. JAMA Intern Med 177(3):368–370, 2017

Grosse SD: Assessing cost-effectiveness in healthcare: history of the $50,000 per QALY threshold. Expert Rev Pharmacoecon Outcomes Res 8(2):165–178, 2008

Hermann RC, Palmer RH: Common ground: a framework for selecting core quality measures for mental health and substance abuse care. Psychiatr Serv 53(3):281–287, 2003

Hood C, Gennuso K, Swain G, et al: County health rankings: relationships between determinant factors and health outcomes. Am J Prev Med 50(2):129–135, 2016

Insel TR: Assessing the economic costs of serious mental illness. Am J Psychiatry 165(6):663–665, 2008

Institute of Medicine, Committee to Design a Strategy for Quality Review and Assurance in Medicare: Medicare: A Strategy for Quality Assurance, Vol I. Edited by Lohr KN. Washington, DC, National Academies Press, 1990

Institute of Medicine: To Err Is Human: Building a Safer Health System. Washington, DC, National Academies Press, 2000

Institute of Medicine: Crossing the Quality Chasm: A New Health System for the 21st Century. Washington, DC, National Academies Press, 2001

Interdepartmental Serious Mental Illness Coordinating Committee: The way forward: federal action for a system that works for all people living with SMI and SED and their families and caregivers. December 13, 2017. Available at: www.samhsa.gov/sites/default/files/programs_campaigns/ismicc_2017_report_to_congress.pdf. Accessed February 4, 2020.

Joint Commission: Specifications Manual for the Joint Commission National Quality Measures, Version 2019A. 2019. Available at: https://manual.jointcommission.org/releases/TJC2019A/assets/Manual/TableOfContentsTJC/TJC_v2019A.pdf. Accessed February 4, 2020.

Joosten EAG, de Jong CAJ, de Weert-van Oene GH, et al: Shared decision-making reduces drug use and psychiatric severity in substance-dependent patients. Psychother Psychosom 78(4):245–253, 2009

Kessler RC, Demler O, Frank RG, et al. Prevalence and treatment of mental disorders, 1990 to 2003. N Engl J Med 352(24):2515–2523, 2005

Knapp M, Mangalore R: "The trouble with QALYs...." Epidemiol Psychiatr Sci 16(4):289–293, 2007

Kudzma EC: Florence Nightingale and healthcare reform. Nursing Sci Q 19(1):61–64, 2006

Lanfredi M, Candini V, Buizza C, et al: The effect of service satisfaction and spiritual well-being on the quality of life of patients with schizophrenia. Psychiatry Res 216(2):185–191, 2014

Lighter DE: Basics of Health Care Performance Improvement: A Lean Six Sigma Approach. Burlington, MA, Jones & Bartlett Learning, 2013

Marseille E, Larson B, Kazi D, et al: Thresholds for the cost-effectiveness of interventions: alternative approaches. Bull World Health Organ 93(2):118–124, 2015

Medicaid and CHIP Payment and Access Commission: Behavioral health in the Medicaid program—people, use, and expenditures, in Report to Congress on Medicaid and CHIP. June 2015. Available at: www.macpac.gov/publication/june-2015-report-to-congress-on-medicaid-and-chip/. Accessed February 4, 2020.

Melek S, Norris D, Paulus J, et al: Potential economic impact of integrated medical-behavioral healthcare: updated projections for 2017. Milliman Research Report, February 2018. Available at: www.milliman.com/insight/Potential-economic-impact-of-integrated-medical-behavioral-healthcare-Updated-projections. Accessed February 4, 2020.

Naylor C, Preety D, Shilpa R, et al: Bringing together physical and mental health: a new frontier for integrated care. Kings Fund, March 2016. Available at: www.kingsfund.org.uk/sites/default/files/field/field_publication_file/Bringing-together-Kings-Fund-March-2016_1.pdf. Accessed February 4, 2020.

Neumann P, Sanders G: Cost-effectiveness analysis 2.0. N Engl J Med 376(3):203–205, 2017

Neumann P, Cohen J, Weinstein M: Updating cost-effectiveness—the curious resilience of the $50,000-per-QALY threshold. N Engl J Med 376(3):203–205, 2014

Organisation for Economic Co-operation and Development: Health at a glance 2017: OECD indications. 2017. Available at: www.oecd-ilibrary.org/social-issues-migration-health/health-at-a-glance-2017_health_glance-2017-en. Accessed February 4, 2020.

Papanicolas I, Woskie LR, Jha AK: Health care spending in the United States and other high-income countries. JAMA 319(10):1024–1039, 2018

Parks J, Svendsen D, Singer P, Foti ME: Morbidity and mortality in people with serious mental illness. The National Association of State Mental Health Program Directors, October 2006. Available at: www.nasmhpd.org/sites/default/files/Mortality%20and%20Morbidity%20Final%20Report%208.18.08_0.pdf. Accessed February 4, 2020.

Porter ME: Value-based mental health care delivery. February 29, 2012. Available at: www.hbs.edu/faculty/Publication%20Files/2012.02.29%20Value-Based%20Mental%20Health%20Delivery_db29fc61-98a3-421d-a734-2c46d2989c73.pdf. Accessed February 4, 2020.

Prieto L, Sacristan J: Problems and solutions in calculating quality-adjusted life years (QALYs). Health Qual Life Outcomes 1:80, 2003

Sanders G, Neumann P, Basu A, et al: Recommendations for conduct, methodological practices, and reporting of cost-effectiveness analyses: second panel on cost-effectiveness in health and medicine. JAMA 316(10):1093–1103, 2016

Substance Abuse and Mental Health Services Administration: Programs: Section 223 demonstration program for certified community behavioral health clinics: quality measures. October 10, 2010. Available at: www.samhsa.gov/section-223/quality-measures. Accessed February 4, 2020.

Substance Abuse and Mental Health Services Administration: SAMHSA's working definition of recovery (HHS Publ No PEP12-RECDEF). 2012. Available at: https://store.samhsa.gov/system/files/pep12-recdef.pdf. Accessed February 4, 2020.

Vigo D, Thornicroft G, Atun R: Estimating the true global burden of mental illness. Lancet Psychiatry 3(2):171–178, 2016

von Neumann J, Morgenstern O: Theory of Games and Economic Behavior. Princeton, NJ, Princeton University Press, 1944

Wharam F, Zhang F, Eggleston M, et al: Diabetes outpatient care and acute complications before and after high-deductible insurance enrollment: a Natural EXperiment for Translation in Diabetes (NEXT-D) study. JAMA Intern Med 177(3):358–368, 2017

Whiteford H, Degenhardt L, Rehm J, et al: Global burden of disease attributable to mental and substance use disorders: findings from the Global Burden of Disease Study 2010. Lancet 382(9904):1575–1586, 2013

2

Evolution of Funding and Quality Control in Health Care

Deepika Sastry, M.D., M.B.A., FAPA

Historical Background

Since the beginning of human civilization, many cultures have regarded mental illness as a type of curse or religious punishment, as evidenced in ancient Egyptian, Indian, Greek, and Roman writings. In the fifth century B.C., Hippocrates, considered the father of Western medicine, was a pioneer in treating people with mental illness by using primitive medications and recommending changes to their environment or occupation. Through most of our history, however, fear, loathing, and ostracism of those afflicted with mental disorders have been predominant. From the Middle Ages through much of the eighteenth century, it was generally believed that individuals with mental illness were demonically possessed, morally weak, or biologically deficient; therefore, various remedies that reflected these beliefs were devised, including balancing bodily fluids, exorcisms, insulin shock therapy, and unhygienic and degrading confinement (PBS 2012).

In the United States, negative attitudes toward mental illness and resulting stigma persisted into the eighteenth century. It was only in the middle to late 1800s that reforms for more humane care of people with mental illness emerged, including moral therapy and provision of shelter, meals, and work opportunities. American activist and educator Dorothea Dix was a champion of such moral treatment reform, calling for "supportive care in kind and calming environments" and lobbying for better institutional living conditions for those with mental illness (Feldman 2012). In the 1850s and 1860s, despite her failure to obtain federal support, Dix tirelessly advocated for the plight of the mentally ill, resulting in the creation of 32 state-funded asylums (aka state hospitals) by the end of the 1870s (PBS 2012).

Beyond the Asylums

Institutionalization was embraced by mental health advocates, families, and communities as a safe and effective treatment for individuals with severe mental illness. In the first half of the twentieth century, asylums were the primary locus of care for people with mental illness who required long-term care or support (Fisher et al. 2009). But in the decades that followed, "insane asylums," as they were pejoratively called, became overwhelmed by an influx of people in need, such as orphans, the indigent, elderly individuals with dementia, and people with psychiatric sequelae of syphilis. The increased demand, poor funding, and understaffing of these facilities led to deterioration in humane care, leaving individuals with mental illness living in confinement with little hope for improvement in their condition.

These attitudes and practices began to change in the early to mid–twentieth century, starting in Europe, when the advent of psychoanalytic theory transformed the concept of mental illness with its focus on the unconscious mind. Developed by physician Josef Breuer and others in the late 1890s for patients with neurosis and what was referred to as "hysteria," psychoanalysis was practiced and developed further by Austrian neurologist Sigmund Freud (Gill 2009). By the 1930s and 1940s, psychoanalytic theories were widely accepted and practiced and disseminated to the United States and beyond. In another development, the serendipitous discovery and use of antipsychotic medication in the 1950s triggered a new era of biological psychiatry. Psychoanalytic techniques and neurologically focused treatment approaches began to legitimize psychiatric treatment, and the success of medications, such as the mood stabilizer lithium (first used in 1948) and the antipsychotic chlorpromazine (first administered in 1952), brought about profound changes in treatment. These medications could be manufactured inexpensively and often provided enough stability to allow patients to return to the community, thus decreasing the need for long-term hospitalizations and lowering the expense of the confinement of people with mental illness in state hospitals.

The Era of Deinstitutionalization

Deinstitutionalization refers to the movement of mental health patients out of state-run facilities and into community living. Ostensibly, deinstitutionalization was intended to improve the conditions for people with mental illness, but it was primarily driven by the desire to cut state government budgets. The number of psychiatric beds available per 100,000 people was 340 in 1955 but only 17 in 2005, reflecting a 95% decrease in a 50-year period (Fuller Torrey et al. 2008). Between 1955 and 1994, roughly 487,000 patients were discharged from state hospitals, reducing the availability of inpatient treatment that provided room and board, socialization, and mental and physical health care. The most rapid rate of deinstitutionalization happened after the passage of Medicaid in 1965 (Mechanic and Rochefort 1990). The trend continued for the next four decades, so that only 14 beds per 100,000 people were available in 2010, which was the same ratio as in 1850 (Amadeo 2018).

Legislation providing federal funding to states to provide community-based services, in addition to the development of efficacious medications, started the decline of state hospitals. This legislation began with the creation of the National Institute of Mental Health (NIMH) in 1948, to "transform the understanding and treatment of mental illnesses through basic and clinical research, paving the way for prevention, recovery, and cure" (National Institute of Mental Health 2013). The Community Mental Health Act of 1963 called for building 2,000 mental health centers in order to provide comprehensive community-based treatment for individuals with serious mental illness (SMI), as well as adults, families, and children dealing with stress (Feldman 2012). In the mid-1960s, the establishment of both Medicaid and Medicare opened new possibilities for eligible low-income adults and families, people age 65 and older, and people with mental health disabilities.

Medicaid was one of the factors that propelled deinstitutionalization. It was also a great financial boon to states because it provided federal funding for community-based treatment, as well as incentives to reduce the census of state hospitals, especially by providing funding for elderly patients with dementia to be discharged to nursing homes (Gronfein 1985). Since 1965, the growth of Medicaid has been tremendous; it is now the single largest payer of mental health services in the United States (Behavioral Health Services 2020). Deinstitutionalization was a gradual process, in large part because much of the infrastructure needed to treat the large institutionalized population was not yet in place (Amadeo 2018). In addition to advances in medications and psychotherapy, psychosocial rehabilitation and social supports were needed for successful community living. The Community Mental Health Center Act led to the construction of mental health centers that were meant to provide 24-hour psychiatric care for individuals with SMI; these centers offered options ranging from inpatient and outpatient services to day treatment programs to crisis intervention. Unfortunately, the federal government provided no funding for staff or programmatic support. Services varied from state to state, but on the whole the community mental health centers did not adequately meet the high demand for these services, again leaving those with SMI to fend for themselves in many cases (Feldman 2012).

Alternative sources of financing for community-based support for individuals with SMI were developed under the auspices of the Social Security Administration (SSA), which provided an expansion of the Social Security Disability Insurance (SSDI) program in the 1970s and creation of the Supplemental Security Income (SSI) program in 1972. SSI is a federal income supplement program funded by general tax revenues to help individuals who are disabled, blind, or at least 65 years old who have little or no income or work history, whereas SSDI is funded through Social Security payroll taxes and pays benefits to those under 65 years of age who have work histories but have a qualifying severe disability. Individuals with psychiatric disabilities constitute the largest subgroup of beneficiaries, even though disability policy was technically not designed for them. SMI tends to be diagnosed earlier in life, which is why these individuals are younger than most other beneficiaries and therefore remain on the rolls for much longer. Also, SMIs are characterized by fluctuating courses, partly as a result of varied responses to treatments and psychosocial interventions, whereas chronic and/or terminal physical illnesses have more steady, longitudinal declines. Individuals with SMI also tend to have comorbid medical illnesses and substance use disorders as well as cognitive deficits; these comorbidities can lead to ongoing, complex disability that necessitates more longitudinal support.

The Community Mental Health Centers Amendments of 1975 allocated additional money for community-based services, such as intensive case management, community outreach, and supportive housing. Nevertheless, there was still not enough federal funding to accommodate the exodus of patients from institutions to the community following the census reduction in or closure of state hospitals. President Jimmy Carter tried to rectify this problem with the Mental Health Systems Act of 1980, which provided grants to better fund and support community mental health centers. However, just a year later, in August 1981, President Ronald Reagan signed the Omnibus Budget Reconciliation Act, which repealed most of the Mental Health Systems Act, thus eliminating many services for people struggling with mental illness (Ford 2015).

State psychiatric hospital closures led to a reduction in the availability of long-term, inpatient treatment facilities. Between 1950 and 2005, there was a 37% decline in state psychiatric hospitals and a 90% reduction in state hospital patients, with the majority of closures occurring in the 1950s–1970s. There are still state-owned psychiatric inpatient beds in every state that are operated for individuals who need a high level of mental health services, but these beds are far fewer than before. As of 2014, there were 188 operational state psychiatric hospitals in the United States, a 42% decline compared with 322 state psychiatric hospitals in 1950 (Lutterman and Manderscheid 2017).

The reduced availability of long-term hospital care has caused many individuals to decompensate, thereby straining emergency departments with patients waiting for acute care beds to open and increasing family and caregiver burden. Although states reduced spending on state-supported hospital beds, costs for some services, such as room and board, were shifted to other lines of state budgets. However, considering this shifting in addition to the subsidies provided by the federal government through Medicaid, it is not clear that there has been an overall decrease in public spending for people with SMI (Frank and Glied 2006). According to 2014 data, of individuals discharged from U.S. hospitals, approximately 13% of those receiving treatment for mental health disorders and 10% of those receiving treatment for substance use disorders are readmitted within 30 days, a finding that is indicative of inadequate development of community services (Kamal 2017).

The Modern Era: Biological Psychiatry and Recovery

In the later part of the twentieth century, the trend toward more biological treatment modalities continued, fostered by the discovery and application of new psychotropic medications ranging from antidepressants such as fluoxetine in the 1980s to atypical antipsychotics such as risperidone and quetiapine in the 1990s and aripiprazole and ziprasidone in the early 2000s. The hope was that medications would be an effective yet inexpensive way to treat mental illnesses. Ironically, in the modern era, the cost of psychotropic medications has skyrocketed, in many cases resulting in the restriction of their use by insurance companies or other payers that administer Medicaid. This limitation can have a significant impact on individuals with chronic mental illness, who require therapy and medications on an ongoing basis. One in six U.S. adults reported taking psychiatric medications at least once in 2013, and nearly 17% of U.S. adults that same year filled one or more prescriptions for psychiatric medications (Moore and Mattison 2017).

However, even the most efficacious medications could not ameliorate the psychosocial impact of severe mental illness and substance use. This recognition led to more widespread use of psychosocial and vocational rehabilitation interventions beginning in the 1970s and continuing through the 2000s.

The Clubhouse model of psychosocial rehabilitation offered people living with mental illness a "restorative environment" and opportunities for friendship, employment, housing, education, and access to medical and psychiatric services and support to maintain their recovery. The first Clubhouse in the United States was Fountain House, established in 1948 in New York City (Clubhouse International 2018). Others followed, each providing an inclusive and welcoming community.

In Clubhouses and other rehabilitation settings, services such as family psychoeducation, supported employment, peer support, and living skills training provided the foundation for member self-determination and the recovery movement. Although these services have a significant impact on participants' quality of life, it is not clear how much they reduce mental health costs. There is evidence that Clubhouse participation can delay and reduce rates of rehospitalization for individuals with SMI; however, those cost savings may be offset by higher levels of intensive mental health services such as case management and residence in a supervised setting (McKay et al. 2018). Further studies with more rigorous methodology are needed to determine the cost-effectiveness and efficacy of rehabilitation activities.

The recovery paradigm was strengthened in 2003 when President George W. Bush's New Freedom Commission on Mental Health issued its comprehensive review of public and private mental health service delivery systems (President's New Freedom Commission on Mental Health 2003). The recovery model for adults with severe mental illness was defined by the Substance Abuse and Mental Health Services Administration (SAMHSA) as "a process of change through which individuals improve their health and wellness, live a self-directed life, and strive to reach their full potential." This approach heralded a new era in behavioral health treatment, one that provided hope for improvement in emotional health, including substance use, and the possibility of effective management and even recovery from mental illness (Substance Abuse and Mental Health Services Administration 2019).

Although this framework has had important implications for the cost and quality of care for individuals with severe mental illness, the transition to a community-based system of care and the recovery paradigm has not been smooth. Rather, it has encountered political, social, and economic potholes within the market-driven health care system of the United States. As noted in a 2005 article, "Efforts to transfer responsibility/costs between and among agencies, states, and the federal government...resulted in confusion, complexity in access to payment of services.... [W]hat developed was lack of consistent national mental health policies...that led to a piecemeal financial system that diffused accountability, encouraged cost shifting, and obscured service responsibility... resulting in vulnerable populations being poorly served or abandoned" (Grazier et al. 2005, p. 549).

Mental Health Costs Post-Deinstitutionalization

In 1971, the United States spent an estimated $8.96 billion on mental health care, making up about 0.84% of the Gross Domestic Product (GDP) that year. The system continued to rely heavily on institutional care, with an estimated 433,000 patients hospitalized for mental illness, which was only a 22% decrease compared with just 16 years earlier in 1955, when there was a peak of 558,000 patients hospitalized with mental illness (Amadeo 2018). Thirty years later, in 2001, mental health care spending was $85.4 billion, nearly 10 times greater than in 1971 but still making up only 0.84% of the year's GDP.

A superficial interpretation of the relatively low GDP share for mental health spending of around 1% over this time is that behavioral health is not a very significant contributor to overall health status. In reality, the picture is much more complex. Spending is not necessarily a reflection of the disability burden or of the true cost related to mental illness and substance use. Insurers in many cases have limited spending on mental health services, and the indirect costs of social services and lost productivity are not included in these calculations. Even with the passage of the Mental Health Parity and Addiction Equity Act in 2008, coverage for behavioral health has not been sufficient. Many people with needs for treatment do not receive it due to expense, accessibility, and stigma associated with a mental health diagnosis. Ultimately, mental health spending has not grown as a share of national income for over 40 years due to the fragmented nature of funding. Much of the costs are indirect, such as decreased worker productivity, loss of income, and increased expenses for a social safety net. People with undertreated or untreated mental illness are also at increased risk of developing medical illnesses such as obesity and cardiovascular disease. As a result, many of its costs are shifted to other areas of the budget that are not captured as "mental health" spending. There is growing recognition that emotional health issues have significant expense associated with them, but there is continuing concern that mental health spending could be curtailed by cost containment efforts when resources are scarce (Frank and Glied 2006).

The shortage of adequate psychiatric treatment has resulted in over 2.2 million patients with severe mental illness not receiving proper care. Nearly one-third of the total homeless population, about 200,000 individuals, suffer from schizophrenia or bipolar disorder. Over 300,000 people with mental illness are in correctional facilities, with 16% of inmates diagnosed with severe mental illness. As of 2014, there were 10 times as many people with SMI in prisons and jails than in hospitals (Amadeo 2018).

Overall, demand for mental health services has been rising, with utilization of mental health care by the noninstitutionalized population increasing by 50% from 1977 to 2006. The 2016 National Survey on Drug Use and Health administered by SAMHSA found that 44.7 million Americans, or nearly one in five adults, reported having a mental illness (Substance Abuse and Mental Health Services Administration 2017). According to the 2015 Kaiser Family Foundation Global Burden of Disease survey, mental health and substance use disorders are the leading cause of disability-adjusted life years (DALYs) and have been rising steadily for the past two decades (Cox and Sawyer 2017). In 2008, mental illnesses resulted in $193 billion in lost earnings in the United States. According to data from the Bureau of Economic Analysis, cited in the same Kaiser Family Foundation survey, noninstitutionalized spending on mental illness in 2013 was $89 billion, with the number of treated mental illness cases growing at an average annual rate of 2.8% from 2000 to 2012.

The Development of Managed Care

Private health insurance has been a significant payer of health care expenses in the United States since the early part of the twentieth century. Although this continues to be the case, rising costs of care have resulted in more active management of treatment delivered by providers, in an attempt to control costs. This oversight of treatment to control costs has come to be known as *managed care*. Medicaid has had an increasing role in the payment of behavioral health treatment and is now the major payer for these services. Because of concern with the high costs of care, most states have now contracted with managed care companies to manage Medicaid services.

Historical Overview

Managed care had its origins in 1973, when the Health Maintenance Organization Act was passed as a means of curbing health care cost inflation. The act provided funding for the creation and expansion of health maintenance organizations (HMOs), medical insurance groups that provide a range of direct health services for a fixed annual fee. These organizations emphasize primary care and prevention. Essentially, an HMO attempts to provide care within its network of employed and contracted professionals and to control access to specialty treatments (Forrest and Reid 1997). As time progressed, HMOs concentrated more and more on this gatekeeping function, and less on the provision of direct care. Eventually, these companies began to focus exclusively on managing treatment within a defined network of providers with a focus on cost control.

By the late 1980s, managed care organizations (MCOs) seemed to be fulfilling their goal of suppressing medical cost inflation via utilization reviews, preauthorization for certain services, hospital preadmission screenings, denial of services, restricted access to specialists, and restricted formularies. Over time, there was public backlash against for-profit MCOs, which restricted access to services in a manner that actually undermined the health and well-being of their subscribers. MCOs were accused of selectively choosing healthy members to keep costs low and avoiding consumers with chronic illnesses and/or disabilities. They were also seen as micromanaging and dictating treatment to physicians and being more focused on the care of illness rather than preventive health care. By 2000, over 1,000 bills were introduced both in Congress and in state legislatures dealing with consumer protection in managed care, and a presidential commission was created to examine the need for future guidelines in this rapidly growing industry (Blendon et al. 1998). The development of the National Committee for Quality Assurance (2020) quality standards for accreditation of health plans began to curb the most egregious restrictions on coverage.

In response to criticism of MCOs, numerous amendments were made to the original Health Maintenance Organization Act and many states passed laws mandating managed care standards. Insurance companies began to offer alternative plans with more comprehensive provider and hospital networks. Despite this, per capita spending on health care in the United States began to increase again in the late 1990s and continued to rise for the next two and a half decades. From 1970 to 2017, per capita health spending increased over 30-fold, from $355 per person in 1970 to $10,739 in 2017. Health care expenditures also outpaced the growth of the U.S. economy by 2.4% since 1970, making up 17.9% of the GDP by 2017 (Kamal and Cox 2018).

Proponents of the managed care industry contend that managed care has reduced unnecessarily long hospital stays, increased provider accountability, improved coordination of care, and promoted use of evidence-based practices. Opponents argue that managed care has not curbed costs, has created financial barriers for consumers (especially those with chronic, complex conditions), has increased administrative burdens for physicians, and has not improved quality overall (Feldman et al. 1998). As of 2017, nearly 90% of Americans are enrolled in some type of managed care plan, including Medicare and Medicaid plans (Centers for Medicare and Medicaid Services 2019). Under the current financing system, MCOs are likely to remain as part of the payment system, but they have not been a solution for the issues of cost or quality of care in the United States. All of these issues have reignited the push for health care reform. The passage of the Patient Protection and Affordable Care Act of 2010 (ACA) represented the most significant regulatory overhaul and expansion of coverage since the passage of Medicare and Medicaid in 1965.

Affordable Care Act

In July 2009, a group of Democrats in the House of Representatives proposed a new plan to reform health care. Nine months later, on March 23, 2010, President Barack Obama signed ACA into law (eHealth Insurance Resource Center 2018). The passage of ACA, which also came to be known as Obamacare, was landmark legislation with three primary goals (Healthcare.gov 2020):

- Make affordable health insurance available to more people. ACA health exchanges were created in each state for people to sign up for and purchase health insurance.
- Expand Medicaid to cover all adults with income below 138% of the federal poverty level by January 1, 2014.
- Support innovative medical care delivery methods designed to lower the costs of health care generally.

ACA built on the Paul Wellstone and Pete Domenici Mental Health Parity and Addiction Equity Act of 2008, which required group health plans and insurers that offer mental health and substance use disorder benefits to provide coverage that is comparable to coverage for general medical and surgical care (United States Department of Labor 2008). Starting in 2014, ACA required all new small group and individual market plans to cover 10 Essential Health Benefit categories, including mental health and substance use disorder services, and to cover them at parity with medical and surgical benefits. In doing so, ACA provided one of the largest expansions of mental health and substance use coverage in over a generation (Beronio et al. 2013).

One of the cornerstones of ACA, as listed above, was the mandated expansion of Medicaid to increase eligibility for all U.S. household incomes up to 138% of the federal poverty level by 2014. However, in 2012, the Supreme Court struck down this mandated expansion, ruling that each state could make its own decision about whether to expand Medicaid. By November 2018, a total of 37 states and the District of Columbia had elected to expand the program (Kaiser Family Foundation 2020). By June 2018, Medicaid covered nearly 70 million Americans and had become the largest and primary source of coverage for low-income and disabled populations in the United States, with children representing the largest share at 48%, nonelderly adults constituting 27%, and seniors and people with disabilities making up the remaining 24% of enrollees (Goldblot 2017).

Impact of the Affordable Care Act

Nearly a decade later, can we say the Affordable Care Act achieved its goals of making health care more affordable and accessible while also improving quality of care? More people did obtain health insurance: 16 million in the first 5 years. The percentage of uninsured in the United States decreased from 16%, or 48 million people in 2010, to 8.8% by 2017. Furthermore, states that expanded their Medicaid programs under ACA have had large reductions in uninsured rates, compared with little or no change in those rates in non-expansion states (Glied et al. 2017). Under ACA, more people have been able to afford health insurance because of federal subsidies. Insurance companies must spend at least 80% of insurance premiums on medical care and service improvements, cannot make unreasonable increases in rates, and cannot impose annual or lifetime coverage limits (Roland 2015). Businesses with more than 50 employees were mandated to offer health insurance and were given tax credits to offset some of this cost. People with preexisting conditions are no longer denied coverage, and young people can stay on their parents' plans until age 26 years. As a result, millions of Americans have benefited from receiving insurance through ACA (Amadeo 2019).

Despite these positive outcomes, ACA has not been without its share of controversies. Starting in 2013, several new taxes were created to pay for ACA, including a rise in the tax rate for those earning over $200,000 as well as taxes on medical device manufactures and pharmaceutical sales. People are paying higher premiums because insurance companies have to provide a wider range of benefits, including covering those with preexisting conditions and chronic illnesses without limits.

Until 2019, ACA mandated health coverage for all citizens, by taxing those who did not have health insurance for at least 9 months out of the year. Elimination of the mandate has had significant impact on premiums and insurers. Some insurance companies are exiting the health care exchanges because of the lack of profitability, reducing options for consumers. In the end, despite the controversies and political battle lines drawn around ACA, it has not really lowered health care costs in the United States. Its legacy will be that it was the first real step on the road toward universal care—the vision of health care in this country as a public service and universal right as opposed to a privilege.

Value and Quality in Health Care

Value has been defined in many different ways over the years, given the myriad of organizational units (hospitals, clinics, health systems) and stakeholders involved in the system. In recent years, an oft-used definition of *value* has been "health outcomes achieved per dollar spent," as discussed by renowned Harvard economist and professor Michael Porter in his famous *New England Journal of Medicine* article (Porter 2010, p. 2477). According to this definition, value in health care depends on two key variables: quality (outcomes) and cost. The remainder of this chapter focuses on quality, including the various ways to define it and the challenge of achieving it.

Historical Overview

The concept of quality in health care appeared as early as the 1850s in the United States. Florence Nightingale, considered the founder of modern nursing, demonstrated in the 1850s that basic sanitation and hygiene standards would lead to decreased mortality of soldiers wounded in the Crimean War. Her association of these previously unrelated ideas led to improved sanitary conditions in hospitals as well as private residences. Another pioneer of the quality concept was Dr. Ernest Codman, a surgeon at Massachusetts General Hospital and faculty member at Harvard Medical School. He kept track of his patients with "End Result Cards," index cards that contained patient demographics, diagnoses, treatments, and outcomes. He emphasized that understanding why treatments were successful was the key to improving the care of future patients. He was a pioneer of evidence-based medicine, including the development of hospital standards of care and strategies to assess health care outcomes. In 1913, Dr. Codman cofounded the American College of Surgeons (ACS), and as the chair of the ACS Committee for Hospital Standardization, he created an "End Result System," adopted by the ACS in 1917. It served as the foundation for basic hospital operating procedures (Chun and Bafford 2014).

By 1952, the Joint Commission on Accreditation of Hospitals, later called the Joint Commission on Accreditation of Healthcare Organizations (JCAHO) (now just The Joint Commission), was created with the collaboration of the American College of Surgeons, American Medical Association, American Hospital Association, American College of Physicians, and Canadian Medical Association. When it implemented a rigorous set of accreditation standards in the 1980s, JCAHO adopted concepts developed by Dr. Avedis Donabedian in his 1966 article, "Evaluating the Quality of Medical Care" (Donabedian 1966/2005). Widely regarded as the founding father of quality in health care and medical outcomes research, Dr. Donabedian defined quality measurement in three areas: structure, process, outcomes (Chun and Bafford 2014). (Donabedian's three-factor model is discussed later in this chapter in the section "Outcome Measurement.")

In 2000, the Institute of Medicine (IOM), a recognized leader and national advisor on health care, published *To Err Is Human: Building a Safer Health System* (Institute of Medicine 2000), which shed light on the nearly 98,000 Americans who die from medical errors each year. This report brought the topic of quality improvement in health care into the light for policy makers, health care administrators, physicians, and other health care workers in the United States. The IOM earlier defined *quality* as "the degree to which health care services for individuals and populations increase the likelihood of desired health outcomes and are consistent with current professional knowledge" (Institute of Medicine 1990, p. 21). The following year, the IOM published *Crossing the Quality Chasm: A New Health System for the 21st Century* (Institute of Medicine 2001). This report lamented the failure of the United States health care delivery system to provide consistent, high-quality medical care, and called for a fundamental redesign of the entire health system. These two IOM reports kick-started efforts by health care organizations large and small to improve the quality of health care in the United States.

Quality Indicators

The IOM definition of *quality* was "a direct correlation between the level of improved health services and the desired health outcomes of individuals and populations" (Health Resources and Services Administration 2011, p. 1). The IOM also developed the following six parameters to define quality in health care from the perspective of organizations delivering care (Institute of Medicine 2001):

- *Safety:* preventing and avoiding actual or potential bodily harm
- *Effectiveness:* providing care processes and achieving outcomes as supported by scientific evidence
- *Patient centeredness:* meeting patients' needs and preferences and providing education and support

- *Timeliness:* obtaining needed care while minimizing delays
- *Efficiency:* maximizing the quality of a comparable unit of health care delivered or unit of health benefit achieved for a given unit of health care resources used
- *Equity:* providing health care of equal quality to those who may differ in personal characteristics other than their clinical condition or preferences for care

To build on the work of the Foundation for Accountability (FACCT), a nonprofit group that believes that "the people who buy and use healthcare should hold the system accountable for its performance," consumer perspectives on health care needs are defined as (Graham 1997):

- *Staying healthy:* avoiding illness and remaining well
- *Getting better:* recovering from an illness or injury
- *Living with illness or disability:* managing an ongoing, chronic condition or dealing with a disability that affects function
- *Coping with the end of life:* dealing with aging, chronic illness, and terminal illness

A patient-centric approach to care was also evident in the Triple Aim, developed by the Institute for Healthcare Improvement in 2007 as a "foundation for organizations and communities to successfully navigate the transition from a focus on health care to optimizing health for individuals and populations" (Institute for Healthcare Improvement 2020b). The three aims are as follows:

- Improving the patient experience of care (including quality and satisfaction)
- Improving the health of populations
- Reducing the per capita cost of health care

In recent years, a fourth dimension has been added: improving the work life of health care practitioners (Bodenheimer and Sinsky 2014). Multiple surveys over the past couple of decades have demonstrated a steady, alarming rise in the rate of physicians reporting signs and symptoms of burnout. Thus, it has become essential to take into account the well-being of health care professionals as a direct correlate to quality of care.

Quality Improvement

Quality improvement (QI) (formerly called *quality assurance* or *quality control*), as defined by the U.S. Department of Health and Human Services'

Health Resources and Services Administration, is the "systematic and continuous actions that lead to measurable improvement in health care services and the health status of targeted patient groups" (U.S. Department of Health and Human Services, Health Resources and Services Administration 2011). Quality is directly linked to an organization's underlying system of care and service delivery approach. To achieve a better or different level of performance and to improve quality, an organization needs to honestly and objectively appraise its current system, identify areas of improvement, commit to implementing these changes, and continuously monitor its performance over time. A QI program involves systematic activities that are structured and implemented by an organization to monitor, assess, and improve its quality of health care. Ideally, a successful QI program should incorporate a focus on the following four key elements: systems and processes, patients' needs and expectations, collaboration as part of a team, and use of data (Massoud 2001).

Systems and Processes

To make improvements, an organization needs to begin by examining its current delivery system and processes, which consist of two components: what is done and how it is done. In other words, the organization considers what type of care is provided and when, where, and by whom it is delivered. Each component can be addressed separately to attain improvement, but the greatest impact for QI occurs when both are addressed simultaneously. Also, QI is most effective if it is personalized to meet the needs of a specific organization's health service delivery system. Simply put:

Resources (Inputs) → Activities (Processes) → Results (Outputs/Outcomes)

Patients' Needs and Expectations

An important measure of quality is the extent to which patients' needs and expectations are met. Factors in this area include access to and availability of health care services, safety, effective communication, coordination of care, patient-centered care, adequate customer support, use of evidence-based practices, and cultural competency.

Collaboration as Part of a Team

A team approach is at the core of QI and is critical in achieving significant and long-lasting improvements. This is particularly true for health care organizations, which are complex, involving multiple disciplines and layered processes. Each team member should have buy-in to a QI initiative, contributing ideas based on his or her own unique skill set. Ideally, a team should incorporate knowledge and experience from varied staff and implement ideas based on a synthesis of this information. However, without the proper infrastructure, including well-defined policies, clear expectations, and strong leadership, even the best QI teams will flounder. It is important for teams to feel supported enough to communicate their ideas openly and freely in order to make effective changes.

Use of Data

Data are absolutely necessary to describe and truly understand how well current systems are working and what happens when changes are applied, as well as to document performance. Most health care organizations have access to considerable data from multiple sources, including electronic health records, practice management systems, external audits, and patient satisfaction surveys. The key is to use these data in a methodical and systematic way, such that a health system can evaluate its current system, identify opportunities for improvement, and monitor performance improvement over time. Data for QI programs should be both quantitative (measurable) and qualitative (observable). Also, standardized performance measures that are nationally or internationally recognized should be used (U.S. Department of Health and Human Services, Health Resources and Services Administration 2011). Examples of such measures used in mental health are screening questionnaires such as the Patient Health Questionnaire–9 (PHQ-9) and the 7-item Generalized Anxiety Disorder scale (GAD-7) to measure depression and anxiety, respectively.

Continuous Quality Improvement

Continuous quality improvement (CQI) is intimately linked to QI but also distinctly different, in that it comprises an ongoing, comprehensive process of identifying, describing, and analyzing strengths and problems, followed by implementing, learning from, and revising solutions. It has roots in the same movement that led to the development of QI but actually originated in the industrial sector, where the focus was on improving the quality of goods by improving the manufacturing process. CQI was popularized through the Toyota Production System (TPS), which was a management philosophy the automaker officially implemented in 1992 as a means of streamlining processes in an effort to reduce waste. TPS emphasized *kaizen* (continuous improvement), following a long-term vision and seeking input from every member of the team involved in the manufacturing process (Toyota 2020).

One of the hallmarks of CQI is its mission to alter the culture of an organization by focusing on process improvement rather than faulting individuals.

It insists on collaboration, trust, communication, respect, and empowerment of both employees and management. Unlike QI, which can be seen as a top-down directive, CQI is much more team oriented and relies on input from all stakeholders to work toward a unified vision for the organization. Another way to look at CQI is as the application of the scientific method to organizational processes to achieve a paradigm shift in a workplace culture; CQI may be easy to envision but difficult to apply (Radawski 1999).

In health care organizations, the application of CQI based on TPS is known as Lean, which was coined by James P. Womack and Daniel T. Jones during their in-depth study of the influential TPS. Lean is a way of thinking about an activity and seeing the waste inadvertently generated by the way the process is organized and then modifying the process as a result (Womack and Jones 1996).

Lean principles have been applied to a number of health care systems throughout the world to improve the following: quality and cost-effectiveness of services for patients, throughput times, and productivity. One of the big challenges has been coordinating the activities of individual professionals on a health care team toward a unified organizational goal. In 1987, JCAHO began changing its quality assurance standards to a CQI framework. Since then, a number of articles have appeared applying the TPS model to health care settings (Chowanec 1994). One model for CQI, as outlined by the Institute for Healthcare Improvement, is the "Plan-Do-Study-Act cycle," as summarized below (Institute for Healthcare Improvement 2020a) and shown diagrammatically in Figure 2–1.

- *Plan:* Develop a plan to test the change.
- *Do:* Carry out the test.
- *Study:* Observe and learn from the consequences.
- *Act:* Determine what modifications should be made to the test.

The process emphasizes the need to repeat and implement the changes on an ongoing basis, as often as necessary. To be effective, this cycle also requires institutional buy-in and active engagement of employees and stakeholders at all levels during the process.

Continuous Quality Improvement Challenges in Health Care

CQI can be effective only if an organization is willing to engage in constant examination and improvement that is aligned with its mission, vision, and values. Given the difficulty of this task, CQI has not always been welcomed with open arms by health care practitioners. Since the 1980s, the United

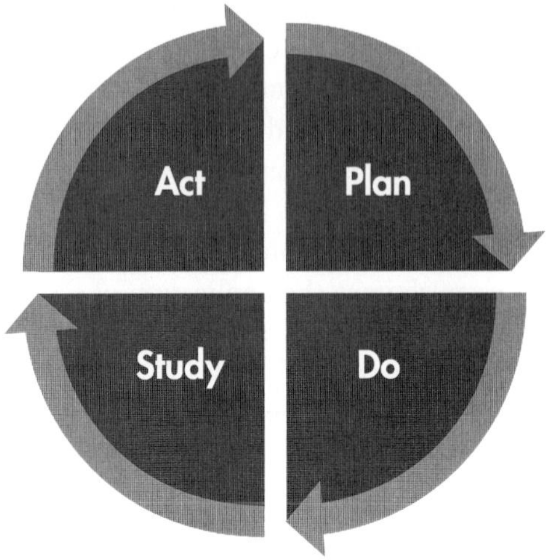

FIGURE 2–1. Plan-Do-Study-Act cycle.

States health care system has been under pressure from government and MCOs to reduce costs and improve quality, while also promoting patient satisfaction and reducing adverse outcomes. Part of the challenge is the coordination of a myriad of independent players on a health care "team." For example, on an inpatient psychiatric unit, the treatment team can consist of attending psychiatrists, nurses, technicians, social workers, psychologists, occupational therapists, residents, and medical students. Getting team members to agree on a singular goal can be akin to herding cats! Expanding the circle reveals other invested parties, including patients, their families, parents (for child and adolescent patients), hospital administrators, utilization review staff, and insurance companies.

Given the vast array of stakeholders, multiple goals arise, including but not limited to quality, patient-centered care, profitability, cost controls, access to innovative treatment, safety, efficacy, and patient and family satisfaction. The trick is to recognize each stakeholder's interest and address it as directly as possible. If this is not done, obtaining buy-in from all team members will be difficult. Without broad participation and a strong and clear vision, CQI initiatives can appear abstract, or just a series of flow diagrams and charts. They may be regarded by staff as an additional task on their to-do list, rather than a potentially powerful tool to create a process change (Chowanec 1994). It is of utmost importance for all members of a CQI initiative to have a shared objective that unites the interests and activities of all stakeholders. Without clarity and communication around a common goal, it is impossible to maintain accountability and solidarity toward improving quality. After all, to quote Dr. Chowanec (1994) in his article "Continuous Quality Improvement: Conceptual Foundations and Application to Mental Health Care," the "best way to herd cats is to get them all to chase after the same mouse" (p. 793).

Outcome Measurement

Every health care system touts its highest quality care and effective staff and services. But how can a system prove that its model is actually the best? The standard for measuring quality in health care organizations is Donabedian's (1966/2005) three-factor model (introduced briefly earlier in the section "Value and Quality in Health Care"):

- **Structure:** Measures an organization's capacity, systems, and processes.
  - *Examples:* ratio of providers to patients, utilization of an electronic health record, number of board-certified physicians on staff
- **Process:** Measures what an organization does to maintain or improve health, either for healthy people or for those diagnosed with a health care condition. Process measures reflect generally accepted recommendations for clinical practice and can help improve health outcomes. Such measures are what are typically seen in public reports of health care quality.
  - *Examples:* percentage of people receiving preventive services such as mammograms or immunizations, percentage of people with diabetes who had their blood sugar tested and adequately controlled
- **Outcomes:** Measures that reflect the impact of the intervention on the health status of patients. Outcome measures are considered the gold standard in measuring quality.
  - *Examples:* percentage of patients who died as a result of surgery (surgical mortality rates), infant mortality rates

Program Evaluation

In public health a common and comprehensive method to assess the efficacy and impact of an intervention is a program evaluation. Very similar to CQI, a program evaluation is a systematic method for collecting, analyzing, and using information to answer questions about projects, policies, and programs (Administration for Children and Families: Office of Planning, Research, and Evaluation 2010). Program evaluations, in addition to incor-

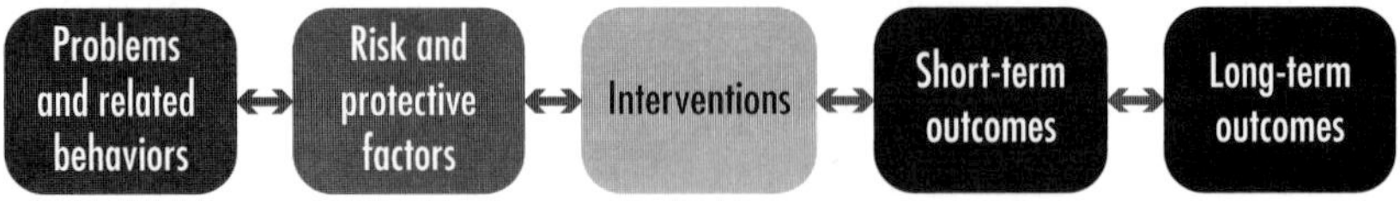
Problems and related behaviors
Risk and protective factors
Interventions
Short-term outcomes
Long-term outcomes

FIGURE 2–2. The logic model.

porating the three elements of the Donabedian model just described, ask the following three questions (Tyrer 2011):

1. Is the treatment/service effective? (Does it serve its purpose?)
2. Is the treatment/service efficacious? (Does it work in day-to-day practice?)
3. Is the treatment/service cost-effective?

Program evaluations include measures of program fidelity, organizational processes, and individual performance. Examples of program evaluation projects in mental health are assessing treatment efficacy of medication and/or psychotherapeutic interventions and determining whether overbooking patients in a community mental health clinic can reduce the cost impact of no-shows. Program evaluations can be quantitative, qualitative, or both. The type of methodology used should be driven by the question being asked.

Qualitative Measures

Qualitative methods focus on the questions how and why, and sources include direct observation of people and processes, interviews (ideally with open-ended questions), and document analysis. One type of qualitative approach is the logic model, which is like an interconnected roadmap to understanding the rationale, or logic, behind a program or process, as shown in Figure 2–2. Understanding how and why the elements of the logic model connect can help an organization visualize whether a process or program in its current form is efficacious and cost-effective.

Another type of qualitative method is examining how a program was implemented. This involves asking questions, such as the following, of staff, patients, community members, and stakeholders:

- Is the program well defined? Easy to utilize?
- Do staff communicate effectively about the purpose of the program?
- What was the journey that led to implementation? What organizational changes were required?

Questions like those above demand detail and clear description. They demonstrate the underlying importance of a qualitative approach in this particular kind of evaluation (Office of Data, Analysis, Research and Evaluation Administration on Children, Youth and Families 2016).

Quantitative Measures

Quantitative methods are more interested in questions involving who, what, where, when, and how many. Any quantitative research instrument should be both valid (i.e., it should measure what it is intended to measure) and reliable (i.e., it should provide repeatable results regardless of the condition). Numeric data can be collected in the form of surveys (using methods such as the Likert scale) or questionnaires. Once obtained, the data can be analyzed statistically. For example, in a program evaluation measuring antidepressant efficacy, two self-reporting scales commonly used for objective symptom assessment are the Hamilton Depression Rating Scale and Beck Depression Inventory (Thornicroft and Bebbington 1996). For a project looking at the impact of physical and mental illnesses on employee productivity, a starting point can be examining existing records that provide information about absentee rates, turnover, injury/accident rates, and disability claims filed. These records should be easily accessible and can help a company find out how much money it is losing because of lost or decreased productivity, and whether it would be more cost-effective to invest in wellness initiatives or change its current process instead of hiring new employees as ways to curb this loss.

Taken together, qualitative and quantitative approaches to outcome measurement help provide context for a problem within an organization and data to develop solutions.

Evidence-Based Practice

The term *evidence-based practice* (EBP) refers to a systematic application of scientific evidence to decision making regarding treatment with individual patients, thus bridging the gap between research and clinical practice (Sur and Dahm 2011). EBP has permeated all fields of health care, including mental health, and has become synonymous with quality. However, in the case of chronic and severe mental illnesses, where the focus has shifted to recovery, there has been some controversy about the use of EBP. Nonetheless, EBPs have been widely embraced by state mental health authorities in the United States. Implementation of EBPs need to be done from a systems perspective, incorporating input from all stakeholders and developing guidelines specific to the organization. Using a CQI approach, EBPs should be reevaluated regularly and modified accordingly (Savage et al. 2012). At a mental health agency, this includes staff ranging from psychiatrist to case manager, with the end user being the consumer of mental health services. On a larger scale, it is important to demonstrate quality and value to those funding the care and the community at large. (For more detail on EBPs, see Chapter 5, "Successful Approaches to Increasing Value.")

Conclusion

This chapter has provided a review of the history of mental health care costs and quality in the United States. We study our past not only to avoid repeating our mistakes but also to imagine what is possible for the future. We still have work to do in terms of destigmatizing mental illness; history has demonstrated that as long as fear of mental illness persists, there will be limited resources, funding, and research devoted to prevention and treatment. Thankfully, the last few decades have seen increased public awareness and advocacy with regard to treatment of psychiatric and substance use disorders. This needs to translate into policy changes and parity. The twenty-first century has ushered in numerous initiatives aimed at improving health care quality, one of the components of value. Health care practitioners emphasize quality, patients want lower costs and convenience, and employers and administrators focus on accountability and costs (University of Utah Health 2017). Reconciling these differences is the missing link in the value equation. As medical innovation continues and accelerates, we need to develop processes that move us toward a more inclusive, transparent, and multidimensional approach to measuring value—one that acknowledges heterogeneous stakeholder interests. Human beings are gravitating toward personalization in every consumer arena, and this is true in health care as well. One need only look at the burgeoning interest in pharmacogenomics in mental health as evidence of this movement.

In other words, treatment and cost benchmarks based on an "average" patient with a given condition will soon be confined to actuarial calculations. In a consumer-centric culture, patients will demand personalized treatment that takes into account their specific needs, which may be related to cost in some cases and efficacy in others (Bright and Linthicum 2018). There is no one-size-fits-all answer to the question of value, either in health care broadly or in psychiatry specifically. Nor is the system we have now equipped to handle a personalized, patient-centric model that is heralded as the future of medicine. This disconnect is the reason it is imperative that all stakeholders come together to seek and find a better approach while staying open-minded and adaptable along the way.

References

Administration for Children and Families, Office of Planning, Research, and Evaluation: The Program Manager's Guide to Evaluation, 2nd Edition. 2010. Available at: www.acf.hhs.gov/sites/default/files/opre/program_managers_guide_to_eval2010_508.pdf. Accessed February 5, 2020.

Amadeo K: Deinstitutionalization, its causes, effects, pros, and cons. November 4, 2018. Available at: www.thebalance.com/deinstitutionalization-3306067. Accessed February 5, 2020.

Amadeo K: 10 Obamacare pros and cons: is Obamacare worth it? January 17, 2019. Available at: www.thebalance.com/obamacare-pros-and-cons-3306059. Accessed February 5, 2020.

Behavioral Health Services: Medicaid.gov: keeping America healthy. 2020. Available at: www.medicaid.gov/medicaid/benefits/bhs/index.html. Accessed February 5, 2020.

Beronio K, Po R, Skopec L, et al: Affordable Care Act will expand mental health and substance use disorder benefits and parity protections for 62 million Americans. Department of Health and Human Services Office of the Assistant Secretary for Planning and Evaluation, ASPE Research Brief, February 2013. Available at: https://aspe.hhs.gov/report/affordable-care-act-expands-mental-health-and-substance-use-disorder-benefits-and-federal-parity-protections-62-million-americans. Accessed February 5, 2020.

Blendon RJ, Brodie M, Benson JM, et al: Understanding the managed care backlash. Health Aff (Millwood) 17(4):80–94, 1998

Bodenheimer T, Sinsky C: From Triple to Quadruple Aim: care of the patient requires care of the provider. Ann Fam Med 12(6):573–576, 2014

Bright J, Linthicum M: Is one answer good enough for all? Defining value in healthcare. American Journal of Managed Care, August 22, 2018. Available at: www.ajmc.com/contributor/innovation-and-value-initiative/2018/08/is-one-answer-good-enough-for-all-defining-value-in-healthcare. Accessed February 5, 2020.

Centers for Medicare and Medicaid Services: Medicaid Managed Care Enrollment and Program Characteristics, 2017. Mathematica Policy Research, Winter 2019. Available at: https://www.medicaid.gov/medicaid/managed-care/downloads/enrollment/2017-medicaid-managed-care-enrollment-report.pdf. Accessed July 27, 2020.

Chowanec S: Continuous quality improvement: conceptual foundations and application to mental health care. Hosp Community Psychiatry 45(8):789–794, 1994

Chun J, Bafford AC: History and background of quality measurement. Clin Colon Rectal Surg 27(1):5–9, 2014

Clubhouse International: What clubhouses do. 2018. Available at: https://clubhouse-intl.org/what-we-do/what-clubhouses-do. Accessed February 5, 2020.

Cox C, Sawyer B: What do we know about the burden of disease in America? Chart Collections: Peterson-KFF Health System Tracker May 22, 2017. Available at: https://www.healthsystemtracker.org/chart-collection/know-burden-disease-u-s/?_sf_s=burden#item-mental-health-circulatory-disorders-leading-causes-disease-burden-u-s. Accessed July 27, 2020.

Donabedian A: An Introduction to Quality Assurance in Health Care. New York, Oxford University Press, 2002

Donabedian A: Evaluating the quality of medical care (1966). Milbank Q 83(4):691–729, 2005

eHealth Insurance Resource Center: History and timeline of the Affordable Care Act. March 5, 2018. Available at: www.ehealthinsurance.com/resources/affordable-care-act/history-timeline-affordable-care-act-aca. Accessed February 5, 2020.

Feldman DS, Novack DH, Gracely E: Effects of managed care on physician-patient relationships, quality of care, and the ethical practice of medicine: a physician survey. Arch Intern Med 158(15):1626–1632, 1998

Feldman JM: History of community psychiatry, in Handbook of Community Psychiatry. Edited by McQuistion H, Sowers W, Ranz J, et al. New York, Springer, 2012, pp 11–18

Fisher WH, Geller JL, Pandiani JA, et al: The changing role of the state psychiatric hospital. Health Aff (Millwood) 28(3):676–684, 2009

Ford M: Cook County Jail, America's largest mental hospital is a jail. The Atlantic, June 8, 2015. Available at: www.theatlantic.com/politics/archive/2015/06/americas-largest-mental-hospital-is-a-jail/395012/. Accessed February 5, 2020.

Forrest C, Reid R: Passing the baton: HMOs' influence on referrals to specialty care. Health Aff (Millwood) 16(6):157–162, 1997

Frank R, Glied S: Changes in mental health financing since 1971: implications for policymakers and patients. Health Aff (Millwood) 25(3):601–613, 2006

Fuller Torrey E, Entsminger K, Geller J, et al: The shortage of public hospital beds for mentally ill persons. 2008. Available at: www.treatmentadvocacycenter.org/storage/documents/the_shortage_of_publichospital_beds.pdf. Accessed February 5, 2020.

Gill MM: Psychoanalysis, Part 1: Proposals for the Future. New York, American Mental Health Foundation, 2009

Glied S, Ma S, Borja A: Effect of the Affordable Care Act on health care access. Commonwealth Fund, May 8, 2017. Available at: www.commonwealthfund.org/publications/issue-briefs/2017/may/effect-affordable-care-act-health-care-access. Accessed February 5, 2020.

Goldblot D: Medicaid: America's largest health insurer. Center for Global Policy Solutions Fact Sheet, July 2017. Available at: http://globalpolicysolutions.org/wp-content/uploads/2017/07/Medicaid-Final.pdf. Accessed February 5, 2020.

Graham J: FACCT (Foundation for Accountability): a large measure of quality. J AHIMA 68(6):41–46, 1997
Grazier KL, Mowbray CT, Holter MC: Rationing psychosocial treatments in the United States. Int J Law Psychiatry 28(5):545–560, 2005
Gronfein W: Incentive and intentions in mental health policy: a comparison of the Medicaid and community mental health programs. J Health Soc Behav 26(3):192–206, 1985
Healthcare.gov: Affordable Care Act (ACA). 2020. Available at: www.healthcare.gov/glossary/affordable-care-act. Accessed February 5, 2020.
Health Resources and Services Administration: Quality Improvement. Rockville, MD, U.S. Dept of Health and Human Services, April 2011. Available at: https://www.hrsa.gov/sites/default/files/quality/toolbox/508pdfs/qualityimprovement.pdf. Accessed July 27, 2020.
Institute for Healthcare Improvement. Tools: Plan-Do-Study-Act (PDSA) worksheet. 2020a. Available at: www.ihi.org/resources/Pages/Tools/PlanDoStudyActWorksheet.aspx. Accessed February 5, 2020.
Institute for Healthcare Improvement: Triple aim for populations. 2020b. Available at: www.ihi.org/Topics/TripleAim/Pages/Overview.aspx. Accessed February 5, 2020.
Institute of Medicine: Medicare: A Strategy for Quality Assurance, Vol 1. Washington, DC, National Academies Press, 1990
Institute of Medicine: To Err Is Human: Building a Safer Health System. Washington, DC, National Academies Press, 2000
Institute of Medicine: Crossing the Quality Chasm: A New Health System for the 21st Century. Washington, DC, National Academies Press, 2001
Kaiser Family Foundation: Status of state action on the Medicaid expansion decision. January 10, 2020. Available at: www.kff.org/health-reform/state-indicator/state-activity-around-expanding-medicaid-under-the-affordable-care-act. Accessed February 5, 2020.
Kamal R: What are the current costs and outcomes related to mental health and substance abuse disorders? Peterson-Kaiser Health System Tracker, July 31, 2017. Available at: www.healthsystemtracker.org/chart-collection/current-costs-outcomes-related-mental-health-substance-abuse-disorders/#item-start. Accessed February 5, 2020.
Kamal R, Cox C: How has U.S. spending on healthcare changed over time? Peterson-Kaiser Health System Tracker, December 10, 2018. Available at: www.healthsystemtracker.org/chart-collection/u-s-spending-healthcare-changed-time/#item-start. Accessed February 5, 2020.
Lutterman T, Manderscheid R:Trends in total psychiatric inpatient and other 24-hour mental health residential treatment capacity, 1970 to 2014. NASMHPD Commissioners Meeting. National Association of State Mental Health Program Directors Research Institute, July 31, 2017. Available at: https://www.nri-inc.org/media/1302/t-lutterman-and-r-manderscheid-distribution-of-psychiatric-inpatient-capacity-united-states.pdf. Accessed July 27, 2020.
Massoud MR: Advances in quality improvement: principles and framework. QA Brief 9(1):13–17, 2001

McKay C, Nugent K, Johnsen M: A systematic review of evidence for the Clubhouse model of psychosocial rehabilitation. Adm Policy Ment Health 45(1):28–47, 2018

Mechanic D, Rochefort DA: Deinstitutionalization: an appraisal of reform. Annual Review of Sociology 16:301–327, 1990

Moore TJ, Mattison DR: Research letter: adult utilization of psychiatric drugs and differences by sex, age, and race. JAMA Intern Medicine, February 2017. Available at: https://jamanetwork.com/journals/jamainternalmedicine/fullarticle/2592697. Accessed February 5, 2020.

National Committee for Quality Assurance: Health plan accreditation. 2020. Available at: www.ncqa.org/programs/health-plans/health-plan-accreditation-hpa. Accessed February 5, 2020.

National Institute of Mental Health: About NIMH. Available at: https://www.nimh.nih.gov/index.shtml. Accessed May 21, 2013.

Office of Data, Analysis, Research and Evaluation Administration on Children, Youth, and Families: Qualitative research methods in program evaluation: considerations for federal staff. May 2016. Available at: www.acf.hhs.gov/sites/default/files/acyf/qualitative_research_methods_in_program_evaluation.pdf. Accessed February 5, 2020.

PBS: Timeline: treatments for mental illness. American Experience, A Brilliant Madness: The Story of Nobel Prize Winning Mathematician John Nash. June 27, 2012. Available at: www.pbs.org/wgbh/americanexperience/features/nash-treatments-mental-illness/. Accessed February 5, 2020.

Porter M: What is value in health care? N Engl J Med 363(26):2477–2481, 2010

President's New Freedom Commission on Mental Health: Achieving the Promise: Transforming Mental Health Care in America: Final Report. Rockville, MD, President's New Freedom Commission on Mental Health, 2003

Radawski D: Continuous quality improvement: origins, concepts, problems, and applications. J Physician Assist Educ 10(1):12–16, 1999

Roland J: The pros and cons of Obamacare. Healthline Newsletter, June 15, 2015. Available at: www.healthline.com/health/consumer-healthcare-guide/pros-and-cons-obamacare. Accessed February 5, 2020.

Savage R, Cornett P, Goodwin N: Program evaluation and quality management, in Handbook of Community Psychiatry. Edited by McQuistion H, Sowers W, Ranz J, et al. New York, Springer, 2012, pp 551–560

Substance Abuse and Mental Health Services Administration: Key substance use and mental health indicators in the United States: results from the 2016 National Survey on Drug Use and Health (HHS Publ No SMA 17-5044, NSDUH Series H-52). 2017. Available at: www.samhsa.gov/data/sites/default/files/NSDUH-FFR1-2016/NSDUH-FFR1-2016.htm. Accessed February 5, 2020.

Substance Use and Mental Health Services Administration: Recovery and recovery support. May 17, 2019. Available at: www.samhsa.gov/find-help/recovery. Accessed February 5, 2020.

Sur RL, Dahm P: History of evidence-based medicine. Indian J Urol 27(4):487–489, 2011

Thornicroft G, Bebbington P: Quantitative methods in evaluation of community mental health services, in Integrated Mental Health Services: Modern Community Psychiatry. Edited by Breakey WR. New York, Oxford University Press, 1996, pp 120–138

Toyota: Toyota production system: company information, vision and philosophy. 2020. Available at: https://global.toyota/en/company/vision-and-philosophy/production-system. Accessed February 5, 2020.

Tyrer P: Research designs and evaluating treatment interventions, in Oxford Textbook of Community Mental Health. Edited by Thornicroft G, Szmukler G, Mueser KT, et al. New York, Oxford University Press, 2011, pp 297–304

University of Utah Health: The state of value in U.S. healthcare. November 2017. Available at: https://uofuhealth.utah.edu/value/#forum. Accessed February 5, 2020.

U.S. Department of Health and Human Services, Health Resources and Services Administration: Quality improvement. April 2011. Available at: www.hrsa.gov/sites/default/files/quality/toolbox/508pdfs/qualityimprovement.pdf. Accessed February 5, 2020.

U.S. Department of Labor: Fact sheet: the Mental Health Parity Act. October 2008. Available at: www.dol.gov/ebsa/newsroom/fsmhparity.html. Accessed February 5, 2020.

Womack JP, Jones DT: Lean Thinking: Banish Waste and Create Wealth in Your Corporation. New York, Simon & Schuster, 1996, pp 15–17

3

The Current System

The Mess We Are In

Wesley E. Sowers, M.D.

It is often said that describing the health care system in the United States is an impossible task because it is not really a system at all—at least not in the way that we usually think about systems. Health care in the United States is delivered through a conglomerate of systems that operate more or less independently with little coordination, communication, or collaboration. In this chapter, we consider how this strange mixture came to be and what some of the forces are that have driven it and kept it in place. Having previously considered the nature of value and ways to measure it in Chapter 1, "Defining and Measuring Value," we scrutinize in this chapter the structures that have been put in place and consider how well they would hold up in a value-driven environment. We then identify those aspects of the system that fall short of our value expectations. This discussion will set the stage for the extensive consideration of alternatives—whether minor tweaks or major revisions—that will occupy most of this book and help us envision a high-value system.

Over the past several decades, the cost of health care in the United States has risen dramatically, far exceeding expenditures of other developed countries. At the same time our population health outcomes have been poor relative to those of other wealthy nations, which spend a considerably lower percentage of their gross domestic product (GDP) on health care. Unlike most other nations, the United States does not consider health care to be a public service, similar to education, policing, or municipal emergency services, to which all residents have access. The exclusion of health care from the domain of public goods and services is largely responsible for the lack of value that we have obtained through the (mis)management of our nation's health.

Many factors impact spending and outcomes, but most of them derive from our reliance on free market forces to govern the delivery of health services. The United States has a long tradition of valuing free enterprise and entrepreneurial interests over governmental regulation and administration (Griffin 2017). Although this has served the U.S. economy well in many cases, the interests of a business do not always coincide with social needs or the development of unified systems to meet them. Competition often creates improved products when companies compete for market shares, but in the health care market, the demand for services is high and resources available to support them are limited, so there is often little incentive to develop products or programs that adequately meet identified needs (Everett et al. 2012). As a result, local, state, and federal programs have gradually been adopted to fill the gaps that market forces have left neglected. The mixture of governmental, private nonprofit, and private for-profit services adds to the complexity of the health care conglomerate, and ultimately negatively impacts our population's health.

Market forces that play an important role in the value equation are examined more closely in some of the chapters that follow (see Chapters 4, 6, 12, and 13). This chapter examines various aspects of our systems that impact outcomes and expenditures and considers how they are related to the political and economic forces that are responsible for them. Organization, administration, financing, focus of care, liability, workforce composition, and waste all contribute to the poor value outcomes that will be considered in greater detail later in this chapter. First, we take a brief look at the evolution of some of the basic elements of the health care services conglomerate.

Historical Considerations

Until the early part of the twentieth century, most health care was a locally based and loosely organized enterprise. Medical science did not have a great deal to offer as effective and proven treatments, and most services were delivered by individual physicians and were paid out of pocket by the recipients of care. Although some private insurers were offering policies, they served a small portion of the population. As medical knowledge expanded, and the cost of care along with it, there were increasing proposals for developing universal health care insurance, but these were consistently thwarted. Unlike in European countries, in the United States there was little support from the working classes or the newly developed medical establishment for a program of universal health care coverage (Gordon 1997). Private insurers also opposed these proposals in fear of losing business as a result (Navarro 1989; Starr 1982). At the turn of the twentieth century, health care spending was estimated to be about 2%–3% of GDP, and it remained under 5% until the 1960s (Catlin and Cowan 2015; Griffin 2017).

The quality of medical care was widely unregulated at the turn of the century. Although the United States had several reputable medical schools, there were few standards for education of physicians that were broadly followed. It was not until the issuance of the Flexner Report in 1910, with its recommendations to follow the European model of medical education and to introduce accountability and standards into medical curricula, that this situation began to change. Other structures for regulation and monitoring the quality of care were developed as the century progressed, not only for education, but also for hospitals and other health care facilities. Accreditation organizations, such as the Joint Commission on Accreditation of Healthcare Organizations (now The Joint Commission) and the Commission on Accreditation of Rehabilitation Facilities, and state licensing standards are examples of the latter (Luce et al. 1994).

Private health insurance began to expand in various forms in the first half of the twentieth century. In the early part of the century, unions began to provide sickness insurance to their members (Murray 2007). In the 1920s and 1930s, some hospitals started to offer prepaid policies enabling consumers who became ill to receive services at a specified hospital. An association of such hospitals was formed, and the Blue Cross Blue Shield nonprofit insurance program eventually evolved from this association (Cunningham and Cunningham 1997). During and after World War II, employer-based insurance began to emerge. Businesses were hard-pressed to meet labor needs, and a wage freeze in the form of the Stabilization Act of 1942 made them look at other methods to attract workers. Health insurance became a nonmonetary form of compensation on which employees did not have to pay taxes. These programs remained intact and grew as veterans returned from the war and the economy expanded. Nevertheless, a significant portion of the population that did not work remained without health care (Numbers 1979). In 1960, about 70% of the population had health insurance, primarily for hospitalization. During this period of the Cold War, efforts to put forward universal health care plans were deemed "socialist" and faced fierce opposition from predominantly anti-communist constituencies, including the medical establishment (Mahar 2006).

In the second half of the twentieth century, medical science and technology began to advance rapidly, as did the cost of services. In the context of the prosperity of the 1960s, President Lyndon Johnson was able to gain passage of legislation establishing Medicare for older adults and people with disabilities and of Medicaid for indigent populations, greatly increasing the number of U.S. residents having some type of insurance (Everett et al. 2012). By 1970, health care expenses climbed to 6.9% of GDP (Catlin and Cowan 2015). Although many people still worked for employers who did not offer insurance, proposals by President Richard Nixon and others to extend employer-based insurance by making it mandatory, with some proposed subsidies, also failed. This approach was revisited with proposals put forth by President Bill Clinton's administration in 1993, but it would be another 17 years before it was eventually adopted with the passage of the Patient Protection and Affordable Care Act of 2010 (ACA), signed into law by President Barack Obama (Griffin 2017; Morrissey 2008).

During the 1980s and 1990s, the cost of care continued to rise sharply. Insurance premiums began a marked climb, and insurers became increasingly restrictive in terms of what coverage they would provide and to whom. People with significant health problems (preexisting conditions) and people who worked independently and were not part of a large risk pool, found it very difficult to find or afford health insurance. Stories began to emerge of families going bankrupt or becoming mired in severe debt due to unexpected illnesses and enormous health expenses (Dranove and Millenson 2006). In 1997, the Clinton administration was able to pass a significant improvement in public health care funding in the form of the Children's Health Insurance Program (CHIP), which assured health care to children up to age 19 who were not otherwise insured. At this time, the "working poor" constituted the largest group of uninsured individuals in the United States—a group that grew to nearly 50 million people by the early years of the new millennium (Morrissey 2008).

It was also during this period that new approaches to providing health care coverage began to evolve. Health maintenance organizations, which emphasized holistic care and prevention, became increasingly common. They were also developed to help control the costs of care, but as they focused on this aspect of their mission, they became increasingly restrictive in terms of approved providers and services. They gradually evolved into managed care organizations (MCOs), focusing on resource management rather than the direct provision of care. These organizations assumed a gatekeeping role for approval of services, effectively usurping the role of providers in deciding medical needs. Profit for these companies was derived from limiting payment for services as much as the companies possibly could (Morrissey 2008). This was a revolutionary development that shook the medical profession and created an adversarial relationship between those who controlled costs and those who delivered care. Ironically, this development added the expense of a micromanagement infrastructure to the already burgeoning cost of care, and although this practice did change some wasteful clinical practices, the attempt to control costs ultimately failed. After a brief respite, costs resumed their historic rise.

Controversy regarding the fragmented collection of health providers and payers in the U.S. health care conglomerate has continued through the early part of the twenty-first century. The rate of increase in spending has slowed, but about 18% of GDP is now devoted to health expenses, and most health economists predict that spending will continue to rise. Passage of the ACA in 2010 began to address some of the problems related to coverage of the working poor and individuals with preexisting conditions, as well as availability of primary care and preventive services (eHealth 2019; Shim et al. 2012), but many problems remained (Buchmueller et al. 2016; Saloner et al. 2017). In 2018, about 10% of the U.S. population, or about 30 million people, remained uninsured, compared with 0%–2% in countries of similar economic status. Even the improvements put in place by the ACA were threatened by a change of the political wind, bringing opponents of the act into power in 2016 (Papanicolas et al. 2018).

This brief review of some of the major developments in the evolution of health care funding in the United States provides a glimpse of the patchwork process that has been responsible for the quilt of our health care landscape. A closer look at health care spending and health outcomes in the United States and other countries, as discussed in the following two sections, should provide a better idea of how this conglomerate has served the U.S. population.

Comparative Health Care Spending

There are many ways in which spending on health care can be monitored, but in almost every way imaginable, the United States spends more than any other high-income country. Sixteen years into the twenty-first century, the United States was spending about $3.3 trillion annually on health care, approaching 18% of GDP, as noted in the previous section. That is over $10,000 per person per year, and these amounts are about twice as much as the average spending of other countries with similar economic conditions (Papanicolas et al. 2018). Spending is expected to continue to rise through the first quarter of the century, and quite probably beyond, if nothing is done to fundamentally change the infrastructure of health care administration in the United States. Although spending for health care in the United

States is high, population health outcomes are no better, and in most areas are worse, than those in the member states of the Organisation for Economic Co-operation and Development (OECD), a broad consortium of countries with developed economies (see Chapter 1, "Defining and Measuring Value"). Before examining health outcomes, we look more closely at the sources of the spending differences.

Data collected to show rates of service use do not indicate that U.S. citizens use services to a significantly greater extent than citizens of other OECD nations, but the cost of the services they do use is much higher. On average, a day of hospitalization in the United States costs about five times as much as it does in France. Surgical procedures, imaging and other diagnostic tests, pharmaceuticals, and medical equipment are all much costlier than in other countries (Papanicolas et al. 2018). For example, per capita spending on drugs in the United States is almost $1,500 per year, compared with an average of less than $800 in other developed countries. Computed tomography (CT) scans are nine times as expensive as the same tests in Canada, and about twice as much as in Australia, its closest cost rival for this test. Bypass surgery often costs up to $75,000 in the United States, which is two to five times the cost of the same surgery in other developed nations (Anderson et al. 2005; Squires 2015). Physician costs are likewise higher than in other countries. Primary care physicians in the United States earn, on average, a little over $200,000 a year, about double the average earnings of physicians in other OECD countries. The disparity for specialists is even greater (Laugesen and Glied 2010). The reasons for these compensation disparities will be considered more closely later in this chapter, but higher earnings are a clear contributor to the excessive spending for health care in this country (Schneider et al. 2017).

The situation is more complex when mental illness and addiction services are considered. Mental health and substance use disorders cause the greatest amount of disease burden of any major category of illness, as measured by the amount of disability that can be attributed to them (typically reported in disability-adjusted life years). Despite this sobering fact, these disorders account for only 7% of total health spending (Kaiser Family Foundation 2020). It may be argued, therefore, that this is one area of health spending that is actually lower than necessary. The United States does not spend significantly more than other countries of similar economic status on behavioral health, but its behavioral health outcomes are significantly worse in most respects, a fact that raises concerns about how money is spent and how it is not (Bricker 2017; Shekhar et al. 2007). Although spending on direct behavioral health services is a relatively small part of total health care spending, there are many ways in which poor mental health has a significant impact on other aspects of health that are not easily measured.

These indirect costs add significant expense to the total cost of other medical services and probably far exceed the direct spending for the treatment of these behavioral illnesses (Roehrig 2016).

Behavioral health services offer fewer opportunities to extract profit from the system than other categories of illness, which have many more high-tech interventions included in their treatment protocols. Nonetheless, the $90 billion spent directly on mental illness and substance use services is a quite formidable sum. Some recent estimates put attributable costs at more than twice that figure, which would make it the costliest of disease categories in the country (Roehrig 2016). Many of the cost disparities examined above between the United States and other countries are observed in behavioral health as well. Pharmaceuticals and procedures such as electroconvulsive therapy and transcranial magnetic stimulation are, on average, almost twice as expensive as those in other similar nations, although the costs are quite variable from country to country. Although psychiatry has typically been one of the U.S. specialties with the lowest compensation (about the same as that of primary care providers), salaries have been rising in recent years because of the high demand for psychiatric services and the short supply of psychiatrists (Naibuzz 2020). The disparity in compensation for physicians in the United States versus those in other wealthy nations holds for psychiatrists as well. U.S. psychiatrists make about twice the income of European psychiatrists.

Health Outcomes

A variety of indicators provide some perspective on a population's health. Commonly used indicators include life expectancy, infant mortality, disease burden, and prevalence of chronic health conditions. Life expectancy in the United States is 78.8 years, about 3 years fewer than the average of 11 other high-income countries. In 2015, U.S. infant mortality rates were about 6 per 1,000 live births, whereas they were 3.6 per 1,000 in those same 11 nations. The disease burden, as measured in disability-adjusted life years per 100,000 population, is about 15% higher in the United States than in comparable countries. Death rates from preventable illnesses related to lack of access to health care (mortality amenable to health care) have also been highest in the United States (Organisation for Economic Cooperation and Development 2019).

Several other indicators can provide a glimpse into the state of the U.S. population's health and difficulties within the services available. The United States has the highest rates of medical errors among comparable countries; the highest percentage of its population with two or more chronic conditions (e.g., diabetes, heart disease, schizophrenia); the highest percentage of residents who are overweight or obese (35.6%); and the highest average number of medications taken regularly among individuals ages 18 and older (Avendano and Kawachi 2014; Papanicolas et al. 2018).

Although the United States has done well with respect to reducing rates of smoking, previously high rates may be contributing to the overall disease burden, especially among the growing older population. The United States also does well with respect to outcomes for care that requires a high degree of technical expertise and equipment. Despite these bright spots, access to care is generally more difficult in the United States, and particularly access to and use of primary care. The number of people who receive care in emergency departments rather than primary care offices is on average much higher in the United States than in comparable countries. People in the United States who have low and middle incomes are less likely to seek care because of cost by a wide margin over those in other countries (Davis and Ballreich 2014; Mettler 2018).

Minorities are more likely to have lower incomes and less likely to have insurance, both of which contribute to the health disparities observed in the United States. According to the Centers for Disease Control and Prevention (2013), infant mortality rates for black Americans are twice those for whites, and blacks are more likely to die prematurely from stroke or cardiovascular disease. Homicide rates are markedly higher as well, and blacks and other minorities fared significantly worse on a number of other health indicators. These disparities based on class and minority status increase the disease burden in the United States and make it more likely that people in these groups will need to use more expensive, high-intensity services when they delay treatment and develop more serious illness, again adding to unnecessary expenditures in U.S. systems (Buchmueller et al. 2016; Centers for Disease Control and Prevention 2013). These findings do not take into account the costs related to the political and social ramifications of these disparities, which may be much more significant (Cutler 2018; Mettler 2018).

Behavioral health indicators reveal many of the same types of disparities. The U.S. mortality rate for mental health and substance use disorders together is 12.0 per 100,000 population, compared with an average of 4.9 per 100,000 population in similarly wealthy countries. The disease burden caused by behavioral health disorders has been rising, up about 25% in the two decades prior to 2015 (Roser and Ritchie 2016; Spaeth-Rublee et al. 2014). The burden attributable to substance use disorders is about 3 times the impact in other comparable nations, and accidental poisoning deaths (including drug overdoses) are 6 times the rate in countries with similar incomes. Suicide rates have increased in the United States over the past two decades, reaching 13 per 100,000 people in 2014, a 24% increase in just over 15 years (Substance Abuse and Mental Health Services Administration 2016). Despite the obviously great need for services, estimates suggest that only a small percentage of people with diagnosable behavioral health disorders actually receive services, either from direct behavioral health services or primary care (Wang et al. 2007). The Epidemiologic Catchment Area study of 1986 estimated this percentage as only 20%. At least 20% of people with mental health diagnoses do not participate in treatment due to cost, access, or stigma-related concerns (Kamal et al. 2017).

The preceding examination of health expenditures and outcomes in the United States, especially in contrast to those of other countries, provides a clear indication of the lack of value the United States has obtained from its health care complex. The public has become increasingly dissatisfied with the quality of health care it receives, as well as the cost and impersonal nature of services. Clinicians have likewise been dissatisfied by the growing stress and pressure to do more in less time, and burnout has become an issue of great concern. The remainder of this chapter considers specific aspects of the system that diminish value outcomes in this country. The forces that create these circumstances and that resist efforts to reform them are also examined.

Factors That Diminish Value Outcomes

Organization of Services

The vast majority of the public, and even most people working in health care, would have a very difficult time describing the U.S. systems of care to someone who might ask. As noted at the beginning of this chapter, the source of this difficulty is the fact that rather than having a single system that covers the entire population, the United States has a conglomerate of systems that serve different constituencies. The quality and cost of coverage vary significantly depending on a variety of factors, including who is paying, whether the person has a public or private sector plan, where in the United States the person lives, and whether the plan is provided by a for-profit or not-for-profit entity. Anyone who has had to choose an insurance plan from an employer's benefit program will likely express bewilderment by the choices of deductibles and copays that are offered, in addition to various options regarding the extensiveness of coverage and the designated network. These options, taken together, determine the price of the plan and often the amount the employee must contribute. How do people decide? How can people predict their needs? There is no acceptable recipe to guide people in this process, and ultimately a large portion of the U.S. public must gamble on their health and the resources to protect it (Morrissey 2008).

Most services in the United States are provided by private entities, which may be either for-profit enterprises or nonprofit organizations. For-profit enterprises are generally paid for the services they provide by private insurance companies through a billing process. Most accept a variety of insurance policies, and many have a preferred provider status with an insurer. It is easy to imagine how complicated these financial arrangements can become, requiring providers to bill various insurers, each with a different process for doing so, and then to bill patients for the portion of each bill that an insurer will not pay (Everett et al. 2012).

Each care provider must develop an internal documentation system for medical records (often a commercial electronic medical record), which may or may not interface with the systems of other providers. When providers are not part of a medical information exchange system and patients are involved with more than one provider, communication can be very slow and cumbersome. Communication is often impeded further by confidentiality standards, which are sometimes obstructive even when patients want their information to be shared. This lack of coherence is in many cases the source of mistreatment, delays in treatment, or redundancy, affecting both the cost and quality of care.

Publicly funded health insurance is also complicated. Medicare, which is coverage for elderly people and for some people with disabilities, is paid for by the federal government through the Centers for Medicare and Medicaid Services (CMS) but administered through a variety of locally contracted insurance companies, called Medicare Administrative Contractors (Centers for Medicare and Medicaid Services 2019). Although Medicare Part A (hospitalization) is free, Part B (doctors' fees and clinical visits) and Part D (medication) have premiums attached. All parts include deductibles. Part C, also known as Medicare Advantage plans, are products developed by private insurance companies that meet or exceed the coverage of the original Medicare (Parts A and B). Part C is optional and typically has higher premiums depending on the additional coverage offered (Centers for Medicare and Medicaid Services 2019; Everett et al. 2012). The basic coverage provided for all enrollees in the original Medicare is not comprehensive, paying only about 80% of expenses; therefore, many recipients feel the need to buy Part C to protect them from uncovered charges. If this explanation seems complex, it is only because Medicare is hard to understand. Choosing the best plan for supplemental care and prescription medication can be challenging. Nevertheless, most participants feel satisfied with Medicare insurance, which is often used as the model for proposals for single-payer universal coverage.

Medicaid is administered by the states, but at least 50% of expenditures for these programs come from the Federal Medical Assistance Percentage (FMAP). States with lower per capita incomes receive a larger match. States may administer Medicaid programs directly or delegate administration to regions or counties. This fairly straightforward arrangement of government insurance has become more complex in recent years as management of Medicaid funds has, in many cases, shifted to MCOs contracted by the states (Everett et al. 2012). When this is the case, Medicaid recipients are often offered choices between qualified MCO plans for their coverage. Benefits are usually fairly consistent for these plans within a particular state, and there are usually no premiums and little or no copays or deductibles. There are federal guidelines governing Medicaid services and fees, but they are fairly broad, and states have considerable flexibility in designing their programs, and therefore benefits vary greatly from state to state. States may also apply for waivers to enact plans that fall outside established CMS parameters. Services are most often provided by private nonprofit organizations, such as community mental health clinics or other publicly funded clinics. Because reimbursement rates are relatively low with Medicaid, many private for-profit organizations do not serve Medicaid recipients (Morrissey 2008).

The Children's Health Insurance Program (CHIP) was enacted in 1997 to cover children whose families are not eligible for Medicaid and are otherwise uninsured. Organized and operated in much the same way as Medicaid, CHIP is also a federally subsidized, state-administered program. Like Medicaid, CHIP is regulated by CMS, but states have considerable flexibility in the design of the program and setting eligibility requirements. Some states operate CHIP as a program separate from Medicaid, whereas others administer their CHIP funding as a Medicaid expansion. About 9.5 million children are insured under this program (Morrissey 2008).

The other major publicly funded health program is the Veterans Health Administration (VHA) system. Serving about 9 million veterans, the VHA system was founded in 1929. Today, the system is organized into 22 regional Veterans Integrated Services Networks that operate 170 medical centers and 1,074 outpatient clinics, many of which have affiliations with U.S. medical schools (Veterans Health Administration 2020). The VHA system operates separately from other health systems in the United States and provides care free of charge to eligible veterans (Oliver 2007).

Since the 2010 passage of ACA, coverage has markedly expanded for U.S. residents, through subsidized insurance for those with low incomes, and small businesses, but even with these programs in place, funding for varying degrees of coverage is available to only about 90% of Americans (Cohen et al. 2019). A large number of people in the United States either cannot afford to or choose not to purchase health insurance because they feel that the price is so great (even for state or federally subsidized insurance exchange plans) that purchasing coverage would require them to sacrifice other essentials. Although ACA imposed an individual mandate requiring all citizens to purchase insurance, subsidies for the working poor seem inadequate for many who are eligible. Also, many of the so-called working poor do not meet eligibility requirements for any of the publicly funded insurance plans or subsidies, and therefore can only hope that they will not get sick. Of course, a substantial number will develop health problems during the time they have no coverage. Many of these individuals delay seeking health care until they are quite ill, at which point they often receive care in hospital emergency departments, which are obliged by law (Emergency Medical Treatment and Active Labor Act of 1986) to address emergency and life-threatening conditions. When these individuals need admission to a hospital, they can be transferred to a public or nonprofit hospital system that will accept them. Those hospitals that accept a large number of indigent patients are eligible to receive disproportionate share hospital payments from federal Medicaid funds (La Couture 2014). Another option for the uninsured is to seek care from a Federally Qualified Health Center; these clinics receive federal subsidies for providing care for this population (DeLeon et al. 2003). For many individuals without insurance, this can be a primary care option that could help them address health conditions before they become severe, but many members of this population are not aware of this option or do not use it.

The conglomerate of systems that provide and pay for care does cover most Americans to some degree, but what is the consequence of relying on this poorly organized network serving different groups of people in different ways? This fragmentation creates barriers to communications and to continuity and integration of care, and subsequently reduces the quality of the experience and health outcomes. There are also implications for the administration of care, which will now be considered.

Administration

A variety of administrative roles and tasks are essential for a health system to function. Developing and maintaining physical facilities, arranging appointments, managing health records, performing accounting duties, and ordering supplies are examples of activities that even the simplest and most coherent health system could not do without. In systems that are complex and incoherent, many administrative activities arise that are not necessary in better organized systems. When multiple payers must be billed for each service provided or each product used in treatment, additional staff and infrastructure are required. Activities related to billing and insurance require a significant investment from agencies providing services. In a managed care environment, a new layer of administration is introduced with regard to review and approval of payments for services and procedures recommended by clinicians. Also, licensing and regulatory reviews are required from multiple sources, and this necessitates additional time and attention from clinical and support staff.

Given this background, it is not surprising that the United States spends an alarming amount on health care administration. It is variously estimated that the United States spends from 25% to 30% of total health expenditures on administrative activities; this is about twice as much as other countries with comparable incomes (Michael 2020). Data vary somewhat depending on how *administrative expense* is defined. For example, if the administrative expenses associated with hospital and nursing home care are left out, the United States spends about 8% on administration, compared with 1%–2% in comparable nations (Papanicolas et al. 2018). In any case, the U.S. system is obviously much costlier to administer. When all administrative expenses are combined, even when lower estimates with recent data are used, the United States is spending about 5% of its GDP, or nearly $1 trillion per year to keep health care systems operating (Cutler 2018). A significant portion of this expense can be attributed to billing- and insurance-related activities, which account for about half of all administrative expenses, or about $500 billion (Jiwani et al. 2014; Sakowski et al. 2009).

Other administrative expense can be attributed to the free market health care industry. The United States is the only country worldwide that has conceived of health care primarily as a business in which lucrative profits can be extracted by companies both large and small. Profits extracted from the overall costs of health care are basically regarded as the cost of doing business (Woolhandler and Himmelstein 2004). That said, there is little doubt that profit motives increase the cost of care without improving its quality, and in many ways profit incentives can be seen as actually reducing quality. Health care firms profit in excess of an estimated $65 billion annually (Ryder 2018). This is a small amount relative to administrative expenses, for example, but the profit motive has implications for the system that are far reaching. The drive for profit is largely responsible for the high prices of U.S. pharmaceuticals, for example, and for the overpricing of other products relative to their cost in other countries. Similarly, the profit motive is contributing to the high cost of physician services, procedures, overtreatment (when clients get more of a billable service than they need), and undertreatment (when clients do not receive all the service elements they need), all of which are significant sources of expense. Also, major businesses beyond those that are most commonly identified—namely, pharmaceuticals and insurance—have developed around health care provision (Berwick and Hackbarth 2012). Many argue, however, that this profit motive is not a bad thing, despite its expense, and that it has been an incentive for the innovation and technological improvements that have been responsible for the superiority of highly technical care in the United States. Although this argument may be valid, it seems that these technological advantages ultimately use resources that would be better spent on improving the population's health overall.

As alluded to above, there are many sources of cost in our system that do not contribute in any positive way to the quality of health in this country. Berwick and Hackbarth (2012) identified elimination of waste as the best opportunity for reducing health expenditures in the United States. They designated the following six categories of waste that impact the U.S. system, and they estimated that these factors make up at least 20%, and possibly as much as 40%, of all health expenditures in 2012:

1. *Failure of care delivery:* Poor quality of care or failure to use best practices results in poor outcomes.
2. *Poor coordination of care:* Care coordination is more difficult in fragmented systems, but failure to carry out such coordination results in complications, readmissions, and increased disability and chronicity.
3. *Overtreatment:* Irrational polypharmacy, redundant diagnostics, unnecessary surgeries or procedures, and unwanted care at the end of life are examples of treatments that are excessive and counterproductive.
4. *Administrative complexity:* Overly prescriptive rules and regulations with lack of consistency across microsystems make inefficient use of clinicians' time and efforts.
5. *Overpricing:* Lack of effective competition and cost transparency result in high prices and profits, which are extracted from the system.
6. *Fraud and abuse:* Overbilling or billing occurs for services that were not actually provided.

They postulate that focusing on the reduction of these sources of waste in the system would be much more effective than attempts to limit spending on direct services through restricted access or reduction of reimbursement rates, which has been the traditional approach (Berwick and Hackbarth 2012; Cutler 2018).

Liability for malpractice is another frequently cited source of waste. Related expenses include indemnity payments, administrative (including legal) expenses, the cost associated with defensive medicine (overtreatment), and the direct and indirect expenses associated with malpractice insurance premiums. A study in 2008 estimated the overall annual liability system cost at $55.6 billion, or 2.4% of health care spending (Mello et al. 2010). This study did not include insurance premiums. Other analyses that have been more inclusive (including insurance premiums, impact on physician payments, documentation) have estimated the contribution to be as high as 9%, or nearly $300 billion in the context of more recent spending data. Relative to other countries grounded in the British legal tradition (Canada, Australia, United Kingdom), rates of litigation were 50% higher in the United States than in its closest comparable country, the United Kingdom, but 3.5 times higher than in Canada. Malpractice awards were slightly higher in the United States than in these comparable countries, but payments per case were actually lower in the United States. There have been highly divergent estimates of the actual costs attributable to defensive medicine, so it is not clear how successful tort reform could be in reducing the cost of health care, but there have been several proposals for such reform. It is worth noting that malpractice expenses play a relatively small role in behavioral health spending (Anderson et al. 2005).

Current Funding of Health Services

As noted in the previous section, billing and insurance issues are the major source of administrative expense in the U.S. system. These issues arise primarily because of the system's predominant reliance on fee-for-service (FFS) reimbursement arrangements for provided services. Financing solutions will be considered in detail in Chapter 6 ("Innovative Financing"), but the consideration of issues adversely affecting value within the current system in the United States would not be complete without discussing the implications of choosing this financing arrangement. Although all financing arrangements create particular incentives to those who hold risk and those who do not, FFS arrangements are most toxic to the value equation (Woolhandler and Himmelstein 2004). Providers are restricted in their options for designing programs to identify specific needs, clinicians feel restricted with regard to diversity in their activities and satisfaction with their roles, and patients feel that they do not have significant relationships with service providers because of limited provider time and attention.

Apart from the obvious problems related to the need to bill payers, which are especially onerous in a fragmented system with multiple payers and providers, FFS arrangements create other incentives for providers and payers that have implications for cost and quality. Entities providing coverage set rates for specific services that they consider necessary and "billable." Although these billable services are often defined through some internal process by payers, they are not necessarily comprehensive or adequate to meet the needs of the populations being served. Providers often are limited to providing services that are billable rather than being able to include all that are necessary, a practice that leads in some cases to undertreatment and in other instances to overtreatment. Providers have an incentive to provide as much billable service as they can, whereas payers have an incentive to limit outlays as much as possible, creating an adversarial relationship that is cumbersome and fraught with complexity (Woolhandler et al. 2003).

Among the disadvantages related to this payment method are that it discourages innovation, flexibility, and creativity by service providers and it does not permit service providers to use their personnel as effectively as they would like to. For example, an outpatient behavioral health provider might see some advantage in using their psychiatrists as a resource in treatment team meetings or in a consulting or supervisory role; however, if these services are not considered billable, it would not be financially viable for the provider to use the psychiatrists in these ways. There are many other examples of how FFS financing is restrictive and cumbersome in designing programs to meet identified needs. In recent years, it has become clear that the integration of primary care and behavioral health offers many advantages (O'Neil and Scheinker 2010). Beyond the grants to pilot these programs, however, it has been difficult to sustain them. This is because funding and billing for behavioral health and physical health services are usually quite distinct in FFS systems, so it is difficult to arrange payment pathways that allow reimbursement of integrated behavioral health services. These are only a few examples of how FFS arrangements indirectly impact the quality of care, satisfaction with services, and cost of care.

Focus of Services

As noted earlier, U.S. health systems do a good job of treating acute illness, and they have abundant access to technological advances that aid in the diagnosis and treatment of acute conditions. Unfortunately, these miraculous interventions are not uniformly accessible to all members of society, but even if these interventions were, they would have very little impact on the overall health of the population. Although the cure or curtailment of disease is often dramatic and astonishing, it is also expensive and may be only partially or transiently effective. As noted earlier in the section "Health Outcomes," the United States has a very high rate of residents with two or more chronic illnesses, which is indicative of a system that delivers too little, too late. The focus on tertiary care eats up a large part of U.S. health care spending and has made it difficult to reserve additional funding for those activities that do have the capacity to significantly improve the population's health outcomes (Grogan 2012). Prevention, including health promotion, and primary care command a relatively small part of the health care budget, and this imbalance has much to do with the poor value realized by the U.S. health care systems.

Prevention

Estimates suggest that spending on prevention varies between 2% and 9% of total health care spending, and the variation seems to depend to a large extent on what types of activities are considered as part of prevention spending (Miller et al. 2012). A full discussion of prevention and its role in a value-based system is provided in Chapter 8 ("Prevention and Health Promotion"), but a brief consideration of the three types of prevention is useful here. *Primary prevention* is defined as activities designed to prevent new cases of disease (the goal is decreased incidence). *Secondary prevention* involves early detection and treatment prior to onset of symptoms, reducing the impact and duration of the disease process (the goal is reduced prevalence). *Tertiary prevention* is basically treatment to reduce morbidity related to an illness (Compton 2012). Generally, tertiary prevention is not included in prevention spending estimates because it is generally accounted for in treatment costs.

Miller and colleagues (2012) divide primary and secondary prevention spending into three categories: 1) personal health care preventive services, which include interventions such as wellness counseling, immunizations, and screening; 2) public health activities that impact the entire population; and 3) prevention research to determine what interventions are most effective. These authors estimate that 8.6% of health care funding is related to these three prevention categories. This estimate drops to 8.3% when the rather minuscule allotment for prevention research is subtracted. The estimate drops further to 5.3% when consideration is limited to primary prevention activities and screening, and to 4.4% when the prevention aspects of primary care are eliminated (these functions are usually factored into the costs of direct medical care). Spending for public health interventions alone amounts to just 3.1% of total health care funding (Miller et al. 2008). Although there is some lack of clarity about what activities are included in public health interventions (Sensenig 2007), these 2008 estimates do not differ significantly from most other attempts to quantify prevention spending.

Regardless of the estimate used, investment in prevention is grossly inadequate relative to its potential to impact the population's health status. For example, to illustrate this in other terms, Grogan (2012) notes that for every dollar spent on health care in the United States, 75 cents is spent on chronic illnesses and only 4 cents on preventing those diseases. It is worth noting that, unlike other areas of health spending where the United States spends considerably more than similar countries, the estimated average for

OECD member nations for prevention spending is only 3% (Gmeinder et al. 2017; Organisation for Economic Cooperation and Development 2017). The undervaluing of prevention continues to be an issue worldwide and is an area in which reallocation of spending could have a significant impact.

Primary Care

Primary care is another area in which considerable improvement is needed (Campbell 2007; Friedberg et al. 2010). Health promotion activities, including education, counseling, monitoring and screening, and immunizations, all occur primarily in the context of primary care. Strong primary care capacity and performance are associated with better health outcomes, yet primary care in the U.S. system is difficult to access and is less capable in many respects than primary care in other developed countries. In addition to having direct health benefits, broad-scale engagement with primary care reduces costs and health disparities (Starfield et al. 2005). There is strong evidence for these outcomes across regions and health systems (Starfield and Shi 2007).

A few factors are influential in the association of primary care and positive health outcomes. Areas in which the supply of and access to primary care physicians are high have better health outcomes on a variety of health measures, and individuals with an identified primary care provider are on average healthier than those without this connection. The United States has fewer primary care providers per 100,000 people than comparable countries and more financial barriers to care. There is also a clear association of outcomes to the quality of primary care; the better the quality of primary care, the better the outcomes achieved (Starfield et al. 2005).

Consultation duration, patient mix, and scope of practice are three indicators that are associated with better quality primary care. The average per capita exposure to a primary care physician in the United States is 29.7 minutes annually, less than half of the per capita exposure in the United Kingdom, New Zealand, and Australia (Campbell 2007). Typically, U.S. primary care practitioners manage a more limited case mix and feel less able to manage chronic and complex conditions, including mental health disorders. Home visits are also much less common in the United States. Primary care physicians' focus on acute conditions limits their capacity to provide care for chronic conditions and prevention activities. Compared with primary care physicians from comparable countries, those in the United States are more likely to feel that the system in which they work needs fundamental reform and that they spend too much time on administrative activities (Schoen et al. 2012).

Another relevant aspect of the U.S. system is that more people receive primary care from specialists, such as obstetrician-gynecologists, pediatricians, and internists, than in most other countries (Bindman et al. 2007). This is in some respects a positive compensation for lack of access to general practitioners such as family practice physicians. However, with the possible exception of pediatrics, this arrangement may also limit the scope of the care provided, particularly with regard to preventive and behavioral health issues. Although psychiatry has at times been regarded as a primary care specialty, in reality few psychiatrists feel comfortable managing simple medical problems or engaging in general health promotion activities, even when their clients are unconnected to primary care, as they often are for a variety of reasons (Sowers et al. 2016). Lack of preparation is likely one of the most important explanations for psychiatrists' discomfort with taking a role in primary care issues. The final subsection of this chapter will consider how the design and experience of medical education support many of the deficits identified in U.S. health care.

Medical Education

This chapter has identified several ways in which the cost of care in the United States is needlessly high, as well as many factors that undermine the quality of care and the population's health. Many aspects of the system's design (or lack thereof) impact this situation, and medical education is one more that can be added to the list. In many ways the system of medical education in the United States adversely affects both cost and quality of care.

As stated earlier in this chapter (see section "Comparative Health Care Spending"), physicians in the United States make about twice as much as their peers in other developed countries. This is true across specialties including psychiatry. What leads to the high valuation of physician services in the United States? It is due in part to how medical education is financed. Because there is little government funding for medical school, a medical education is very costly and well beyond the means of most applicants. As a result, most students need to borrow money to pay for their education. The average debt accumulated by graduates from U.S. medical schools is about $200,000 (Gil et al. 2013). This amount is more or less equivalent to the mortgage on a modest home in many parts of the country and is a daunting burden for someone beginning a career. This burden causes many physicians to seek lucrative positions after their graduation and has contributed to the high percentage of physicians in specialties, subspecialties, and private practices, as opposed to primary care, although there is some evidence that this is not the major consideration for career selections (Gil et al. 2013). Nonetheless, the burden also creates incentives for physicians, particularly those in technical and surgical specialties, to perform more procedures than evidence from outcomes would support. One additional factor adding to the cost physicians contribute to health care spending is the limited production of medical graduates, creating a relative shortage of physicians, and therefore a high demand for physician services (Association of American Medical Colleges 2018). This shortage has resulted in an escalation in physician compensation, particularly in psychiatry, which has risen sharply in recent years.

In light of these facts, it becomes clear that the U.S. system of medical education has implications beyond the direct compensation of physicians for the overall spending on health care and indirectly supports many of the factors identified earlier which contribute to the high cost of health care. These factors include the overuse of expensive technology, the excessive performance of questionably effective surgeries and procedures, the limited supply of primary care physicians, and a focus on acute rather than chronic care and preventive activities. In psychiatry, the use of a complex diagnostic system, with questionable validity and reliability, also contributes to cost (due to overtreatment) and erodes quality (through the prescription of inappropriate care) (see Chapter 11, "An Expanded Role for Psychiatry").

The content of medical school education has implications for the quality of health care in the United States. Medical school curricula tend to focus on the evolution of disease and the treatment of disease, rather than health and its preservation (Garr et al. 2000; Taylor and Moore 1994). Young adults who enter medicine are often inspired by the dramatic reversals of disease processes as depicted in television and films, and reported in news and social media. Doctors who are involved in the high-profile activities of fighting rare or severe diseases enjoy greater prestige than those who toil in the trenches providing primary care. At the same time, research funding is heavily weighted toward finding cures for acute-onset diseases, such as cancer or infections, and for the treatment of chronic conditions, such as diabetes or schizophrenia, whereas funding for prevention research is hard to come by (Health Affairs 2012). Because research funding supports the institutions and the careers of faculty who participate in medical education, it is little wonder that medical schools have skewed curricula toward disease processes.

The discussion of prevention and health promotion in the preceding subsection emphasized the value of these activities to population health. The shortage of primary care providers and the lack of preparation of the medical workforce to provide preventive care are major factors in the poor outcomes achieved in U.S. health care. Because training is embedded in a system governed by market forces, institutions providing it often have financial interests that partially dictate clinical rotations in the curricula.

One glaring example of this situation is in the training of psychiatrists. Accreditation standards require that 6 months of the 4-year curriculum be spent in general medical training. The interests of caring for psychiatric patients with co-occurring physical health issues would best be served if that 6 months were spent in primary care settings. Instead, with few exceptions, aspiring psychiatrists spend 6 months in hospital settings, caring for patients with acute illnesses. This arrangement serves the interests of the institution, which benefits from the low expense of care provided by house staff and the higher rate of Medicare support for inpatient services. However, this practice leaves psychiatrists ill prepared to address physical health issues that have a significant impact on the mental health of the people they serve.

Overall, public health, prevention and health promotion, and training rotations in community settings make up only a small part of medical education, and this minimization of such content has an adverse effect on population health (Finkel 2012). Despite growing recognition that this imbalance in the focus of education has to change, few advances have yet been made toward this goal. There have been several experiments in curriculum structure and in the reduction of debt for medical graduates. For example, New York University is now providing free tuition for all enrolled medical students in an attempt to free them from financial concerns in planning their careers (Weisman 2018). The outcome of this endeavor will be of interest in light of some evidence that debt has a limited impact on career choices (Gil et al. 2013). More focused incentives for entering primary care and serving in underserved areas may have more favorable results. A full consideration of workforce development for psychiatric care is provided in Chapter 12 ("Psychiatric Workforce Development").

Conclusion

This chapter has focused on the issues in the current conglomerate of services and payers that adversely affect the value derived from health care in the United States. Most of these issues permeate the entire health care landscape in the United States, encompassing the psychiatric care that is the main focus of this book. Because it is difficult to separate mental health from overall health, the difficulties encountered in the delivery or quality of mental health care has a significant impact on population health and health care spending. The psychiatric workforce is stressed and employed inefficiently, and most psychiatrists are ill prepared to take responsibility for reducing waste and promoting health as aggressively as needed. Most of the remainder of this book is focused on finding solutions to these issues that have negatively impacted the value obtained from health care services, leaving the United States with a "system" that is the most expensive in the world despite delivering health outcomes that are inferior to those in comparable countries that spend much less.

References

Anderson GF, Hussey PS, Frogner BK, et al: Health spending in the United States and the rest of the industrialized world. Health Aff (Millwood) 24(4):903–914, 2005

Association of American Medical Colleges: GME funding and its role in addressing the physician shortage. May 29, 2018. Available at: https://news.aamc.org/for-the-media/article/gme-funding-doctor-shortage. Accessed February 6, 2020.

Avendano M, Kawachi I: Why do Americans have shorter life expectancy and worse health than do people in other high-income countries? Ann Rev Public Health 35:307–325, 2014

Berwick DM, Hackbarth AD: Eliminating waste in U.S. health care. JAMA 307(14):1513–1516, 2012

Bindman AB, Forrest CB, Britt H, et al: Diagnostic scope of and exposure to primary care physicians in Australia, New Zealand, and the United States: cross sectional analysis of results from three national surveys. BMJ 334(7606):1261, 2007

Bricker E: Healthcare costs are rising, but where is the money going? Compass Navigating Healthcare Blog, Healthcare Trends, 2017. Available at: www.compassphs.com/blog/healthcare-costs-are-rising-but-where-is-the-money-going. Accessed February 6, 2020.

Buchmueller TC, Levinson ZM, Levy HG, et al: Effect of the Affordable Care Act on racial and ethnic disparities in health insurance coverage. Am J Public Health 106(8):1416–1421, 2016

Campbell JL: Provision of primary care in different countries. BMJ 334(7606):1230–1231, 2007

Catlin AC, Cowan CA: History of health spending in the United States, 1960–2013. November 19, 2015. Available at: www.cms.gov/Research-Statistics-Data-and-Systems/Statistics-Trends-and-Reports/NationalHealthExpend-Data/Downloads/HistoricalNHEPaper.pdf. Accessed February 6, 2020.

Centers for Disease Control and Prevention: Health disparities and inequalities report—United States. MMWR Suppl 62(3):1–187, 2013

Centers for Medicare and Medicaid Services: What is a MAC. December 13, 2019. Available at: www.cms.gov/Medicare/Medicare-Contracting/Medicare-Administrative-Contractors/What-is-a-MAC.html. Accessed February 6, 2020.

Cohen RA, Terlizzi EP, Marinez ME: Health insurance coverage: early release of estimates from the national health interview survey, 2018, National Center for Health Statistics. May 2019. Available at: https://www.cdc.gov/nchs/data/nhis/earlyrelease/insur201905.pdf. Accessed June 24, 2020.

Commonwealth Fund: The Commonwealth Fund 2014 international health policy of older adults in eleven countries. November 2014. Available at: www.commonwealthfund.org/sites/default/files/documents/___media_files_publications_in_the_literature_2014_nov_pdf_1787_commonwealth_fund_2014_intl_survey_chartpack.pdf. Accessed February 6, 2020.

Compton M: Public health, prevention and community psychiatry, in Handbook of Community Psychiatry. Edited by McQuistion HL, Sowers WE, Ranz JM, et al. New York, Springer Science & Business Media, 2012, pp 37–44

Cunningham R III, Cunningham RM Jr: The Blues: A History of the Blue Cross and Blue Shield System. DeKalb, IL, Northern Illinois University Press, 1997, pp 25–53

Cutler D: What is the U.S. health spending problem? Health Aff (Millwood) 37(3):493–497, 2018

Davis K, Ballreich J: Equitable access to care—how the United States ranks internationally. N Engl J Med 371(17):1567–1570, 2014

DeLeon PH, Giesting B, Kenkel MB: Community health centers: exciting opportunities for the 21st century. Professional Psychology: Research and Practice 34(6):579–585, 2003

Dranove D, Millenson M: Medical bankruptcy: myth versus fact. Health Aff (Millwood) 25(2):579–585, 2006

eHealth: History and timeline of the Affordable Care Act (ACA). October 31, 2019. Available at: https://resources.ehealthinsurance.com/affordable-care-act/history-timeline-affordable-care-act-aca. Accessed February 6, 2020.

Everett A, Sowers WE, McQuistion HL: Financing of community behavioral health services, in Handbook of Community Psychiatry. Edited by McQuistion HL, Sowers WE, Ranz JM, et al. New York, Springer Science and Business Media, 2012, pp 50–59

Finkel ML: Integrating the public health component into the medical school curriculum. Public Health Rep 127(2):145–146, 2012

Friedberg MW, Hussey PS, Schneider EC: Primary care: a critical review of the evidence on quality and costs of health care. Health Aff (Millwood) 29(5):766–772, 2010

Garr DR, Lackland DT, Wilson DB: Prevention, education and evaluation in U.S. medical schools. Acad Med 75(7 Suppl):S145–S146, 2000

Gil JA, Waryasz GR, Liu D, et al: Influence of medical student debt on the decision to pursue careers in primary care. R I Med J 99(7):19–21, 2013

Gmeinder M, Morgan D, Mueller M: How much do OECD countries spend on prevention? OECD Health Working Papers, No 101. December 15, 2017. Available at: www.oecd-ilibrary.org/social-issues-migration-health/how-much-do-oecd-countries-spend-on-prevention_f19e803c-en. Accessed February 6, 2020.

Gordon C: Why no national health insurance in the U.S.? The limits of social provision in war and peace, 1941–1948. Journal of Policy History 9(3):277–310, 1997

Griffin J: The history of healthcare in America. JP Griffin Group, March 7, 2017. Available at: www.griffinbenefits.com/employeebenefitsblog/history_of_healthcare. Accessed February 6, 2020.

Grogan CM: Prevention spending. J Health Polit Policy Law 37(2):329–342, 2012
Health Affairs: The prevention and public health fund. Health Affairs Health Policy Brief, February 23, 2012. Available at: www.healthaffairs.org/do/10.1377/hpb20120223.98342/full. Accessed February 6, 2020.
Jiwani A, Himmelstein D, Woolhandler S, et al: Billing and insurance-related administrative costs in United States' health care: synthesis of micro-costing evidence. BMC Health Serv Res 14:556, 2014
Kaiser Family Foundation: Peterson-Kaiser health system tracker, health status, OECD health statistics. 2020. Available at: www.healthsystemtracker.org/?sfid=4356&_sft_category=access-affordability,health-well-being,spending,quality-of-care. Accessed February 6, 2020.
Kamal R, Cox C, Rousseau D: Costs and outcomes of mental health and substance use disorders in the U.S. JAMA 318(5):415, 2017
La Couture B: Primer: the Disproportionate Share Hospital (DSH) program: American action forum. August 21, 2014. Available at: www.americanactionforum.org/research/primer-the-disproportionate-share-hospital-dsh-program. Accessed February 6, 2020.
Laugesen MJ, Glied SA: Higher fees paid to U.S. physicians drive higher spending for physician services compared to other countries. Health Aff (Millwood) 30(9):1647–1656, 2010
Luce J, Bindman AB, Lee PR: A brief history of health care quality assessment and improvement in the United States. West J Med 160(3):263–268, 1994
Mahar M: Money-driven medicine: the real reason health care costs so much. BMJ 333(7566):504, 2006
Mello M, Chandra A, Gawande AA, et al: National costs of the medical liability system. Health Aff (Millwood) 29(9):1569–1577, 2010
Mettler S: The Government-Citizen Disconnect. New York, Russell Sage Foundation, 2018
Michael E: A third of US health care spending stems from administrative costs. Healio January 6, 2020. Available at: www.healio.com/news/primary-care/20200106/a-third-of-us-health-care-spending-stems-from-administrative-costs. Accessed June 20, 2020.
Miller G, Roehrig C, Hughes-Cromwick P, et al: Quantifying national spending on wellness and prevention, in Beyond Health Insurance: Public Policy to Improve Health (Advances in Health Economics and Health Services Research, Vol 19). Edited by Helmchen L, Kaestner R, Lo Sasso A. Bingley, UK, Emerald Group Publishing, 2008, pp 1–24
Miller G, Roehrig C, Hughes-Cromwick P, et al: What is currently spent on prevention as compared to treatment? in Prevention vs. Treatment: What's the Right Balance? Edited by Faust H, Menzel E. New York, Oxford University Press, 2012, pp 37–55
Morrissey M: History of health insurance in the United States, in Health Insurance, 2nd Edition. Chicago, IL, Health Administration Press, 2008, pp 3–21
Murray JE: Origins of American Health Insurance: A History of Industrial Sickness Funds. New Haven, CT, Yale University Press, 2007, pp 65–87

Naibuzz: Ten countries with the highest psychiatrist salaries. Available at: https://naibuzz.com/countries-with-the-highest-psychiatrist-salaries. March 2, 2020. Accessed June 2020.

Navarro V: Why some countries have national health insurance, others have national health services, and the United States has neither. Soc Sci Med 19(3):383–404, 1989

Numbers RL: The third party: health insurance in America, in The Therapeutic Revolution: Essays in the History of Medicine, Edited by Vogal HG, Rosenberg CE. Philadelphia, PA, University of Pennsylvania Press, 1979, pp 177–200

Oliver A: The Veterans Health Administration: An American success story? Milbank Q 85(1):5–35, 2007

O'Neil D, Scheinker D: Wasted health spending: Who's picking up the tab? Health Aff (Millwood) 29(9):1569–1577, 2010

Organisation for Economic Cooperation and Development: Health at a Glance 2017: OECD indicators. 2017. Available at: www.oecd.org/els/health-systems/Health-at-a-Glance-2017-Chartset.pdf. Accessed February 6, 2020.

Organisation for Economic Cooperation and Development: Health at a Glance 2019: OECD indicators. 2019. Available at: www.oecd.org/els/health-systems/Health-at-a-Glance-2019-Chartset.pdf. Accessed June 2020.

Papanicolas I, Woskie LR, Jha AK: Health care spending in the United States and other high-income countries. JAMA 319(10):1024–1039, 2018

Roehrig C: Mental disorders top the list of the most costly conditions in the United States: $201 billion. Health Aff (Millwood) 35(6):1130–1135, 2016

Roser M, Ritchie H: Burden of disease. Our World in Data 2016. Available at: https://ourworldindata.org/burden-of-disease. Accessed June 19, 2020.

Ryder B: Which firms profit most from America's health care system? The Economist, May 15, 2018. Available at: www.economist.com/business/2018/03/15/which-firms-profit-most-from-americas-health-care-system. Accessed February 6, 2020.

Sakowski JA, Kahn JG, Kronick RG, et al: Peering into the black box: billing and insurance activities in a medical group delivering on global health. Health Aff (Millwood) 28(4):w544–w554, 2009

Saloner B, Bandara S, Bachhuber M, et al: Insurance coverage and treatment use under the Affordable Care Act among adults with mental and substance use disorders. Psychiatr Serv 68(6):542–548, 2017

Schneider EC, Sarnak DO, Squires D, et al: Mirror, mirror 2017: international comparison reflects flaws and opportunities for better U.S. health care. The Commonwealth Fund, July 2017. Available at: https://interactives.commonwealthfund.org/2017/july/mirror-mirror. Accessed February 6, 2020.

Schoen C, Osborn R, Squires D, et al: Survey of primary care doctors in ten countries shows progress in use of health information technology, less in other areas. Health Aff (Millwood) 31(12):2508–2516, 2012

Sensenig AL: Refining estimates of public health spending as measured in national health expenditures accounts: the United States experience. J Public Health Manag Pract 13(2):103–114, 2007

Shekhar S, Thornicroft G, Knapp M, et al: Resources for mental health: scarcity, inequity, and inefficiency. Lancet 370(95):878–889, 2007

Shim R, Koplan C, Langheim F, et al: Health care reform and integrated care: a golden opportunity for preventive psychiatry. Psychiatr Serv 63(12):1231–1233, 2012

Sowers W, Arbuckle M, Shoyinka S: Guidelines for primary care provided by psychiatrists. Community Ment Health J 52(4):379–386, 2016

Spaeth-Rublee B, Pincus HA, Silvestri F, et al: Measuring quality of mental health care: an international comparison. Int J Environ Res Public Health 11(10):10384–10389, 2014

Squires D: U.S. health care from a global perspective: spending, use of services, prices, and health in 13 countries. October 8, 2015. Available at: www.commonwealthfund.org/publications/issue-briefs/2015/oct/us-health-care-global-perspective. Accessed February 6, 2020.

Starfield B, Shi L: Commentary: Primary care and health outcomes: a health services research challenge. Health Serv Res 42(6 Pt 1):2252–2256, 2007

Starfield B, Shi L, Macinko J: Contribution of primary care to health systems and health. Milbank Q 83(3):457–502, 2005

Starr P: Transformation in defeat: the changing objectives of national health insurance, 1915–1980. Am J Public Health 72(1):78–88, 1982

Substance Abuse and Mental Health Services Administration: Behavioral health spending and use accounts, 1986–2014 (HHS Publ No SMA-16-4975). Rockville, MD, Substance Abuse and Mental Health Services Administration, 2016

Taylor WC, Moore T: Health promotion and disease prevention: integration into a medical school curriculum. Med Educ 28(6):481–487, 1994

Veterans Health Administration: Providing health care for veterans. Updated July 13, 2020. Available at: https://www.va.gov/health. Accessed July 27, 2020.

Wang P, Aguilar-Gaxiola S, Alonso J: Use of mental health services for anxiety, mood, and substance disorders in 17 countries in the WHO world mental health surveys. Lancet 370(9590):841–850, 2007

Weisman J: NYU is making its medical school free. What a waste. Slate, August 20, 2018. Available at: https://slate.com/business/2018/08/nyu-medical-school-plans-free-tuition-for-all-what-a-waste-of-money.html. Accessed February 6, 2020.

Woolhandler S, Himmelstein DU: The high costs of for-profit care. CMAJ 170(12):1814–1815, 2004

Woolhandler S, Campbell T, Himmelstein DU: Costs of health care administration in the United States and Canada. N Engl J Med 349(8):768–775, 2003

4

Social Determinants of Health

Kyle E. Rodenbach, M.D.

In the preamble to its constitution, the World Health Organization defines *health* as "a state of complete physical, mental and social well-being and not merely the absence of disease or infirmity" (World Health Organization 1946). This definition is noteworthy for two reasons: 1) it defines *health* as a state of complete rather than partial well-being and 2) it highlights the notion that health is not simply the absence of illness. Indeed, health is an active process and a goal in itself. Systems that wish to provide high-value services must constantly pursue population health.

There is extensive literature concerning the various social determinants of health as well as policy initiatives to address them. One might ask why these social variables have drawn so much attention and why they are considered by many to be more important than other aspects of health and health care, such as research for new treatments or the development of new pharmaceuticals. The social determinants of health are important because they contribute significantly to morbidity and mortality and are potentially modifiable. Commonly referred to as the "causes of the causes," social determinants include both basic needs (water, food, shelter, health care, and income) and the root causes that drive unequal access to them (discrimination, poverty, income inequality, and adverse life experiences). Resulting health disparities indicate a lack of equality in the distribution of social goods that most democratic nations have, at least ostensibly, articulated interest in ameliorating. If this is in fact true, then there should be a moral imperative to eliminate these disparities in order to create the egalitarian society that democracy implies. Additionally, continuing to spend on the downstream effects of social disparities rather than invest in social equality itself results in extremely expensive, yet ineffective, systems of health care, such as that developed in the United States.

The Organisation for Economic Co-operation and Development, or OECD, was founded in 1961 with goals that included the comparison of international policies to solve social, economic, and environmental challenges. Review of available data related to social spending, health care spending, and health care outcomes is particularly relevant here. The OECD Web site publishes data from each member country in graphic form for a variety of health indicators. The following discussion draws from these indicators, which are easily accessible via the OECD site (https://data.oecd.org).

Among the 36 OECD nations, the United States continues to outspend all other members on per capita health care yet ranks in the bottom half for life expectancy from birth, ninth for per capita suicide rate, and third for percentage of adults who are overweight or obese. However, increased U.S. health care spending does not translate into improved health. Additionally, despite a large and seemingly robust economy, taxation in the United States is low compared to that in other OECD nations, ranking in the bottom quartile for overall collected tax revenue as a percentage of gross domestic product (GDP). Because of low rates of wealth and service redistribution in the United States, the country ranks fourth for percentage of adults living below the poverty line and sixth for income inequality. Moreover, in overall social spending—defined as cash benefits, direct provision of goods and services, and tax breaks with social purposes—the United States ranks in the bottom half of OECD nations, specifically in the bottom five for unemployment spending and in the bottom 10 for incapacity spending (disability, sickness, and injury).

Although it is exceedingly difficult to definitively link redistribution of wealth and increased spending on social services to decreased health care spending and improved population health, closer examination of data from other OECD nations supports a correlation. The United States, Switzerland, Luxembourg, and Norway, in that order, spend the most per capita on health care. Of those four countries, all but the United States have significantly better than average ratings for life expectancy from birth, ranking in the top 10 of OECD nations. Like the United States, these nations also have large economies, ranking in the top 10 in overall GDP. Why would an industrialized nation such as the United States with a similarly large economy and high levels of health care spending experience significantly worse health outcomes than these other nations? Although there are no definitive data, the fact that Switzerland, Luxembourg, and Norway rank significantly higher than the United States in terms of tax revenue collected and significantly lower in income inequality may explain part of the discrepancy.

Additionally, OECD data tend to contradict the notion that having a large economy and spending large amounts on health care are required for population health. Israel, Spain, Italy, and Australia, for example, are notable for spending less than half per capita on health care compared with the United States while still ranking in the top 10 for life expectancy from birth. Additionally, nations ranking highest in overall social spending, such as France, Belgium, Finland, Denmark, and Italy, continue to surpass the United States in life expectancy at birth and life expectancy at age 65. Additionally, Denmark is the only nation in that group ranking in the top 10 for health care spending, suggesting that social spending in other areas may produce better health outcomes than spending on health care itself. Italy, for example, spends roughly one-third of what the United States spends per capita on health care but is often considered to be one of the healthiest nations in the world.

Although social determinants of health are relevant to all fields of medicine, this chapter discusses the social determinants of mental health based on the available evidence. Disparities in basic needs are addressed first, followed by discussion of the underlying causes of inequality, such as discrimination, poverty, and adverse childhood experiences. This is followed by discussion of incentives for change, as well as the role of psychiatrists and other stakeholders in implementing solutions. The social determinants of health are relevant to discussions of cost and quality because, as will be discussed, failure to address them seriously hinders delivery of high-quality, cost-effective mental health services to the impacted populations. Solutions to these problems will require increased clinical attention, clinician and patient advocacy, and substantial financial support from relevant stakeholders, including local and federal governments. Continued failure to address social disparities will perpetuate a system of wasteful, ineffective health care and continued decline in the health of average Americans.

Basic Needs

Food and Nutrition

Food insecurity encompasses a broad spectrum of deficiencies ranging from profound hunger and starvation to a troubling but less dire phenomenon of running low on food toward the end of the month. Although mental health providers practicing in certain parts of the world may encounter the psychiatric conditions associated with starvation and severe malnutrition (e.g., Wernicke's encephalopathy, dementia associated with pellagra), practitioners in industrialized countries will more commonly encounter food insecurity as contributing to mental illness in more subtle ways. An extensive literature also exists examining correlations between poor diet and numerous chronic medical conditions, such as the metabolic syndrome (a clustering of conditions generally including high blood pressure, central obesity determined by waist circumference or waist-to-hip ratio, elevated cholesterol, elevated triglycerides, and diabetes). This literature is not discussed in great detail here, although it is worth noting that medical comorbidity is an independent and incremental risk factor for development of depression and indirectly contributes to psychiatric illness by affecting one's ability to engage in enjoyable and fulfilling activities (Read et al. 2017).

The relationship between food insecurity and physical and mental illness is complex. In terms of physical health, for example, food insecurity has been linked to obesity rather than low body weight, particularly in women (Dinour et al. 2007; Siefert et al. 2001). Evidence suggests that diets comprising calorie-dense, nutrient-deficient foods may be associated with higher levels of inflammatory markers and altered immune system function, possibly mediating the link between food insecurity, obesity, and chronically poor health (Gowda et al. 2012). Whether these high-inflammatory states contribute to mental illness appears less clear. There does, however, appear to be a clear and compelling link between food insecurity and depressive disorders, particularly in women, but also in adolescents of both sexes.

Heflin and colleagues (2005) prospectively examined self-report data of depressive symptoms from female welfare recipients in an urban Michigan county over a 3-year period while controlling for other known social confounders such as stressful life circumstances (homelessness, utility shutoffs), domestic violence, and perceived discrimination. Their findings suggest that food insufficiency in this population is a strong and independent risk factor for meeting criteria for major depressive disorder. Related findings suggest that a similar relationship exists for women living in rural communities in the United States (Huddleston-Casas et al. 2009). Interestingly, in the rural population examined, the relationship between food insufficiency and depression was bidirectional (food insufficiency contributed to depression, and depression contributed to food insufficiency), suggesting, again, that the relationship between food insecurity and mental illness is complex. Multifaceted policy interventions may be required to interrupt this cycle. Other investigators have confirmed that depression itself may exacerbate food insufficiency by limiting a person's capacity to maintain employment and generate income to support a healthy diet (Lent et al. 2009).

Although the majority of research in this area has studied adult female welfare recipients, a significant body of evidence suggests similar links between food insufficiency and behavioral disturbances in children and adolescents in low-income families (Weinreb et al. 2002). Food insufficiency also appears to be an independent risk factor for depressive disorders and suicidality in adolescents. Alaimo and colleagues (2002) analyzed data from the Third National Health and Nutrition Examination Survey to examine the correlation between depressive symptoms and food insufficiency in a representative sample of adolescents. The findings suggested that food insufficiency was associated with depressive symptoms and positive responses (high risk) on suicide ratings. Low family income was not itself associated with suicidal ideation, suggesting an independent role for food insufficiency in the development of psychopathology beyond the effects of low socioeconomic status in general. Additionally, other data suggest that food insufficiency, particularly lack of breakfast, may be associated with worsened cognitive performance in school-age children (Hoyland et al. 2009).

Together, these findings suggest a strong and independent link between food insufficiency and mental health, particularly depressive disorders, in women and adolescents in the United States. Data on adult males are not robust, although a similar relationship may exist. As discussed above, the relationship is likely mediated by multiple biological and social factors and intermediates, may be bidirectional, and may add to the negative effects associated with low socioeconomic status in general.

Housing

Similar to food insecurity, housing instability is defined by a spectrum of difficulties ranging from "street" homelessness to consistent but substandard living conditions. Unstable housing poses numerous threats to a patient's ability to engage in psychiatric treatment by affecting often overlooked yet fundamental aspects of recovery. These include being able to maintain regular sleep-wake cycles, having a safe place to store psychotropic medications, avoiding exposure to drugs and alcohol, and having a stable address where one can receive mail and phone calls. Making use of social services without access to Internet, phone, or a consistent mailing address can make interrupting a period of homelessness especially difficult. Unstable housing and housing quality have been shown to negatively impact mental health in a variety of ways.

Although it is commonly accepted that homeless individuals suffer mental illness and drug and alcohol dependence at greater rates than the general population, these relationships have proved difficult to quantify. Fazel and colleagues (2008) addressed this question by conducting a systematic review of available data in Western countries and found prevalence rates among

5,684 homeless individuals of 12.7% for psychotic illness, 11.4% for major depression, 23.1% for personality disorder, 37.9% for alcohol dependence, and 24.4% for drug dependence, with a significant degree of study heterogeneity for all conditions. These rates are similar to those occurring in the general population of other Western countries, which confirms a significantly higher rate of psychiatric illness in homeless individuals. Although few studies have examined the cause-effect relationship between homelessness and mental illness, one survey examining the temporal relationship between onset of mental illness and onset of homelessness found that in the majority of cases, mental illness preceded the onset of homelessness, with the possible exception of alcohol use disorder in the male homeless population (North et al. 1998).

As a group, homeless individuals tend to have significant challenges in using ambulatory care for health problems. They have higher utilization rates of acute care services, including emergency departments, compared to individuals with more stable housing. They also have significant difficulty in adhering to prescribed treatment for a variety of reasons, including difficulties with accessing care and medications due to lack of insurance (Kushel et al. 2001).

Once begun, a cycle of homelessness may be extremely difficult to interrupt, especially for individuals with severe mental illness. Some authors have recommended specially tailored social programs to help high-risk individuals. People returning to the community from prisons or psychiatric hospitals and those aging out of the foster care system are examples of groups at risk for homelessness in the absence of careful planning (Fazel et al. 2014). Avoiding the onset of homelessness in these high-risk groups may be a key step in preventing the synergistic and cyclical relationship between homelessness, mental illness, and drug and alcohol dependence, which ultimately leads to costly treatments for advanced illnesses.

Whereas available data suggest that homelessness is a common result of and contributor to mental illness, some studies have highlighted the relationship between poor-quality housing and the development and exacerbation of mental health problems. This line of inquiry follows a robust body of evidence documenting the association between poor-quality housing and development of numerous physical illnesses, including lead poisoning, asthma, and injuries, particularly among children (Krieger and Higgins 2002). Indeed, after adjusting for periods of homelessness based on self-report, residential transience (defined as two or more moves in the past 6 months) has been shown to be significantly associated with higher rates of depressive symptoms in men and women (Davey-Rothwell et al. 2008).

A study of an urban population of women across 20 U.S. cities examined multiple aspects of deficient housing and found that after controlling for other confounders, such as interpersonal violence and economic hardship, housing disarray (dark interior, noise, overcrowded and unclean conditions) was associated with higher rates of depression (Suglia et al. 2011). As expected, housing instability, defined as two or more moves in the past 2 years, was also associated with depression and with screening positive for generalized anxiety disorder symptoms. Interestingly, housing deterioration, defined as structural deficits such as peeling paint, holes in walls, or holes in floors, was not associated with either depression or anxiety symptoms in this population of urban women. Other studies, however, have found associations between structural housing deficits and adverse mental health outcomes. The existence of dampness and mold in the home, for example, has been shown to be independently associated with depressive symptoms, a relationship that may be mediated by lack of perceived control over one's living conditions (Shenassa et al. 2007).

Income and Employment

In modern society, income is a basic need. For a person without a stable source of income, obtaining basic resources such as food, water, and shelter is not possible. Sources of income vary and may include contributions from public sources such as social security or welfare, contributions from social supports such as family members or friends, and personal income generated via employment. The term *living wage* commonly refers to the hourly rate that permits full-time employees to meet their basic needs. At this time the federal minimum wage is insufficient to meet the basic needs of individuals in many locations. As of 2014, a total of 140 municipalities in the United States, including New York, Los Angeles, Chicago, Boston, and San Francisco, had enacted living wage legislation to augment the federal minimum wage. Some research suggests that these policies may have unintended consequences, however, such as promoting the preferential hiring of more skilled workers and reducing overall employment hours, thereby harming the poor, unskilled workers the legislation hoped to help (Lamman 2014). Further refinement of these policies is required to ensure that the interventions benefit the intended individuals.

Some nations (Finland, Switzerland, Namibia, Kenya) have gone further by experimenting with pilot programs that implement a universal basic income, which is unconditionally paid to all individuals and not tethered to employment. One such pilot program, called MINCOME, was conducted in Manitoba, Canada, between 1974 and 1979. Although the project itself was not systematically analyzed for health outcome data, a quasi-experimental approach was later used by Forget (2011) to show that the community in which the guaranteed income pilot was implemented had reduced rates of hospitalizations, especially for mental health problems, accidents, and injuries, compared with a matched control group. Interpretation of results is limited by the fact that not all individuals in the community participated in the MINCOME pilot; however, the results were nevertheless promising.

As the most desirable means to income, stable employment permits access to a variety of other social determinants of health, such as food security, housing security, and insurance coverage, as well as a sense of personal fulfillment and dignity. Unemployment has been independently linked to adverse mental health outcomes, a relationship that has been reinforced by analyses conducted after the most recent economic recession. Along with access to food, health care, housing, and education, employment frequently headlines in local and national elections and is an important modifiable determinant of mental health in the United States. As with previously discussed determinants, employment deficiencies encompass a spectrum of difficulties ranging from total joblessness to a situation in which a worker is considered underemployed in terms of hours, pay, or abilities.

Underemployment has received significantly less attention than unemployment in political campaigns, statistics reporting, and public policy initiatives, but it is worthy of discussion because of its impact on health outcomes. Underemployment remains operationally defined and may include a variety of deficits such as low hours, low pay, or general discontent due to an undesirable work environment. In some circumstances, it is economically advantageous for patients to collect welfare rather than work available jobs due to low pay, low hours, or lack of child care. The mental health implications of underemployment have not been well investigated, and most results are cross-sectional rather than longitudinal in nature. However, the few available studies suggest the existence of links with adverse mental health outcomes that warrant further investigation (Dooley 2003).

Compared with the effects of underemployment on mental health, the effects of job loss and unemployment on mental health are better studied and more consistent. This line of inquiry was initiated during the Great Depression of the 1930s, and there has been renewed interest during and after the Great Recession in the early 2000s. A large survey of more than 2 million adults in New Zealand, for example, correlated suicide rates with employment status during the 3 years following the 1991 census. Unemployed men and women ages 25–64 experienced significantly higher odds of suicide compared with employed individuals. Additionally, after the researchers controlled for other socioeconomic confounders, being unmarried and being unemployed remained significant predictors of suicide risk. Coexisting mental illness was estimated to explain about half of the association (Blakely et al. 2003).

Similarly, troubling results were reported in the United States following the Great Recession. Although the suicide rate in the United States had been rising steadily between 1999 and 2007, one group reported a significant increase in the suicide rate during the recessionary period between 2007 and 2010, to which they attributed an excess of 4,750 deaths due to suicide (Reeves et al. 2012). Additionally, taking advantage of state-level variation in generosity of benefits, other researchers have reported lower suicide rates in U.S. states that provide more generous unemployment benefits compared to those that do not (Cylus et al. 2014). Additionally, although unemployment is known to be a population-level risk factor for suicide, the risk may correlate significantly with the duration of unemployment, particularly beyond the first 5 weeks (Classen and Dunn 2012). Mass layoffs may also result in localized increases in suicide rates, particularly for men.

The frequency with which unemployed Americans use alcohol and other substances is a common source of political and social controversy. Some conservative politicians have advocated making welfare benefits contingent on urine drug screening, and some conservative states have actually piloted programs to this effect. Underlying these policies is a significant yet complicated correlation between alcohol or substance use and unemployment. In the 1980s, investigators began recognizing the complexity of the interactions between drinking behavior and job loss, which had previously been conceptualized primarily as the former resulting from the latter (Forcier 1988). In a more recent large review of more than 130 relevant studies of the association between unemployment and substance use that revealed several important trends, Henkel (2011) reported evidence that problematic use of substances tends to increase the likelihood of unemployment and decrease the chances of finding and keeping a job. Henkel also identified unemployment as a significant risk factor for substance use, development of a substance use disorder, and increased risk for relapse after drug and alcohol treatment.

Access to Mental Health Care

Access to health care is a problem in the United States for a variety of reasons, which include, among others, lack of insurance, poor-quality insurance, inadequate provider availability, transportation barriers, and lack of cultural competence among providers. Accessing mental health care on an outpatient basis is a particularly formidable challenge. Scheduling and attending an outpatient mental health appointment requires, at a minimum, access to a phone, a list of providers with contact information, active health insurance, proof of insurance, proof of identity, and transportation to and from the appointment. Satisfying these requirements while living with a severe mental illness and/or substance use disorder is obviously extremely difficult. If an appointment is scheduled, the wait time may be several months, by which point the condition for which a patient is seeking treatment may have worsened, possibly leading to loss of employment, loss of housing, loss of insurance, and the development of a comorbid condition. It is not uncommon in this system for patients with few other options to present to urgent care centers and hospital emergency departments with mental health complaints that could have been addressed on an outpatient basis prior to a stage of crisis. Many of these critiques apply to health care in general; however, access to mental health care is particularly poor in most regions of the country, even in regions where access to medical services in general is fairly good.

Data suggest that in addition to overall psychiatric workforce shortages, lack of willingness of the existing workforce to work with disenfranchised populations reduces the latter's access to mental health care. Physician-level trends in provider shortages include factors such as unequal distribution of psychiatrists across the country, fewer hours worked overall, and decline in direct patient care activities (Scully and Wilk 2003). Additionally, when compared with other specialists, psychiatrists were found to be significantly less likely to accept private insurance, with an overall decline of such practice of 17% since 2005–2006. Acceptance rates for Medicare and Medicaid were similarly lower for psychiatrists than other medical specialists (Bishop et al. 2014).

Although limited engagement by psychiatrists in public sector work may be one factor limiting access, characterizing the other factors impeding access is difficult to accomplish. Quantifying the need for psychiatric services is methodologically complex for several reasons. Primary care physicians, for example, can reasonably supply some psychiatric care, but the pattern for doing so may vary regionally. It may be difficult to determine, therefore, how many patients in a particular region would truly need a psychiatrist without also knowing the practice patterns of the family doctors in the region. Demand has increased, because of some reduction in the stigma associated with seeking care for mental health problems and to the closure of state-run institutions, but it is difficult to quantify. Overall, there is little dispute that the nation needs more psychiatrists. An analysis based on data from 2006 suggested, for example, that after correcting for primary care substitution, 25.9 psychiatrists per 100,000 individuals would be required to meet existing needs in the United States (Konrad et al. 2009). This estimate is almost double the estimate published by the Graduate Medical Education National Advisory Committee in 1980. It also far exceeds current supply, which was recently estimated to be 9.35 psychiatrists per 100,000 individuals on average across the United States (Merritt Hawkins 2018).

Although community care has been an important public goal for more than 50 years, accessing mental health care in the community can be exceedingly difficult, particularly in underserved areas. An investigation of access to mental health care in Boston found the situation to be rather abysmal

(Boyd et al. 2011). Study personnel posed as patients with coverage from Blue Cross Blue Shield of Massachusetts Preferred Provider Organization, the largest insurer in the state. Investigators contacted 64 sites and reported they had been seen in local emergency departments for depression and were advised to obtain outpatient appointments for follow-up within 2 weeks. Of the contacted sites, 12.5% offered appointments, but only 6.2% offered these within the 2-week window. The fact that these individuals reported having private insurance makes the results even more surprising.

In addition to initial scheduling, wait time can be an important impediment to receiving adequate care. In fact, some authors have found a strong and linear relationship between appointment delay and the likelihood of a cancellation or no-show to an initial mental health appointment (Gallucci et al. 2005). Additionally, wait times vary considerably based on geographic location and population served. Gallucci and colleagues (2005), for example, surveyed 5,901 consecutive patients contacting a Johns Hopkins Bayview Medical Center community psychiatry clinic and found wait times of 3.5 ± 3.2 days for adults and 6.2 ± 5.7 days for adolescents. These wait times are far shorter than typical. A similar study (Steinman et al. 2015) revealed wait times averaging 50 days (interquartile range: 29–81 days) for researchers posing as parents of an adolescent in metropolitan and rural areas across Ohio. Wait times were greater than 70 days on average in some regions, including northwest rural Ohio and the core county for Columbus. Because of these regional variances, the average wait time for an adult or child seeking mental health care across the United States is currently unknown.

Difficulty in accessing mental health services is not equally distributed across all demographics in the United States. The problem is more severe for minority and other at-risk populations. One large study (N=15,762) of individuals in the 48 contiguous United States found that Mexican American and African American populations were significantly less likely to receive any type of psychotherapy for depression compared with non-Latino whites, even though they had similar rates of depression (González et al. 2010). Other studies have reported similar findings suggesting that non-Hispanic whites are more likely than Hispanics or African Americans to receive needed care for alcohol and mental health problems (Wells et al. 2001). Addressing racial disparities in access to care will be a key step in improving overall access to mental health services.

Evidence suggests that removing barriers to access has a positive impact. Increased funding of community health centers and Medicaid expansion under the Affordable Care Act of 2010 (ACA) have yielded promising results in this regard. It has long been established that availability of public insurance programs such as Medicaid permits individuals with severe mental illness to engage with specialty mental health services at significantly higher rates than those who are uninsured (McAlpine and Mechanic 2000). A recent study in the post-ACA era confirmed that compared with people with continuous Medicaid coverage, people with gaps in insurance coverage during a 12-month period were more likely to have difficulty in obtaining care, including obtaining prescription drugs and completing outside referrals (Seo et al. 2019). One study in Oregon reported lower rates of depression following experimental expansions of Medicaid (Baicker et al. 2013).

Education

Although both availability and quality of education undoubtedly influence mental health in numerous ways, limited research has been conducted on the direct correlations between education and mental health outcomes. It is worth noting that theoretically a certain degree of educational attainment permits an individual to obtain other important social determinants, such as employment, housing, food, and health care, which are positively associated with better mental health. Likewise, lack of quality education tends to perpetuate the cycle of poverty and associated social disparities. These downstream effects undeniably impact mental health; however, definitive data for independent statistical associations between educational attainment and negative mental health outcomes are minimal.

School dropout has long been recognized as a social problem, because it reduces the skilled workforce, compromises national innovation and competition, and leads to increased rates of crime and incarceration. More recently, school dropout has been recognized as a public health problem rather than a purely moral, social, or political issue, which is promising. A literature review by Freudenberg and Ruglis (2007) indicated that education has downstream impacts on health, including access to safer, healthier neighborhoods; access to health insurance and health care; access to healthier foods; and improved social support. Because educational attainment tends to be lower in certain minority groups, members of those groups may be more likely to experience these adverse circumstances.

Root Causes

Race, Privilege, and Discrimination

The United States has a long and troubling history of racial and ethnic discrimination in social policy and health care. Soon the nation will mark the fiftieth anniversary of the 1972 revelation of the Tuskegee syphilis study, which began in 1932. Conducted by the Public Health Service, the study monitored African American males to learn the natural history of untreated syphilis, even well after treatment with penicillin became the standard of care. The Tuskegee study serves as an egregious example of racial devaluation and discrimination in health care that has plagued minority populations throughout U.S. history. Although some writers have argued that the Tuskegee study was a major cause of the pervasive mistrust that African Americans have for the medical community (Alsan and Wanamaker 2018), others have noted that this mistrust derives from much broader personal, community, and historical experiences with discrimination and mistreatment (Gamble 1997).

Unfortunately, even decades before the Tuskegee study, racial discrimination had been pervasive in clinical care throughout the U.S. South, as well as other parts of the country. By affecting access to basic needs such as adequate food and nutrition, housing, employment, and education, racial discrimination is a root cause of poor mental health. It is also an independent risk factor for adverse mental health outcomes for U.S. minorities. Because most of the available literature has focused on the plight of African Americans, this is the population highlighted in this section, although similar relationships likely exist for other marginalized groups (e.g., LGBTQ, Native Americans, people with disabilities).

Racial bias in diagnosis and treatment may result in inappropriate or misguided mental health care for minority populations. For example, one well-designed study in this area built on an existing body of evidence suggesting the overdiagnosis of schizophrenia spectrum illnesses in African Americans by controlling for relevant confounders, including age, sex, income, treatment location, education, and the presence or absence of serious affective disorder (Gara et al. 2012). The authors found, after controlling for the confounding variables, that African American patients continued to have significantly higher rates of schizophrenia diagnoses compared with non-Latino whites. The authors point out that there are no epidemiological data suggesting racial differences in the prevalence of schizophrenia and highlight premature diagnostic closure as a possible reason for overdiagnosing African Americans with psychotic illnesses rather than affective psychoses. The implications of this type of misdiagnosis are significant and include overtreatment with potentially harmful antipsychotic medications, failure to treat an underlying affective disturbance, and engendering of the difficult-to-quantify distress associated with receiving an erroneous diagnosis of schizophrenia, which typically carries a worse prognosis than an affective disorder.

A separate but related line of inquiry has shown that the perception of discrimination itself is independently associated with negative mental health outcomes in African Americans. Brown and colleagues (2000) used longitudinal data from the National Survey of Black Americans (NSBA) to show that the experience of racial discrimination at an early age was associated with high levels of psychological distress at follow-up years later. In another finding, a high level of psychological distress at an early age was not associated with higher rates of reported discrimination at follow-up.

Additionally, the nature of the discrimination does not need to be egregious to have a negative impact on mental health. One research group, for example, has shown that everyday experiences of discrimination are associated with development of social anxiety disorder, regardless of race (Levine et al. 2014). A systematic review of available publications reporting associations between racial and ethnic discrimination and mental health identified three additional studies reporting positive associations with depression and 20 additional studies reporting positive associations with nonspecific measures of psychological distress (Williams et al. 2003).

Despite the significant burden of psychiatric illness in minority communities, little has been done to reduce the disparities in health outcomes and access to mental health care, and recent evidence suggests that the gap is not narrowing (Cook et al. 2017). Reasons for this are multifactorial and may include stigma within minority communities, transportation barriers, financial barriers, and insurance barriers, as well as underlying differences in perception of need for mental health treatment in minority communities (Breslau et al. 2017).

Racial and ethnic minorities continue to face significant challenges in maintaining mental health in the United States. History of mistreatment by the medical establishment and the continued experience of discrimination from individuals, communities, and institutions both contribute to reduced utilization of health services among minority groups. Additionally, the psychological distress associated with discrimination itself continues to have a negative impact on the mental well-being of minorities. Unfortunately, despite increased interest from advisory groups such as the Institute of Medicine, which published *Unequal Treatment* in 2003 to provide guidance for ameliorating racial and ethnic disparities in health care, substantive changes have not occurred. Renewed initiatives will need to focus on reducing stigma, improving access to public insurance with prescription drug coverage, and improving trust between mental health providers and community members.

In this context of a long and troubling history of structural racism in the United States came an event that set off a period of social unrest and activism in May and June of 2020, not seen since the 1960s and 1970s. The nationwide protests followed the killing of an African American man, George Floyd, while being restrained by a policeman with a knee on his neck for over 8 minutes, cutting off his airway. Deaths of this kind at the hands of police had occurred numerous times in the past but had rarely penetrated the public consciousness to the same extent or elicited the same degree of outrage. It seems that a unique combination of factors (the capture of the event on video and the widespread distribution of the video to the public, growing discontent with an increasingly confrontational and provocative president, the social inequalities brought to light by the coronavirus pandemic of 2020, and the particularly egregious nature of the killing itself) coalesced to mobilize the public outcry. At the time of this writing, it is unclear whether this activism around the elimination of structurally entrenched racism will be sustained and pave the way for meaningful change. It is clear, however, that racial discrimination and the disparities that result have had decidedly negative consequences for the population's health and well-being and that corrections must occur if the country hopes to overcome them (Gamble 1997; Williams et al. 2003).

Poverty and Economic Inequality

Economic hardship can have profound implications for a patient's ability to pursue wellness. In fact, most practitioners familiar with treating impoverished individuals will understand that for this population of patients, wellness is considered a luxury. Indeed, when individuals and families are experiencing difficulty in maintaining basic needs such as access to food, housing, running water, and electricity, seeking care for mental health problems frequently occupies a lower position on the list of priorities. Although poverty itself increases risk of mental illness, it also limits access to mental health care.

Whether or not poverty is an intergenerational phenomenon has actually generated substantial debate in the sociology community since the 1950s. The idea that "hard work" and pulling oneself "up by the bootstraps" leads to prosperity has been prominent in American lore since its foundation. If that is not the case, the validity of the "American Dream" is called into question (Corcoran 1995). Unfortunately, success stories appear to be exceptions to the rule. Despite the existence of abundant literature placing blame on confounders such as family factors, neighborhood factors, receipt of welfare, and other noneconomic factors, Corcoran (1995) demonstrates that even after accounting for these factors, regardless of the specific mediating mechanisms, parental economic resources overwhelmingly predict children's economic outcomes. Children born into poverty have great difficulty reaching higher socioeconomic status (SES) as adults due to the multitude of factors working against them.

The relationship between poverty and mental illness has been well established. After controlling for confounders, a large (N=34,653) U.S. study reported increased incidence of mood disorders for participants with household incomes below $20,000 compared with those with household incomes above $30,000 over a 3-year period (Sareen et al. 2011). Additionally, after controlling for the presence of baseline disorders, the authors found that a decrease in household income during the study was associated with increased incidence of mood, anxiety, or substance use disorders. Other researchers have reported similar associations between socioeconomic factors and suicide. Li and colleagues (2011), for example, reported on socioeconomic factors contributing to suicide rates in addition to the more proximal risk factor of having a psychiatric disorder in adult men and women. Associations between adverse socioeconomic conditions and mental health have also been reported in children (Yoshikawa et al. 2012).

Interestingly, some researchers have reported that in addition to the absolute degree of economic hardship experienced by a family, income inequality within a population may have important implications for adverse mental health outcomes. This theory was articulated by Pickett and Wilkinson (2009) in their controversial text *The Spirit Level: Why Greater Equality Makes Societies Stronger*. They suggest that while absolute economic deprivation of individuals is associated with mental illness, relative deprivation within a community is also an important factor. Messias and colleagues (2011), for example, examined the correlation between depressive symptoms, major depression, and income inequality by comparing these parameters across 43 U.S. states. Income inequality was quantified using the Gini coefficient, which ranges from 0 (maximum equality) to 1 (maximum inequality) and provides an estimate of the degree of economic inequality in a population. After adjusting for age over 65, having a college degree, and per capita income, the researchers found income inequality to be positively associated with both depressive symptoms and major depression in the population studied. A longitudinal study found positive associations between depression and income inequality in women but not in men using state-level data in a similar fashion (Pabayo et al. 2014). Whether income inequality affects men and women differently requires further study. Others have reported similar associations between income inequality and child well-being on a cross-sectional basis (Pickett and Wilkinson 2007).

Explaining the existence of poverty and social inequality is a politically polarizing task. Liberals have argued that centuries of systemic racism, oppression, selective incarceration, and other forms of social control have resulted in the economic gap in American society. Conservatives have argued that those factors may have played some historical role, but continued dependence on welfare and other social services will only perpetuate the problem. Costello and colleagues (2003) report on an intriguing social experiment to this effect. The authors analyzed data from a representative sample of 1,420 rural children ages 9–13, one-quarter of whom were American Indian, over an 8-year period. Interestingly, halfway through the study, a casino opened, resulting in American Indian families receiving an annual income supplement. This created three economic classes of children: persistently poor, ex-poor, and never-poor. Prior to the opening of the casino, persistently poor and ex-poor children reported more psychiatric symptoms overall compared with the never-poor. After the casino opening, behavioral symptoms declined in the ex-poor children but not in the persistently poor. There was no observed reduction in emotional symptoms, possibly due to short follow-up duration or factors other than poverty that contributed to persistence of these symptoms. The authors concluded that at least for behavioral symptoms in children, increases in family income result in symptom reduction. Whether these results can be extrapolated to adults or to other types of psychiatric and substance use disorders remains to be seen.

Deprived Neighborhoods and Toxic Shared Environments

Driving end to end through any major U.S. city often reveals glaring disparities in localized areas of poverty and neighborhood-level deterioration and deprivation. Commonly referred to as the "bad parts of town," the housing in these areas is old and in disrepair, street signs are covered in graffiti, schools look like abandoned factory buildings, and instead of supermarkets there are corner stores that invariably sell tobacco, alcohol, and lottery tickets rather than produce. The infrastructure in these areas is dated, and children are exposed to higher levels of various environmental toxins, including air pollution and lead. In recent years, researchers have attempted to quantify the adverse health consequences associated with living in such areas.

On a neighborhood level, access to different sources of food is directly correlated with important indicators of physical health. Larson and colleagues (2009), for example, conducted a systematic review of 54 studies published between 1985 and 2008 in the United States examining links between access to food and physical health. Results indicated that neighborhood residents with better access to supermarkets, limited access to convenience stores, and limited access to fast-food restaurants had healthier diets and lower levels of obesity. Additionally, findings suggested that across the United States, residents of low-income, minority, and rural neighborhoods were most often affected by poor access to supermarkets and healthy foods.

While the relationship between access to quality food and adverse physical health outcomes has garnered significant attention in the public health literature, the relationship between neighborhood deprivation and adverse mental health outcomes has received less attention. However, the literature is growing and has important implications for changes in public policy. Evans (2003) reviewed important relationships between different aspects of the built environment and mental health while recognizing the inherent difficulty in drawing independent associations and firm conclusions from these relationships. Overcrowding in residential areas, for example, and loud exterior noise sources, such as airports, have been shown to elevate levels of psychological distress but not necessarily severe mental illness. Additionally, inadequate access to natural light has been shown to increase depressive symptoms. A sense of lack of personal control over these circumstances may also have important implications for one's sense of mental well-being.

For various methodological reasons, however, these relationships are difficult to separate from confounding variables, such as internal or structural characteristics of dwellings, and are difficult to study longitudinally or to quantify in a reliable manner. Available results do suggest, however, that improvements in neighborhood conditions may be associated with improvements in mental health for those remaining in the neighborhood over time (Dalgard and Tambs 1997). Additionally, one fastidiously designed study in north London showed positive associations between the prevalence of depression and recent construction (post-1969) of dwellings as well as dwellings with deck access (British term describing multi-level, row-style dwellings in which front doors open onto a shared walkway with limited private space) (Weich et al. 2002). These associations persisted after the study authors controlled for socioeconomic status and internal characteristics of the dwellings, suggesting that characteristics of the built environment may be independently associated with adverse mental health outcomes. Why newer construction might be associated with higher rates of depression remained unclear to the authors.

Different aspects of the shared and built environment may have significant effects on the mental health and development of children as well. Jackson and Tester (2008), for example, draw a clear distinction between child development in previous eras, in which children had intimate interactions with the natural world and peers, and the current era, in which children predominately have interactions with the built environment (the insides of houses, schools, vehicles, and commercial facilities) and are increasingly isolated from neighborhood playgrounds and developmentally appropriate social interactions. Indeed, urban social planning has typically involved building low-cost, high-rise buildings for low-income individuals, and these buildings are typically in geographically undesirable locations, such as near interstate highways, airports, or public rail systems.

Adverse Childhood Experiences

The experiencing of unfortunate developmental circumstances and traumatic exposures, cumulatively termed *adverse childhood experiences* (ACEs), profoundly impacts the development of psychiatric symptoms later in life. Early life circumstances, including relationships with siblings and parents, memories of home and school experiences, frightening or traumatic experiences, and exposure to poverty, parental joblessness, incarceration, or substance use, all contribute to these symptoms. The importance of these early childhood experiences is well established in the literature because they are now universally recognized social determinants of mental health.

In the Adverse Childhood Experiences Study (ACE Study), the Centers for Disease Control and Prevention (CDC) and the Kaiser Permanente Health Maintenance Organization (HMO) collected data from over 17,000 Kaiser HMO participants between 1995 and 1997 to examine relationships between childhood experiences and adult health and behaviors (Centers for Disease Control and Prevention 2019). ACEs were categorized as abuse (emotional, physical, sexual), household challenges (mother treated violently, substance abuse in the household, mental illness in the household, parental separation or divorce, incarceration of a household member), and neglect (emotional, physical) during the first 18 years of life. The study revealed that exposure to ACEs has dramatic effects on subsequent health and well-being later in life.

Overall, nearly two-thirds of the CDC-Kaiser ACE Study participants reported at least one ACE, with more than 20% reporting three or more. Additionally, authors observed a graded dose-response relationship between ACEs and negative outcomes (Centers for Disease Control and Prevention 2019). Specific outcomes studied included physical injuries (traumatic brain injuries, fractures, burns) (Felitti et al. 1998); mental illness (depression, anxiety, suicide, posttraumatic stress disorder) (Anda); maternal health (unintended pregnancy, pregnancy complications, fetal death) (Dietz et al. 1999); infectious disease (HIV, sexually transmitted diseases) (Hillis et al. 2000); chronic disease (cancer, diabetes) (Brown et al. 2010); risky behaviors (alcohol and drug abuse, unsafe sex) (Dube et al. 2002); and opportunities in later life (education, occupation, income) (Anda et al. 2004). The ACE study has generated scores of publications, a selection of which are cited above. Following is a more detailed discussion of findings most pertinent to mental health.

Perhaps the most troubling adverse mental health outcome for providers, patients, and families is suicide. Dube et al. (2001) reported that in the CDC-Kaiser ACE study population, the lifetime prevalence of a suicide attempt was 3.8% overall. Those participants with zero ACEs had a 1.1%

prevalence of attempted suicide. Compared with participants with zero ACEs, those with seven or more ACEs were found to have 31.1 higher odds of attempting suicide (95% confidence interval, 20.6–47.1). This relationship was found to be partially mediated by depressed affect, illicit drug use, and self-reported alcoholism. Overall, for each additional ACE, the authors found the risk of suicide attempts to increase by approximately 60%.

The CDC-Kaiser ACE study was also particularly revealing in terms of the pervasive negative impact of household alcoholism on mental health (Anda et al. 2002). Among the 20% of study respondents who reported parental alcohol abuse, the risk of having had exposure to all of the remaining ACEs was significantly increased. Additionally, the number of ACEs experienced was found to have a graded relationship to personal alcoholism and depression in adulthood, independent of parental alcohol abuse. Regardless of the number of ACEs experienced, the prevalence of alcoholism was higher among those reporting parental alcohol abuse. These results strongly suggest that targeting household alcohol abuse may have far-reaching impacts on the mental health of children in the household. Similar graded dose-response relationships were reported between ACEs and the initiation of drug use in adolescence, addiction, and parenteral drug use (Dube et al. 2003), as well as for the development of depressive disorders in adulthood (Chapman et al. 2004).

Reducing exposure to ACEs requires identifying and targeting their underlying causes. Although treatment of parental mental illnesses and substance use disorders will certainly improve the mental health outcomes of children and adolescents, a better strategy seeks to prevent parental mental health and substance use problems from developing at all. In large part, ACEs result from the previously discussed disparities and are best understood as intermediates between root causes and overt psychopathology. Addressing the root causes will reduce exposure to these harmful intermediates.

Recommendations

Incentives for Change

This chapter describes how social disparities adversely impact mental health in the United States. In many cases, social determinants are the predisposing, precipitating, and perpetuating causal factors of physical and mental illnesses. The existence of these disparities is an issue of social injustice, but regardless of one's political views regarding this issue, on the basis of the data reviewed herein, it is difficult to deny the impact that social factors have on health. Ignoring them can only lead to lost revenue via taxes for other social services and related costs such as Social Security Disability Insurance and health care spending. If not simply because it is the right thing to do, Americans should take interest in social reform because it makes economic sense.

In a recent review on the topic, Nichols and Taylor (2018) use economic theory to explain why health care stakeholders have few immediate incentives to address the social determinants of health, thus partially explaining how and why these disparities continue. The authors discuss the example of an elderly patient who lives on the third floor of a building that does not have an elevator. This patient cannot get from the third-floor apartment to the ground floor in order to travel to an outpatient clinic appointment because her family members work during normal business hours and are not available to assist her. As a result, the patient does not get to the clinic regularly and eventually can no longer obtain refills of her medications. Providers are unable to make house calls or to bill for remote communication to such a patient. Without the necessary medications, the patient's health will deteriorate to the point that emergency services are required. By this point, her condition will likely be severe enough to require hospitalization. The hospital will treat the patient until she is again in a condition that permits outpatient care and discharge her home as soon as that threshold is crossed. However, the patient is still living in the same apartment and still unable to attend outpatient appointments, so the cycle repeats. The cost of multiple ambulance trips, emergency department visits, and hospitalizations likely exceeds the cost of providing a different apartment or assisted transportation to outpatient care by tens of thousands of dollars. In the absence of tailored incentives to address the underlying cause of the problem and make these simple changes, the system continues to pay a high price for poor outcomes.

Interventions that would address the relevant social determinants in this example include improved funding for accessible, low-income housing for seniors; more paid time off for non-salaried workers to assist family members; and improved financial incentives for providing in-home health services. Perhaps the least costly approach in this case would be to focus on investing in nonemergency medical transportation services, and this is the approach discussed in detail by the authors. They argue that the economic issues relevant for the social determinants of health are the same as those for other public goods, such as law enforcement, national defense, or sewer systems. It is impractical and inefficient for private entities to invest in providing these services unless there is sustainable funding for them to do so. Usually, government must contribute to supporting public goods. Health care is unique in the sense that it is not an entirely government-run enterprise, such as national defense. The presence of individual stakeholder interests in the health care system without consistent oversight and coordination from a single governing body permits the fragmented and inefficient system that exists today.

In their article, Nichols and Taylor (2018) go on to offer a unique solution, borrowing from game theory and the Vickrey-Clarke-Groves mechanism, with the goal of optimizing outcomes while actually minimizing government intervention. The Vickrey-Clarke-Groves mechanism was popularized in the 1970s as a way to solve the economic problem of disparate individual stakeholder interests, despite mutually shared goals, without excessive reliance on government. In the proposed model, an external entity, or "trusted broker," facilitates bidding from the interested parties in terms of how much they would be willing to contribute for a shared beneficial outcome, which in this case is reduction of a social determinant deficit.

Not all outcomes would necessarily be monetary. Improved quality of care, for example, could be assigned value in this model. Alternatively, external incentives could be introduced in order to monetize value, as is already being done in small ways in the U.S. system with the shift from fee-for-service to quality-driven care. The key, of course, is in convincing stakeholders (hospitals, emergency departments, community health centers, insurance companies, providers) that the return is worth the investment. This could be handled via the inclusion of side payments, or "tax" in the language of the model, which helps ensure that all stakeholders gain.

In the example above, for example, the hospital has no intrinsic interest in spending money on patient transportation to and from outpatient clinic appointments. The hospital, however, could be enticed via a side payment. In fact, Medicare has already employed a similar strategy via reimbursement adjustments for 30-day readmissions, effectively incentivizing hospitals to have interest in patients doing well after discharge, at least for 30 days. Stakeholders, in other words, invest in the amelioration of social determinants of health in a collaboration that is likely to yield a mutually satisfactory return on investment, after inclusion of the side payments. Acting as individual entities, the stakeholders would have little economic interest in remedying social disparities. Together, however, the authors argue that their individual interests are balanced and they are able to reach a mutually satisfactory solution via cooperation with and coordination by the "trusted broker." Although not explicitly explored in the article, government influence via tax breaks, reimbursement adjustments, and other strategies of monetizing quality would likely be a potent addition to this coordinated approach.

Role of Psychiatrists and Other Stakeholders

Although the sorts of interventions just discussed would require cooperation of large entities such as public and private insurance providers, corporate and community health care systems, and local and federal governments, individual providers can enact change via other means. Providers can direct attention to social factors by including, in routine mental health assessments, questions about basic needs (access to food, shelter, income, and health care) and root causes of deficits in basic needs (discrimination, income inequality, poverty, and adverse experiences). Additionally, after identifying social factors, providers can incorporate them into the treatment plan by considering the current impact they will have on care and strategizing to reduce their influence. These interventions might include preferential selection of low-cost medications, referral for mental health service coordination, referral for mobile medication services, completion of disability paperwork, and/or referral for occupational and vocational rehabilitation programs. In communities where these services do not exist, physicians must advocate for their implementation.

In addition to increasing clinical focus on social determinants of mental health, providers must take the lead in advocating for the social reforms their patients require. This advocacy might include forming alliances with other like-minded clinicians, undertaking quality improvement projects within their health care systems, starting new programs for treating disenfranchised populations, and lobbying relevant stakeholders, including insurance companies, hospitals, health systems, and legislators. Clinicians have personal experience treating individuals with adverse social circumstances while occupying a privileged social role. Physicians in particular must take advantage of this role by advocating for their patients in the ways outlined above. Physicians also have the ability to encourage patients to advocate for themselves via numerous mechanisms, such as writing letters to important stakeholders, canvassing, lobbying, and joining local chapters of organizations such as the National Alliance on Mental Illness. Via a coordinated and calculated approach, these problems are solvable. The first step, of course, is convincing naysayers of their importance.

Conclusion

This chapter has reviewed and evaluated available evidence to show that social disparities negatively impact mental health. To improve the cost-effectiveness and quality of care provided in the United States, reducing social disparities should be a priority. Economic trends in other developed nations suggest that social spending is associated with improved population health and that positive health indicators do not necessarily correlate with more health care spending. The United States has been vastly outspending other developed countries, with poor results and glaring health disparities.

From both ethical and financial perspectives, all Americans should be concerned with the current state of the system. Change will require cooperation from stakeholders with disparate individual interests and advocacy by patients, clinicians, and families. Through careful evaluation of programs and policies, strategic planning can ensure that the system obtains improved outcomes. Through a joint effort, the quality of mental health care in the United States can be improved. The process starts by recognizing the common interest in eliminating social disparities, and emphasizing their amelioration should be a public health priority.

References

Alaimo K, Olson CM, Frongillo EA: Family food insufficiency, but not low family income, is positively associated with dysthymia and suicide symptoms in adolescents. J Nutr 132(4):719–725, 2002

Alsan M, Wanamaker M: Tuskegee and the health of black men. Q J Econ 133(1):407–455, 2018

Anda RF, Whitfield CL, Felitti VJ, et al: Adverse childhood experiences, alcoholic parents, and later risk of alcoholism and depression. Psychiatr Serv 53(8):1001–1009, 2002

Anda RF, Felitti VJ, Fleisher VI, et al: Childhood abuse, household dysfunction, and indicators of impaired worker performance. Perm J 8(1):30–38, 2004

Anda RF, Brown DW, Felitti VJ, et al: Adverse childhood experiences and prescribed psychotropic medications in adults. Am J Prev Med 32(5):389–394, 2007

Baicker K, Taubman SL, Allen HL, et al: The Oregon experiment—effects of Medicaid on clinical outcomes. N Engl J Med 368(18):1713–1722, 2013

Bishop TF, Press MJ, Keyhani S, et al: Acceptance of insurance by psychiatrists and the implications for access to mental health care. JAMA Psychiatry 71(2):176–181, 2014

Blakely TA, Collings SCD, Atkinson J: Unemployment and suicide. Evidence for a causal association? J Epidemiol Community Health 57(8):594–600, 2003

Boyd JW, Linsenmeyer A, Woolhandler S, et al: The crisis in mental health care: a preliminary study of access to psychiatric care in Boston. Ann Emerg Med 58(2):218–219, 2011

Breslau J, Cefalu M, Wong EC, et al: Racial/ethnic differences in perception of need for mental health treatment in a U.S. national sample. Soc Psychiatry Psychiatr Epidemiol 52(8):929–937, 2017

Brown DW, Anda RF, Felitti VJ, et al: Adverse childhood experiences and the risk of lung cancer. BMC Public Health 10:20, 2010

Brown TN, Williams DR, Jackson JS, et al: "Being black and feeling blue": the mental health consequences of racial discrimination. Race and Society 2(2):117–131, 2000

Centers for Disease Control and Prevention: About the CDC–Kaiser ACE Study. April 2, 2019. Available at: www.cdc.gov/violenceprevention/childabuseand-neglect/acestudy/about.html. Accessed February 9, 2020.

Chapman DP, Whitfield CL, Felitti VJ, et al: Adverse childhood experiences and the risk of depressive disorders in adulthood. J Affect Disord 82(2):217–225, 2004

Classen TJ, Dunn RA: The effect of job loss and unemployment duration on suicide risk in the United States: a new look using mass-layoffs and unemployment duration. Health Econ 21(3):338–350, 2012

Cook BL, Trinh NH, Hou SS, et al: Trends in racial-ethnic disparities in access to mental health care, 2004–2012. Psychiatr Serv 68(1):9–16, 2017

Corcoran M: Rags to rags: poverty and mobility in the United States. Annual Review of Sociology 21(1):237–267, 1995

Costello EJ, Compton SN, Keeler G, et al: Relationships between poverty and psychopathology: a natural experiment. JAMA 290(15):2023–2029, 2003

Cylus J, Glymour MM, Avendano M: Do generous unemployment benefit programs reduce suicide rates? A state fixed-effect analysis covering 1968–2008. Am J Epidemiol 180(1):45–52, 2014

Dalgard OS, Tambs K: Urban environment and mental health: a longitudinal study. Br J Psychiatry 171:530–536, 1997

Davey-Rothwell MA, German D, Latkin CA: Residential transience and depression: does the relationship exist for men and women? J Urban Health 85(5):707–716, 2008

Dietz PM, Spitz AM, Anda RF, et al: Unintended pregnancy among adult women exposed to abuse or household dysfunction during their childhood. JAMA 282(14):1359–1364, 1999

Dinour LM, Bergen D, Yeh MC: The food insecurity–obesity paradox: a review of the literature and the role food stamps may play. J Am Diet Assoc 107(11):1952–1961, 2007

Dooley D: Unemployment, underemployment, and mental health: conceptualizing employment status as a continuum. Am J Community Psychol 32(1–2):9–20, 2003

Dube SR, Anda RF, Felitti VJ, et al: Childhood abuse, household dysfunction, and the risk of attempted suicide throughout the life span: findings from the Adverse Childhood Experiences Study. JAMA 286(24):3089–3096, 2001

Dube SR, Anda RF, Felitti VJ, et al: Adverse childhood experiences and personal alcohol abuse as an adult. Addict Behav 27(5):713–725, 2002

Dube SR, Felitti VJ, Dong M, et al: Childhood abuse, neglect, and household dysfunction and the risk of illicit drug use: the Adverse Childhood Experiences Study. Pediatrics 111(3):564–572, 2003

Evans GW: The built environment and mental health. J Urban Health 80(4):536–555, 2003

Fazel S, Khosla V, Doll H, et al: The prevalence of mental disorders among the homeless in western countries: systematic review and meta-regression analysis. PLoS Med 5(12):e225, 2008

Fazel S, Geddes JR, Kushel M: The health of homeless people in high-income countries: descriptive epidemiology, health consequences, and clinical and policy recommendations. Lancet 384(9953):1529–1540, 2014

Felitti VJ, Anda RF, Nordenberg D, et al: Relationship of childhood abuse and household dysfunction to many of the leading causes of death in adults. The Adverse Childhood Experiences (ACE) Study. Am J Prev Med 14(4):245–258, 1998

Forcier MW: Unemployment and alcohol abuse: a review. J Occup Med 30(3):246–251, 1988

Forget EL: The town with no poverty: using health administration data to revisit outcomes of a Canadian guaranteed annual income field experiment. University of Manitoba, February 2011. Available at: https://web.archive.org/web/20170126003728/http://public.econ.duke.edu/~erw/197/forget-cea%20%282%29.pdf. Accessed February 9, 2020.

Freudenberg N, Ruglis J: Reframing school dropout as a public health issue. Prev Chronic Dis 4(4):A107, 2007

Gallucci G, Swartz W, Hackerman F: Impact of the wait for an initial appointment on the rate of kept appointments at a mental health center. Psychiatr Serv 56(3):344–346, 2005

Gamble VN: Under the shadow of Tuskegee: African Americans and health care. Am J Public Health 87(11):1773–1778, 1997

Gara MA, Vega WV, Arndt S, et al: Influence of patient race and ethnicity on clinical assessment in patients with affective disorders. Arch Gen Psychiatry 69(6):593–600, 2012

González HM, Vega WA, Williams DR, et al: Depression care in the United States: too little for too few. Arch Gen Psychiatry 67(1):37–46, 2010

Gowda C, Hadley C, Aiello AE: The association between food insecurity and inflammation in the U.S. adult population. Am J Public Health 102(8):1579–1586, 2012

Heflin CM, Siefert K, Williams DR: Food insufficiency and women's mental health: findings from a 3-year panel of welfare recipients. Soc Sci Med 61(9):1971–1982, 2005

Henkel D: Unemployment and substance use: a review of the literature (1990–2010). Curr Drug Abuse Rev 4(1):4–27, 2011

Hillis SD, Anda RF, Felitti VJ, et al: Adverse childhood experiences and sexually transmitted diseases in men and women: a retrospective study. Pediatrics 106(1):E11, 2000

Hoyland A, Dye L, Lawton CL: A systematic review of the effect of breakfast on the cognitive performance of children and adolescents. Nutr Res Rev 22(2):220–243, 2009

Huddleston-Casas C, Charnigo R, Simmons LA: Food insecurity and maternal depression in rural, low-income families: a longitudinal investigation. Public Health Nutr 12(8):1133–1140, 2009

Institute of Medicine: Unequal Treatment: Confronting Racial and Ethnic Disparities in Health Care. Washington, DC, The National Academies Press, 2003

Jackson RJ, Tester J: Environment shapes health, including children's mental health. J Am Acad Child Adolesc Psychiatry 47(2):129–131, 2008
Konrad TR, Ellis AR, Thomas KC, et al: County-level estimates of need for mental health professionals in the United States. Psychiatr Serv 60(10):1307–1314, 2009
Krieger J, Higgins DL: Housing and health: time again for public health action. Am J Public Health 92(5):758–768, 2002
Kushel MB, Vittinghoff E, Haas JS: Factors associated with the health care utilization of homeless persons. JAMA 285(2):200–206, 2001
Lamman C: The economic effects of living wage laws. Fraser Institute, January 2014. Available at: www.fraserinstitute.org/sites/default/files/economic-effects-of-living-wage-laws.pdf. Accessed February 9, 2020.
Larson NI, Story MT, Nelson MC: Neighborhood environments: disparities in access to healthy foods in the U.S. Am J Prev Med 36(1):74–81, 2009
Lent MD, Petrovic LE, Swanson JA, et al: Maternal mental health and the persistence of food insecurity in poor rural families. J Health Care Poor Underserved 20(3):645–661, 2009
Levine DS, Himle JA, Abelson JM, et al: Discrimination and social anxiety disorder among African-Americans, Caribbean blacks, and non-Hispanic whites. J Nerv Ment Dis 202(3):224–230, 2014
Li Z, Page A, Martin G, et al: Attributable risk of psychiatric and socio-economic factors for suicide from individual-level, population-based studies: a systematic review. Soc Sci Med 72(4):608–616, 2011
McAlpine DD, Mechanic D: Utilization of specialty mental health care among persons with severe mental illness: the roles of demographics, need, insurance, and risk. Health Serv Res 35(1 Pt 2):277–292, 2000
Merritt Hawkins: The silent shortage: a white paper examining supply, demand, and recruitment trends in psychiatry. 2018. Available at: www.merritthawkins.com/uploadedFiles/MerrittHawkins/Content/News_and_Insights/Thought_Leadership/mhawhitepaperpsychiatry2018.pdf. Accessed February 9, 2020.
Messias E, Eaton WW, Grooms AN: Economic grand rounds: income inequality and depression prevalence across the United States: an ecological study. Psychiatr Serv 62(7):710–712, 2011
Nichols LM, Taylor LA: Social determinants as public goods: a new approach to financing key investments in healthy communities. Health Aff (Millwood) 37(8):1223–1230, 2018
North CS, Pollio DE, Smith EM, et al: Correlates of early onset and chronicity of homelessness in a large urban homeless population. J Nerv Ment Dis 186(7):393–400, 1998
Pabayo R, Kawachi I, Gilman SE: Income inequality among American states and the incidence of major depression. J Epidemiol Community Health 68(2):110–115, 2014
Pickett KE, Wilkinson RG: Child wellbeing and income inequality in rich societies: ecological cross sectional study. BMJ 335(7629):1080–1086, 2007

Pickett KE, Wilkinson RG: The Spirit Level: Why Greater Equality Makes Societies Stronger. New York, Bloomsbury Press, 2009

Read JR, Sharpe L, Modini M, et al: Multimorbidity and depression: a systematic review and meta-analysis. J Affect Disord 221:36–46, 2017

Reeves A, Stuckler D, McKee M, et al: Increase in state suicide rates in the USA during economic recession. Lancet 380(9856):1813–1814, 2012

Sareen J, Afifi TOP, McMillan KA, et al: Relationship between household income and mental disorders: findings from a population-based longitudinal study. Arch Gen Psychiatry 68(4):419–427, 2011

Scully JH, Wilk JE: Selected characteristics and data of psychiatrists in the United States, 2001–2002. Acad Psychiatry 27(4):247–251, 2003

Seo V, Baggett TP, Thorndike AN, et al: Access to care among Medicaid and uninsured patients in community health centers after the Affordable Care Act. BMC Health Serv Res 19(1):291, 2019

Shenassa ED, Daskalakis C, Liebhaber A, et al: Dampness and mold in the home and depression: an examination of mold-related illness and perceived control of one's home as possible depression pathways. Am J Public Health 97(10):1893–1899, 2007

Siefert K, Heflin CM, Corcoran ME, et al: Food insufficiency and the physical and mental health of low-income women. Women Health 32(1–2):159–177, 2001

Steinman KJ, Shoben AB, Dembe AE, et al: How long do adolescents wait for psychiatry appointments? Community Ment Health J 51(7):782–789, 2015

Suglia SF, Duarte CS, Sandel MT: Housing quality, housing instability, and maternal mental health. J Urban Health 88(6):1105–1116, 2011

Weich S, Blanchard M, Prince M, et al: Mental health and the built environment: cross-sectional survey of individual and contextual risk factors for depression. Br J Psychiatry 180:428–433, 2002

Weinreb L, Wehler C, Perloff J, et al: Hunger: its impact on children's health and mental health. Pediatrics 110(4):e41, 2002

Wells K, Klap R, Koike A, et al: Ethnic disparities in unmet need for alcoholism, drug abuse, and mental health care. Am J Psychiatry 158(12):2027–2032, 2001

Williams DR, Neighbors HW, Jackson JS: Racial/ethnic discrimination and health: findings from community studies. Am J Public Health 93(2):200–208, 2003

World Health Organization: Preamble to the Constitution of the World Health Organization as adopted by the International Health Conference, New York, June 19–22, 1946. Available at: www.who.int/governance/eb/who_constitution_en.pdf. Accessed February 10, 2020.

Yoshikawa H, Aber JL, Beardslee WR: The effects of poverty on the mental, emotional, and behavioral health of children and youth: implications for prevention. Am Psychol 67(4):272–284, 2012

5

Successful Approaches to Increasing Value

Jorge R. Petit, M.D.
Mark Graham, LCSW
Amanda Semidey, LCSW

Many evidence-based and innovative clinical practices have demonstrated improved outcomes and associated cost-effectiveness despite the low value delivered by the U.S. health care system overall. Unfortunately, community-based health and human services have not always had access to adequate funding for these effective practices beyond their pilot phases. As a result, they are not widely disseminated, broadly implemented, or consistently followed by practitioners, leaving a gap between the science and practice in the community (Institute of Medicine 2003; Lehman et al. 2004; Melnyk et al. 2005; Wallen et al. 2010). This chapter focuses on these best practices and a growing movement toward generating practice-based evidence, which recognizes the importance of achieving an impact on real-world outcomes. The chapter also describes programs that organize care and respond to population needs in ways that enhance the quality of care and reduce the cost of delivering them, such as continuum of care coordination, health homes, and crisis services. The discussion here sets the stage for the consideration of how these practices can be implemented more broadly in Part II, "Where We Want to Go: Systems Interventions," and Part III, "Where We Want to Go: Professional Interventions."

Evidence-Based Practices

Public health and services research, epidemiology, and emerging technologies have all been essential in expanding the knowledge base and translating interventions into clinical practice (Ammerman et al. 2014). Evidence-based practices (EBPs) are approaches that emphasize scientifically grounded decision making. They are based on data collection that reflects outcomes related to a specific intervention or program. They are intended to improve services delivered and to minimize unsound or unproven practices (Coopey et al. 2006; Institute of Medicine 2003; Tannenbaum 2005). The implementation of evidence-based care hinges on an investment in quality at all levels of an organization so that the current best evidence, along with clinical expertise, will provide service recipients with adequate information to assert their values and preferences in the decision-making process (Melnyk et al. 2005; Sackett et al. 2000).

Studies have demonstrated that clinical practice guidelines, protocols, and standards based on evidence can lead to increased consistency in the care delivered, enhanced patient satisfaction, improved outcomes, and increased provider satisfaction (Swinkels et al. 2002). The implementation of EBPs into daily clinical practice has been slow but has recently been accelerating.

The adoption of EBPs results in greater standardization of clinical practice. Programs choosing only those interventions or treatments that are empirically supported have consistently better outcomes than those that do not do so. Development of EBPs has relied on results generated from controlled experimental designs. Although these experimental designs may lead to inadequate attention to questions related to the scale and application in real-world settings (Gone 2015), the gold standard for an EBP remains the randomized controlled trial (RCT) (Isaac and Franceschi 2008). RCTs are studies that attempt to limit the influence of elements in the environment on the outcome of the study. When these studies are done properly, only the effects of the identified treatment or intervention are accountable for observed changes in the outcomes.

Some experts cite a time lag of upwards of 17 years for "research evidence, including much that never gets published, to be translated into practice," depending on the way in which translation, dissemination, and delivery of this research to practitioners is conducted (Ammerman et al. 2014, p. 48). To disseminate clinically sound and scientifically based behavioral health practices in the areas of prevention, treatment, and recovery support services, the Substance Abuse and Mental Health Services Administration (2014) created the National Registry of Evidence-based Programs and Practices. This registry was replaced in 2018 by an enhanced resource when the Evidence-Based Practices Resource Center was launched (Substance Abuse and Mental Health Services Administration 2020). This resource center makes available, for a broad range of audiences, a collection of scientifically based resources, including Treatment Improvement Protocols, toolkits, resource guides, clinical practice guidelines, and other science-based resources, and it provides communities and clinicians with easy access to EBPs for their clinical settings. The Assertive Community Treatment (ACT) model is one such practice identified in the EBP Resource Center.

An Evidence-Based Program: Assertive Community Treatment

Deinstitutionalization was at its height across the United States during the early 1970s. Care in the community had become widely recognized and accepted as being more humane and appropriate than care in large mental health institutions and, after the passage of Medicaid in 1965, as being much less costly for the states (Test 1979). As institutions rushed to transition people into the community, the supports the people would need for sustained tenure there did not keep pace with the demand for them. There were complaints that even the newly established facilities created after the passage of the Community Mental Health Act of 1963 were not using their resources to adequately address the needs of these new arrivals with serious mental illness (SMI). Preexisting and newly created services were often inadequate for this population. The lack of appropriate planning and services for those being discharged from short-term psychiatric hospital stays often resulted in high readmission rates. This recidivism was also recognized as a serious challenge.

The ACT model was developed in the early 1970s, at the Mendota Mental Health Institute (MMHI) in Madison, Wisconsin, to address the hospital system's high readmission rates. The MMHI team examined the functioning of their mental health system to develop strategies to assist discharged patients in making a successful transition back to the community. Recognizing that the intensive support people received in institutional settings decreased dramatically at discharge, the team proposed that for people with behavioral health issues, community care should maintain the same level of intensity as hospital care, by acting like a hospital without walls. In response to the service deficiencies identified in their evaluation, MMHI developed the Program of Assertive Community Treatment (PACT), which has since been widely adopted across the United States and internationally. It is now more commonly known as ACT. ACT teams serve individuals with SMI who are living in the community. Coordinated professional care and treatment is provided in the individual's home or other community settings. The program offers a broad range of services to meet each individual's unique personal needs, reduce symptoms, and promote recovery. Its overarching goal is to enable patients to live successfully and autonomously in the community and reduce the need for hospitalization.

ACT teams are multidisciplinary, often including some combination of nurses, social workers, vocational specialists, case managers, substance abuse counselors, wellness coaches, psychiatrists, and peers. Through their pooled knowledge and experience, team members can better address an individual's comprehensive needs and help the individual continue in community living (Wisconsin Department of Health Services 2019). Team members have a small caseload ratio of 1:10 to ensure that the individuals receiving care get the most attentive treatment possible. Although individuals have an identified point person on the team assigned to each of them, they ultimately have interaction with and are supported by all team members. As clients' symptoms improve and worsen, the ACT team is able to decrease or increase the intensity of services and support as needed. When clients achieve prolonged stability, they can graduate to less intensive supportive housing and community services.

Since the late 1970s, the ACT model has been widely replicated and adapted (Deci et al. 1995). Teams now serve unique populations, such as chronically homeless, deaf, or justice-involved individuals. These distinct populations can be accommodated without significantly impacting fidelity to the model. However, some of the requirements and regulations, designed by states to maintain fidelity to the ACT model, can be onerous for sponsoring organizations with limited resources. For example, ACT teams in some states are expected to see patients a minimum of six times a month or to have them meet with a psychiatrist at least once a month, regardless of their clinical status and stability. Team members often feel that these requirements override clinical judgment and reduce their capacity to respond to those patients with the greatest need. These prescriptive regulatory requirements may ultimately undermine quality when the intensity of interaction is being determined by something other than the patient's actual level of need.

Generating Practice-Based Evidence

Even though EBPs have advanced the practice of mental health services, there is some controversy regarding their application in various situations. The movement toward EBPs and the emphasis on empirically supported treatments and services has limited the development of interventions that are rooted in clinical practice experience with positive impacts on treatment benefits. Today's public health care challenges are complex and require partnerships and interventions that are rooted in the community and have worked well in real-world practice (Ammerman et al. 2014). In some instances, managed care organizations (MCOs) have required a rigid adherence to certain EBPs, even when EBPs may not fit the context in which they are implemented. This lack of flexibility reduces providers' ability to address the variability of need in the type and duration of care. The MCOs have been accused of using rigid requirements and exclusion criteria as part of cost containment strategies (Cummings 2000; Oss 2002).

There is growing acceptance that effectiveness rather than efficacy is most important in determining a program's success. *Efficacy* is demonstrated through the study of an intervention in controlled conditions, such as in RCTs, as described earlier. *Effectiveness*, on the other hand, is demonstrated through consistent production of desired outcomes under a variety of circumstances and variables that will be encountered in "real-world" settings. Developing effective programming requires an understanding of the population, the community, and the local health environment (Green and Glasgow 2006). As opposed to EBPs, *practice-based evidence* originates on the practice level and incorporates the perspectives of those delivering the interventions as well as the recipients of those services (Ammerman et al. 2014; Viswanathan et al. 2004). Practice-based approaches may be more easily replicated and sustained across different settings and circumstances.

The 2001 Institute of Medicine report *Crossing the Quality Chasm* identified the need to move beyond evidence as defined by RCTs and to include "the identification of best practices in the design of care processes" (p. 147) and better disseminate and integrate these practices into clinical practice. The complexity of behavioral health care issues treated in the public sector calls for innovative research designs that will ascertain whether or not an intervention is effective. Some difficulties in conducting such research include the chronic or recurrent nature of many serious mental health conditions, multiple comorbidities, poor adherence to treatment and medication regimens, and the overlay of social determinants of health. RCTs can be modified to have a greater focus on effectiveness than on efficacy, their traditional focus, so that they can be employed in complex community settings.

Such modifications can generate outcome data from real-world settings, which have implications for both practice and policy. These modified approaches might include one or more of the following: 1) selecting clinically relevant alternative interventions to compare, 2) including a diverse population of study participants, 3) recruiting participants from heterogeneous practice settings, and 4) collecting data on a broad range of health outcomes (Ammerman et al. 2014; Tunis et al. 2003).

The 2010 Patient Protection and Affordable Care Act continued movement toward achieving the Triple Aim (i.e., improving patient experience of care, improving health of population, reducing per capita cost of health care; Berwick et al. 2008), which resulted in the establishment of the independent, nonprofit research organization known as Patient-Centered Outcomes Research Institute (https://www.pcori.org). This institute was established to fund research that can help patients and those who care for them to make better-informed decisions about the daily health care choices they face.

Practice-Based Evidence Programming: Pathway Home

Successful transitions from inpatient care to the community often demand navigating a complex, fragmented health care system (Petit et al. 2018). This has proven particularly challenging for individuals with SMI, especially those returning to the community from lengthy state hospital admissions. In an innovative response to those challenges, a group of New York City's largest nonprofit organizations developed and piloted a transition program called Pathway Home (PH). Using a multidisciplinary approach and adaptation of Critical Time Intervention (e.g., a model designed to prevent recurrent homelessness among persons with severe mental illness by enhancing continuity of care during transition from institution to community living) (Herman et al. 2007), PH has significantly improved community outcomes after long-term inpatient stays (Petit et al. 2018). The PH model is a time-limited intervention that mobilizes support for vulnerable individuals during periods of transition. The PH program focuses on treatment-related issues and social determinants of health that are drivers of preventable readmissions and emergency department visits at a time that is widely considered to be the most critical in a patient's care—the months after a hospital discharge (Herman et al. 2007).

The PH approach advocates for predischarge engagement. To ensure that this occurs, the teams offer immediate response to new referrals and include a member engagement specialist (MES). Different referral sources receive a same-day receipt of referral, and an inpatient engagement session occurs within 48 hours. PH does not conduct initial extensive comprehensive assessments; rather, assessment is viewed as ongoing. The initial contact is focused on the identification of just one need that is important to the participant and can be easily resolved. Multiple, duplicative assessments are considered to be unnecessary and actually off-putting for patients, leading to high patient disengagement. PH develops and promotes a Guided Conversation approach. Used by the MES and other trained staff, the PH Guided Conversation promotes member engagement and has resulted in increased enrollment rates (Petit et al. 2018). The Guided Conversations focus on planned prompts, active listening, and skillfully chosen discussion topics to enable members to feel heard and in control of their care. Although casual in appearance, these conversations actually cover the topics of traditional assessments without paper in hand and rote questioning. The MES then completes assessments back at the office with the information received through the Guided Conversation and uses the assessments as the foundation for more comprehensive assessments in the community. When patients are able to tell their story rather than merely check boxes on a form, the result is increased participation in care.

Another key to PH's success is that a team member is present on the day a patient is discharged from the hospital to ensure that discharge plans are understood, medication is filled, anxieties are addressed, and the community destination is safe and secure. The PH team's ongoing care focuses on facilitating community reintegration and ensuring active engagement with medical and specialty care and social services. Accompanying patients to their initial behavioral health and primary care appointment ensures that Healthcare Effectiveness Data and Information Set measures for follow-up after hospitalization are met while improving patient outcomes (Petit et al. 2018). Teams in PH, as in other complex care management programs, have a lower than average staff-to-patient ratio, which allows the teams to flexibly meet with patients several times each week for several hours at a time during the first few intensive months of care. The PH model facilitates a personal connection in which patients receive understanding and personalized care, leading to increased involvement in health goals and satisfaction with the health care system.

Preliminary review of PH outcome data shows high rates of adherence to aftercare medical and behavioral appointments at 30 and 90 days (88% and 100%, respectively) and decreased readmissions to inpatient behavioral settings (89% of patients upon completion of the 9-month intervention had not been readmitted) (Petit et al. 2018). These data provide an early evidence base supporting the effectiveness of the program. PH demonstrates how community-based care transition interventions can improve health outcomes and reduce avoidable costs, enabling patients to live healthier, happier lives. The model is also an innovative example of the generation of practice-based evidence in which programming designed to operate in a patient's natural environment is evaluated. It is also a part of the continuum of community-based care coordination services that is transforming health systems, which will be considered later in this chapter.

Enhancing the Value of Services for Individuals With Complex Needs

It has been well documented that chronic illness represents a major burden to both general medicine and behavioral health treatment facilities. As a result, "all states…are facing crushing financial and public health challenges" (Smith et al. 2013, p. 831). Medicaid enrollees with comorbid mental health conditions receive a lower quality of care for chronic conditions such as diabetes and have a mortality rate that is up to four times higher than the general population (Unützer et al. 2013). Individuals with SMI and/or substance use disorders are less likely to follow a treatment plan accurately, more often have repeated and lengthy hospitalizations, and have an increased likelihood of homelessness and incarceration. These individuals are also twice as likely to have incomes under 133% of the federal poverty level and are at higher risk of being uninsured for a full year or more (Garfield et al. 2011). Studies suggest that only half receive mental health services, and those who do often fail to take medication as prescribed. These conditions reflect poor engagement in care and unmet treatment needs. They often result in emergency department recidivism and higher rates of psychiatric hospitalization, resulting in huge health care expenses (Smith and Sederer 2009).

The need for community-based services for people with complex health conditions is growing. Garfield and colleagues (2011) estimated that by the end of 2019, when the authors expected the Affordable Care Act to be fully implemented, 3.7 million individuals with SMI would have gained coverage, and nearly one-quarter (24.1%) of those individuals would have been residing in the community (in noninstitutionalized settings). Many individuals with SMI already fall through the cracks due to inadequate engagement or poor retention in treatment services (Smith et al. 2013). It is critical that these challenges be addressed with more effective services. Connecting these individuals to care and establishing their stability in the community will become a critical factor in a high-performance health care system (Gauthier et al. 2006). One effective approach is the development of a full spectrum of care coordination services and methods for the selection of the most appropriate level of service for each individual (Smith et al. 2013). Community-based care coordination services will become an important element of a value-driven system of care regardless of the evolution of the health care systems in the years ahead.

Care Coordination Continuum

The mental health field has struggled with defining *care management*, *case management*, and *care coordination*. These terms are often used interchangeably or synonymously (there are over 40 distinct definitions of *care coordination* and related concepts), leading to significant confusion in describing them. The common thread running through these concepts is the importance of communication across the mosaic of services provided by the many stakeholders that may be involved in a patient's health care. This basic concept is an integral component of any health care system attempting to achieve the Triple Aim of improving patients' experience of care, improving population health, and reducing costs (Berwick et al. 2008). Care coordination, as defined by the Agency for Healthcare Research and Quality, is "the deliberate organization of patient care activities between two or more participants (including the patient) involved in a patient's care to facilitate the appropriate delivery of health care services" (McDonald et al. 2007, p. 5). The agency emphasizes the need for "marshaling of personnel and other resources needed to carry out all required patient care activities," which is "often managed by the exchange of information among participants responsible for different aspects of care" (McDonald et al. 2007, p. 5). Care coordination also creates opportunities to maximize resources, helps to avoid duplication of services, and facilitates comprehensive planning of services in the community.

Care coordination has been used to enhance health and human services in the United States for more than a century. It is often provided by different professional disciplines, but for the most part by nurses and social workers. In many cases paraprofessionals with a bachelor's degree or other specialized training may fill these roles. Regardless of the discipline, the goal has been, and continues to be, the coordination of complex, fragmented services to meet the needs of the patients while reducing the costs of care by using resources wisely. Well-coordinated care is the cornerstone of successfully maintaining an individual with complex needs in the community (Schoen et al. 2011). Working collaboratively with the individual in the coordination of their care and the development of their care plan and goals, as well as including the perspectives of their care network, is at the heart of care coordination approaches. For many years planners have recognized that a variety of populations, such as older adults and people with learning disabilities, can benefit from better coordination of their care. Success in these efforts leads to reduced reliance on emergency services and long-term hospital care, resulting in a significant reduction in health care spending. Research suggests that improving treatment adherence could lower Medicaid hospital days by 13.1%, with over $100 million in annual savings for the national Medicaid system (Smith and Sederer 2009).

There is growing recognition that care coordination activities offering flexibility in their intensity are advantageous. For example, models of lower-intensity traditional case management have a more narrow and targeted scope of focus on a particular problem area, while models offering a more intensive care management approach have a more comprehensive, dynamic, and person-centered array of activities to support recovery (Table 5–1).

Another way to conceptualize the spectrum of care coordination is as a range of intensity from "light-touch" interventions (brief, time-limited approaches similar to traditional case management) to "high-touch" interventions (more intense, comprehensive, long-term approaches, similar to higher-intensity care management models) (Center for Health Care Strategies 2007). Care coordination should be tailored to the needs of patients with widely varying health and social conditions.

Person-centered care approaches have led practitioners and researchers to recognize that traditional case management (too siloed and narrow in scope) does not sufficiently meet the needs of all segments of the population. The United Kingdom Department of Health noted that community care coordination means providing the right level of intervention and support to enable people to achieve maximum independence and control over their lives (Øvretveit 1993). Similarly, "determining the right dose of the right intervention with the right individual at the right time in the right location" is at the center of achieving successful outcomes (Hasselman 2013, p. 5).

One example of a light-touch care coordination program is the New York State Department of Health's Delivery System Reform Incentive Payments. This 30-day care transition program employs care managers to follow up with patients for a month following discharge to ensure attendance at outpatient appointments. The program serves both medical and behavioral health patients and assures inpatient treatment teams that their efforts to arrange aftercare and hospital discharge planning will be supported in the community. A more comprehensive discussion of high-touch care coordination follows.

TABLE 5–1. Case management versus care management

	Case management	Care management
Definition	Process of assessment, planning, facilitation, care coordination, evaluation, and advocacy for options and services to meet a client/patient's and family's health needs.	Comprehensive identification of medical needs, behavioral health needs, and factors of social determinants of health impacting an individual's ability to gain access to, connect with, or remain engaged in the health care system.
		Promising team-based, patient-centered approach designed to assist patients and their support systems in managing medical and behavioral health conditions, particularly chronic health conditions, more effectively. Currently a leading practice in managing the health of a defined population.
Intensity	Traditionally, a fee-for-service structure with a required number of visits (e.g., four face-to-face contacts per month) irrespective of the member's current functioning, need, or acuity. Fee for service encourages most providers to offer maximum services, regardless of whether they are necessary or optimal.	Intersection between the client/patient and the health care system documented in the client/patient's plan of care with ongoing and periodic reassessment.
Scope	Targeted processes designed to address one aspect of general disease management exclusively.	Practice based on three core concepts: patient education, coordination of services and resources, and self-management.
		Addresses the multifaceted social, developmental, educational, and financial needs of individuals with complex medical and behavioral health.
Staffing	Primarily social workers and nurses (with some mental health counselors).	Diverse staff, including social workers, nurses, psychologists, gerontologists, and providers from other health-related fields.

TABLE 5–1. Case management versus care management *(continued)*

	Case management	Care management
History	Case management began with Medicaid and Medicare demonstration projects in the early 1970s but has since become common in all developed countries, although the implementation of these models varies greatly based on health care systems, philosophy, and geography.	A more episodic approach that has developed into a leading practice-based strategy for managing population health.
Goal	Aim is to improve health status for a focused set of predetermined diseases or conditions based on process measures in an attempt to manage cost and address overutilization of services.	Aims are to promote better quality of life, maintain independence to the extent possible, improve communication among those involved in client/patient's care, ensure that the client/patient's needs are met and his or her goals are achieved, and provide education to the client/patient and family members. Emphases are on population health, data analytics, and improved health outcomes with intention to reduce health care costs.
Focus	Approach centered on client/patient, but with limited focus on medical, legal, and financial issues.	Holistic, client/patient- and family-centered approach inclusive of addressing social determinants of health; understanding underlying client/patient-family dynamics; and advocating for client's needs and maximum benefits (i.e., from an insurer).
Limits	Agency defines the limits/scope of work. Typically, provider will be managing a specific disease, issue, condition, or event, and focus may be constrained by regulations, policies, and funders.	Client/patient defines the scope of work (based on a care plan that is developed with his or her input).

Source. Antonelli et al. 2009; Care Management 2018; Center for Health Care Strategies 2007.

Innovative Intensive Care Coordination Approaches

Although some light- and moderate-touch care coordination programs have been successful, there remains a segment of the population with more complex needs (e.g., multiple chronic illnesses) that require more intensive care coordination approaches. These individuals with complex needs are often known as "super-utilizers" (Hasselman 2013). The failure of traditional case management approaches to meet the needs of these individuals is demonstrated by their higher health care expenses and justice system involvement. Adults with SMI account for a disproportionate percentage of these super-utilizers, so a person-centered, intensive care coordination approach is a key to support them in the community (Schoen et al. 2011). These types of programs are costly because they rely on a highly trained staff, but the money saved by reducing the use of more expensive emergency department and hospital services usually offsets those expenditures. Across the United States a series of innovative care management programs are being developed, researched, and replicated to address the needs of this cohort.

These innovative care management programs and services extend beyond medical issues to address patients' psychosocial circumstances, which often affect their ability to follow treatment recommendations and achieve a healthier lifestyle (Hong et al. 2014). To explore how Medicaid could advance models for this high-need group of patients, the Center for Health Care Strategies and the National Governors Association held a Super-Utilizer Summit in 2013. An outcome of the summit was the formation of the National Center for Complex Health and Social Needs. The objective was to coalesce the emerging field of complex care coordination by bringing together experts in the field to develop, test, and scale new models of team-based integrated care coordination.

High-Touch Care Coordination: Hotspotting

The innovative care management approach of "hotspotting" super-utilizers of hospital systems is credited to Dr. Jeff Brenner and his work in Camden, New Jersey, which gained national recognition through a *New Yorker* magazine article (Gawande 2011). Dr. Brenner used data to map neighborhoods that had a disproportionate share of patients with high utilization of costly medical services. With the support of local hospitals, Dr. Brenner and his team were able to mine claims data to identify these super-utilizers. Through intensive care management efforts, they successfully addressed the needs of these individuals and enhanced their support networks and, in doing so, reduced hospital admissions and lowered medical costs (Hasselman 2013).

The Camden Core Model applies many of the principles outlined previously for supporting people with SMI to a medically needy population. Frequently, these individuals who are in and out of hospitals also have associated mental health issues. In much the same way that Pathway Home facilitated transition to stable community living (see earlier section "Practice-Based Evidence Programming: Pathway Home"), the Camden Core Model emphasizes the importance of an "authentic healing relationship" between the care team and the patient as a means to support behavioral change (Camden Coalition of Healthcare Providers 2016). The team also attends medical and psychiatric outpatient appointments with a client to better understand the patient's perspective, any possible obstacles to treatment, and the patient's medication regimen (Camden Coalition of Healthcare Providers 2016).

Outcomes showed that by helping individuals manage their social, medical, and behavioral needs, these complex care management interventions successfully impacted the harmful and costly cycle of repeated and avoidable hospitalizations. The Camden Coalition measured the long-term effect of their intervention on the first 36 super-utilizers they worked with. The group averaged 62 hospital and ER visits per month prior to joining the program. After 3 months of enrollment in the program, the super-utilizer group averaged 37 hospital and emergency room visits per month, which represents a 40% reduction in visits. Their hospital bills averaged \$1.2 million per month before enrollment in the program and just over \$0.5 million per month after participation in the program, a 56% reduction in hospital costs (Gawande 2011).

The Camden teams benefit greatly from real-time data provided by participating hospitals and through the use of a citywide health information exchange that flags patients who have been admitted to a hospital at least twice in the past 6 months. This information collection is the means of identifying those who might benefit from this type of program. In adaptations of the model, although information may not be immediately available, hospital teams rely on the collection of similar data to identify patients. Data include the number of hospital admissions in the past 6 months and various social determinants of health, such as housing, transportation, and food security. This model is an example of an integrated care program to meet both physical and psychiatric needs of a population with complex conditions through the use of a high-intensity care coordination strategy.

Community-Based Care: Health Homes

In 1963, the Community Mental Health Act "set out to revolutionize services for individuals with serious mental illness by emphasizing community life grounded in social and vocational pursuits" (Smith and Sederer 2009, p. 528). Individuals with SMI had not been receiving adequate community-based services; some studies indicated that approximately 50% did not receive any mental health treatment at all (Kessler et al. 1998; Smith and Sederer 2009). The Patient-Centered Medical Home (PCMH) emerged as an innovative service that would begin to remedy this situation. This was an approach that recognized "the need for a single repository of medical records to promote communication and collaborative treatment among care providers" (Smith and Sederer 2009, p. 529).

The PCMH can be designed to meet the needs of the various populations it serves. A light-touch PCMH may be provided through the primary care physician's office for the health care of all the patients in the practice. A high-touch PCMH serves patients who have chronic illnesses or other complex medical and behavioral issues, who see multiple providers, and who are frequently poorly connected to needed services (Peikes et al. 2009). This discussion first focuses on moderate- and low-touch PCMHs serving those with relatively uncomplicated health needs, and subsequently considers high-touch iterations of the PCMH, and particularly the Medicaid Health Home (MHH) model.

Improving health and well-being in patients with complicated needs requires unique knowledge of all the issues impacting the individual and the full array of available local community-based services. Expertise in social services, ongoing persistent patient engagement, family support, advocacy, and motivational interviewing skills, as well as time and resources to provide crisis intervention, are needed. Patients with complex medical needs may have several different providers in the course of a year. These providers may be "incompletely aware of each other's care, often prescribing incompatible or contraindicated treatments or providing conflicting advice." Often, no single physician or provider is designated to be responsible for coordinating the individual's health care goals (Peikes et al. 2009).

By 2007, medical practices and health care networks began to develop PCMHs nationwide, using the National Committee for Quality Assurance standards as a framework to evaluate quality. Development of the electronic health record enabled various treatment providers to record goals, medical interventions, and progress (Bates and Bitton 2010). During this same time, the *Joint Principles of the Patient-Centered Medical Home*, published collaboratively by the American Academy of Family Physicians, American Academy of Pediatrics, American College of Physicians, and American Osteopathic Association (2007), put forth the following objectives for PCMHs:

- Enhanced access to care for patients
- Ongoing relationship between patients and personal physicians

- Whole-person orientation in assessment and care delivery
- Team-based approach to care
- Coordinated and integrated care
- Commitment to quality and safety

The PCMH model relies on primary care providers (PCPs) to work effectively with other providers involved with their patients (American Academy of Family Physicians, American Academy of Pediatrics, American College of Physicians, and American Osteopathic Association 2007). With access to data and health information technology, PCPs could share information with specialty care providers, furthering the goal of continuity of care, family engagement, and stakeholder accountability. The PCMH was designed to address the delivery gaps in primary care systems, exacerbated by communication challenges and the limited infrastructure supports available to small practices. This model best serves a population that has moderately complex service needs that often include emotional health issues such as depression, anxiety, or substance misuse.

People with more complex medical and behavioral health problems are better served by high-touch PCMHs that have greater resources available and a broader treatment team. It is important to recognize that individuals with SMI and significant medical problems are less likely than the general population to engage with a PCP without additional supports (Smith and Sederer 2009). In the high-touch PCMH model, individuals with SMI usually establish their primary treatment alliance with someone on their behavioral health treatment team (Smith and Sederer 2009), who then coordinates with the PCP and other service providers to address the full spectrum of the individuals' needs.

The Affordable Care Act established the option for states to develop health homes for Medicaid recipients. The Medicaid Health Home (MHH) program is partly funded by the federal government to help states pay for more complex care management for people with multiple chronic conditions. As a form of a moderate- to high-touch PCMH, MHHs seek to coordinate complex medical and behavioral health needs with services and enhanced access to care. The MHH combines care coordination services with the social supports these patients require. Twenty-one states and the District of Columbia have launched MHH programs, and more than 1 million individuals are enrolled nationwide (Citizens Budget Committee 2018).

The MHH is one example of this transition, enhancing community-based service delivery with an emphasis on optimizing outcomes and delivering care more efficiently. Addressing known risk factors with person-centered approaches and community-based care coordination, the MHH supports a more integrated model of service delivery that equips providers to respond in a timely manner to critical events. It shifts the practice standard from discrete, disconnected services to collaborative ones that address all of an individual's chronic health conditions (Mechanic 2012). The MHH model is based on a whole-person approach, encompassing comprehensive care management, integration of physical and behavioral health care, and links to nonclinical supports (U.S. Department of Health and Human Services 2017).

Medicaid has allowed states to develop payment innovations to subsidize care coordination services in MHHs, which were not previously reimbursed (Mechanic 2012). States have flexibility in designing their programs for MHH care coordination services, including determining how these services are defined and reimbursed. States develop the eligibility criteria and targeted medical and/or behavioral health conditions to be addressed. States such as Iowa and Missouri have implemented MHHs via their preexisting Primary Care Health Homes. Iowa demonstrated an average of 15% cost savings related to lower emergency department utilization and even greater reductions in use by patients who continued their enrollments for at least 1 year. Missouri specialized its MHH to focus on SMI and has expanded the service to serve approximately 19,000 individuals (Citizens Budget Committee 2018).

So far, North Carolina has achieved the largest enrollment of the states with MHH programs, with more than 525,000 enrollees. North Carolina's strategy was to serve a broad network of potentially eligible individuals. Other states, focusing on a narrower criterion, such as SMI or HIV/AIDS populations, have achieved more modest enrollments. Whereas other states such as New Mexico and Connecticut limited their eligible population for enrollment, Washington State rolled out its MHH statewide in 2017, covering more than 35 counties with a strategy to provide services to a broad array of chronic conditions and mental health diagnosis (Citizens Budget Committee 2018).

Regardless of their variations, MHH programs have as their overall goal a less fragmented delivery system with a holistic perspective. Care coordination is the intervention that supports continuity of care across various settings and disciplines (U.S. Department of Health and Human Services 2017). A gradual shift is occurring from the traditional fee-for-service model, with restrictive Medicaid regulations, to new financing models that allow more comprehensive funding for needed services such as care coordination (James and Poulsen 2016).

Patient-Centered Medical Homes: New York State Medicaid Health Homes

In 2009, New York State's total Medicaid expenditures surpassed $54 billion, with nearly 13% attributed to behavioral health conditions. After adjustment for population size, New York State's Medicaid program is one of the most expensive in the nation across geriatric, adult, child, and disabled populations (Citizens Budget Committee 2016). In 2011, New York State Governor Andrew Cuomo convened a Medicaid Redesign Team (MRT) with over 389 projects, each with the specified goal of reducing utilization/costs and improving outcomes for persons with mental illness, substance use disorders, and/or chronic conditions.

In 2012, New York State's MRT decided to implement the MHH option as one of its major initiatives. Medicaid expansion under the Affordable Care Act was supported by a federal fund match of 90% during its first 2 years (Spillman et al. 2014).

In New York State, MHHs were designated as the hubs for the delivery of care coordination services. Previously existing care coordination programs and their respective enrollees transitioned to MHHs in the early wave of New York State's implementation strategy (Citizens Budget Committee 2018). The conversion and placement of these programs under the umbrella of MHHs enabled a greater emphasis on outcomes. Flexible, individualized treatment plans were emphasized. At the local level, community providers collaborated to develop MHHs to provide care coordination. Since the launch of MHHs in New York State in 2012, the program has enrolled over 175,000 individuals. Initial outcomes demonstrated "long-run cost savings for many with complex conditions" (Citizens Budget Committee 2018).

Findings documented by the New York Health Home Coalition suggest that between 2014 and 2016, MHHs reduced preventable emergency department visits by 19% statewide. During the same period MHHs contributed to the reduction in potentially preventable medical inpatient readmissions by 20%, dramatically decreased nursing facility utilization by 53%, and decreased inpatient psychiatric utilization by 26% (New York Health Home Coalition 2020). Beyond these outcomes specific to New York State, most MHHs across the country have identified better access to nonclinical services, such as housing and employment services. According to the Citizens Budget Committee (2018), "the policy question is not whether [Health Homes] 'work.' [Health Homes] do work and should be sustained; they are making a contribution toward promoting the triple aim." The MHHs are one example of a cost-effective strategy to meet the long-term needs of individuals with complex health conditions.

Continuum of Crisis Services

There is a paramount need for a continuum of services in the community to address behavioral health emergencies. If an array of crisis services can be well organized, comprehensive, and seamlessly integrated, costs can potentially be decreased through reductions in emergency department visits and avoidable hospitalizations. Improved outcomes, greater patient satisfaction, and more efficient utilization of community-based supports and services should be obtained.

Many states have developed a continuum of crisis intervention services to provide less expensive, community-based alternatives to the use of hospital-based care. State and local behavioral health authorities have explored various funding mechanisms to support these services, including Medicaid waivers, arrangements with payers, and grants. The research base on the effectiveness of crisis services is growing, and some states now have experience with different payment mechanisms to support a comprehensive crisis system (Substance Abuse and Mental Health Services Administration 2014).

The development of a continuum of community-based behavioral health crisis services needs to be an integral part of the delivery models. A comprehensive continuum incorporates many systems, including health, legal, social services, and community and personal safety, extending beyond the point of contact (Technical Assistance Collaborative 2005). The primary goal of these services is to stabilize and improve psychological symptoms of distress and to engage individuals in the most appropriate interventions to address the problems that led to the crisis. The Substance Abuse and Mental Health Services Administration (2014) has described several core crisis services:

1. **Telephone Crisis Services:** Skilled professionals provide appropriate triage and dispositions. Crisis hotlines provide immediate support and facilitate referrals to medical, health care, and community support services, and promote problem-solving and coping skills via telephone (or even text or online chat) to individuals who are experiencing distress. These hotlines may use secure Web interfaces to provide an initial assessment and access to large data sets, enabling immediate referral to appropriate crisis care.
2. **Mobile Crisis Teams (MCTs):** These teams have the ability to respond quickly to a behavioral health crisis in the community. They provide acute mental health crisis stabilization and psychiatric assessment services to individuals within their own homes and in other sites outside of traditional clinical settings. The main objectives of MCTs are to provide rapid response, assessment, and resolution of the crisis situations. MCTs have been deployed in urban, rural, and even frontier areas.
3. **Peer Crisis Services:** These services are designed as a respite model that provides safety, relief, and recovery in an environment more like a

home than an institution. Peer crisis services are an alternative to a psychiatric emergency department and are operated primarily by people who have experience living with a mental illness. Peer crisis services are intended to be shorter term than traditional crisis residential services, but may extend up to several days, if needed.

4. **Crisis Residential Services:** These services are designed to prevent or ameliorate a behavioral health crisis and reduce acute symptoms of mental illness by providing continuous 24-hour observation and supervision for individuals who are not at imminent risk of harm. These services are intended for individuals who do not require inpatient services. These crisis residential services are often referred to as respite services, providing a safe environment removed from the environment in which the crises evolved.
5. **Emergency Care Services:** These may exist in a variety of forms, ranging from urgent behavioral care/walk-in centers, to crisis observation and stabilization settings, to full-service, hospital-based psychiatric emergency services. They provide individuals in distress with immediate assessment and disposition in a protected environment. When patients present in agitated states or with imminent risk of harm to themselves or others, these services help deescalate, provide urgent care (including detoxification), and arrange transitions to other elements of the service system as the situation evolves. Unnecessary hospitalizations are avoided whenever possible.

Conclusion and Recommendations

This chapter has considered a range of services that improve outcomes and reduce the costs of care. The principles of providing a comprehensive continuum of service options and care coordination are at the core of these services. Nevertheless, the full realization of these programs across all systems of care are limited by multiple systemic and individual barriers but are of critical importance as the needed reforms of the current system are advanced.

Psychiatrists clearly play a vital role in the provision of the services described in this chapter. Although most of these services do not depend on psychiatrists to prescribe medications, these system-level transformations and adoption of effective programs require broad knowledge of biological, psychological, and sociological factors, which makes psychiatrists a well-suited group to deliver these services. Moreover, team-based delivery of care is an important component of the effective practices that have been considered, and psychiatrists are integral parts of those teams. Psychiatrists' specific roles within these teams are considered further in Chapters 11 ("An Expanded Role for Psychiatry") and 12 ("Psychiatric Workforce Development").

Clearly, no one-size-fits-all strategy can work when it comes to effectively managing the delivery of community-based care. This is especially true in attempting to meet the needs of the most vulnerable populations most effectively. Incorporating services that have established effectiveness, such as the evidence-based practices and practice-based evidence described in the beginning of this chapter, provides a sound base for achieving desired outcomes. An array of service options will provide the best results and increased patient and provider satisfaction. Care coordination services, all along the continuum described in this chapter, are a requisite for meaningfully advancing population health and movement toward value-based care. They span health, behavioral, and social determinants to ensure that individuals are receiving the right care at the right time in the right dosage. It is only in this way that a continued focus on optimizing health system performance will be achieved.

References

American Academy of Family Physicians, American Academy of Pediatrics, American College of Physicians, American Osteopathic Association: Joint principles of the Patient-Centered Medical Home. May 2007. Available at: www.acponline.org/system/files/documents/running_practice/delivery_and_payment_models/pcmh/demonstrations/jointprinc_05_17.pdf. Accessed February 11, 2020.

Ammerman A, Smith TW, Calancie L: Practice-based evidence in public health: improving reach, relevance, and results. Annu Rev Public Health 35:47–63, 2014

Antonelli RC, McAllister JW, Popp J: Making care coordination a critical component of the pediatric health system: a multidisciplinary framework. The Commonwealth Fund, May 2009. Available at: https://doc.uments.com/d-making-care-coordination-a-critical-component-of-the-pediatric.pdf. Accessed February 11, 2020.

Bates DB, Bitton A: The future of health information technology in the Patient-Centered Medical Home. Health Aff (Millwood) 29(4):614–621, 2010

Berwick DM, Nolan TW, Whittington J: The Triple Aim: care, health, and cost. Health Aff (Millwood) 27(3):759–769, 2008

Camden Coalition of Healthcare Providers: COACH Manual: The Camden Coalition of HealthCare Providers. November 2016. Available at: www.camdenhealth.org/wp-content/uploads/2017/04/COACHManual_FINAL_WithAppendix_Dec2016.pdf. Accessed February 11, 2020.

Care Management: Implications for medical practice, health policy, and health services research. August 2018. Available at: www.ahrq.gov/professionals/prevention-chronic-care/improve/coordination/caremanagement/index.html. Accessed February 11, 2020.

Center for Health Care Strategies: Care management definition and framework. 2007. Available at: www.chcs.org/resource/care-management-definition-and-framework. Accessed February 11, 2020.

Citizens Budget Committee: What ails Medicaid in New York? And does the Medicaid Redesign Team have a cure? May 2016. Available at: https://cbcny.org/sites/default/files/media/files/REPORT_MEDICAID_05232016_1.pdf. Accessed February 11, 2020.

Citizens Budget Committee: Options for enhancing New York's health home initiative: a discussion paper. Citizens Budget Committee. May 1, 2018. Available at: https://cbcny.org/research/options-enhancing-new-yorks-health-home-initiative. Accessed February 11, 2020.

Coopey M, Nix MP, Carolyn CM: Translating research into evidence-based nursing practice and evaluating effectiveness. J Nurs Care Qual 21(3):195–202, 2006

Cummings N: The first decade of managed behavioral health care: what went right and what went wrong. Critical Strategies: Psychotherapy in Managed Care 1(1):19–38, 2000

Deci PA, Santos AB, Hiott DW, et al: Dissemination of assertive community treatment programs. Psychiatr Serv 46(7):676–678, 1995

Garfield RL, Zuvekas SH, Lave JR: The impact of national health care reform on adults with severe mental disorders. Am J Psychiatry 168(5):486–494, 2011

Gauthier AK, Davis K, Schoenbaum SC: Commentary—Achieving a high-performance health system: high reliability organizations within a broader agenda. Health Serv Res 41(4 Pt 2):1710–1720, 2006

Gawande A: The hot spotters. The New Yorker, January 24, 2011. Available at: www.newyorker.com/magazine/2011/01/24/the-hot-spotters. Accessed February 11, 2020.

Gone JP: Reconciling evidence-based practice and cultural competence in mental health services: introduction to a special issue. Transcult Psychiatry 52(2):139–149, 2015

Green LW, Glasgow RE: Evaluating the relevance, generalization, and applicability of research: issues in external validation and translation methodology. Eval Health Prof 29(1):126–153, 2006

Hasselman D: Super-Utilizer Summit: common themes from innovative complex care management programs. Center for Health Care Strategies, October 2013. Available at: www.chcs.org/resource/super-utilizer-summit-common-themes-from-innovative-complex-care-management-programs/. Accessed February 11, 2020.

Herman D, Conover S, Felix A, et al: Critical Time Intervention: an empirically supported model for preventing homelessness in high risk groups. J Prim Prev 28(3–4):295–312, 2007

Hong CS, Siegel AL, Ferris TG: Caring for high-need, high-cost patients: what makes for a successful care management program. The Commonwealth Fund, Issue Brief, August 2014. Available at: www.commonwealthfund.org/sites/default/files/documents/___media_files_publications_issue_brief_2014_aug_1764_hong_caring_for_ high_need_high_cost_patients_ccm_ib.pdf. Accessed February 11, 2020.

Institute of Medicine: Crossing the Quality Chasm: A New Health System for the 21st Century. Washington, DC, National Academies Press, 2001

Institute of Medicine: Health professions education: a bridge to quality, in Committee on the Health Professions Education Summit. Edited by Greiner AC, Knebel E. Washington, DC, National Academies Press, 2003

Isaac CA, Franceschi A: EBM: evidence to practice and practice to evidence. J Eval Clin Pract 14(5):656–659, 2008

James BC, Poulsen GP: The case for capitation. Harvard Business Review, July 2016. Available at: https://hbr.org/2016/07/the-case-for-capitation. Accessed February 11, 2020.

Kessler RC, Olfson M, Berglund PA: Patterns and predictors of treatment contact after first onset of psychiatric disorders. Am J Psychiatry 155(1):62–69, 1998

Lehman AF, Goldman HH, Dixon LB: Evidence-based mental health treatments and services: examples to inform public policy. Millbank Memorial Fund, June 2004. Available at: www.milbank.org/wp-content/files/documents/2004lehman/2004lehman.html. Accessed February 10, 2020.

McDonald KM, Sundaram V, Bravata DM, et al: Closing the quality gap: a critical analysis of quality improvement strategies (Vol 7: Care Coordination). Technical Reviews, No 9.7. Agency for Healthcare Research and Quality, June 2007. Available at: www.ncbi.nlm.nih.gov/books/NBK44015/. Accessed February 10, 2020

Mechanic D: Seizing opportunities under the Affordable Care Act for transforming the mental and behavioral health system. Health Aff (Millwood) 31(2):376–382, 2012

Melnyk BM, Fineout-Overholt E, Stetler C, et al: Outcomes and implementation strategies from the first U.S. Evidence-Based Practice Leadership Summit. Worldviews Evid Based Nurs 2(3):113–121, 2005

New York Health Home Coalition: Health home outcomes. 2020. Available at: https://hhcoalition.org/what-are-health-homes/outcomes. Accessed February 11, 2020.

Oss M: Market Share in the United States, 2002–2003: Open Minds Yearbook of Behavioral Health and Employee Assistance Program. Gettysburg, PA, Open Minds, 2002

Øvretveit J: Coordinating Community Care: Multidisciplinary Teams and Care Management. Philadelphia, PA, Open University Press, 1993

Peikes D, Chen A, Schore J, et al: Effects of care coordination on hospitalization, quality of care, and health care expenditures among Medicare beneficiaries: 15 randomized trials. JAMA 301(6):603–618, 2009

Petit JR, Graham M, Granek B: Pathway Home: an innovative care transition program from hospital to home. Psychiatr Serv 69(8):942–943, 2018

Sackett D, Strauss S, Richardson W: Evidence-Based Medicine: How to Practice and Teach EBM, 2nd Edition. Edinburgh, Churchill Livingstone, 2000

Schoen C, Osborn R, Squires D, et al: New 2011 survey of patients with complex care needs in eleven countries finds that care is often poorly coordinated. Health Aff (Millwood) 30(12):2437–2448, 2011

Smith TE, Sederer LI: A new kind of homelessness for individuals with serious mental illness? The need for a "mental health home." Psychiatr Serv 60(4):528–533, 2009

Smith TE, Erlich MD, Sederer LI: Integrating general medical and behavioral health care: the New York State perspective. Psychiatr Serv 64(9):828–831, 2013

Spillman BC, Richardson E, Spencer A, et al: Evaluation of the Medicaid Health Home Option for Beneficiaries With Chronic Conditions: Final Annual Report—Year Two. Washington, DC, Urban Institute, Office of The Assistant Secretary for Planning and Evaluation, U.S. Department of Health and Human Services, June 2014. Available at: https://aspe.hhs.gov/execsum/evaluation-medicaid-health-home-option-beneficiaries-chronic-conditions-final-annual-report-year-two. Accessed January 2020.

Substance Abuse and Mental Health Services Administration: Crisis services: effectiveness, cost- effectiveness, and funding strategies (HHS Publ No SMA-14-4848). 2014. Available at: https://store.samhsa.gov/system/files/sma14-4848.pdf. Accessed April 5, 2019

Substance Abuse and Mental Health Services Administration: Evidence-Based Practices Resource Center. 2020. Available at: www.samhsa.gov/ebp-resource-center. Accessed February 10, 2020.

Swinkels A, Albarran JW, Means RI, et al: Evidence-based practice in health and social care: where are we now? J Interprof Care 16(4):335–347, 2002

Tannenbaum SJ: Evidence-based practice as mental health policy: three controversies and a caveat. Health Aff (Milwood) 24(1):163–173, 2005

Technical Assistance Collaborative: A community-based comprehensive psychiatric crisis response service. 2005. Available at: www.tacinc.org/media/13106/Crisis%20Manual.pdf. Accessed February 11, 2020.

Test MA: Continuity of care in community treatment. New Directions for Mental Health Services 1979(2):15–23, 1979

Tunis SR, Stryer DB, Clancy CM: Practical clinical trials: increasing the value of clinical research for decision making in clinical and health policy. JAMA 290(12):1624–1632, 2003

Unützer J, Harbin H, Schoenbaum M, et al: The collaborative care model: an approach for integrating physical and mental health care in medicaid health homes. Center for Health Care Strategies, May 2013. Available at: www.chcs.org/resource/the-collaborative-care-model-an-approach-for-integrating-physical-and-mental-health-care-in-medicaid-health-homes. Accessed February 11, 2020.

U.S. Department of Health and Human Services: Evaluation of the Medicaid Health Home Option for beneficiaries with chronic conditions: evaluation of outcomes of selected health home program. Annual report—year five. U.S. Department of Health and Human Services, Assistant Secretary for Planning and Evaluation, Office of Disability, 2017. Available at: https://aspe.hhs.gov/system/files/pdf/258871/HHOption5.pdf. Accessed February 11, 2020.

Viswanathan M, Ammerman A, Eng E, et al: Community-based participatory research: assessing the evidence: summary, in AHRQ Evidence Report Summaries. Agency for Healthcare Research and Quality, August 2004. Available at: www.ncbi.nlm.nih.gov/books/NBK11852/. Accessed February 11, 2020.

Wallen GR, Mitchell SA, Melnyk B, et al: Implementing evidence-based practice: effectiveness of a structured multifaceted mentorship programme. J Adv Nurs 66(12):2761–2771, 2010

Wisconsin Department of Health Services: MMHI: program of assertive community treatment. October 2, 2019. Available at: www.dhs.wisconsin.gov/mendota/programs/pact.htm. Accessed February 11, 2020.

Part II

Where We Want to Go

Systems Interventions

6

Innovative Financing

Incentivizing Value

Sosunmolu O. Shoyinka, M.D., M.B.A.

The U.S. health care system is among the most advanced in the world. It is also, however, the most expensive in the developed world, accounting for 18% of the gross domestic product in 2017 (Centers for Medicare and Medicaid Services 2019c). U.S. health care expenditures are over $3 trillion annually (Moses et al. 2013). Reasons for the rising cost of health care include an aging population, changing disease prevalence, inadequate investment in social services, emphasis on expensive medical interventions, and high clinician and administrative fees (Branning and Vater 2016). Unfortunately, health outcomes have not reflected the level of this expenditure (Sawyer and McDermott 2019). In behavioral health, access to and quality of care remain pressing concerns (Cohen Veterans Network, National Council for Behavioral Health 2018).

To comprehend why health systems function the way they do, one must understand how they are funded. Because payment essentially serves as a reward or reinforcement for specific behaviors by providers, services typically reflect what is paid for and how that payment is structured. Although other incentives can motivate providers to deliver desired care, financial incentives are often the simplest and most direct way to do so. Funding mechanisms are therefore a useful lever in making changes to how care is delivered. Indeed, many of the successes and challenges of the U.S. health care system can be tied to funding. As we shall see in this chapter, value in health care (the benefit derived vs. the cost of inputs) is tied to the more fundamental question of societal values (what the collective society determines to be important and is willing to invest resources in).

This chapter provides an overview of health funding in the United States. It focuses on dominant funding mechanisms and recent efforts to improve them, considers efforts to align payment with quality, and concludes with a vision of the future of behavioral health financing. The historical underpinnings of the current health care financing system are covered in Chapter 2 ("Evolution of Funding and Quality Control in Health Care").

Values Underlying Health Care Financing in the United States

Health care must be paid for. As the expense of health care has grown in recent years, it has become impractical for all but the very rich to pay for their needs out of pocket. As a result, all people need some form of assistance to pay for the costs of their care when it is needed. This raises questions: How should health care be paid for? Who should pay for it? There are a number of issues that must be resolved by whatever entity pays for care: What should be paid for? How much should be paid for? Should payment ever be withheld or stopped? And who should make those decisions? The resolution to these questions will have a significant impact on both the quality and the cost of care.

At the core of health care financing is a fundamental value judgment: Should health care be a right or a commodity? The answer to this question determines how a nation chooses to fund the care of its citizens. If health care is a fundamental right, then all citizens will be covered through some financing mechanism or other, regardless of social status or ability to pay. If, on the other hand, it is a commodity, then standard business principles (including profit making) will drive who gets it, how it is paid for, and how it is delivered. There would be no guarantee that all citizens would have some form of health insurance.

A study of other developed nations' funding of health care shows that in most, health care is considered a fundamental right of all citizens. Although the ways in which other nations choose to finance health care differ, individuals' ability to pay and profit generation are not primary considerations (Bodenheimer and Grumbach 2016). In the United States, cultural values of consumer choice and self-determination, physician autonomy, reliance on market forces, and entrepreneurship have had a significant impact on the evolution of how health care is paid for. Because these values implicitly govern policy making, they shape the way health care is financed and delivered. Furthermore, these values are often in conflict with each other. For example, satisfying the value of individual or physician autonomy may conflict with ensuring the value of cost containment. Such conflicts may explain the seeming incoherence of U.S. health care policy, which has resulted in a system that still struggles with access and quality (Prester 1992). In contrast, other developed nations' health care systems deliver better access and quality at lower expenditure; arguably, this is traceable to different values, which have evolved different policies. Clear distinctions between the systems of these other nations and those of the United States include the central role of the government in the design, financing, administration, and oversight of these systems (resulting in low administrative overhead in nations such as Canada) and the view of health care as a social right of all citizens.

In the United States, there has been significant resistance from a variety of sources to government oversight and financing of health care. Despite this resistance, health care financing is now a mixture of private, for-profit, and nonprofit insurers and a slowly growing role of government-sponsored insurance programs for specific segments of the population. Nonetheless, 8%–10% of the population remains uninsured, 10 times higher than in any other developed nation (Cohen et al. 2018). Conflicting values of social responsibility and the primacy of private enterprise create a tension that is crucial to understanding the lack of value in our systems of care. Even the payment/insurance mechanisms that are in place are poorly suited to meet the needs of many of those who are most ill. Understanding the forces that have shaped most aspects of services currently in place in the United States will also be key to creating a vision for the future financing of health care in the United States, which will be discussed at the conclusion of this chapter.

Overview of Current Health Care Financing Systems

Fee-for-service (FFS) payment is the primary method for covering the costs of providing care to individuals with health problems in the United States, accounting for 71% of health care spending in 2016 (Rama 2017). In this system, the payer, whether private or governmental, establishes a set of services that are covered or "billable" and sets a rate of compensation for each of the services in that set. In many cases, compensation is influenced by which type of professional is providing the service. Third-party payers (entities that serve as intermediaries between service users and providers to manage and pay for health care expenses) collect premiums (or taxes in the case of government plans) and provide payments on behalf of the insured. Providers bill the third-party payer for services delivered, and the insured users often pay a predetermined portion of the cost of services received.

The advantage of FFS arrangements is that there is accountability that services are actually being provided. One concern with FFS arrangements is that they incentivize providers to prioritize volume over outcomes; the more of a billable service that is provided, the more a provider is paid—regardless of the outcome of the care provided. Another critique of the FFS system is that it reduces providers' ability to find innovative and individualized responses to clients' needs. Because services are limited to what can be reimbursed, certain services may not be provided, either because they cannot be billed for or because reimbursement is so low that it is not financially rewarding for providers to make them available.

The major elements of FFS systems are discussed in the following subsections. These include service users, health care providers, insurers or third-party payers, private insurance plans, insurance exchanges, government-sponsored insurance plans.

Service Users

Service users generally refers to persons seeking medical care for various conditions. In behavioral health, other terms historically used have included *patient*, *consumer*, *participant*, and sometimes *client*.

Health Care Providers

Health care providers include all parties involved in caring for a patient, including hospitals, health centers, physicians, dieticians, pharmacists, nurse practitioners, nurses, respiratory and physical therapists, speech pathologists, care coordinators, billers, coders, and support staff. Providers of care are diverse in terms of the range of services they offer and their reasons for doing so. They may be organized on a continuum from single practitioners to multispecialty group practices to large-scale enterprises such as hospitals or corporations. Private practices providing mental health treatment are essentially small businesses, run on a for-profit basis in most cases. Various professionals may be involved in private practices, which sometimes operate on direct cash payments from patients but in most cases bill insurers on behalf of their patients. Many health care entities such as hospitals, freestanding clinics, and community mental health centers operate as not-for-profit 501(c)(3) entities. Although these entities often derive the majority of their revenue from fee-for-service billing of third-party payers, they also may receive other sources of funding such as charitable contributions and grants.

Insurers or Third-Party Payers

An insurance company (third party) is an agent that serves as an intermediary between the patient (first party) and the provider (second party). For a set price, insurers act on behalf of first parties to guarantee payment for a defined set of "covered" health-related services, products, and care. These companies may pay all or part of expenses incurred when an individual is engaged in health care. Third-party payers ensure that the potential cost of treatment for future illness will be paid if an individual pays a premium for this protection. Another entity, such as an employer, may pay the premium on employees' behalf, as is often the case in the United States. Through complex calculations, actuaries project the likely costs that will be incurred by the people they cover and set premiums at a rate that ensures that their income will exceed their expenses. This is accomplished when a large number of both healthy and ill individuals have their premiums pooled, so that young healthy individuals subsidize the expenses of older and less healthy members (American Academy of Actuaries, Individual and Small Group Markets Committee 2017).

Private Insurance Plans

Privately funded coverage is provided primarily through employer-sponsored plans in the United States. With employment-based health insurance, employers usually pay most of the premium that purchases health insurance for their employees. Employees often pay part of the premium as well, usually in the form of a salary deduction. Insurance plans with greater choice, lower out-of-pocket contributions (deductibles and copays), and more covered services tend to be more expensive than those with restricted networks, higher out-of-pocket charges, and fewer covered services.

Private insurance plans are most often for-profit entities. As such, they need to maintain financial health and satisfy investors. These goals require that they control costs and limit utilization of services; to some degree, this puts them in conflict with quality imperatives. Expenses have been limited through the use of medication formulary restrictions, restrictive medical necessity criteria, and onerous preauthorization processes for services. Some companies have resisted the provision of coverage parity for mental health and have been tempted to preferentially fund short-term treatments that stabilize episodes of crisis for people with chronic conditions rather than invest in long-term solutions (*Wit v. United Behavioral Health* 2019). Although this approach may be less costly for the payer in the short term, it does not promote long-term recovery for individuals with chronic conditions. These shortcomings have a significant impact on psychiatric care and outcomes, particularly for severe, chronic, and persistent mental illnesses (Glick et al. 2011); this is because such conditions (e.g., schizophrenia) often require sustained, coordinated multimodal treatment. These conditions are similar to other chronic and persistent medical conditions, such as cardiac failure, diabetes, cancer, renal disease, and autoimmune conditions. Although little evidence is available to support limiting treatment for mental illnesses to short-term episodic treatment, substantial evidence exists to show that long-term pharmacotherapy, psychotherapy, and psychosocial treatments can alter the course of illness (Kreyenbuhl et al. 2010).

The National Committee for Quality Assurance (NCQA) sets quality standards for health care insurance companies (National Committee for Quality Assurance 2020). Compliance with these standards allows insurance companies to become accredited by NCQA and provides some assurance that they are giving adequate attention to quality of care, providing some needed balance to this system.

Table 6–1 lists the four major types of plans that exist for managing payments and services (Kongstvedt 2013). For the purposes of this chapter, I will focus on health maintenance organizations.

Insurance Exchanges

An insurance exchange functions as an insurance marketplace where individuals, businesses, and families can compare the costs of various types of plans and make an informed choice about which to purchase. Individuals who are self-employed or not covered by their employer may purchase insurance via these exchanges. Insurers in the exchanges offer several types of plans with variable degrees of coverage and cost sharing. Individuals with lower incomes may be eligible for subsidies from the federal government. These exchanges pool the risk of participating individuals to offer coverage at a lower rate than had been available to individuals purchasing independently in the past. People can choose from a range of government-standardized health care benefit plans offered by private insurers participating in the exchange. Subsidies, in the form of premium tax credits and cost-sharing reductions for purchasers, are available to individual purchasers on a sliding scale according to income. Small businesses may be eligible for small business health insurance tax credits when they purchase coverage for their em-

TABLE 6–1. Health plan types and their characteristics

Type of plan	Network restriction	Relative cost of care/out-of-pocket requirement	PCP gatekeeper role
Health maintenance organization (HMO)	Yes	Low if within network	Yes; PCP coordinates care
Preferred provider organization (PPO)	Yes: cost of care fully covered for in-network but can go out of network at higher cost	More expensive; copays and deductibles are higher; can go out of network at higher cost	More flexible; PCP referral not required for access to specialists
Point of service plan: combined HMO and PPO features	Yes, but can go out of network (more expensive)	Lower copays than PPOs, no annual deductibles for PCP and preventive care services; deductible required for out-of-network providers	PCP required for coordination of care
Indemnity plan	None	Higher premiums, deductibles, and copays	Not required

Note. PCP=personal care provider.
Source. Based on Kongstvedt 2013.

ployees through the exchange (Centers for Medicare and Medicaid Services 2020b; Internal Revenue Service 2019).

The original version of the Patient Protection and Affordable Care Act of 2010 was designed to create large risk-sharing pools by mandating coverage for all citizens. States were offered the option of organizing these exchanges themselves, but many states declined this option and deferred to the federal government to establish them (French et al. 2016). This mandate was eliminated through court action (*Texas v. United States* 2018), and as a result, younger, healthier individuals often opted out of the plans and premiums were not reined in as originally envisioned.

Government-Sponsored Insurance Plans

Government-sponsored insurance plans include all tax-supported insurance provided through federal, state, and local government programs. Some examples are Medicare, Medicaid, the federal insurance exchanges, Children's Health Insurance Program (CHIP), Veterans Administration, Indian Health Service, and insurance of last resort. These are all hybrid programs jointly funded by federal and/or state funds, along with some individual out-of-pocket contributions.

Medicare

Medicare Part A covers hospital-based care for adults ages 65 and older and people with disabilities. It is funded through Social Security taxes paid to the government by employers and employees. Medicare Part B pays for physician services, and Part D covers prescription drugs. Parts B and D are paid for by federal taxes and small monthly premiums from beneficiaries (Centers for Medicare and Medicaid Services 2020a).

Medicaid

Medicaid provides insurance for low-income Americans and is jointly funded and administered by the federal and state governments (Medicaid.gov 2020). It was significantly expanded in most states under the Affordable Care Act, which funds the majority of coverage (90%) for additional enrollees. It is available to all citizens and legal residents with family income below 133% of the federal poverty line in the expansion states. There is a great deal of variation in coverage across states due to a Supreme Court ruling that states would not be required to participate in the Medicaid expansion (Ix 2013). Unfortunately, this has left many impoverished Americans uninsured.

Children's Health Insurance Program

CHIP is health insurance for uninsured children whose parents make too much money to qualify for Medicaid (Medicaid.gov 2020). Eligibility limits for CHIP vary by state but are generally limited to low-income families whose income is too high to qualify the entire family for Medicaid. Pregnant women with low incomes and children of state employees may also qualify.

Veterans Administration

Individuals who served in the U.S. military, National Guard, or Reserves may qualify for Veterans Administration (VA) health care benefits, as long as they served for a designated amount of time and their discharge or release was under conditions other than dishonorable. VA benefits provide access to comprehensive health care services for enrolled individuals. Most veterans have no out-of-pocket costs, although some may have small copayments for health care or prescription drugs. All services are prepaid (Erickson-Hurt et al. 2017; U.S. Department of Veterans Affairs 2019).

Indian Health Service

The Indian Health Service (IHS; https://www.ihs.gov/) is a single, comprehensive federal health system that provides direct medical and public health services to Native Americans and Alaska Natives. IHS is funded directly by the federal government. An Office of Quality aims to strengthen IHS's capacity to meet accreditation standards and improve processes that ensure safety and patient satisfaction.

Insurance of Last Resort

Because health care needs are often unpredictable and the cost of care is beyond the ability of most families to pay, those who cannot afford to buy health insurance, or who choose to use their resources otherwise, make up the majority of the uninsured in this country. The uninsured group also includes undocumented immigrants and some individuals who have a criminal record. In many states, health insurance benefits, including for public/government insurance such as Medicaid, are suspended or terminated for individuals who become incarcerated. Benefits can be reinstated after release, but reinstatement is often delayed. When uninsured individuals become ill, they are generally cared for through publicly funded programs. This care, however, is often not accessed until an illness is quite severe, at which point more expensive resources are needed than would have been necessary if early diagnosis and treatment had been available (McWilliams 2009).

Many uninsured or underinsured individuals are served through Federally Qualified Health Centers (FQHCs). FQHCs receive federal Health Center Program grant funding through a prospective payment system (see description of prospective payments in the following section) to improve the health of underserved and vulnerable populations. These include homeless people, migratory and seasonal agricultural workers, and residents of public housing. Other funding sources include Medicaid, Medicare, private insurance, and sliding scale patient fees. FQHC services offered include primary and preventive care, behavioral health treatment, subsidized pharmacy services, and dental care (Health Resources and Services Administration 2018).

Certified Community Behavioral Health Clinics (CCBHCs) constitute a new class of federally subsidized providers charged with providing comprehensive primary care services to populations being served in behavioral health settings. Similar to FQHCs, CCBHCs base prospective payments on the anticipated costs of serving their complex patient population. CCBHCs may provide direct services or contract with partner organizations to provide some of the required services, which include 24-hour crisis care, evidence-based treatments, care coordination, and primary health care (Substance Abuse and Mental Health Services Administration 2016).

Core Concepts in Financing Arrangements

Having reviewed the major elements of FFS systems in the preceding section, we can now consider some of the attempts that have been made to make up for the deficits of FFS financing. Other methods of compensation include various forms of bundled payments, prospective payments, and pay-for-performance arrangements. These and other models have been employed by payers with the common goal of incentivizing cost-effective, quality care. A central goal of value enhancement in health care is to fundamentally realign incentives to reward the provision of high-quality, cost-effective care. Value-based reimbursement has become a core strategy for achieving this in the current financing environment (Joynt Maddox et al. 2017). Regardless of how health care is financed, becoming familiar with some key concepts related to the design of financing arrangements will be helpful to providers.

Risk

Assuming risk means accepting financial responsibility to operate within available resources and liability for any expenses that exceed them. Private insurers take on risk in exchange for the opportunity to make a profit. Through actuarial calculations, they project what their costs are likely to be and set premiums at a level that creates revenue that exceeds that figure. One of the major threats to those bearing risk is unanticipated costs from catastrophic events or unexpectedly high utilization. Most private insurers purchase reinsurance policies from the government to safeguard against catastrophic loss. Risk can also be assumed by government entities or by providers. The location of risk significantly impacts service design and utilization. When providers assume partial or total risk, they have greater freedom to design services in more efficient and effective ways. However, some form of accountability for outcomes is needed when for-profit providers accept risk to ensure that services are not unduly limited (Henkel and Maryland 2015).

Incentives

The term *incentives* in the context of financing arrangements refers to the use of strategies and techniques that reward desired practices and outcomes while discouraging (or not rewarding) undesired practices and outcomes, often through fiscal and other penalties. For example, productivity-based incentives (as in FFS systems) may hinder well-intentioned efforts to improve quality, whereas incentives aimed at the provision of good outcomes may result in higher spending if cost limitations are not in place.

Carve-Outs

Behavioral health carve-outs refer to a funding mechanism whereby states set aside the entire budget for funding behavioral health care apart from the rest of (general, physical) health care. Carve-outs were created to protect funding for behavioral health services by preventing this funding from being diminished when competing for resources with physical health care in carved-in systems (Mandros 2017). Managed Care Organizations for Behavioral Health (MCO-BHs) contract with payers or health plans to assume financial risk and responsibility for management of behavioral health care. Operating independently from enrollees' general medical insurance, MCO-BHs maintain their own provider networks and coverage rules. Although MCO-BHs often pay providers via a fee-for-service arrangement, alternative payment models, such as delegated risk payment mechanisms (see section "Future of Behavioral Health Financing" later in this chapter), are increasingly being developed throughout the country.

Data Collection and Analysis

Data collection and analyses are integral to measuring both quantitative and qualitative outcomes in health care. They can show what impact occurred in response to an intervention, and to what degree. They are particularly important in value-based contracting (discussed later in this section) and actuarial processes. Ideally, providers and payers would agree on measures and indicators of quality, methods for data collection and analyses, interpretation of data, and the benchmarks for measuring outcomes. Reaching agreement has been challenging, particularly in profit-driven behavioral health systems, because payers, providers, and service recipients often have distinct interests. The complex nature of behavioral health makes it difficult to identify quality indicators that capture all stakeholders' interests, as pointed out in Chapter 1.

Value

Value refers to the benefit derived from money invested. A full discussion of value is provided in Chapter 1 ("Defining and Measuring Value"), but a brief review of some of its nuances is relevant here. It is important to note that there are multiple stakeholders with multiple perspectives on value. Parties in the transaction or relationship may define *value* differently but also usually agree on at least a few core aspects of the benefit to be gained from the transaction or interaction.

In health care, the parties usually agree on the mutually desired outcome of improved health and wellness. However, individuals seeking health care may define and perceive value very differently from how the system delivering care views it. For the individual, quality care may refer to relief from troubling symptoms, speed and ease of access to care, improved physical or emotional functioning, or a simple feeling of being cared for. Other measures that impact the consumer's sense of quality may be the degree of service integration, ease of communication with providers, clarity of instructions, amount of family inclusion, and the cultural sensitivity of care.

When they are governed by profit, private payers and providers may focus on the cost aspect of the value equation, such as revenue during the fiscal year, stock price, or market share rather than outcome or quality. Nonprofit organizations are more likely to emphasize nonmonetary quality indicators, such as measures of patient satisfaction, patient safety, timeliness, and patient centeredness (Agency for Healthcare Research and Quality 2018; Newgard et al. 2017).

Value-Based Reimbursement

Value-based reimbursement (VBR) refers to payment mechanisms that are structured to reward the delivery of high-quality care (i.e., mutually agreed-upon health care *outcomes*) rather than simply reimbursing services provided. By rewarding providers for both efficiency and effectiveness, VBR advances the triple aims of providing better care for individuals, improving population health, and reducing health care costs (Berwick et al. 2008). A key aspect of VBR is the sharing of risk by provider and payer. Performance based risk-sharing incentivizes service providers to focus on improving quality and outcomes rather than revenue-focused and crisis oriented episodic care. Additionally, VBRs allow the development of critical supportive services, such as comprehensive care coordination, that are essential aids to recovery processes. These services are usually not fully covered under fee-for-service reimbursement arrangements.

Bundled Payments

Bundling involves calculating costs of all predetermined service inputs (including ancillary costs and services) for treatment of a medical condition, which is then billed at a single pre-negotiated rate. This billing structure encourages efficiency in service planning since it simplifies payment and clarifies what providers can expect to be paid. One of the simplest forms of bundled payments are "per diem" payments for intensive treatment settings such as hospitalizations and residential treatments. A set reimbursement rate is established to cover all provided services per person, per day (Quinn et al. 2017).

Prospective Payments

Prospective payments are made in advance of service delivery. They are projected from usage history. Payment amounts are calculated from the resources historically needed to treat a particular condition. Classification systems such as diagnosis-related groups (DRGs) are frequently used for this purpose (Krinsky et al. 2017).

Episode-of-Care Payments

Episode-of-care payments, also known as episode-based payments or case rates, involve the reimbursement of health care providers based on cost projections for an episode of care (Yuan et al. 2017). The foundational construct for this payment mechanism is the DRG, which classifies patients into clinical categories based on diagnoses, age, gender, wellness, and expected treatment. Reimbursement is based on average costs of treatment calculated for each DRG. Although often paid retrospectively, payments can also be prospective. The recovery course can be highly variable with psychiatric illnesses, and therefore episodic bundling can be risky for the provider because it depends on the case mix that arrives. If providers are confronted with a large number of complex, poorly responsive individuals, the bundled payments may not be sufficient to cover expenses. This can be mitigated by ensuring that actuarial analyses consider the complexity of the population that the provider treats and adjusting the bundled payments accordingly. Ambulatory Payment Classification is a form of the DRG applied in outpatient settings.

Capitation

Within a capitation arrangement, risk-bearing entities (providers or managed care organizations [MCOs]) contract with a payer (government or insurer) to receive fixed, predetermined payments for each member (per capita, per month), regardless of care provided or its intensity (Yuan et al. 2017).

Global Payments

With global payments, in a manner similar to the capitation and prospective payment models, large multispecialty provider groups or health care systems receive a fixed prepayment for all care for defined enrollee groups over a specified time period. This prepayment covers all treatment, including diagnostic tests, prescription drugs, and clinical services. Global payments may be used for a variety of programs, such as hospice, home health care, partial hospital, and care coordination. Payments are risk-adjusted to reflect the health status of the group on whose behalf the payments are made. Accountable Care Organizations (ACOs) are other entities that receive global payments.

Quality Measurement

Quality metrics are integral to determining value (e.g., for value-based reimbursement). Payers and insurers need objective benchmark standards (metrics) against which aggregate outcomes (quality) can be measured. In general medicine, there are quantifiable laboratory or physical examination values that delineate health status for hypothyroidism, pregnancy, hypertension, glycemic control, obesity, cholesterol, and many other health indices. It is therefore relatively straightforward to measure quality of care (e.g., whether blood pressure treatment results in normalized blood pressure values). These clear cutoffs, however, do not exist for behavioral health conditions. Therefore, measuring quality (and thereby determining value) in behavioral health relies on proxy or inexact measures (Kilbourne et al. 2018). Examples include measures of treatment response, process, functional outcomes, and functional outcomes.

Treatment Response Measures

Treatment response may be measured by symptom quantification, which is accomplished using standardized questionnaire data. A myriad of such questionnaires have shown reliability and validity. Examples include the Patient Health Questionnaire–9 (Kroenke et al. 2001) and the Beck Depression Inventory (Beck et al. 1996). These measures attempt to track response to treatment and can be useful when paired with functional outcome measures (discussed next).

Functional Outcome Measures

Sigmund Freud famously defined *mental health* as “the ability to love and work,” meaning that daily functioning is a good approximation of recovery from mental illness or addiction. Functional outcomes can be measured by rating scales, such as the Daily Living Activities Scale, a validated tool assessing activities of daily living areas impacted by mental illness or disability (Scott and Presmanes 2001), and the World Health Organization Disability Assessment Scale 2.0 (World Health Organization 2018).

Process Measures

Process measures assess adherence to treatment processes that influence health outcomes. Examples of such processes are 7-day follow-up after hospitalization and initiation and engagement in treatment. The Healthcare Effectiveness Data and Information Set (HEDIS; National Committee for Quality Assurance 2020) is a measure of initiation and engagement in treatment that monitors whether adolescents and adults with an episode of alcohol or other drug dependence had inpatient or outpatient treatment within 14 days of their initial diagnosis and two additional treatments within 30 days of the first visit. Hospital readmission rates are also commonly used as process measures. Another measure is adherence to antipsychotic medication by individuals diagnosed with schizophrenia. Although these processes are important for health care delivery, they cannot measure treatment efficacy (Claxton et al. 2015).

HEDIS

The NCQA's HEDIS (Healthcare Effectiveness Data and Information Set) performance measures are considered the gold standard for measuring quality of care and tracking population health. Comprising 90 measures across six domains of care, these metrics capture and quantify performance by individual clinicians, health care organizations, and health plans. They facilitate benchmarking against a national standard. Domains include Effectiveness of Care, Access/Availability of Care, Experience of Care, Utilization and Risk Adjusted Utilization, Health Plan Descriptive Information, and Measures Collected Using Electronic Clinical Data Systems (National Committee for Quality Assurance 2020). Although these measures are fairly unambiguous in general medicine, they have been harder to define in behavioral medicine. Over the past few years, NCQA has worked toward the development of quality measures for behavioral health (National Committee for Quality Assurance 2020).

Alternative Payment Models

Innovations that tie payment to quality outcomes have been a major focus of value enhancement strategies. These alternative payment models (APMs) include prospective payment arrangements with case-mix adjustments, global or program funding, pay-for-performance (P4P), shared savings, capitated payment models, and full-risk advanced payment models (Burwell 2015; Mayes 2011). They leverage measurement-based care and technology, foster flexibility in care delivery, and aim to contain costs. Several APMs focus specifically on behavioral health services (Mauri et al. 2017). Various types of APMs are considered in the following subsections.

Pay-for-Performance Incentive Program

Under P4P incentive programs, providers can earn an incentive payment by demonstrating a measurable improvement in clinical targets, usually in addition to routine reimbursement models such as FFS arrangements. Because the incentive is usually in addition to the usual rate, there is little risk to the provider. The payment can be used to incentivize very specific services or outcomes, such as preventive screening, enhancing patient satisfaction, or achieving certain quality outcomes. Although there are fewer objective measures in behavioral health than in other areas of health care, P4P has been tied to HEDIS measures, such as 7- or 30-day follow-up after hospitalization or screening for diabetes and antidepressant medication adherence (Kilbourne et al. 2010; Unützer et al. 2012).

Shared Savings

Shared savings programs incentivize providers under FFS arrangements to lower cost of care by improving coordination of care to meet quality metrics. Actual spending is calculated against projected spending for a wide range of health services and settings. Pharmacy, laboratory, radiology, and pharmaceutical utilizations are analyzed to determine whether or not savings were realized. When specific cost and quality benchmarks are realized, the provider can "share" in the savings with its payer (Ouayogodé et al. 2017).

MACRA and MIPS

The Medicare Access and CHIP Reauthorization Act of 2015 (MACRA) potentially transforms health care practices by establishing new payment methodologies for Medicare beneficiaries. MACRA and the Merit-based Incentive Payment System (MIPS), the measurement component of MACRA, create an incentive for physicians to utilize measurement in routine care delivery. MIPS specifies measurement requirements for providers. Currently, providers must submit data on six quality measures that are approved by the

Centers for Medicare and Medicaid Services. This system creates a monetary incentive for providers to track and demonstrate improved quality of care (Centers for Medicare and Medicaid Services 2019a).

Accountable Care Organizations

ACOs typically comprise a group of services and programs contained within a large medical center or a consortium of health care provider organizations that contract with a payer to serve defined patient populations while meeting specific quality and cost benchmarks over a set period of time. Essentially, an ACO assumes responsibility and financial risk for an assigned beneficiary population previously reimbursed through an FFS arrangement. Accountability for quality of care is required and monitored through the establishment of outcome benchmarks. A shared risk and/or savings arrangement is often part of the funding scheme. If the ACO can provide care at a lower cost than the predetermined threshold, all or part of the savings is retained by the organization. With full risk arrangements, when costs exceed the threshold, the ACO bears the loss.

Alternative Payment Models for Mental Health

A variety of payment mechanisms have been proposed for individuals with serious mental illness (SMI) who have high service utilization and require multiple supports and/or care coordination. SMI is defined as a mental, behavioral, or emotional disorder resulting in serious functional impairment, which substantially interferes with or limits one or more major life activities. Models proposed for persons with SMI usually blend all needed services and cover the costs of behavioral and physical health, care coordination, medication, and all ancillary services (Mauri et al. 2017). A capitated rate often includes costs of both inpatient and outpatient care.

One example of this all-inclusive bundled rate financing is the specialized case rate for serious mental illness. This is the model used by the city of Baltimore, Maryland, and in the Health and Recovery Plan (HARP) in New York State. Under the Baltimore model, 350 individuals with extremely high utilization (a state hospital admission lasting greater than 6 months, more than 7 emergency room visits, or more than 4 acute inpatient psychiatric admissions in a year) are enrolled in a specialized service plan (Mauri et al. 2017). The city contracts with two providers to assume all care for this population at a capitated annual rate that includes up to 30 days of inpatient treatment per year. Metrics tracked include housing, employment, incarceration, and patient satisfaction. In New York State's HARPs, MCOs are paid an enhanced rate to cover services (New York State Office of Mental Health 2020).

Alternative Payment Models for Addiction Treatment

Like the APMs for mental health treatment, APMs for addiction treatment bundle costs of addiction treatment, including service coordination. They save money long term by facilitating care coordination, improving engagement, and promoting flexibility in treatment, thus reducing long-term costs related to recidivism or complications of delayed treatment. Examples include the following:

- *Single case rates for each level of addiction treatment intensity:* Case rates are used to pay for each level of care (detoxification, rehabilitation, partial hospitalization, and intensive outpatient), delegating risk to providers and eliminating the need for concurrent reviews.
- *Patient-Centered Opioid Addiction Treatment Payment (P-COAT):* P-COAT is an APM designed to incentivize the utilization of medication assisted treatment (MAT) by eliminating barriers such as prior authorization and FFS billing. Bundled payments under this model cover three phases of care: patient assessment and treatment planning, initiation of MAT, and maintenance of MAT. These bundles cover medication, psychological treatment, and coordination of social services necessary to remain in treatment following initiation. For individuals who drop out or terminate treatment early, monthly payments for maintenance of MAT are made to the team to facilitate reengagement (American Society of Addiction Medicine 2018).

Next-Generation Health Care Financing Models

Further innovations in paying for health care services are being considered and piloted for the enhancement of value in health care, but these are not currently widely available. Two innovative models are described.

Value-Based Insurance Design

Value-Based Insurance Design (V-BID) (Centers for Medicare and Medicaid Services 2019b; Choudhry et al. 2010) aims to increase consumer adherence with recommended care guidelines by aligning consumer out-of-pocket costs with the potential clinical benefit of certain health services and medications. For example, graduated copays may incentivize use of preventive services such as smoking cessation, cancer screening, or medication for chronic conditions (e.g., hypertension) over curative services such as surgery. Because copays for curative services are more expensive relative to preventive care, members are motivated to use the less expensive preventive services.

Health Maintenance Organizations Incorporating Socioeconomic Determinants of Health

Some HMOs, such as Kaiser Permanente and Geisinger Health System, are beginning to incorporate community health programs that target social determinants. By focusing on preventive care, these plans realize savings in the form of avoided costs of downstream care for complex and advanced conditions. Examples of services paid for include housing, healthy nutrition, employment, and programs that prevent mental illness and addiction. In a for-profit environment, these arrangements are a hard sell to companies that cover a population that is transient, because they will not necessarily benefit from long-term cost savings achieved through prevention.

Future of Behavioral Health Financing

APMs represent piecemeal attempts to address the ineffectiveness of FFS and profit-driven systems to create value in health care. They attempt to bridge the conflict between the values of health care as social insurance and health care as a commodity. Although well intended, these mechanisms have not produced significant improvements in value overall. FFS reimbursement models are still dominant. The single most critical factor needed to drive change is a sustainable financing model. Future sustainable funding mechanisms must ensure equitable, adequate funding of behavioral health services that are quality driven. The system must have sufficient resources to allow providers of care to have some flexibility in planning services for improved outcomes. The ability to measure the impact of care is central to both quality and cost containment. In other words, funding must be tied to quality metrics in order to calculate value. The following subsections describe foundational principles for developing future financing models that support behavioral health and value.

No Health Without Mental Health

Abundant evidence indicates that mental illness and other behavioral health conditions have a unique, pervasive, and disproportionate impact on health across all strata of society. This occurs for a variety of reasons, including reductions in self-care, treatment participation, and adherence to a care plan, as well as functional decline. Both acute and chronic medical conditions have poorer outcomes when comorbid with behavioral health conditions. Behavioral health treatment should be included in coverage provided through any financial arrangement and be accessible to all members of society (Prince et al. 2007).

Access

Access to quality health services remains challenging in the United States. Over 60% of rural counties do not have access to any behaviorally trained clinicians (New American Economy 2017). Financing arrangements must provide incentives for clinicians to serve neglected populations and must support the role of technology in addressing personnel shortages. Poverty dramatically impacts ability to pay for treatment, travel to appointments, coordinate care, and maintain stable housing (Cohen Veterans Network, National Council for Behavioral Health 2018).

Delegated Risk and Bundling Mechanisms

Shifting some or all of the financial risk to providers may offer the greatest opportunity for flexibility with accountability in health care. Various types of bundled payments accomplish this when tied to measurable outcomes. Bundling has the potential to enhance quality by allowing providers the leeway to customize services as needed.

Efficiency

Integration of services reduces redundancies and simplifies administration. Integrated financing streams and licensing will also increase efficiency. There must be incentives to reduce barriers to consolidations of fragmented services.

Analytics and Informatics

Analytics (i.e., data collection and analysis for actionable insights) is the backbone of health financing and population health management. Analytics can be used to isolate segments of the population, identify cost trends, and predict future utilization. This process facilitates targeted interventions and further analysis, potentially reducing waste and improving efficiency. Furthermore, technologies can revolutionize data management by facilitating information sharing in health care. The capacity to store information about transactions in a secure and indelible way must be supported by financing plans. These technologies can reduce fragmentation, thereby improving integration and reducing cost. Meaningful outcome metrics that address the values of all stakeholders can be tracked and monitored. Analytics will be an important element of efforts to enhance quality.

Socioeconomic Determinants

Proactively addressing health at a population level through integration of financing for health and social spending will be necessary to reduce the impact of socioeconomic determinants. Inclusion of measures to ensure that basic needs are met as part of medical necessity criteria is one step in that direction, but financing plans will need to develop incentives to promote primary prevention as well (Geisinger Medical Center 2020; Philadelphia Department of Behavioral Health and Intellectual disAbility Services 2020).

Conclusion

A Vision for the Future

This chapter has considered the impact of various financing arrangements on health and well-being. Current systems that are profit driven have not been effective in delivering high value for the U.S. population's health. Various approaches to overcome this weakness are not widely implemented and have not had a significant impact on health outcomes. We now consider how some of these approaches might be incorporated into a financing scheme that would deliver value that is more in line with that of other developed countries. Given the broad societal impact of behavioral health conditions on society and the health care system, behavioral health interventions must be an integral element in the coverage provided by this system. A single-payer model that reduces opportunities for profit to be extracted from available resources will be the most efficient way to accomplish this goal. Universal coverage that ensures a full spectrum of care must be available for all citizens.

Single-source payment will simplify administration, reduce waste, and allow more resources to be directed to services. Administrative agents can be overseen by mental health boards at federal, state, or local levels. These entities would employ analytics to track quality, access, and costs. These oversight bodies should comprise an array of stakeholders, including service users, family members, providers, administrators, and community representatives. In the city of Philadelphia, for example, an arrangement of this type is used to govern the city's not-for-profit MCO-BH, which is overseen by a board of directors under the auspices of the county mental health authority (Community Behavioral Health 2020; Philadelphia Department of Behavioral Health and Intellectual disAbility Services 2020).

Funding for the health care system would be derived from taxes if the predominant payer is governmental, replacing the premiums now collected by private plans. If nongovernmental entities remain part of the financing system, a blended model might be financed through employee and employer contributions in addition to government contributions. Consumer contributions through graduated cost-sharing arrangements could be used to incentivize prevention and primary care and discourage the overuse of tertiary interventions. This concept is already being implemented in some U.S. jurisdictions (e.g., in Denver, Colorado, through Caring for Denver; http://caring4denver.org).

Ensuring High-Value Psychiatric Care

Even in a single-payer system, a framework may be needed for assuring that behavioral health is prioritized appropriately. This type of intentional prioritization is needed because of the persistence and pervasiveness of stigma (including that among clinicians and within treatment settings) and a general lack of knowledge about behavioral health treatment. A "mental health fund" that essentially carves out a portion of the health care budget would be one way to ensure that behavioral health services remain funded to the extent necessary. Bundled payments offer the best framework for flexibility and innovation when paired with quality benchmarks for accountability. Segmentation analysis (categorization of portions of the population) could be used to develop tiers of risk (e.g., low, moderate, and high complexity). Assignments could be based on a combination of medical and behavioral health variables, social determinants, historical use of services, and predicted costs. Bundled payments to providers could then be adjusted based on population/case complexity to reduce incentives to cherry-pick, likely showing bias to serve those with the fewest needs. The Baltimore SMI global payment covers medical and behavioral health care, legal fees, housing, income support, and wraparound and case management services; it is an excellent example of this model (Centers for Medicare and Medicaid Services 2018).

In the current system, inpatient and residential psychiatric and addiction treatment is funded on a per diem or diagnosis-related group basis. This practice creates a perverse incentive for hospitals and patients to "overuse" these services when reimbursement is not linked to outcomes. Prospective, capitated payments tied to specific measurable outcomes for defined populations would shift these incentives. Accountable Care Organizations serving a defined "catchment area" would help align payment and outcomes by rewarding wise use of resources. Savings could be shared with contracted outpatient and supportive service providers to encourage community-based solutions for behavioral health issues.

For most individuals with mental health conditions, community-based services offer the greatest source of ongoing treatment and supports. Community-based treatment encompasses a wide array of services, such as medication management, psychotherapy, family psychoeducation, and psychosocial rehabilitation. Other community-based services include supportive services that aim at restoring and maximizing function, such as recovery-oriented case management, supported employment, and supportive housing. These services must be supported by any financing arrangement. Tiered capitated payments, adjusted for risk and complexity, will offer the greatest flexibility for both quality of outcomes and cost containment. Outcome metrics should focus on recovery-related goals and functioning, rather than process measurement alone.

Health care financing is crucial to the provision of health care because it provides a strong incentive for providers to deliver both evidence-based and innovative care. Current models represent a compromise between the basic premises of health care as a right versus a commodity. Because of the disproportionate and broad impact of behavioral health on society, mental health must be prioritized along with other critical public health interventions as a right for all citizens. Although it is extremely difficult to measure quality and value in behavioral medicine, several metrics exist today that are useful for evaluating both the process and the impact of service delivery. Historically, rate-adjusted bundled payments tied to metrics offer the best blend of flexibility, accountability, and cost containment. Various applications of these principles are needed in crafting the health care financing and reimbursement mechanisms of the future.

References

Agency for Healthcare Research and Quality: Understanding quality measurement: Child Health Toolbox. October 2018. Available at: www.ahrq.gov/professionals/quality-patient-safety/quality-resources/tools/chtoolbx/understand/index.html. Accessed February 12, 2020.

American Academy of Actuaries, Individual and Small Group Markets Committee: An evaluation of the individual health insurance market and implications of potential changes. January 2017. Available at: www.actuary.org/sites/default/files/files/publications/Acad_eval_indiv_mkt_011817.pdf. Accessed February 12, 2020.

American Society of Addiction Medicine: Patient-Centered Opioid Addiction Treatment (P-COAT): alternative payment model (APM). 2018. Available at: www.asam.org/docs/default-source/advocacy/asam-ama-p-coat-final.pdf?sfvrsn=447041c2_2. Accessed February 12, 2020.

Beck AT, Steer RA, Brown GK: Beck Depression Inventory–II Manual. San Antonio, TX, Psychological Corporation, 1996

Berwick DM, Nolan TW, Whittington J: The Triple Aim: care, health, and cost. Health Aff (Millwood) 27(3):759–769, 2008

Bodenheimer T, Grumbach K: Healthcare in four nations, in Understanding Health Policy: A Clinical Approach, 7th Edition. Edited by Fielding A, Davis K. New York, Lange Medical Books/McGraw-Hill, 2016, pp 169–184

Branning G, Vater M: Healthcare spending: plenty of blame to go around. Am Health Drug Benefits 9(8):445–447, 2016

Burwell SM: Setting value-based payment goals—HHS efforts to improve U.S. health care. N Engl J Med 372(10):897–899, 2015

Centers for Medicare and Medicaid Services: Opportunities to design innovative service delivery systems for adults with a serious mental illness or children with a serious emotional disturbance. November 13, 2018. Available at: www.medicaid.gov/federal-policy-guidance/downloads/smd18011.pdf. Accessed February 12, 2020.

Centers for Medicare and Medicaid Services: MACRA: the Medicare Access and CHIP Reauthorization Act of 2015. November 18, 2019a. Available at: www.cms.gov/medicare/quality-initiatives-patient-assessment-instruments/value-based-programs/macra-mips-and-apms/macra-mips-and-apms.html. Accessed February 12, 2020.

Centers for Medicare and Medicaid Services: Medicare general information. November 13, 2019b. Available at: www.cms.gov/Medicare/Medicare-General-Information/MedicareGenInfo/index.html. Accessed February 12, 2020.

Centers for Medicare and Medicaid Services: National health expenditure 2017. December 5, 2019c. Available at: www.cms.gov/research-statistics-data-and-systems/statistics-trends-and-reports/nationalhealthexpenddata/nhe-fact-sheet.html. Accessed February 12, 2020.

Centers for Medicare and Medicaid Services: Medicare Advantage Value-Based Insurance Design Model. February 12, 2020a. Available at: https://innovation.cms.gov/initiatives/vbid. Accessed February 12, 2020.

Centers for Medicare and Medicaid Services: Overview of SHOP: health insurance for small businesses. Available at: www.healthcare.gov/small-businesses/choose-and-enroll/shop-marketplace-overview. 2020b. Accessed February 12, 2020.

Choudhry NK, Rosenthal MB, Milstein A: Assessing the evidence for value-based insurance design. Health Aff (Millwood) 29(11):1988–1994, 2010

Claxton G, Cox C, Gonzalez S, et al: Measuring the quality of healthcare in the U.S. Peterson-KFF, Health System Tracker, September 10, 2015. Available at: www.healthsystemtracker.org/brief/measuring-the-quality-of-healthcare-in-the-u-s/#. Accessed February 12, 2020.

Cohen RA, Martinez ME, Zammitti PZ: Health insurance coverage: early release of estimates from the National Health Interview Survey, January–March 2018. National Center for Health Statistics National Health Interview Survey Early Release Program, August 2018. Available at: www.cdc.gov/nchs/data/nhis/earlyrelease/Insur201808.pdf. Accessed February 12, 2020.

Cohen Veterans Network, National Council for Behavioral Health: America's Mental Health: October 10, 2018. Available at: www.cohenveteransnetwork.org/wp-content/uploads/2018/10/Research-Summary-10-10-2018.pdf. Accessed February 12, 2020.

Community Behavioral Health: CBH leadership and board of directors. January 2020. Available at: https://cbhphilly.org/about-us/cbh-leadership-and-board-of-directors. Accessed February 12, 2020.

Erickson-Hurt C, McGuirk D, Long CO: Healthcare benefits for veterans: what home care clinicians need to know. Home Healthc Now 35(5):248–257, 2017

French MT, Homer J, Gumus G, et al: Key provisions of the Patient Protection and Affordable Care Act (ACA): a systematic review and presentation of early research findings. Health Serv Res 51(5):1735–1771, 2016

Geisinger Medical Center: Community health needs assessment. 2020. Available at: www.geisinger.org/-/media/OneGeisinger/pdfs/ghs/about-geisinger/chna/gmc/chna-booklet-gmc-gsach-102014.pdf?la=en. Accessed February 12, 2020.

Glick ID, Sharfstein SS, Schwartz HI: Inpatient psychiatric care in the 21st century: the need for reform. Psychiatr Serv 62(2):206–209, 2011

Health Resources and Services Administration: What is a health center? November 2018. Available at: https://bphc.hrsa.gov/about/what-is-a-health-center/index.html. Accessed February 12, 2020.

Henkel RJ, Maryland PA: The risks and rewards of value-based reimbursement. Front Health Serv Manage 32(2):3–16, 2015

Internal Revenue Service: Small business health care tax credit and the SHOP marketplace. May 3, 2019. Available at: www.irs.gov/affordable-care-act/employers/small-business-health-care-tax-credit-and-the-shop-marketplace. Accessed February 12, 2020.

Ix M: National Federation of Independent Business v. Sebelius: the misguided application and perpetuation of an amorphous coercion theory. Maryland Law Review 72(4), 2013. Available at: https://digitalcommons.law.umaryland.edu/mlr/vol72/iss4/18. Accessed February 12, 2020.

Joynt Maddox JKE, Sen AP, Samson LW, et al: Elements of program design in Medicare's value-based and alternative payment models: a narrative review. J Gen Intern Med 32(11):1249–1254, 2017

Kilbourne AM, Keyser D, Pincus HA: Challenges and opportunities in measuring the quality of mental health care. Can J Psychiatry 55(9):549–557, 2010

Kilbourne AM, Beck K, Spaeth-Rublee B, et al: Measuring and improving the quality of mental health care: a global perspective. World Psychiatry 17(1):30–38, 2018

Kongstvedt PR: Essentials of Managed Health Care, 6th Edition. Sudbury, MA, Jones & Bartlett Learning, 2013, pp 17–30

Kreyenbuhl J, Buchanan RW, Dickerson FB, et al: The Schizophrenia Patient Outcomes Research Team (PORT): updated treatment recommendations 2009. Schizophr Bull 36(1):94–103, 2010

Krinsky S, Ryan AM, Mijanovich T, et al: Variation in payment rates under Medicare's inpatient prospective payment system. Health Serv Res 52(2):676–696, 2017

Kroenke K, Spitzer RL, Williams JB: The PHQ-9: validity of a brief depression severity measure. J Gen Intern Med 16(9):606–613, 2001

Mandros A: Medicaid behavioral health carve-outs—11 remain. January 16, 2017. Available at: www.openminds.com/market-intelligence/executive-briefings/are-we-watching-the-demise-of-the-behavioral-health-carve-out. Accessed February 12, 2020.

Mauri A, Harbin S, Unützer J, et al: Payment reform and opportunities for behavioral health: alternative payment model examples. Scattergood Foundation, September 2017. Available at: www.scattergoodfoundation.org/wp-content/uploads/yumpu_files/Scattergood_APM_Final_digital.pdf. Accessed February 12, 2020.

Mayes R: Moving (realistically) from volume-based to value-based health care payment in the USA: starting with Medicare payment policy. J Health Serv Res Policy 16(4):249–251, 2011

McWilliams JM: Health consequences of uninsurance among adults in the United States: recent evidence and implications. Milbank Q 87(2):443–494, 2009

Medicaid.gov: Children's Health Insurance Program (CHIP). 2020. Available at: www.medicaid.gov/chip/index.html. Accessed February 12, 2020.

Moses H 3rd, Matheson DHM, Dorsey ER, et al: The anatomy of health care in the United States. JAMA 310(18):1947–1964, 2013

National Committee for Quality Assurance: HEDIS measures and technical resources. 2020. Available at: www.ncqa.org/hedis/measures/. Accessed February 12, 2020.

New American Economy: The silent shortage: how immigration can help address the large and growing psychiatrist shortage in the United States. 2017. Available at: http://research.newamericaneconomy.org/wp-content/uploads/2017/10/NAE_PsychiatristShortage_V6-1.pdf. Accessed July 5, 2020.

Newgard CD, Fu R, Heilman J, et al: Using Press Ganey provider feedback to improve patient satisfaction: a pilot randomized controlled trial. Acad Emerg Med 24(9):1051–1059, 2017

New York State Office of Mental Health: Health and recovery plans (HARPs). 2020. Available at: www.omh.ny.gov/omhweb/bho/harp.html. Accessed February 12, 2020.

Ouayogodé MH, Colla CH, Lewis VA: Determinants of success in shared savings programs: an analysis of ACO and market characteristics. Healthc (Amst) 5(1–2):53–61, 2017

Philadelphia Department of Behavioral Health and Intellectual disAbility Services: Division of Community Behavioral Health (CBH). 2020. Available at: https://dbhids.org/cbh. Accessed February 12, 2020.

Prester R: A values framework for health system reform. Health Aff (Millwood) 11(1):84–107, 1992

Prince M, Patel V, Saxena S, et al: No health without mental health. Lancet 370(9590):859–877, 2007

Quinn AE, Hodgkin D, Perloff JN, et al: Design and impact of bundled payment for detox and follow-up care. J Subst Abuse Treat 82:113–121, 2017

Rama A: Policy Research Perspectives: Payment and delivery in 2016: the prevalence of medical homes, accountable care organizations, and payment methods reported by physicians. American Medical Association, October 2017. Available at: www.ama-assn.org/sites/ama-assn.org/files/corp/media-browser/public/health-policy/prp-medical-home-aco-payment.pdf. Accessed February 12, 2020.

Sawyer B, McDermott D: How does the quality of the U.S. healthcare system compare to other countries? Peterson-KFF Health System Tracker March 28, 2019. Available at: www.healthsystemtracker.org/chart-collection/quality-u-s-healthcare-system-compare-countries/#item-start. Accessed February 12, 2020.

Scott RL, Presmanes WS: Reliability and validity of the Daily Living Activities Scale: a functional assessment measure for severe mental disorders. Research on Social Work Practice 11(3):373–389, 2001

Substance Abuse and Mental Health Services Administration: Criteria for the demonstration program to improve community mental health centers and to establish certified community behavioral health clinics. May 2016. Available at: www.samhsa.gov/sites/default/files/programs_campaigns/ccbhc-criteria.pdf. Accessed February 12, 2020.

Texas v United States, December 14, 2018. Available at: https://oag.ca.gov/system/files/attachments/press-docs/211-texas-order-granting-plaintiffs-partial-summary-judgment.pdf. Accessed February 12, 2020.

Unützer J, Chan Y, Hafer E, et al: Quality improvement with pay-for-performance incentives in integrated behavioral health care. Am J Public Health 102(6):e41–e45, 2012

U.S. Department of Veterans Affairs: VA benefits and healthcare. October 25, 2019. Available at: https://www.va.gov/health/. Accessed February 12, 2020.

Wit v United Behavioral Health, February 28, 2019. Available at: www.courtlistener.com/recap/gov.uscourts.cand.277588/gov.uscourts.cand.277588.418.0.pdf. Accessed February 12, 2020.

World Health Organization: WHO Disability Assessment Schedule 2.0 (WHODAS 2.0). Available at: www.who.int/icidh/whodas. June 14, 2018. Accessed February 12, 2020.

Yuan B, He L, Meng Q, et al: Payment methods for outpatient care facilities. Cochrane Database Syst Rev 3(3), 2017

7

Integration of Services

Manish Sapra, M.D., M.M.M.
George Alvarado, M.D.

***Integrated care* has** become a buzzword in the health care industry. Although it can mean a variety of things based on what is being "integrated," this term generally denotes bringing different health care services together to provide accessible, efficient, and patient-centered care. Integrated care has been defined by the World Health Organization (2016) as "an approach to strengthen people-centered health systems through the promotion of the comprehensive delivery of quality services across the life-course, designed according to the multidimensional needs of the population and the individual and delivered by a coordinated multidisciplinary team of providers working across settings and levels of care" (p. 4).

Typically, society in general and health care in particular have erroneously divided the body from the mind. For the last few decades, there has been growing awareness of the prevalence of comorbid medical and mental illnesses, and the negative effects of such comorbidities on clinical outcomes and costs of providing services (Melek et al. 2014). Beyond these issues, comorbid illnesses make an already difficult to access mental health care system even harder to navigate. In a broad sense, integrated care is conceptualized as a system of care in which professionals from a variety of disciplines collaborate and coordinate to improve clinical outcomes and operational efficiencies. Some of the key features of integrated systems include defined clinical pathways or protocols, unified clinical records, ease of communication between providers, simplified financing arrangements, and comprehensive data collection for tracking outcomes. Integrated care programs focus on the "whole" person's needs (social, psychological, and medical) and strive to provide person-centered treatment (Reed et al. 2005).

Effective integrated care programs provide outcomes that are superior to treatment as usual. These outcomes include easier access, improved patient experience and satisfaction, decreased medical errors, improved clinical outcomes, decreased administrative costs, and decreased expense overall (Katon et al. 2003; Substance Abuse and Mental Health Services Administration–HRSA Center for Integrated Health Solutions 2014; Vickers et al. 2013). Integrated care may also lead to improvement in provider experience. Integrated systems are particularly effective for improving access to evidence-based, comprehensive care for all health issues in destigmatized settings (Center for Substance Abuse Treatment 2007).

In this chapter, *integrated care* refers to any effort that improves the delivery of health care by coordinating elements of care or administration of care for medical illness, mental health, substance use, and social needs. *Integration of services* does not necessarily mean structural integration, but rather refers to the development of processes via collaboration and coordination between disciplines to provide person-centered treatment for the "whole person." Integrated care comes with its own challenges, and these will be highlighted in this chapter. The chapter concludes with a discussion on measuring outcomes and its relevance to quantifying the value of integration.

Scope of Integrated Care Principles

The fragmentation within the U.S. health care system makes it very difficult for people with comorbid mental health, physical health, or substance use conditions to obtain services that address all these issues in a single setting. Consequently, these individuals often find themselves bouncing back and forth between narrowly focused providers with uncoordinated, and often contradictory, treatment plans. Billing restrictions in fee-for-service (FFS) financing and even in some non-FFS arrangements discourage the provision of holistic care.

Pioneering efforts to provide integrated care began for persons with "dual disorders" (co-occurring mental illness and addictions) in the late 1980s. These conditions often interacted in ways that increased the morbidity associated with each. Because these illnesses so frequently coexist, many providers began to develop programs to treat these issues concurrently in the same setting and with the same treatment team, rather than treating them in series (i.e., stabilizing one condition before addressing the second) or in parallel (i.e., providing concurrent care but in different settings with different providers). It became clear that outcomes were much improved when an integrated model was used (Brunette et al. 2008; Torrey et al. 2002). As a result, development and availability of these programs grew; professional training programs began to expand the scope of their curricula; and in assessment protocols, co-occurring disorders became an expectation rather than an afterthought. Despite these changes, many systems still struggled with anachronistic administrative structures, such as distinct regulatory and licensing requirements, that made the implementation of these programs more difficult. Nonetheless, for people with co-occurring disorders, opportunities for integration of care for substance use and mental health care continue to grow (Brunette et al. 2008). The recent development of the opioid epidemic has fueled the growth of integrated services in clinical settings.

Although siloed treatment programs were particularly counterproductive arrangements for people with co-occurring mental health and substance use conditions, there are many other instances in which more than one type of need exists within a single individual. A number of other "silos" of care that have existed for a single class of conditions or a particular population have likewise made navigation and treatment planning insufficient and difficult. Since the early 2000s, the integration of physical health care and emotional health care has become a dominant movement in the health care system, and that integration is the main focus of this chapter. However, there are many other areas in which integration principles apply, as discussed in the next paragraph.

Services for persons with intellectual disabilities have usually been separate from mental health services, despite frequent co-occurrence. Prevention activities have often been separated from treatment settings. Services for children and adolescents have generally been divided from adult services in a way that makes transitions difficult. Behavioral health services in jails and prisons have had little interface with community-based services. Social circumstances play a key role in health outcomes, but as with other fragmented services, funding streams are separate (McGovern 2014). For example, improvement in the availability of low-income housing may lead to a decrease in unnecessary psychiatric hospitalizations or improvement in engagement in outpatient care for patients with mental illnesses. However, currently in the United States, states usually administer housing resources through social services departments, whereas states' departments of health fund medical care. These separate funding streams do not align well for generating cost-effective outcomes: for example, budget cuts in a low-cost housing program may create savings for the social service department but may lead to higher medical costs in the health budget. Blended funding approaches would enable providers to develop integrated care programs more easily.

These are a few examples of differentiated systems for which integration efforts would be beneficial. The remainder of this chapter examines efforts to apply these principles to health care for people with comorbid physical and emotional health care needs.

Background: Integration of Physical and Behavioral Health Care

Early attempts to integrate physical and behavioral health services began in the 1980s at a few programs around the county. In the next couple of decades, models were developed by a several organizations, including the Veterans Administration, Federally Qualified Health Centers (FQHCs), and health systems such as Kaiser Permanente and Intermountain Healthcare. Revelations about the high costs related to untreated chronic diseases, in addition to the morbidity associated with those illnesses, were among the major influences on those developments. Other reasons for this increased attention to integrated care during this early part of the twenty-first century are also worth highlighting. There has been an "access issue" in that behavioral health care may be difficult to access for the general population because of the limited supply of behavioral health providers, stigma associated with mental health and substance use conditions, and limited coverage of these services by insurers. In addition, there was a growing awareness of the prevalence of medical comorbidity in patients with serious mental illnesses (SMIs) and increased mortality for these individuals compared with the general population (Liu et al. 2017). These increased mortality and morbidity rates for people with severe mental illness was a jarring epidemiological discovery.

Arising from this heightened awareness and recognition of need, several other models for expanding sources for the provision of behavioral health care came into play. In medical settings, screening tools and safer medications enabled primary care clinicians to be more comfortable prescribing for behavioral health conditions. The introduction of the chronic care model for disease management was another development that furthered this agenda (Pollack et al. 2012). Important elements of the model are self-management of health maintenance needs with motivational support and the use of clinical information systems (Wagner et al. 2001). The model relies on holistic concepts of health and improved, collaborative, interactions between informed patients and providers. At about the same time, University of Washington researchers developed a collaborative care model (CCM) to assist primary care providers (PCPs) to manage their patients with behavioral health issues. The CCM, originally developed for the treatment of depression, provided psychiatric supervision and consultation to PCPs (Unützer et al. 2002) and has since been used for a variety of conditions in various settings. A meta-analysis and systematic review of collaborative chronic care models concluded that these models "can improve mental and physical outcomes for individuals with mental disorders across a wide variety of care settings, and they provide a robust clinical and policy framework for care integration" (Woltmann et al. 2012, p. 790).

In addition to the improved understanding of effective care for chronic illnesses, value-driven initiatives, such as Patient-Centered Medical Home (PCMH) and Medicare Accountable Care Organizations (ACOs), created new possibilities for integration of behavioral health services in primary care settings. These developments have allowed providers to administer services that would not have been compensated in the past. Multiple payers have recently started reimbursing care management activities related to behavioral health integration. In 2017, the Centers for Medicare and Medicaid Services (CMS), the federal agency that administers the Medicare and Medicaid programs, began reimbursing services provided by behavioral health clinicians separately in medical settings (Press et al. 2017). The new reimbursement codes for the Physician Fee Schedule were created to pay for collaborative care management, an approach to behavioral health integration that is primarily based on the University of Washington's CCM model, mentioned above. Using these new codes, PCPs can bill each month for care management services provided by a behavioral health worker in the practice (Press et al. 2017).

The ACO is a model developed through the Patient Protection and Affordable Care Act of 2010 to provide care for a defined population (Busch et al. 2016). In this model, a health care organization takes financial risk for providing this care, with incentives aligned to encourage a holistic approach to care for patients with high health care needs. The ACO model addresses behavioral health disorders from a population health perspective (i.e., improving health outcomes of the defined population). Because patients with behavioral health comorbidities have significantly higher health costs, the ACO model offers great potential to improve outcomes (Melek et al. 2014). Unfortunately, among ACOs developed so far, there have been limited efforts to implement integrated strategies to address behavioral health issues (Shields-Zeeman et al. 2019). One of the reasons could be that very few ACOs have preexisting experience with providing integrated care. To encourage ACOs to adopt integrated approaches, wide-ranging incentives to improve investment in behavioral health care delivery are needed. Medicare ACO contracts have incorporated behavioral health screenings as a quality measure, but greater attention to behavioral health indicators is needed among the many quality measures set up for ACOs (Busch et al. 2016).

The PCMH model is organized around Pollack and colleagues' (2012) chronic care model, described above, which includes care management services, such as providing self-management tools, patient education, behavior modification, and social interventions. The PCMH model encourages behavioral health integration through the use of a behavioral health workforce in the primary care settings, information sharing, care coordination, and evidence-based practices for screening and monitoring behavioral health conditions (National Committee for Quality Assurance 2020). Psychiatrists are well suited to provide leadership in these programs because they can provide clinical education and consultation on setting up these collaborative services and ensure that evidence-based practices are used in treating behavioral health conditions. Chronic care principles are quite similar to the core components of recovery-oriented care provided by psychiatrists in community-based settings (Chung et al. 2016). The PCMH model is discussed in greater detail in Chapter 5 ("Successful Approaches to Increasing Value").

Current State of Behavioral Health in Primary Care

For many reasons, individuals with behavioral health issues often do not receive the care they need. An analysis of the National Ambulatory Medical Care Survey found an overall depression screening rate of only 4.2%, with even lower rates among African Americans and older adults (Akincigil and Matthews 2017). Even when screening and patient engagement do occur, referrals to outpatient behavioral health care are cited as common challenges, due in part to provider shortage, stigma, and insurance coverage issues (Cunningham 2009). Completion rates for referrals have been shown to be consistently low, with less than one-third of identified referrals actually making it to their outpatient visit (Hacker et al. 2014). Even for those who do make it to their behavioral health visit, follow-up communication between PCP and behavioral health provider is rare to nonexistent. Overly stringent interpretations of the Health Insurance Portability and Accountability Act of 1996 and the protection of information related to psychotherapy undoubtedly contribute to these communication breakdowns. Thus, screening can take on the character of a Pandora's box for the PCP, creating more challenges than solutions. Few resources have been available to assist the PCP, who is already pressed for time, in the management of identified behavioral health problems. The U.S. Preventive Services Task Force (2009) acknowledges this lack of resources by recommending depression screening for adults when staff supports are in place. In the absence of these supports, routine problems regularly escalate to the point of an emergency department visit or inpatient admission, or are never addressed at all.

Despite the problems associated with getting behavioral health treatment in primary care settings, PCPs are the foremost prescribers of psychotropic medication, writing up to 60% of these prescriptions, most commonly for anxiolytics and antidepressants (Mark et al. 2009). Unfortunately, because of the challenges previously described, prescribing patterns can be far from best practice in terms of accurate diagnosis, treatment initiation, dosing, symptom monitoring, and follow-up (Mojtabai and Olfson 2011). Training of PCPs in the management of common mental health concerns has historically been lacking, and they have little time, opportunity, or incentive for expanding these skills. Similarly, psychiatric training has not included time in primary care settings, with integrated experience typically coming almost exclusively from inpatient consultation-liaison work.

Although these barriers would seem to refute contentions that more behavioral health needs should be addressed in primary care settings, there are several factors that constitute a primary care "advantage" for behavioral health treatment. Included among these is the relatively low barrier to access, compared with wait times to see a psychiatrist or therapist in a mental health center (Cama et al. 2017; Steinman et al. 2015). Furthermore, patients who have an established or longitudinal relationship with a PCP can more easily discuss mental health concerns without feeling stigmatized. This is particularly true for people with chronic illnesses and for children, who have established patterns of engagement with their providers. PCPs can provide screening and early identification of a variety of mental health concerns, particularly depression and anxiety, both highly prevalent in the population served by primary care (Agency for Healthcare Research and Quality 2013; Kroenke et al. 1994). In people with chronic physical illness, rates of mental health issues can be up to 2–3 times higher than in the general population, further advancing the advantage of the PCP option (Agency for Healthcare Research and Quality 2013; Lin et al. 2004; Sutor et al. 1998). The question then becomes how systems can make use of these advantages while avoiding the deterrents to high-quality services described earlier. Integrated and collaborative care models attempt to answer that question.

Frameworks for Implementation of Integrated Care

The highly fragmented system of care that has been in place—with poor quality and outcomes, poor patient experience, and low overall value—requires transformation. For most health systems, this will be no small task. Given the heterogeneity of provider attitudes, practice attributes, and behavioral health resources, it is clear that one size will not fit all. Methods to provide a framework to organize different approaches to meet diverse needs are helpful.

Four Quadrant Model

Developed by the National Council for Community Behavioral Healthcare, the Four Quadrant Model (Figure 7–1) provides a framework for identifying and planning physical and mental health services for populations with varying physical and behavioral health acuity (Mauer 2009). As described by Mauer, "Each quadrant considers the behavioral health and physical health risk and complexity of the population and suggests the major system elements that would be utilized to meet the needs of a subset of the population" (p. 23). Populations are defined by the degree (high or low) of physical and behavioral health needs. Quadrant I describes those individuals with less severe physical health (PH) and behavioral health (BH) concerns, Quadrant II encompasses those with elevated behavioral health concerns (e.g., SMI), Quadrant III comprises those with elevated physical health concerns (e.g., chronic illness), and Quadrant IV describes those who have elevated physical and behavioral health issues. Within this framework, primary care behavioral health integration would typically occur in quadrants with low behavioral health needs, namely Quadrants I (low BH/low PH) and III (low BH/high PH), with the implication that the treatment of those with more severe behavioral health needs would best be met in a specialized behavioral health setting.

Of note, primary care integration can also occur in Quadrant II (high BH/low PH), as exemplified by the various "reverse integration" approaches, in which primary care services are set up in outpatient behavioral health settings, as reviewed later in this chapter (see subsection "Colocated Models for Integration"). Primary care integration may also occur in Quadrant IV (high BH/high PH), as exemplified by the Unified Primary Care Behavioral Health model, also discussed later in this chapter (see subsection "Colocated Models for Integration"). It is important to note that assignment to a particular quadrant is not static and can in fact change over time,

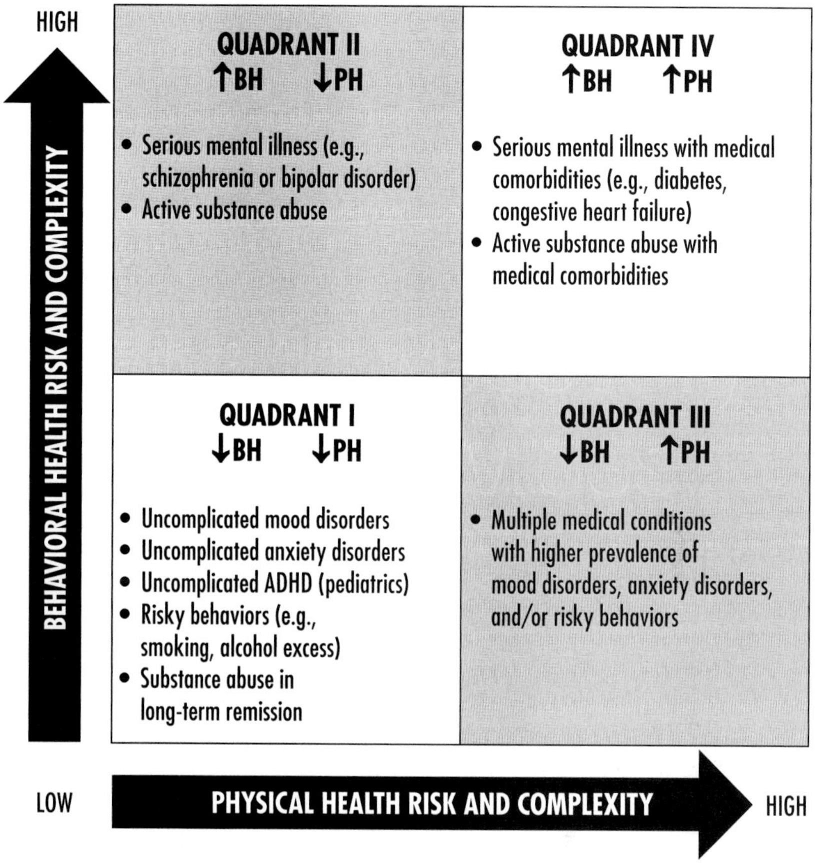

FIGURE 7–1. The Four Quadrant Model.

Note. ADHD=attention-deficit/hyperactivity disorder; BH=behavioral health; PH=physical health.

Source. Adapted from Mauer B: *Behavioral Health/Primary Care Integration and the Person-Centered Healthcare Home.* National Council for Community Behavioral Healthcare, 2009. Available at: www.integration.samhsa.gov/BehavioralHealthandPrimaryCareintegrationandthePCMH-2009.pdf. Accessed February 19, 2020.

because individual behavioral and physical health needs may shift in response to treatment.

Integration Continuum

Looking specifically at the primary care setting, the Substance Abuse and Mental Health Services Administration (SAMHSA) developed a standard classification to describe service integration (Table 7–1; Heath et al. 2013).

TABLE 7–1. Classification of integrated services

Minimal collaboration	Basic collaboration at a distance	Basic collaboration onsite	Close collaboration/ Partly integrated	Fully integrated
Separate systems	Separate systems	Separate systems	Some shared systems	Shared systems and facilities in a seamless biopsychosocial web
Separate facilities	Separate facilities	Same facilities	Same facilities	In-depth appreciation of roles and culture
Rare communication	Periodic focused communication, mostly written	Regular communication, occasionally face to face	Face-to-face consultation; coordinated treatment plans	Collaborative routines that are regular and smooth
Little appreciation of each other's culture	Viewing each other as outside resources	Separate appreciation of each other's role	Basic appreciation of each other's role and culture	Conscious influence sharing based on situation and expertise
	Little understanding of each other's culture or sharing of influence	Mental health has more influence	Collaborative routines difficult; time and operation barriers	
			Influence sharing	

Source. Adapted from Heath et al. 2013.

It consists of a continuum ranging from minimal collaboration to fully integrated practice settings.

In contrast to the Four Quadrant Model, which is grouped according to population needs, the SAMHSA model is organized around practice characteristics, which can then be applied to a variety of populations. Specifically, it focuses on the physical proximity of primary care and behavioral health services, as well as the degree of actual practice integration between the two, including communication workflows, electronic health records, and practice culture (Doherty et al. 1996).

Chung and colleagues (2016) have further refined this integration continuum, with a specific focus on a practice's "size, location, and resources," to help operationalize steps to actual implementation. Their approach has a particular focus on small-and medium-size practices. Degrees of implementation (preliminary, intermediate, and advanced) are assessed across several different domains, including 1) case finding, screening, and referral; 2) ongoing care management; and 3) information tracking and exchange.

Structural Models of Integration

With the rapid proliferation of integrated care models and research, an exhaustive review is beyond the scope of this chapter. For the purpose of this discussion, we utilize the structural groupings of 1) coordinated, 2) colocated, and 3) collaborative, adapted from the classification originally developed by Blount (2003). We review representative models in each grouping and describe how they relate to the frameworks outlined in the preceding section. Finally, given the extensive literature for collaborative models in particular, we take a closer look at the evidence supporting CCM.

Coordinated Consultation Models

In coordinated consultation models, the mental health provider, typically a psychiatrist, serves as a consultant. Cases can be presented to the psychiatrist, or patients can be seen in person, and then the psychiatrist makes recommendations for treatment. In this model, the PCP is ultimately responsible for carrying out those recommendations. The interactions between the psychiatrist and the PCP can be conducted by telephone or in person. Face-to-face evaluations of patients by the psychiatrist are usually reserved for the most challenging cases. A good example of this model is the Massachusetts Child Psychiatry Access Program, which provides telephonic specialty child psychiatry consultation and care coordination and has provided support to over 95% of the pediatric practices in the state (Straus and Sarvet 2014). Project TEACH, operating in New York State, provides a similar service for pediatric providers (https://projectteachny.org). Telepsychiatry has emerged as an option for remote patient evaluations and consultation, although further research is required on effective application in the primary care setting (Hilty et al. 2018). While generally falling on the lower end of the SAMHSA integration continuum (see Table 7–1), such models could be applied to populations across the four quadrants (see Figure 7–1), particularly in the management of more severely ill patients residing in areas with few to no psychiatric resources.

Strengths of these consultation models include the relative ease of implementation, as there is no requirement for additional space (although in the case of telepsychiatry, there is a need for appropriate equipment and connectivity). Barriers include uptake of the service, particularly if there is no preexisting relationship with the psychiatrist, and the fact that PCPs may be reluctant to collaborate with or take recommendations from a physician with whom they are not familiar (Collins et al. 2010). Underlying this reluctance may be issues of training, time, scope of practice, and stigma, all of which speak to the practice culture and motivation for integration, and may vary widely from provider to provider. Furthermore, once a patient's behavioral health need has been identified, PCPs can still struggle with connections to outpatient care, particularly when the patient requires a higher level of care than can be managed in the primary care setting (Straus and Sarvet 2014). For this reason, some consultation models also include brief care management support, although these team members are only as effective as the behavioral health service system in which they operate.

Colocated Models for Integration

Colocation likely represents the most heterogeneous grouping, with respect to both the populations that can be served by these models (i.e., those in Quadrants I–IV) and the degree of service delivery integration (i.e., SAMHSA continuum). The basic model of colocation typically consists of a behavioral health provider agency setting up clinical services in or directly adjacent to a primary care practice to deliver traditional mental health services such as psychotherapy or medication management. The physical proximity between the two providers likely decreases the "access" concern. The patients are typically in Quadrants I and III, although patients with more severe presentations from Quadrants II and IV could be served as well. Care planning, clinical workflows, and administrative functions may be shared with medical providers, but unlike the CCMs, coordination and comanagement are neither inherent to this model nor required for it to function (Collins et al. 2010). The extent to which these clinical and administrative functions are integrated can be variable. In the best case scenario, there is meaningful integration with conduits for communication and record sharing. On the other end of the spectrum, these services still function like siloed systems (AIMS Center 2019). A comparison of the relative effectiveness of the CCM and the colocated model indicated a greater reduction in follow-up scores on the Patient Health Questionnaire–9 (PHQ-9) at 12 weeks of treatment in the collaborative intervention (33%) compared to the colocated intervention (14%) (Blackmore et al. 2018). Furthermore, by functioning in a traditional mental health clinic mold, colocated services can easily encounter capacity issues, which can undermine one of the central objectives of expanding access to care (Collins et al. 2010). That said, all successful colocation arrangements increase accessibility, opportunities for communication, and on-site consultation, which can serve as a foundation for eventual full integration between providers.

The Unified Primary Care and Behavioral Health model (UPCBH) represents a fully integrated, colocated service. Bringing together a full array of physical and behavioral clinical services, as well as administrative functions and financing, the model falls firmly in the fully integrated category of the SAMHSA continuum (Collins et al. 2010). Although designed primarily to target the needs of patients with SMI (i.e., those in Quadrants II and IV), the model can serve patients in any quadrant. Despite being relatively sparse, evidence for the model has been positive, demonstrating a reduced likelihood of emergency department visits, improved physical health status, and improved continuity of care (Druss et al. 2001). To date, this model has been implemented in FQHCs and Veterans Health Administration programs. FQHCs were established in 1991 and receive subsidies through CMS to provide comprehensive care in underserved areas. Many of these centers are certified to provide behavioral health services and directly employ psychiatrists and other behavioral health professionals along with PCPs (Center for Medicare and Medicaid Services 2019).

Reverse integration—that is, the establishment of primary care services in mental health facilities—has emerged as another model of colocation. Particular strengths of this approach include comprehensive physical and behavioral health management in one location, this time with the behavioral health clinic as the primary "hub." Like the UPCBH model, this approach holds particular promise for individuals with severe mental illness, who typically have a much higher burden of physical illness, as well as poor adherence to medication and outpatient care. As in traditional colocation models, the degree of integration can vary, ranging from simple physical proximity all the way to meaningful clinical and administrative integration. In a review of reverse integration models, the Millbank Memorial Fund found that those sites that incorporated a fully integrated care model (i.e., joint treatment planning, electronic health records, etc.) improved their patients' use of preventive and medical services (Gerrity 2014).

The reverse integration approach has created issues around billing and sustainability. In 2018, SAMHSA created demonstration projects in several states to address those issues. The Certified Community Behavioral Health Clinics (CCBHCs) receive subsidies for integrating physical health care services in a manner similar to FQHCs that integrate behavioral health. The CCBHC model effectively creates a "one-stop shop" for clients typically in Quadrants II and IV, potentially providing much better outcomes for persons with SMI who have difficulty engaging with PCPs. Beyond standard clinical services, CCBHCs are paid an enhanced rate through Medicaid to perform nine core services, which include crisis intervention, substance use disorder (SUD) services, targeted case management, psychiatric rehabilitation services, and peer and family support services, as well as primary care (National Council for Behavioral Health 2017).

Collaborative Care Models

CCMs have emerged as the most widely known and disseminated of the integrated care models. In the most basic iteration of CCMs, physical health and mental health professionals work together toward developing a collaborative care plan to meet the needs of a specific patient. Typically, a PCP and a behavioral health care clinician work together in the primary care practice, supported by a supervising psychiatrist, usually by telephone; however, opportunities for in-person evaluation and telepsychiatry exist as well, with unique billing codes associated with each. Despite the various versions of collaborative care used across different settings and populations, a number of common elements can clearly be observed. To guide implementation fidelity, Raney (2015) developed a set of Core Principles of Effective Collaborative Care, summarized below.

1. *Team-based, coordinated care:* The core team typically consists of a PCP, care manager, and supervising psychiatrist. The role of the care manager can be filled by a variety of disciplines, including a registered nurse, PhD, or licensed clinical social worker, and duties include assessment, treatment, and coordination of care, depending on the nature of the patient's needs. The care manager works closely with the PCP and practice, typically consulting with the psychiatrist during supervision or as crises arise.
2. *Evidence-based care:* Evidence-based treatments and protocols are incorporated to address specific disease states. This is in contrast to usual behavioral health treatment in primary care, in which idiosyncratic in-

terventions may be used, or poorly coordinated care may be experienced due to the dearth of psychiatric resources and support available to most practices.

3. *Measurement-based care:* Data collection is used to develop clear, condition-specific treatment targets and outcomes, typically measured using a validated tool. For example, PHQ-9 is often used as a screening method for depression, as well as a way to provide continuous tracking of progress toward recovery. Results are tracked over time with a registry, to ensure that patients do not get lost to follow-up. This process allows for a stepped-care approach, with an escalating intensity of interventions for patients not responding to initial treatment.
4. *Population-based care:* The health outcomes of a specific group of patients are managed. This group can be defined in a variety of ways, using different clinical and demographic criteria (e.g., depressed older adults). Crucial to this approach is a thorough understanding of the needs of the population in question, as these directly impact health and well-being. Typically, populations of interest for intervention include groups with largely unmet or partially met needs who are significantly driving up medical costs.
5. *Accountability:* Outcomes related to clinical effectiveness, patient experience, and cost are tracked and reported for the identified population of interest over time. Performance on these measures can be linked to fiscal compensation, reflecting varying degrees of provider risk (see Chapter 6, "Innovative Financing").

With respect to the Four Quadrant Model (see Figure 7–1), CCM would typically be useful for patients in Quadrants I (low BH/low PH) and III (low BH/high PH). CCM also would generally be considered to be at the high end of the SAMHSA integrated services continuum (partly or fully integrated) (see Table 7–1), given the necessity for close communication and coordination around the elements described above.

Evidence for the Collaborative Care Model

Behavioral health integration in the primary care setting has been a major focus of health care reforms. As a result, integration models and research have proliferated. In one review, Huffman and colleagues (2014) identified over 600 articles pertaining to integration of behavioral health and physical health. Their review, which focused on 67 of the most salient studies, informs much of the discussion in what follows.

Foundational studies demonstrated effectiveness in the treatment of depression for older adults in the primary care setting (Bruce et al. 2004), most notably for the IMPACT (Improving Mood—Promoting Access to Collaborative Treatment) model, developed by Unützer and colleagues (2002) at the University of Washington. The authors described a randomized controlled trial of 1,801 patients, age 60 and older with major depressive disorder, dysthymia, or both, whose depression was treated in a primary care setting. The intervention arm consisted of 12 months of access to a depression care manager. Working with a PCP and supported by a supervising psychiatrist, the care manager could offer education, care coordination, and help with medication administration, as well as time-limited Problem-Solving Treatment. About 45% of patients in collaborative care were found to have a 50% reduction in symptoms from initial assessment, compared with only 19% of those in usual care. Long-term outcomes showed that those in the collaborative care arm continued to fare better than controls at 18 and 24 months after intervention (Hunkeler et al. 2006). Meta-analyses of collaborative care for depression and anxiety have indicated effectiveness in several domains, including reduction of depression symptoms, adherence to treatment, and satisfaction with care (Gilbody et al. 2006; Thota et al. 2012).

Collaborative care for depression in people who have other chronic health conditions has also been effective, as various studies have demonstrated. Positive effects on depression symptoms have been shown in patients with cardiac disease, diabetes, cancer, HIV, and chronic pain (Curran et al. 2011; Davidson et al. 2010; Dobscha et al. 2009; Ell et al. 2008; Lin et al. 2004; Rollman et al. 2009; Strong et al. 2008). Several studies have also looked at combined mental and physical health outcomes, most notably the TEAMcare trial (Kathol et al. 2010). Compared with patients receiving usual care, patients who received collaborative care management for both depression and chronic illness (i.e., diabetes or heart failure) showed lower depression levels and lower cholesterol, blood pressure, and hemoglobin A_{1c} levels at 12 months.

Given the evidence that approximately half of behavioral health conditions present before age 14 years, integrated treatment approaches to pediatric mental health represent a significant opportunity to positively impact this population. Unfortunately, study of integrated care for this population has lagged behind that for adults, in part due to diagnostic and therapeutic variations found among children across the developmental lifespan. As such, it is not simply a matter of transposing the CCM to a different setting; new approaches to screening, engagement, and intervention, involving both children and their parents, are required. Although approaches to adolescent depression and anxiety may have some overlap with interventions for adults, interventions for the same conditions in young children have significant differences, requiring distinct screening tools and treatment models.

Other conditions, such as attention-deficit/hyperactivity disorder (ADHD) or similar disruptive behaviors, which are highly prevalent in the pediatric setting, have no clear analogue in the adult literature and require modified models for collaboration. That said, the core elements of CCM provide a sufficiently flexible framework to address various pediatric issues. A meta-analysis of pediatric integrated care models indicated the overall effectiveness of this approach across a variety of different integration models (Asarnow et al. 2015). Of the models studied, CCM was found to have the strongest effects on targeted diagnoses and symptoms, in comparison to other models that included consultative models, colocated models, and telephone coaching. Conditions addressed by studies using CCM included depression, anxiety, and ADHD. All of the collaborative care trials used two evidence-based therapy approaches: cognitive-behavioral therapy and medication algorithms. Five-year outcomes for pediatric behavioral health integration using a transdiagnostic CCM demonstrated improvements in access, quality, and patient satisfaction while not substantially increasing costs (Walter et al. 2019).

Common Challenges for Integration

Given the heterogeneity of integration models, coupled with the broad variation with health system resources, it is little surprise that a host of challenges should arise with respect to effective implementation. In the development of an implementation strategy, these challenges are essential to consider in order to realize the promise of increased value inherent to the enterprise of behavioral health integration. Although numerous resources have been developed to address implementation issues (AIMS Center 2019; Ratzliff 2014; Substance Abuse and Mental Health Services Administration–HRSA Center for Integrated Health Solutions 2016), relatively few address the ongoing success and sustainability of integrated programming. Specifically looking at the primary care setting, a number of common themes arise, which are summarized below.

Space and Other Physical Resources

Among the most common—and most challenging—issues are physical space constraints, which can at times present an immutable barrier to implementation, particularly for colocated or collaborative models. Once a space has been identified, there are often questions regarding the appropriateness of the space, particularly with respect to privacy and safety. Other concrete concerns, such as computer access and electronic health record connectivity, may pose a significant barrier in smaller practices but are less common in larger practices and health systems.

Practice Culture

Given the default culture of fragmented physical and behavioral health care, cultural change will pose a challenge in nearly all settings, and the primary challenge is provider engagement. Instead of considering behavioral health as part of their primary care mission, PCPs may view it as "another thing to do" in an already overburdened practice environment. Therefore, demonstrating the value of behavioral health resources as collaborators in addressing these issues and meaningfully assisting their patients is crucial to catalyzing this cultural change. Team-building activities, including meet and greets and recurring case conferences, can be very useful in this regard. Physician "champions" for integration can also be helpful drivers of cultural changes.

Workforce

Aside from psychiatrists and psychiatric nurse practitioners, much of the behavioral health workforce has not had training or professional experience in medical settings. Recruitment of candidates who can be comfortable working in a nontraditional setting is essential for advancing integration, particularly for colocated and collaborative models. For example, the pace of the medical practice, with frequent interruptions and potential crises, may be quite different from the steady cadence of outpatient behavioral health work and the traditional therapeutic frame. Also, the therapeutic interventions themselves can often be more time limited and focused, and this may be a contrast to the longer-term time frames practiced by most clinicians in behavioral health settings. Psychiatrists may also need to make an adjustment in regard to making recommendations for patients whom they have not seen directly but are only hearing about in supervision.

Screening and Outcome Measurement (Workflow)

Providers in the culture of usual care may feel overburdened or unprepared to add additional screening protocols and outcome measurement, much less to track them with fidelity over time. In this regard, it makes sense to introduce these changes gradually, with one measurement-based workflow as a starting point. Even once change is established, tracking the collected data and using it to drive care poses another challenge. Registries and other electronic health records can be essential in this regard, but they are ultimately only as good as the quality of the data input and the accuracy of its interpretation. Given the inevitable tendency for variation or "drift" in originally specified models and workflows, it is essential to develop outcome measures and targets for monitoring over time. To date, the CCM likely has the clearest defined outcome measures, particularly with respect to depression and anxiety.

Sustainability

As discussed earlier in this chapter (see "Background: Integration of Physical and Behavioral Health Care"), new payment mechanisms are emerging to aid with reimbursement, particularly for collaborative care services. Nevertheless, developing operational efficiencies to maintain program viability is an ongoing challenge. Initial considerations include both practice volume and payer mix. Low referral rates, even within otherwise large practices, can similarly stymie sustainability and must be monitored and addressed. Process and outcome reporting, such as screening, time spent, and clinical improvement, may be required as well, though requirements often vary across plans, further contributing to process complexity. In short, to achieve sustainability, close collaboration among practice clinicians, especially in regard to "back office" functions such as scheduling, billing, and data/analytics, is necessary. To this extent, addressing the challenges presented earlier in this section is essential for achieving practice alignment and driving high performance of integration efforts and long-term success.

Integrating Substance Use Interventions Into Primary Care

Affecting more than one in seven individuals nationwide, alcohol and SUDs are present in a large proportion of the primary care population, with one large study indicating 24% incidence of risky drinking, 5% for problem drinking, 3% for alcohol dependence, and 3% for illicit drug use (Cherpitel and Ye 2008). Like comorbid mental health concerns, comorbid SUD can significantly impact individual health and chronic disease management and contribute to the development of additional disease burden (U.S. Department of Health and Human Services 2000). A less promising similarity with mental health integration is the extent to which the potential for SUD intervention often outpaces the degree to which these services are actually accessible and available in real-world settings. Issues such as stigma, provider training, workflows, referral resources, and communication, discussed at length in earlier sections, similarly impact meaningful integration of SUD services.

Nevertheless, the national focus on SUDs, particularly in the wake of the opioid crisis, has accelerated efforts to improve access to treatment and effectiveness of services. Primary care is viewed as integral to these efforts, as reflected in the emphasis on SUD integration in the Patient-Centered Medical Home model (Druss and Mauer 2010). Enhanced billing practices for providers, particularly for Screening, Brief Intervention and Referral to Treatment (SBIRT) interventions, have similarly helped with accelerating implementation (Substance Abuse and Mental Health Services Administration 2017). The U.S. Preventive Services Task Force (2019) has similarly promoted screening and intervention for alcohol in primary care as a recommended best practice.

Screening, Brief Intervention and Referral to Treatment Model

SBIRT has emerged as one of the more widely disseminated models for approaching SUDs and has been applied to a variety of populations and clinical settings. A core element of the model is *substance abuse screening*, typically with standardized tools such as the Alcohol Use Disorders Identification Test—Concise (AUDIT-C) or the Drug Abuse Screening Test (DAST). Screening categorizes risk level into no risk, risky use, and active SUDs. *Brief intervention* is meant to foster engagement in treatment following a positive screen. Brief intervention employs a motivational approach; the patient's readiness to change is assessed, and goals are established in accord with the patient's level of readiness (Substance Abuse and Mental Health Services Administration 2017). *Referral to treatment* varies, based on each patient's identified intensity of need and readiness. Providing up-to-date referral information for accessible and clinically appropriate services is a crucial step in this process. Because a dearth of high-quality SUD services can create a bottleneck in effective linkage, developing a network of providers in a geographic region is essential to addressing the needs of this population.

On the basis of a review of the evidence, the U.S. Preventive Services Task Force issued updated guidance in 2004, recommending the use of brief primary care–based interventions to identify and address alcohol misuse (Whitlock et al. 2004). For patients at risk for increased morbidity and mortality due to their patterns alcohol consumption but who do not meet criteria for alcohol dependence, both primary care screening and brief behavioral counseling were supported by "good evidence" of their effectiveness in primary care. Recently, these recommendations have been expanded to include the identification and treatment of other drug use problems for adults age 18 and older (U.S. Preventive Services Task Force 2019).

Medication-Assisted Treatment

Beyond screening and brief assessment, medication-assisted treatment (MAT) for alcohol and opioid use disorders expands the potential for SUD treatment within the primary care setting. Once considered an intervention of last resort, MAT is now seen as an effective way to reduce harm and engage people in treatment (Heinzerling et al. 2016). It is easily made available in communities with otherwise limited access to SUD treatment. MAT is increasingly viewed as an option that reduces barriers to access and capitalizes on its nonjudgmental and anonymous application. Once identified with programs such as SBIRT, MAT can be initiated without a broad referral base. At the same time, significant concerns about and opposition to MAT remain—primarily concerns that providers will be further overburdened, while patients will be undertreated and not receive appropriate supportive services in the form of individual, group, and other supportive services. This intervention is described further in Chapter 17 ("Addiction Treatment and Harm Reduction").

Conclusion

Integrated care has been shown to be effective in several dozen randomized clinical trials and is widely considered an effective strategy for improving behavioral health–related outcomes both in primary care populations and in patients receiving services in traditional mental health clinics (Press et al. 2017; Woltmann et al. 2012). Studies have also documented improved patient satisfaction and quality of life with integrated care relative to treatment as usual (Reed et al. 2016).

New reimbursement codes for Collaborative Care Management and Behavioral Health Integration set up by the Centers for Medicare and Medicaid Services, and increasingly recognized by many other payers, provide a business incentive to invest in integrated care models (Carlo et al. 2018). Another opportunity for financial support for integrated care is improvement in quality measures. Many payers incentivize performance in Healthcare Effectiveness Data and Information Set measures (see Chapter 6, "Innovative Financing"). These quality measures increasingly take into account behavioral health conditions in general medical health settings.

Examples of these measures include screening and follow-up for depression, or initiation and engagement for substance use.

As experience with value-based purchasing matures, improvements of integrated care models are expected. Improvements in outcomes, costs, and patient experience will drive further adoption and sustainability of integrated care. Experienced health systems such as Intermountain Healthcare have published reports about the impact on total health care costs when integrated services are in place (Reiss-Brennan et al. 2016). Individuals with co-occurring medical and behavioral health conditions incur high health care spending compared to those with only medical conditions. Targeting improvement in behavioral health outcomes for this population suffering from comorbid medical conditions is thus an area of opportunity for providers in value-based payment models such as Accountable Care Organizations (Busch et al. 2016).

The value proposition for integrated care has many elements beyond the financial impact. Access to care and improved behavioral health outcomes are important to many stakeholders (e.g., employers and the patients receiving the care). Integrated care adds value by increasing recognition of behavioral health care in primary care settings and improving access to care. In pediatric settings, integration can help with prevention and early intervention. The key opportunity in setting up an integrated care program is transformation of the delivery system. It will be an important element in providing holistic, person-centered approaches to care and in pursuing the Quadruple Aim (see Chapter 1, "Defining and Measuring Value").

Acknowledgment

The authors wish to acknowledge Megan Grella for her assistance with proofreading, arranging references, and formatting tables.

References

Agency for Healthcare Research and Quality: A framework for measuring integration of behavioral health and primary care. 2013. Available at: https://integrationacademy.ahrq.gov/products/ibhc-measures-atlas/framework-measuring-integration-behavioral-health-and-primary-care. Accessed August 8, 2019.

AIMS Center: Implementation guide. 2019. Available at: http://aims.uw.edu/collaborative-care/implementation-guide/lay-foundation. Accessed February 19, 2020.

Akincigil A, Matthews S: National rates and patterns of depression screening in primary care: results from 2012 and 2013. Psychiatr Serv 68(7):660–666, 2017

Asarnow JR, Rozenman M, Wiblin J, et al: Integrated medical-behavioral care compared with usual primary care for child and adolescent behavioral health: a meta-analysis. JAMA Pediatr 169(10):929–937, 2015
Blackmore MA, Carleton KE, Ricketts SM, et al: Comparison of collaborative care and colocation treatment for patients with clinically significant depression symptoms in primary care. Psychiatr Serv 69(11):1184–1187, 2018
Blount A: Integrated primary care: organizing the evidence. Families, Systems, and Health 21(2):121–133, 2003
Bruce ML, Ten Have TR, Reynolds CF III, et al: Reducing suicidal ideation and depressive symptoms in depressed older primary care patients: a randomized controlled trial. JAMA 291(9):1081–1091, 2004
Brunette M, Asher D, Whitley R, et al: Implementation of integrated dual disorders treatment: a qualitative analysis of facilitators and barriers. Psychiatr Serv 59(9):989–995, 2008
Busch A, Huskamp H, McWilliams M: Early efforts by Medicare accountable care organizations have limited effect on mental illness care and management. Health Aff (Millwood) 35(7):1247–1256, 2016
Cama S, Malowney M, Smith AJB, et al: Availability of outpatient mental health care by pediatricians and child psychiatrists in five U.S. cities. Int J Health Serv 47(4):621–635, 2017
Carlo AD, Unutzer J, Ratzliff ADH, et al: Financing for collaborative care—a narrative review. Curr Treat Options Psychiatry 5(3):334–344, 2018
Center for Medicare and Medicaid Services: Federally qualified health center. 2019. Available at:www.cms.gov/Outreach-and-Education/Medicare-Learning-Network-MLN/MLNProducts/downloads/fqhcfactsheet.pdf. Accessed February 19, 2020.
Center for Substance Abuse Treatment: Understanding evidence-based practices for co-occurring disorders (DHHS Publ No SMA-07-4278). COCE Review, Paper 5, 2007. Available at: https://secure.addictioncounselorce.com/articles/101548/OP5-Practices-8-13-07.pdf. Accessed February 19, 2020.
Cherpitel CJ, Ye Y: Drug use and problem drinking associated with primary care and emergency room utilization in the U.S. general population: data from the 2005 National Alcohol Survey. Drug Alcohol Depend 97(3):226–230, 2008
Chung H, Rotanski N, Glassberg H, et al: Advancing integration of behavioral health into primary care: a continuum-based framework. United Hospital Fund, 2016. Available at: https://uhfnyc.org/publications/publication/advancing-integration-of-behavioral-health-into-primary-care-a-continuum-based-framework. Accessed February 19, 2020.
Collins C, Heuson DL, Munger R, et al: Evolving models of behavioral health integration in primary care. Milbank Fund, 2010. Available at www.milbank.org/wp-content/uploads/2016/05/Evolving-Models-of-BHI.pdf. Accessed on February 19, 2020.
Cunningham PJ: Beyond parity: primary care physicians' perspectives on access to mental health care. Health Aff (Millwood) 28(3):w490–w501, 2009

Curran GM, Pyne J, Fortney JC, et al: Development and implementation of collaborative care for depression in HIV clinics. AIDS Care 23(12):1626–1636, 2011

Davidson KW, Rieckmann N, Clemow L, et al: Enhanced depression care for patients with acute coronary syndrome and persistent depressive symptoms: coronary psychosocial evaluation studies randomized controlled trial. Arch Intern Med 170(7):600–608, 2010

Dobscha SK, Corson K, Perrin NA, et al: Collaborative care for chronic pain in primary care: a cluster randomized trial. JAMA Intern Med 301(12):1242–1252, 2009

Doherty WJ, McDaniel SH, Baird MA: Five levels of primary care/behavioral healthcare collaboration. Behav Healthc Tomorrow 5(5):25–27, 1996

Druss BG, Mauer BJ: Health care reform and care at the behavioral health-primary care interface. Psychiatr Serv 61(11):1087–1092, 2010

Druss BG, Rohrbaugh RM, Levinson CM, et al: Integrated medical care for patients with serious psychiatric illness: a randomized trial. Arch Gen Psychiatry 58(9):861–868, 2001

Ell K, Xie B, Quon B, et al: Randomized controlled trial of collaborative care management of depression among low-income patients with cancer. J Clinic Oncol 26(27):4488–4496, 2008

Gerrity M: Integrating primary care into behavioral health settings: what works for individuals with serious mental illness. Milbank Memorial Fund, 2014. Available at: www.milbank.org/publications/integrating-primary-care-into-behavioral-health-settings-what-works-for-individuals-with-serious-mental-illness. Accessed February 19, 2020.

Gilbody S, Bower P, Fletcher J, et al: Collaborative care for depression: a cumulative meta-analysis and review of longer-term outcomes. Arch Intern Med 166(21):2314–2321, 2006

Hacker KA, Penfold RB, Arsenault LN, et al: Behavioral health services following implementation of screening in Massachusetts Medicaid children. Pediatrics 134(4):737–756, 2014

Heath B, Wise RP, Reynolds KA: Review and proposed standard framework for levels of integrated healthcare. Substance Abuse and Mental Health Services Administration–HRSA Center for Integrated Health Solutions, 2013. Available at: www.integration.samhsa.gov/integrated-care-models/a_standard_framework_for_levels_of_integrated_healthcare.pdf. Accessed February 13, 2020.

Heinzerling KG, Ober AJ, Lamp K, et al: SUMMIT: procedures for medication-assisted treatment of alcohol or opioid dependence in primary care. RAND, 2016. Available at: www.integration.samhsa.gov/clinical-practice/mat/RAND_MAT_guidebook_for_health_centers.pdf. Accessed February 19, 2020.

Hilty DM, Rabinowitz T, McCarron RM, et al: An update on telepsychiatry and how it can leverage collaborative, stepped, and integrated services to primary care. Psychosomatics 59(3):227–250, 2018

Huffman JC, Niazi SK, Rundell JR, et al: Essential articles on collaborative care models for the treatment of psychiatric disorders in medical settings: a publication by the Academy of Psychosomatic Medicine Research and Evidence-Based Practice Committee. Psychosomatics 55(2):109–122, 2014

Hunkeler EM, Katon W, Tang L, et al: Long term outcomes from the IMPACT randomized trial for depressed elderly patients in primary care. BMJ 332(7536):259–263, 2006

Kathol RG, Butler M, McAlpine DD, et al: Barriers to physical and mental condition integrated service delivery. Psychosom Med 72(6):511–518, 2010

Katon W, Von Korff M, Lin E, et al: Improving primary care treatment of depression among patients with diabetes mellitus: the design of the Pathways Study. Gen Hosp Psychiatry 25(3):158–168, 2003

Kroenke K, Spitzer RL, Williams JB, et al: Physical symptoms in primary care. Predictors of psychiatric disorders and functional impairment. Arch Fam Med 3(9):774–779, 1994

Lin EH, Katon W, Von Korff M, et al: Relationship of depression and diabetes self-care, medication adherence, and preventive care. Diabetes Care 27(9):2154–2160, 2004

Liu NH, Daumit GL, Dua S, et al: Excess mortality in persons with severe mental disorders: a multilevel intervention framework and priorities for clinical practice, policy, and research agendas. World Psychiatry 16(1):30–40, 2017

Mark TL, Levit KR, Buck JA: Datapoints: psychotropic drug prescriptions by medical specialty. Psychiatr Serv 60(9):1167, 2009

Mauer B: Behavioral health/primary care integration and the person-centered healthcare home. National Council for Community Behavioral Healthcare, 2009. Available at: www.integration.samhsa.gov/BehavioralHealthandPrimaryCareintegrationand thePCMH-2009.pdf. Accessed February 19, 2020.

McGovern L: The relative contribution of multiple determinants to health outcomes. Health Affairs, Health Policy Brief, 2014. Available at: www.healthaffairs.org/do/10.1377/hpb20140821.404487/full. Accessed February 13, 2020.

Melek SP, Norris DT, Paulus J: Economic impact of integrated medical behavioral healthcare. Milliman American Psychiatric Association Report, 2014

Mojtabai S, Olfson M: Proportion of antidepressants prescribed without a psychiatric diagnosis is growing. Health Aff (Millwood) 30(8):1434–1442, 2011

National Committee for Quality Assurance: Distinction in behavioral health integration. 2020. Available at www.ncqa.org/programs/health-care-providers-practices/patient-centered-medical-home-pcmh/distinction-in-behavioral-health-integration. Accessed February 13, 2020.

National Council for Behavioral Health: What is a CCBHC? 2017. Available at: www.thenationalcouncil.org/wp-content/uploads/2017/11/What-is-a-CCBHC-11.7.17.pdf. Accessed February 13, 2020.

Pollack DA, Raney LE, Vanderlip ER: Integrated care and psychiatrists, in Handbook of Community Psychiatry. New York, Springer Science+Business Media, 2012, pp 163–175

Press MJ, Howe R, Schoenbaum M, et al: Medicare payment for behavioral health integration. N Engl J Med 376(5):405–407, 2017

Raney L: Integrating primary care and behavioral health: the role of the psychiatrist in the collaborative care model. Am J Psychiatry 172(8):721–728, 2015

Ratzliff A: Organized, evidence-based care supplement: behavioral health integration. Safety Net Medical Home Initiative, 2014. Available at: www.safetynetmedicalhome.org/sites/default/files/Executive-Summary-Behavioral-Health-Integration.pdf. Accessed February 19, 2020.

Reed GM, Kihlstrom JF, Messer SB: What qualifies as evidence of effective practice? Patient values and preferences, in Evidence Based Practices in Mental Health: Debate and Dialogue on Fundamental Questions. Edited by Norcross JC, Beutler L, Levant R. Washington, DC, American Psychological Association, 2005, pp 31–40

Reed SJ, Shore KK, Tice JA: Effectiveness and value of integrating behavioral health into primary care. JAMA Intern Med 176(5):691–692, 2016

Reiss-Brennan B, Brunisholz KD, Dredge C, et al: Association of integrated team-based care with health care quality, utilization, and cost. JAMA 316(8):826–834, 2016

Rollman BL, Belnap BH, LeMenager MS, et al: Telephone-delivered collaborative-care for treating post-CABG depression: a randomized controlled trial. JAMA 302(19):2095–2103, 2009

Shields-Zeeman L, Lewis C, Gottlieb L: Social and mental health care integration. JAMA Psychiatry June 19, 2019 [Epub ahead of print]

Steinman KJ, Shoben AB, Dembe AE, et al: How long do adolescents wait for psychiatry appointments? Community Ment Health J 51(7):782–789, 2015

Straus JH, Sarvet B: Behavioral health care for children: the Massachusetts Child Psychiatry Access Project. Health Aff (Millwood) 33(12):2153–2161, 2014

Strong V, Waters R, Hibberd C, et al: Management of depression for people with cancer (SMaRT oncology 1): a randomised trial. Lancet 372(9632):40–48, 2008

Substance Abuse and Mental Health Services Administration: Coding for screening and brief intervention reimbursement. U.S. Department of Health and Human Services, 2017. Available at: www.samhsa.gov/sbirt/coding-reimbursement. Accessed August 15, 2019.

Substance Abuse and Mental Health Services Administration–HRSA Center for Integrated Health Solutions: Essential elements of effective integrated primary behavioral health terms. 2014. Available at: www.integration.samhsa.gov/workforce/team-members/Essential_Elements_of_an_Integrated_Team.pdf. Accessed February 13, 2020.

Substance Abuse and Mental Health Services Administration–HRSA Center for Integrated Health Solutions: A Quick Start Guide to Behavioral Health Integration for Safety-Net Primary Care Providers. Rockville, MD, U.S. Department of Health and Human Services, 2016

Sutor B, Rummans TA, Jowsey SG, et al: Major depression in medically ill patients. Mayo Clin Proc 73(4):329–337, 1998

Thota AB, Sipe TA, Byard GJ, et al: Collaborative care to improve the management of depressive disorders: a community guide systematic review and meta-analysis. Am J Prev Med 42(5):525–538, 2012

Torrey WC, Drake RE, Cohen M, et al: The challenge of implementing and sustaining integrated dual disorders treatment programs. Community Ment Health J 38(6):507–521, 2002

Unützer K, Katon W, Callahan CM, et al: Collaborative care management of late-life depression in the primary care setting: a randomized controlled trial. JAMA 288(22):2836–2845, 2002

U.S. Department of Health and Human Services: Special report to the U.S. Congress on alcohol and health. 2000. Available at: https://pubs.niaaa.nih.gov/publications/10report/intro.pdf. Accessed February 19, 2020.

U.S. Preventive Services Task Force: Alcohol misuse: screening and counseling. 2004. Available at: www.uspreventiveservicestaskforce.org/Page/Document/RecommendationStatementFinal/alcohol-misuse-screening-and-counseling-2004. Accessed February 19, 2020.

U.S. Preventive Services Task Force: Screening for depression in adults: U.S. Preventive Services Task Force recommendation statement. Ann Intern Med 151(11):784–792, 2009

U.S. Preventive Services Task Force: Illicit drug use, including nonmedical use of prescription drugs: screening. 2019. Available at: www.uspreventiveservicestaskforce.org/Page/Document/draft-recommendation-statement/drug-use-in-adolescents-and-adults-including-pregnant-women-screening. Accessed February 19, 2020.

Vickers KS, Ridgeway JL, Hathaway JC, et al: Integration of mental health resources in a primary care setting leads to increased provider satisfaction and patient access. Gen Hosp Psychiatry 35(5):461–467, 2013

Wagner EH, Austin BT, Davis C, et al: Improving chronic illness care: translating evidence into action. Health Aff (Millwood) 20(6):64–78, 2001

Walter HJ, Vernacchio L, Trudell EK, et al: Five-year outcomes of behavioral health integration in primary care. Pediatrics 144(1), 2019

Whitlock EP, Polen MR, Green CA, et al: Behavioral counseling interventions in primary care to reduce risky/harmful alcohol use by adults: a summary of the evidence for the U.S. Preventive Services Task Force. Ann Intern Med 140(7):557–568, 2004

Woltmann E, Grogan-Kaylor A, Perron B, et al: Comparative effectiveness of collaborative chronic care models for mental health conditions across primary, specialty, and behavioral health care settings: systematic review and meta-analysis. Am J Psychiatry 169(8):790–804, 2012

World Health Organization: Integrated care models: an overview. Health Services Delivery Programme, 2016. Available at: www.euro.who.int/__data/assets/pdf_file/0005/322475/Integrated-care-models-overview.pdf. Accessed February 13, 2020.

8

Prevention and Health Promotion

Peter L. Chien, M.D., M.A.

An ounce of prevention equals a pound of cure.
Ben Franklin

We as health professionals intuitively know that we should invest in early stage prevention. Compared with treating an illness and its effects, prevention is more effective and efficient, and it provides high satisfaction. It is the ultimate in medical value. The question is how to prevent illness. When prevention works, one may not know that a problem would otherwise have occurred. Effective prevention hides its methods and disguises its value. Even in prevention's most proven forms, the sting of a needle and fear of side effects may be more prominent than the treacherous disease that was avoided.

In mental health, the questions regarding prevention are multiplied. If we do not fully understand the scientific mechanisms behind brain dysfunction, how can we prevent them before they occur? Might we have to wait for further understanding of the brain for effective mental health prevention?

Luckily, prevention in mental health has been proven possible through a public health approach to promote mental health and address risk and protective factors. This chapter first explores this approach to prevention and then provides examples and evidence of the prevention of mental health disorders.

Key Concepts in Prevention

Primary, Secondary, and Tertiary Prevention

One traditional way to conceptualize prevention is to distinguish primary, secondary, and tertiary prevention. Primary prevention occurs prior to the onset of illness, secondary prevention occurs with early identification and treatment of a disease process, and tertiary prevention avoids disability or rehabilitates function in an ongoing disease process (Caplan 1964).

All three goals are important, yet this classification problematically obscures the distinction between prevention and treatment. For example, treatment of depression into remission might fit the category of both secondary and tertiary prevention, as well as potentially the primary prevention of later anxiety or substance use disorders. To distinguish prevention from treatment, the Institute of Medicine (1994) designated the term *prevention* to mean only primary prevention, referring to those interventions that reduce the occurrence of new cases. This definition, which will be used from this point forward in this chapter, focuses preventive thinking, interventions, and funding on the potentially underemphasized area of stopping the onset of disease, while still allowing for the previously classified secondary and tertiary preventive interventions to be discussed in rigorous discussions about treatment.

Universal, Selective, and Indicated Prevention

Primary preventive interventions can be further subdivided based on how people are targeted (Gordon 1983):

- *Universal interventions* are targeted to an entire population.
- *Selective interventions* are targeted to particular groups at risk for a disease.
- *Indicated interventions* target individuals identified as at risk for a disorder, through known vulnerabilities, combinations of risk factors, or early signs of developing a problem.

In an integrated care setting with the target population being those who attend the primary care office, a universal intervention would target everyone in the office regardless of their perceived risk. For the prevention of depression, a universal intervention might be to encourage everyone to exercise regularly, which is potentially protective against depression (Harvey et al. 2018). A selective intervention might be to offer peer telephone support to postpartum women, a high-risk group for depression (Dennis and Dowswell 2013), and an indicated intervention could be to offer group or individual therapy to people who have subthreshold scores on depression screening instruments (van't Veer-Tazelaar et al. 2009). Further discussion of interventions that may prevent depression will be discussed later in the chapter, but first we explore a public health approach to prevention.

A Public Health Framework for Prevention

Risk and Protective Factors

Prevalent approaches to prevention rely on public health principles. One way this happens is through modifying risk factors or bolstering protective factors. In cardiology, for example, the renowned Framingham cohort study identified previously unknown risk and protective factors for coronary artery disease. From this work, people now know that smoking, high blood pressure, and elevated cholesterol are important risks for heart disease. Health care providers calculate Framingham Risk Scores based on this information to predict chances for future cardiovascular disease (D'Agostino et al. 2013).

Even as we have increasingly understood the pathophysiology of atherosclerosis, the mainstay of primary prevention today has remained the limitation of modifiable risk factors such as smoking and high cholesterol and the enhancement of protective factors through regular exercise and healthy diets. These preventive techniques have even more impact than subsequent strategies developed through a better understanding of atherosclerosis (Frohlich and Quinlan 2014).

In the additional case of infectious diseases, best preventive practices rely on modifying risk and protective factors. In a classic public health example, John Snow observed that the cases in the London cholera outbreak of 1854 centered around the Broad Street water pump. He removed the handle from the water pump, and the cholera epidemic subsided. Before knowledge of the cholera bacterium, he prevented infection by constraining the contaminated water as a risk factor. Even though a vaccine for cholera is available today, the best preventive strategies remain good sanitation and clean water supplies to reduce exposure to the bacteria.

These examples show that prevention through a public health approach can be effective whether or not the underlying pathophysiology of a disease is understood. Prevention based on risk and protective factors continues to be prominent, in many cases, even after further scientific understanding.

Similarly, further understanding of mental health disorders may importantly advance preventive and treatment options. We do not need to wait, however, to practice prevention of mental health disorders. Interventions addressing known risk and protective factors are effective strategies for prevention.

Mental Health Promotion

One might think of mental health much like one thinks of physical health or fitness. We can always strive for better physical health and fitness regardless of whether we have physical illness. This is both a worthy goal in itself and also effective prevention. For example, physical activity and fitness are protective factors against dozens of illnesses and chronic diseases (Booth et al. 2012).

Similarly, rather than being merely the absence of disease, mental health is a positive attribute that can be developed (World Health Organization 2002). Ways to promote mental health include, for example, "enhancing individuals' ability to achieve developmentally appropriate tasks (developmental competence) and a positive sense of self-esteem, mastery, well-being, and social inclusion and to strengthen their ability to cope with adversity" (National Research Council and Institute of Medicine 2009, p. 66). Other ways include enhancing an individual's ability to realize their potential, contribute to the community, productively work, engage in activities, enjoy life, and deal with its challenges (Galderisi et al. 2015).

Mental health promotion is one of the most effective ways to prevent a multitude of mental, emotional, and behavioral disorders (Kern et al. 2017; National Research Council and Institute of Medicine 2009) and is an important public mental health strategy (Kalra et al. 2012). One possible way to visualize the opportunities for prevention and health promotion is shown in Figure 8–1. This diagram helps us visualize a timeline of when preventive strategies can be used in relation to risk factors and symptoms. Selective and indicated interventions are timed in relation to the development of risk factors. Universal strategies are most effective early, prior to the onset of risk factors, yet may be effective at different times. Particularly efforts that develop protective factors and mental health promotion can help prevent mental health disorders at any time. They are visualized as a protective shield that can strengthen at all times.

A Developmental Framework

The public health approach described in this chapter allows us to promote age-appropriate developmental competence as a way of helping to prevent mental health problems. Keeping youth and adults on track with the skills, development, and understanding that they need at each age is a common pathway to prevent many mental, emotional, and behavioral disorders. At each developmental stage, we also have to prevent, limit, and address important risk factors, while promoting protective factors, at both individual and community levels. Several common risk and protective factors span different age groups.

Youth development is especially important in the prevention of mental health disorders because half of all mental, emotional, and behavioral disorders start by age 14, and three-quarters start by age 24 (Kessler et al. 2005). A robust and growing literature shows that addressing risk and protective factors and promoting whole child development, skill building, and strong relationships are effective in promoting prevention (National Research Council and Institute of Medicine 2009). "Indeed the major strides in prevention have largely come from a perspective focused on systematically building competency, not correcting weakness" (Seligman and Csikszentmihalyi 2014). Example preventive interventions at each developmental stage are discussed below.

This discussion of development and the example interventions follow a number of general principles of preventive practice for mental health:

1. Promote mental wellness and youth development.
2. Mitigate risk factors and enhance protective factors, at individual and community levels.
3. Think developmentally.
4. Intervene earlier if possible.
5. Work across institutions—such as school, communities, churches, and health care providers.

In the following subsections, we discuss mental health promotion at each developmental stage, present prominent risk factors to development, suggest protective factors that support youth, and give examples of preventive interventions that may take place at each stage. Many considerations span different developmental stages.

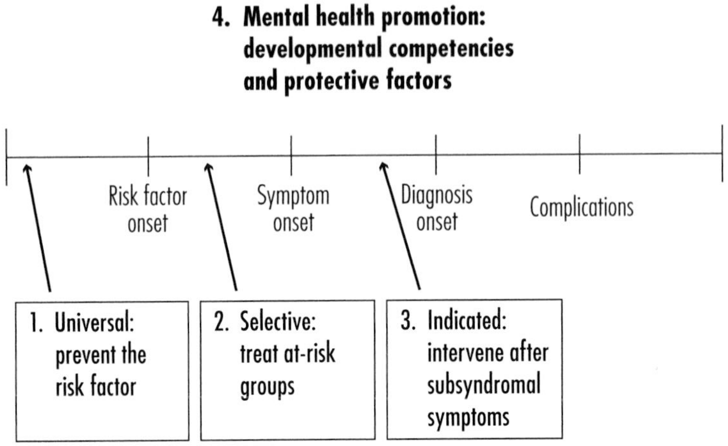

FIGURE 8–1. Four ways of primary prevention.

Prenatal Period

Brain development begins about 3 weeks after conception, followed by development of a rudimentary central and peripheral nervous system by week 8, with rapid growth in cortical, subcortical, and connective pathways continuing beyond birth (Stiles and Jernigan 2010). During the prenatal stage, brain development relies on the general health of the mother. Maternal factors such as maintaining healthy blood pressure and sugar, managing moods and mental health, and having adequate nutrients such as folate all contribute to fetal development.

Risk factors during the prenatal period include nutritional deficiencies and exposure to toxins, such as heavy metals; teratogenic substances; and certain infectious diseases. These risk factors, modifiable at individual and community levels, have impacts when present. For example, fetal alcohol syndrome is estimated to cause between 1% and 5% of children in the United States (May et al. 2018) to have both behavioral and cognitive problems. Lead or heavy metal exposures can also lead to cognitive and behavioral problems (National Scientific Council on the Developing Child 2006). Exposure to infectious diseases, such as toxoplasmosis or the flu, may disrupt brain development and predispose children to mental health disorders. Undernourished mothers have children who are at significantly higher risk of having mental, behavioral, or emotional disorders (Weir 2012).

An additional environmental risk factor is violence in the household, whether verbal, emotional, or physical, because this leads to increases in preterm births, with resultant increases in psychological and behavioral disorders in children (Bailey 2010). Unplanned or unwanted pregnancies can also delay or jeopardize timely prenatal medical care and be an overall risk factor for poorer mental health in the children (Hayatbakhsh et al. 2011).

Protective factors in the prenatal period include family, relational, and medical support. These help support a healthy pregnancy, assure proper maternal nutrition, and prevent undue emotional or mental health stresses. On a community level, protective factors for expecting mothers include easily available access to prenatal care, adequate housing, food supplies, and pregnancy resources.

Example Intervention

One particularly effective intervention starting during the prenatal period is the Nurse-Family Partnership (www.nursefamilypartnership.org). Specially trained nurses visit first-time expectant mothers in their homes starting early in pregnancy and continue through the child's second birthday. The program aims to develop a trusting relationship between the nurses and first-time mothers. This partnership allows medical support and guidance for a healthy pregnancy and then through infancy into the toddler years. The nurses additionally help the mothers envision futures for both their children and themselves. Mothers get support in navigating school, work, relationship, and family responsibilities.

This program has provided positive outcomes for both women and children. Outcomes have included less cigarette smoking and hypertension during pregnancy and fewer preterm births. Families experience less child abuse and neglect. Benefits of the program have been reported in multiple studies, including a 15-year follow-up which showed a 50% reduction in abuse and neglect reports (Olds et al. 1997).

Even though the visits end at age 2 years, children later show improved language development and impulse control, and better academic achievement through the first 6 years of elementary school (Kitzman et al. 2010). Benefits for mothers included less dependence on welfare and government assistance, greater employment, and fewer pregnancies within 18 months of a previous birth, which portends better pregnancy outcomes (Miller 2015). Benefits were highest for at-risk populations such as low-income, unmarried women, and unclear for others. This makes the Nurse-Family Partnership most practical as a selective or indicated intervention for those families most at risk (Donelan-Mccall et al. 2009).

Infancy and Early Childhood

Infants and young children need sufficient nutrition and caregiving to meet physical, communication, and social milestones. A nurturing relationship with one or more adult caregivers is particularly important at this age to provide care and a sense of safety.

Unfortunately, new mothers and fathers are both at risk for postpartum depression and other mental health problems. Biological changes, increased stress, disrupted routines and relationships, and initial difficulty connecting with an infant or young child all pose risks to engaged caregiving, which in turn puts the child at risk.

Adverse childhood experiences are another important set of risk factors. The 10 adverse childhood experiences to be prevented if possible are physical abuse, verbal abuse, sexual abuse, physical neglect, emotional neglect, parental separation, living with a family member with a mental illness, living with a family member with a substance use disorder, having a family member who is incarcerated, and exposure to domestic violence. Each additional adverse life experience increases a child's risk for mental and emotional disorders, substance use, physical health problems, and poorer academic and occupational outcomes. For example, children who have five or more adverse childhood experiences are 7–10 times more likely to use illicit drugs and develop addiction (Felitti et al. 1998).

Possible interventions to address these risk factors include income and food support for families in need and accessible, high-quality child care. The successful treatment of parental mood disorders, if present, alleviates this additional risk to children (Weissman et al. 2006). Also, teaching and modeling positive behaviors for children and parents can make an impact.

Example Intervention

The Incredible Years (www.incredibleyears.com), a combined parent-school intervention, targets preschool and elementary school children at risk for behavioral problems. In the curriculum, parents learn to interact positively with their children and use noncritical disciplinary techniques such as time-outs. Teachers learn effective classroom management techniques, create prosocial classroom environments, and convey social and emotional lessons to the children. Significant outcomes include more nurturing and less harsh parenting, reduced parental depression, better school classroom management, better child social skills and emotion management, children with less aggressive or antisocial behavior, and improved academic success (Reid et al. 2003).

Childhood and School-Age Years

Young children continue to develop competencies: learning in school, handling social situations, making friends, following rules, and showing prosocial behavior. Additionally, they are learning to express emotions, develop self-efficacy, and show understanding and empathy. Risks continue to be undernourishment, adverse childhood experiences, and instability in the caregiving or family situation. Protective factors include consistent, positive discipline; extended family support; getting along with peers; and safe, effective schools.

Example Interventions

The Triple P—Positive Parenting Program is a successful example of an intervention for preventing behavioral and emotional problems in children and teenagers (www.triplep.net/glo-en/home). This program focuses on influencing the social and emotional skills of parents on a variety of levels (Sanders et al. 2000). As a form of universal prevention, mass media information focuses on effective parenting and solutions to common child-rearing problems. Parents also get brief advice from parenting support systems (e.g., pediatricians) and may request information for specific common parenting challenges (e.g., feeding, bedtime strategies, toileting), as a form of selective prevention. Also, parents who have children with more problematic behaviors such as aggression or defiance can learn specific social and emotional parenting skills to deal with these behaviors in 12 one-hour sessions, accomplishing an indicated prevention.

Triple P reduces parental depression and anxiety and decreases children's behavioral problems, which have been maintained at 2 years of follow-up (Ireland et al. 2003). These results have been replicated in multiple groups of children, including children with attention-deficit/hyperactivity disorder. In addition, Triple P has reduced child maltreatment and out-of-home placements for children (Prinz 2016).

In another approach, the Seattle Social Development Project simultaneously involved parents, teachers, and school children. It focused on parenting, classroom management, and children's social competence and showed sustained, interdisciplinary outcomes. Fifteen years later, program participants had more educational attainment, better civic engagement, and fewer mental health disorders and lifetime sexually transmitted diseases compared with control subjects. Participants showed sustained positive directional patterns for 27 of the 28 tracked outcomes across school, work, community, health, mental health, crime, and sexual behaviors (Hawkins et al. 2008).

Adolescence

Adolescents navigate changing physical development while trying to develop a positive sense of self. They independently challenge themselves to make more complicated decisions, develop a moral sense, and control and cope with intense emotions—all while trying to remain socially connected to peers and others (Guerra and Bradshaw 2008). Community protective factors that can facilitate these developmental tasks include positive and safe school and developmental settings that provide opportunities for adolescents to belong and possible mentors. Teaching concrete skills to adolescents and families is one way to address some of the risks adolescents can face—ineffective coping, persistent negative emotions, antisocial behavior, and substance use.

Example Intervention

The Adolescent Transitions Program works with middle schools to provide parenting support via a family resource center. The program strengthens family management skills of encouragement, limit setting, problem solving, and communication patterns. It showed sustained effects, over a 5-year follow-up period, of reduced substance use, fewer arrests, better school attendance, and improved academic performance (Dishion and Kavanagh 2005). A cost-effectiveness study showed a 400% return on investment; for every dollar spent, there were benefits of $5.02 across multidisciplinary systems (Aos et al. 2004).

Early Adulthood

Young adults explore their identities through love, work, and worldview, with an increasing sense of decision making, self-sufficiency, and financial independence. Risks include antisocial behavior, substance use, and fewer competencies in school or workplace. Protective factors include developing autonomy, future orientation, and strong relationships within the family. Communities can embrace young adults through opportunities for exploration in school and work and support systems for people struggling in school or work.

Example Interventions

Known effective interventions for young adults include efforts to reduce substance use and intervene after early signs of a mental health disorder. Below we present interventions for the prevention of depression that are largely targeted to adolescents and young adults with risk factors or early symptoms of depression. Figure 8–2 provides an expansion and summary of the previous discussion of preventive interventions that can be effective at various developmental levels.

Developmental Framework Summary

Prevention in mental health emphasizes a public health, developmental, whole child approach. Focusing on youth and adult development, with attention to risk and protective factors, provides a common strategy to prevent a diverse range of emotional, behavioral, and mental health disorders. We do not deny the role that biological factors play; indeed, we continually learn more about combinations of genes that pose risks, through gene-environment interactions, for a variety of mental health disorders (European Network of National Networks studying Gene-Environment Interactions in Schizophrenia et al. 2014; Lohoff 2010). This discussion, however, focuses on risk and protective factors and developmental course as potentially modifiable pieces toward the goals of prevention and mental health promotion.

Prevention of Depression

The previous subsection focused on efforts to promote age-appropriate developmental competence as a way of preventing mental health disorders. Another way to approach prevention is to examine particular mental health problems and how to prevent them. For example, effective strategies in preventing major depressive disorder could make a significant difference, especially given that the lifetime prevalence is 1 in 6 people in the United States (Kessler et al. 2005).

Risks for major depressive disorder include dysfunctional parenting and family interactions; personality and temperament; cognitive vulnerabilities; internal and external stress, including negative life events; poor interpersonal relationships; and subsyndromal depressive symptoms. Additional societal risk factors include poverty, violence, and cultural factors (Craighead et al. 2017). Protective factors include social skills, problem-solving skills, stress management skills, prosocial behavior, and social support.

Given these risk and protective factors, what indicated, selective, and universal strategies might prevent a depressive disorder prior to onset? Are there ways to build strengths, skills, and resiliency in the face of risks and early symptoms? Approaches that have shown considerable promise in prevention studies include cognitive-behavioral programs, interpersonal therapy, and family educational interventions for individuals at risk. These

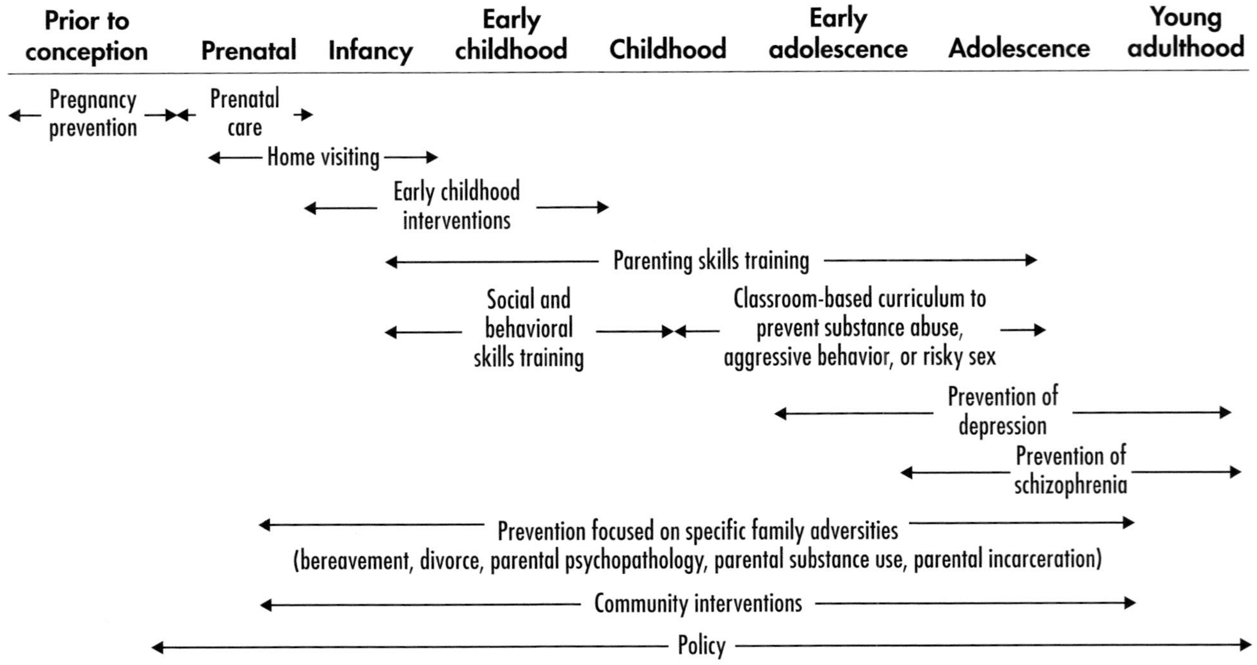

FIGURE 8–2. Preventive interventions by developmental phase.

Source. Reprinted from National Research Council and Institute of Medicine Committee on the Prevention of Mental Disorders and Substance Abuse Among Children, Youth, and Young Adults: *Research Advances and Promising Interventions: Preventing Mental, Emotional, and Behavioral Disorders Among Young People: Progress and Possibilities.* Washington, DC, National Academies Press, 2009. Copyright © 2009 National Academy of Sciences, Courtesy of the National Academies Press.

interventions prevent people from developing the symptoms and dysfunction that lead to onset of major depressive disorder.

Indicated Interventions

Several approaches have shown efficacy in work with individuals at high risk of depression and those showing early symptoms. The Penn Resilience Program was found effective with youth ages 10–13 years who were considered at risk for depression based on their self-reports of parental conflict and depressive symptoms. Participants were selected in part through looking for negative self-evaluations, dysfunctional attitudes, poor interpersonal problem solving, and low expectations for self-performance. The program taught cognitive-behavioral strategies to address cognitive vulnerabilities, and problem-solving and coping skills to deal with stresses. Meta-analyses of its dozens of studies showed decreases in depressive symptoms and reduced onset of depressive disorders when used in an indicated manner for individuals at high risk and showing early symptoms (Hetrick et al. 2015). These results were sustained through at least 12 months of follow-up (Craighead et al. 2017).

Other efficacious, indicated interventions to prevent depression include using cognitive-behavioral therapy (CBT) for adolescents (Clarke et al. 1995) and interpersonal therapy for postpartum women (Dennis and Dowswell 2013). Delivering CBT through an Internet-delivered therapy format (Muñoz et al. 2010) and delivering it in an integrated primary care setting to prevent late-life depression (van't Veer-Tazelaar et al. 2009) show initial promise and are examples of further interventions being studied.

Selective Interventions

Techniques just described for use in indicated interventions have potential to be effective as selective interventions for high-risk groups. Studies have shown effectiveness in particular for two groups: women in the perinatal period and children of depressed parents.

Women at risk for depression in the perinatal period include those with current subsyndromal depressive symptoms; a history of depression; psychosocial risk factors such as low income, recent intimate partner violence, or single parenthood; or mental health factors such as elevated anxiety or a history of significant negative life events. All such women are encouraged to seek CBT or interpersonal therapy that has convincing evidence of preventive effect and moderate certainty of net benefit (U.S. Preventive Services Task Force et al. 2019).

Other interventions in the perinatal period, such as physical activity, education, pharmacotherapy, dietary supplements, and health system interventions, have some limited or mixed evidence of efficacy. Home visits by a nurse, flexible postnatal midwife visits, and peer postnatal telephone support and screening also have shown initial promise as psychosocial interventions (Dennis and Dowswell 2013).

Interventions for children of depressed parents also have shown efficacy. For example, Family Talk provided psychoeducation to parents on the effects of parental depression on children and ways the parents could respond; it also taught children about depression and the effect it could be having on their parents (Beardslee et al. 2003). Incorporating protective factors such as understanding, encouragement of self-reflection, and stronger relationships between parents and children, Family Talk has demonstrated significant gains in behaviors and attitudes toward depression for parents and understanding of the illness by children. The intervention resulted in decreases in depressive symptoms and overall increases in family functioning, which were sustained for more than 4 years (Beardslee et al. 2007). Family Talk has been effectively adapted for use with inner-city, single-parent, minority families (Podorefsky et al. 2001); with Latino families (D'Angelo et al. 2009); in Head Start programs (Beardslee et al. 2009); and in a variety of programs in Europe (Solantaus et al. 2009). Mediating factors for effectiveness were conversations between parents and children about depression and improvements in parents' functioning.

Another way to benefit the children of depressed mothers is to treat the mother's depressive symptoms into remission. This intervention decreases symptoms of depression and psychopathology in the children (Weissman et al. 2006) and correlates with increased functioning in the children (Wickramaratne et al. 2011).

Universal Interventions

As discussed earlier in this chapter, developmental approaches focused on parenting and development of children's social and emotional skills improved a number of outcomes, including emotion regulation and depressive symptoms. Some interventions, such as Triple P, had universal components; however, several programs, such as the Nurse-Family Partnership, were effective as selective or indicated interventions but not as universal interventions. The Penn Resilience Program also showed effects in an indicated subpopulation of at-risk youth but no overall effect when studied as a universal intervention (Spence and Shortt 2007).

Although indicated and selective strategies have promising evidence for the prevention of depression in at-risk individuals and groups, no rigorous evidence currently shows effectiveness for the universal, population prevention of depression (van Zoonen et al. 2014). With few studies dedicated to universal prevention, however, it is difficult to make a conclusion at this time. Researchers of universal preventive efforts for depression may not have used the right approach, studied a large enough sample, or included long enough follow-up to detect a significant effect. An alternative possibility is that cognitive-behavioral and skill-building interventions are effective for high-risk youth but not for a universal population.

Health Promotion

Interest is growing in health promotion strategies for the prevention of depression and other mental illnesses. In a large cohort study of 11 years, exercise of at least 1 hour a week reduced new incidence of depression by one-third, mediated potentially by increased parasympathetic activity, greater perceived social support, and a decreased onset of comorbid physical illnesses (Harvey et al. 2018).

Other efforts emphasize the importance of nutrition. Unhealthy diets consistently seem to correlate with worse mental health in children and adolescents (O'Neil et al. 2014). Nutrient deficiencies are a risk factor for the development of depression, and supplementation of nutrients such as omega-3 fatty acids, *S*-adenosyl methionine, *N*-acetylcysteine, and vitamins B and D may impact and even prevent depression for some people. Healthier diets, such as the Mediterranean diet, also may be protective for new-onset depression (Sarris et al. 2015). Although the effects of diet for mental health still need to be confirmed, an integrated approach that includes physical activity and healthy diets would likely be more effective than isolated approaches (Berk and Janka 2019). Other health promotion efforts include educating people about getting sufficient micro- and macronutrients, eating gut-healthy foods, and participating in mindfulness practices or other positive psychological strategies.

Prevention of Depression Summary

The overall effect of programs to prevent depression could be a 21% decrease in the incidence of depressive disorders in targeted intervention groups (van Zoonen et al. 2014). Given the high prevalence, morbidity, and cost of depressive disorders, further action to prevent depression is needed. As Craighead and colleagues (2017) concluded, "Based on the preceding summaries of outcomes, we should begin to disseminate CBT and family-based programs as a major public health initiative. Both the international consortium on the prevention of depression...and others...have strongly suggested such an effort" (p. 86). Early screening for risk factors and subsyndromal symptoms may help direct increasingly large numbers of people to effective, targeted interventions. These indicated and selective prevention measures of providing cognitive flexibility, behavioral options and tools, and family psychoeducation to at-risk youth are usually delivered in group settings, at relatively low costs. Even if only a few individuals in an intervention group are able to avoid a later depressive disorder, those few avoid the high interdisciplinary costs of a depressive disorder and its decades of potential morbidity. This outcome also looks favorable when analyzed by the cost of reducing disability. For example, using group-based psychological instruction for the prevention of adolescent depression costs about $5,000 (Australian dollars) and psychological treatment for postpartum depression costs about $15,000 (Australian dollars) per depression-free year. Both of these figures indicate highly cost-effective interventions (Mihalopoulos et al. 2011).

Cost-Effectiveness of Programs

Another way to look at economic benefits is to examine the cost savings of preventing mental health disorders. For example, for every $1 spent on the Seattle Social Development Project, an estimated $3 was saved that otherwise would have been spent on health and mental health problems, disability payments, juvenile justice expenses, or employment expenses such as short-term disability. The same analysis showed that the Adolescent Transitions Program saved $5 per dollar spent on the program (Aos et al. 2004).

These analyses highlight the economic savings from prevention. The cost of mental, emotional, and behavioral disorders for young people—taking into account the costs of mental health and health services, productivity, and crime—was estimated at $247 billion in 2007 (National Research Council and Institute of Medicine 2009). This estimate does not include indirect costs, such as the cost to families for caring for a child with mental illness. Programs that prevent these disorders reduce these costs.

Programs with sustained effects over many years continue to accrue these savings over the lifetimes of the youths affected. The Seattle Social Development Project saved an estimated $10,000 per youth involved in the program (Aos et al. 2004). With outcomes sustained over at least 15 years (Hawkins et al. 2008), these initial savings continue to grow every year of additional sustained outcomes.

Given the positive population health possibilities of prevention, the value and cost savings across interdisciplinary systems, and the positive experiences for both patients and providers, prevention is a pure expression of the

Quadruple Aim in health care (see Chapter 1, "Defining and Measuring Value," for more about the Quadruple Aim). A robust and growing evidence base shows that prevention in mental health is possible, primarily through a focus on youth development and mental health promotion. Evidence for indicated, selective, and universal strategies for prevention of mental health disorders is also growing.

Implementing Prevention and Mental Health Promotion

Even with the cost and health benefits of prevention, implementation of its evidence base will only happen with intentional efforts. Many barriers exist, including funding and aligning more efforts toward preventive and health promotion principles. Government, community, and individuals all can play an important role.

On a public policy level, government should reduce known risks and increase protective factors for mental health disorders. Mental and emotional well-being is an explicit priority of the U.S. national prevention strategy (National Prevention Council 2012), and actions could include promoting healthy and safe communities, including opportunities for physical activity and healthy foods, as well as improving the quality of the environment and limiting exposure to toxic heavy metals and air pollution.

Reducing the rates or stresses of poverty would address another common risk factor for many mental and emotional disorders (National Research Council and Institute of Medicine 2009). Policies such as tenant rental assistance, active labor market policies, and a living wage ordinance are examples of how government can alleviate the effects of poverty (Komro et al. 2013). Additionally, youth development programs for children rated the highest level of evidence for lowering the stresses of poverty due to the outcomes of fewer anxiety, depressive, and conduct problems in children; they also create better long-run educational and employment outcomes for the children involved.

Governments should provide ample funding for these evidence-based, high-quality health promotion and preventive efforts, with the knowledge that doing so would produce value in both health outcomes and savings. For example, public support of the Nurse-Family Partnership, authorized through the U.S. Department of Health and Human Services, has shown positive impacts for mothers, child development, and reduction of adverse childhood experiences for children in multi-site studies (Miller 2015). Programs like this can be funded, expanded, and improved for greater impact.

Effective community implementation of evidence-based programs depends on funding, in addition to community factors such as knowledgeable and organized community leaders and a coalition of engaged community stakeholders (Shapiro et al. 2015). Ideally, communities also need to adapt programs for their particular cultural, linguistic, and socioeconomic demographics. One example of an approach that accomplishes this is the Communities That Care program (www.communitiesthatcare.net), which starts with the creation of a community prevention board to survey community assets and identify prevention priorities. Based on community-chosen goals, a menu of evidence-based prevention programs is developed to address the relevant risk factors and protective factors present in the community. This process has fared well in multi-year process and outcome evaluations. Results included substantially less youth substance abuse, violence, and antisocial behavior through at least age 21, for several years after direct participation in program interventions (Oesterle et al. 2018).

Community implementation of evidence-based mental health promotion and prevention practices faces a number of obstacles. Successful implementation requires "coordinated change at system, organization, program, and practice levels" (Fixsen et al. 2005, p. vi). Challenges at any of these levels could jeopardize desired outcomes. Inconsistent government funding, unsupportive policies or regulations, lack of community investment, poor leadership or organization at community institutions, or high turnover among program staff have all been implementation obstacles faced by communities. Prevention is not always a core expertise of community institutions, and most evidence-based prevention programs do not have sufficient if any technical assistance for communities (Greenberg 2004). Capacity building for prevention at all of these policy, community, and individual levels should be a priority as part of realizing the benefits of an evidence-based prevention agenda.

Short of fully adopting or funding evidence-based programs, communities can also strive to encourage common principles among evidence-based prevention approaches. Examples include the following (National Research Council and Institute of Medicine 2009):

- Reducing youth exposure to harsh discipline, abuse, and neglect
- Positive reinforcement of prosocial behavior
- Acceptance and encouragement in family, school, and community settings
- Supportive environments with nurturance
- Techniques such as praise notes, peer-to-peer tutoring, and caregiver training to create nurturing environments
- Adequate sleep, diet, and exercise, and television viewing limits aimed toward positive health outcomes

Although these principles have not been studied in isolation, each is a reasonable approach based on themes from many different evidence-based inquiries.

Behavioral Kernels

Recent efforts have also tried to separate specific preventive behaviors for individuals or groups. These could be practiced whether part of broader prevention efforts or not, without needing the infrastructure of a community-based effort or the funding of an evidence-based program.

Common behavioral kernels, distilled from evidence-based prevention programs, have been identified that can be used in home, school, or community settings. Examples for parents to use at home include positive reinforcement, positive discipline such as time-outs, and encouragement of youth self-monitoring. Cooperative playground games at school and positive notes home from teachers have reduced aggression, a common risk factor for many mental and emotional disorders. Embry and Biglan (2008) identified 52 of these discrete, actionable, behavioral kernels from common themes in multiple evidence-based programs.

Separating behavioral kernels from proprietary, evidenced-based program materials allows them to be more accessible for dissemination. Public mental health strategies can then advertise behavioral kernels similarly to the promotion of health strategies, such as vaccines or child car seats. This type of action may allow public mental health strategies to counter well-funded advertising for mental health risk factors such as alcohol and tobacco.

These materials, if enough institutions, groups, and people used them, could have a broader population effect, similar to a behavioral vaccine. People practicing positive mental health strategies would model them for others. As norms shifted, fewer youths might engage in risky behaviors such as aggression or substance use. This type of change could lead to the "herd immunity" effect of vaccines by changing the culture and peer pressure with which youth respond (Embry 2011).

Health care and mental health professionals can particularly benefit from knowing and practicing individual actions for prevention and mental health promotion. In addition, sharing behavioral prevention strategies with the many people we serve could amplify the impact of such practices.

Prevention Training

Reaching medical professionals early during their training is strongly desired but presently not well done. Medical students start with positive attitudes toward the importance and effectiveness of preventive interventions (Bellas et al. 2000), and academic associations, medical schools, and medical educators all recognize the importance of teaching prevention and population health strategies (Garr et al. 2004). Yet, surveys consistently show that as medical students learn more about disease and pathophysiology, their attitudes toward prevention deteriorate during medical training (Kershaw et al. 2017).

An emphasis on the health benefits of behavioral kernels could be analogous to teaching exercise medicine. Promoting physical exercise, when presented well, is enthusiastically embraced by medical students for both themselves and their patients (Jones et al. 2013). Promoting behavioral kernels could similarly allow discrete actions for mental health promotion to be widely known. Trainees could learn by practicing kernels that promote their well-being, such as taking omega-3 fatty acids, aerobic activity, proper rest, and progressive muscle relaxation. Like exercise, these could be important tools for providers, given the high rates of provider burnout (West et al. 2018), as well as for patients.

In the absence of strong government or community adoption of mental health promotion and prevention principles, individuals can try to practice behavioral kernels. From the inside out, individuals can create positive mental health cultures, and influence the settings where they live and work. By spreading this knowledge to the patients we serve, greater population effects, such as healthy youth development and the prevention and reduction of substance use, are possible.

Relevance of Prevention for Psychiatrists and Mental Health Professionals

Our primary charge as mental health professionals is to work with individuals already showing symptoms of illness. Although our day-to-day experience may not routinely require work with people prior to the onset of illness, in broadening the view of our work, there are many possible connections to prevention.

We strive to create mental health in our work, an effort that makes preventive strategies directly relevant. In seeing someone suffering from depressive symptoms, we naturally try to prevent further dysfunction from substance use. We try to reduce the impact of mental illness on relationships to mitigate the stresses on family and friends, potentially lowering their risk of mental health problems.

An especially important goal is that we use our prevention expertise toward overall population mental health. Prevalence rates for mental health disorders are high; it is estimated that approximately 1 in 5 children and adults suffer annually from at least one mental health disorder (Substance Abuse and Mental Health Services Administration 2016). Because half the people with a mental health disorder in the United States did not receive treatment in the previous year (Stockman 2012), we cannot achieve overall population health solely through care in our offices. We need to use our expertise to advocate for effective, preventive strategies that could reduce the burden of mental illness.

The following are suggested preventive principles for the practicing mental health clinician:

- Reach people as early as possible, ideally when they are at risk or are showing early symptoms of a disorder.
- Encourage integrated partnerships with primary care physicians. This is one way to screen and catch people with early mental health signs and symptoms.
- In work with children, encourage their developmental competencies. Use preventive strategies for children at risk, such as children of parents with mental illness.
- Work in systems—with primary care physicians, health-outreach community organizations, schools, churches, and juvenile justice systems.
- Promote whole health and mental wellness, such as healthy living, emotion management, and healthy parenting.
- Promote discrete behavioral kernels to people you serve for mental health promotion, child development, or behavior change.
- Encourage health-promoting actions, such as exercise, healthy diet, smoking cessation, recreation, meditation, and so forth.
- Think about the support systems for the people you see. Treating symptoms into remission may prevent onset of illness in a relative. Family members may benefit from understanding relevant services for them.
- Advocate for policy addressing public health risk factors, such as poverty and exposure to violence, which are common mental health risk factors.

Through concrete ways of linking our practice to family, systems, and health promotion, there are many ways to implement prevention in our daily work. Some evidence-based preventive strategies can even be office based, such as having group meetings for subsyndromal adolescents or treating parental depression with family psychoeducation to reduce risk for the children.

Vision of the Future—A Public Health Approach

Prevention's tenets require us to follow proven ways to support mental health and prevent mental health problems. Current evidence points to approaches such as access to early prenatal care, pre- and postpartum supports for mothers, high-quality child care and schools, parenting programs and supports, school social and emotional strength building, and more.

Our responsibility to the population's mental health calls for creating routine access to proven preventive interventions and addressing risk and protective factors at different stages of development. Our social policies should address the common ills of poverty, violence, discrimination, and social isolation. They should support vibrant schools and communities and commit necessary resources in support of healthy children and families. Our community institutions should support multiple points of entry for youth to learn appropriate developmental, communication, and relationship skills. Our individual actions should align with common behavioral actions that tend to promote mental health.

Prevention is the best value in medicine. Prevention is cost-effective by saving health care and other social costs. With robust evidence that prevention is achievable, prevention provides what both patients and providers desire by preserving health and mental health. The value is indisputable; the question is one of values. Can we reorganize ourselves to provide more of our resources toward youth development and the promotion of mental health for all? Are we willing to reduce the stresses of abuse, neglect, and poverty and to invest more in programs and approaches for high-risk youth? Can the mental health professional community promote health, practice behavioral kernels, and encourage systematic ways to intervene earlier?

The vision for an intentional future based on prevention shows us a proven path to promoting youth and human development. Although obstacles exist, our children deserve all of our efforts.

References

Aos S, Lieb R, Mayfield J, et al: New study outlines benefits and costs of prevention and early intervention programs for youth. Washington State Institute for Public Policy, 2004. Available at: www.wsipp.wa.gov/ReportFile/881/Wsipp_Benefits-and-Costs-of-Prevention-and-Early-Intervention-Programs-for-Youth_Summary-Report.pdf. Accessed February 20, 2020.

Bailey B: Partner violence during pregnancy: prevalence, effects, screening, and management. Int J Womens Health 2:183–197, 2010

Beardslee WR, Gladstone TRG, Wright EJ, et al: A family-based approach to the prevention of depressive symptoms in children at risk: evidence of parental and child change. Pediatrics 112(2):e119–e131, 2003

Beardslee WR, Wright ETJ, Gladstone TR: Supplemental material for long-term effects from a randomized trial of two public health preventive interventions for parental depression. J Fam Psychol 21(4):703–713, 2007

Beardslee WR, Avery MW, Ayoub C, et al: Family Connections: helping early Head Start/Head Start staff and parents address mental health challenges. Zero to Three Journal 29:34–42, 2009

Bellas PA, Asch SM, Wilkes M: What students bring to medical school. Am J Prev Med 18(3):242–248, 2000

Berk M, Janka FN: Diet and depression—from confirmation to implementation. JAMA 321(9):842–843, 2019

Booth FW, Roberts CK, Laye MJ: Lack of exercise is a major cause of chronic diseases. Compr Physiol 2(2):1143–1211, 2012

Caplan G: Principles of Preventive Psychiatry. Foreword by Robert H. Felix. New York, Basic Books, 1964, pp 26–27

Clarke GN, Hawkins W, Murphy M, et al: Targeted prevention of unipolar depressive disorder in an at-risk sample of high school adolescents: a randomized trial of a group cognitive intervention. J Am Acad Child Adolesc Psychiatry 34(3):312–321, 1995

Craighead WE, Beardslee W, Johnson R: Prevention of depression and bipolar disorder, in Treating and Preventing Adolescent Mental Health Disorders: What We Know and What We Don't Know, 2nd Edition. Edited by Evans DL, Foa EB, Gur RE, et al. New York, Oxford University Press, 2017, pp 69–88

D'Agostino RB Sr, Pencina MJ, Massaro JM, Coady S: Cardiovascular disease risk assessment: insights from Framingham. Glob Heart 8(1):11–23, 2013

D'Angelo EJ, Llerena-Quinn R, Shapiro R, et al: Adaptation of the preventive intervention program for depression for use with predominantly low-income Latino families. Fam Process 48(2):269–291, 2009

Dennis C-L, Dowswell T: Psychosocial and psychological interventions for preventing postpartum depression. Cochrane Database Syst Rev (2):CD001134, 2013

Dishion TJ, Kavanagh K: Intervening in Adolescent Problem Behavior: A Family Centered Approach. New York, Guilford, 2005

Donelan-Mccall N, Eckenrode J, Olds DL: Home visiting for the prevention of child maltreatment: lessons learned during the past 20 years. Pediatr Clin North Am 56(2):389–403, 2009

Embry DD: Behavioral vaccines and evidence-based kernels: nonpharmaceutical approaches for the prevention of mental, emotional, and behavioral disorders. Psychiatr Clin North Am 34(1):1–34, 2011

Embry DD, Biglan A: Evidence-based kernels: fundamental units of behavioral influence. Clin Child Fam Psychol Rev 11(3):75–113, 2008

European Network of National Networks studying Gene-Environment Interactions in Schizophrenia; van Os J, Rutten BP, et al: Identifying gene-environment interactions in schizophrenia: contemporary challenges for integrated, large-scale investigations. Schizophr Bull 40(4):729–736, 2014

Felitti VJ, Anda RF, Nordenberg D, et al: Relationship of childhood abuse and household dysfunction to many of the leading causes of death in adults. Am J Prev Med 14(4):245–258, 1998

Fixsen D, Naoom S, Blase K, et al: Implementation Research: A Synthesis of the Literature. Tampa, FL, University of South Florida, Louis de la Parte Florida Mental Health Institute, National Implementation Research Network, 2005

Frohlich E, Quinlan P: Coronary heart disease risk factors: public impact of initial and later-announced risks. Ochsner J 14(4):532–537, 2014

Galderisi S, Heinz A, Kastrup M, et al: Toward a new definition of mental health. World Psychiatry 14(2):231–233, 2015

Garr DR, Lackland DT, Wilson DB: Prevention education and evaluation in U.S. medical schools. Acad Med 75(7 Suppl):S14–S21, 2004

Gordon R: An operational classification of disease prevention. Public Health Rep 98(2):107–109, 1983

Greenberg MT: Current and future challenges in school-based prevention: the researcher perspective. Prev Sci 5(1):5–13, 2004

Guerra NG, Bradshaw CP: Linking the prevention of problem behaviors and positive youth development: core competencies for positive youth development and risk prevention. New Dir Child Adolesc Dev 2008(122):1–17, 2008

Harvey SB, Overland S, Hatch SL, et al: Exercise and the prevention of depression: results of the HUNT cohort study. Am J Psychiatry 175(4):28–36, 2018

Hawkins JD, Kosterman R, Catalano RF, et al: Effects of social development intervention in childhood 15 years later. Arch Pediatr Adolesc Med 162(12):1133–1141, 2008

Hayatbakhsh MR, Najman JM, Khatun M, et al: A longitudinal study of child mental health and problem behaviours at 14 years of age following unplanned pregnancy. Psychiatry Res 185(1–2):200–204, 2011

Hetrick S, Cox G, Merry S: Where to go from here? An exploratory meta-analysis of the most promising approaches to depression prevention programs for children and adolescents. Int J Environ Res Public Health 12(5):4758–4795, 2015

Institute of Medicine: Reducing Risks for Mental Disorders: Frontiers for Preventive Intervention Research. Washington, DC, National Academies Press, 1994

Ireland JL, Sanders MR, Markie-Dodds C: The impact of parent training on marital functioning: a comparison of two group versions of the Triple P-Positive Parenting Program for parents of children with early onset conduct problems. Behavioural and Cognitive Psychotherapy 31:127–142, 2003

Jones PR, Brooks JHM, Wylie A: Realising the potential for an Olympic legacy; teaching medical students about sport and exercise medicine and exercise prescribing. Br J Sports Med 47(17):1090–1094, 2013

Kalra G, Christodoulou G, Jenkins R, et al: Mental health promotion: guidance and strategies. Eur Psychiatry 27(2):81–86, 2012

Kern ML, Park N, Romer D: The positive perspective on youth development, in Treating and Preventing Adolescent Mental Health Disorders: What We Know and What We Don't Know, 2nd Edition. Edited by Evans DL, Foa EB, Gur RE, et al. New York, Oxford University Press, 2017, pp 543–570

Kershaw G, Grivna M, Elbarazi I, et al: Integrating public health and health promotion practice in the medical curriculum: a self-directed team-based project approach. Front Public Health 5:193, 2017

Kessler RC, Berglund P, Demler O, et al: Lifetime prevalence and age-of-onset distributions of DSM-IV disorders in the National Comorbidity Survey Replication. Arch Gen Psychiatry 62(6):593–602, 2005

Kitzman HJ, Olds DL, Cole RE, et al: Enduring effects of prenatal and infancy home visiting by nurses on children. Arch Pediatr Adolesc Med 164(5):412–418, 2010

Komro KA, Tobler AL, Delisle AL, et al: Beyond the clinic: improving child health through evidence-based community development. BMC Pediatr 13:172, 2013

Lohoff FW: Overview of the genetics of major depressive disorder. Curr Psychiatry Rep 12(6):539–546, 2010

May PA, Chambers CD, Kalberg WO, et al: Prevalence of fetal alcohol spectrum disorders in 4 U.S. communities. JAMA 319(5):474–482, 2018

Mihalopoulos C, Vos T, Pirkis J, et al: The economic analysis of prevention in mental health programs. Ann Rev Clin Psychol 7:169–201, 2011

Miller TR: Projected outcomes of Nurse-Family Partnership home visitation during 1996–2013, USA. Prev Sci 16(6):765–777, 2015

Muñoz RF, Cuijpers P, Smit F, et al: Prevention of major depression. Annu Rev Clin Psychol 6:181–212, 2010

National Prevention Council: National Prevention Council action plan. 2012. Available at: www.surgeongeneral.gov/priorities/prevention/2012-npc-action-plan.pdf. Accessed February 20, 2020.

National Research Council and Institute of Medicine Committee on the Prevention of Mental Disorders and Substance Abuse Among Children, Youth, and Young Adults: Research Advances and Promising Interventions: Preventing Mental, Emotional, and Behavioral Disorders Among Young People: Progress and Possibilities. Washington, DC, National Academies Press, 2009

National Scientific Council on the Developing Child: Early exposure to toxic substances damages brain architecture: working paper number 4. 2006. Available at: https://developingchild.harvard.edu/resources/early-exposure-to-toxic-substances-damages-brain-architecture. Accessed February 20, 2020.

Oesterle S, Kuklinski MR, Hawkins JD, et al: Long-term effects of the Communities That Care trial on substance use, antisocial behavior, and violence through age 21 years. Am J Public Health 108(5):659–665, 2018

Olds DL, Eckenrode J, Henderson CR, et al: Long-term effects of home visitation on maternal life course and child abuse and neglect. JAMA 278(8):637–643, 1997

O'Neil A, Quirk SE, Housden S, et al: Relationship between diet and mental health in children and adolescents: a systematic review. Am J Public Health 104(10):e31–e42, 2014

Podorefsky DL, McDonald-Dowdell M, Beardslee WR: Adaptation of preventive interventions for a low-income, culturally diverse community. J Am Acad Child Adolesc Psychiatry 40(8):879–886, 2001

Prinz RJ: Parenting and family support within a broad child abuse prevention strategy. Child Abuse Negl 51:400–406, 2016

Reid MJ, Webster-Stratton C, Hammond M: Follow-up of children who received the Incredible Years intervention for oppositional-defiant disorder: maintenance and prediction of 2-year outcome. Behavior Therapy 34(4):471–491, 2003

Sanders MR, Markie-Dadds C, Tully LA, et al: The Triple P-Positive Parenting Program: a comparison of enhanced, standard, and self-directed behavioral family intervention for parents of children with early onset conduct problems. J Consult Clin Psychol 68(4):624–640, 2000

Sarris J, Logan AC, Akbaraly TN, et al: Nutritional medicine as mainstream in psychiatry. Lancet Psychiatry 2(3):271–274, 2015

Seligman MEP, Csikszentmihalyi M: Positive psychology: an introduction, in Flow and the Foundations of Positive Psychology: The Collected Works of Mihaly Csikszentmihalyi. New York, Springer, 2014, pp 279–298

Shapiro VB, Hawkins JD, Oesterle S: Building local infrastructure for community adoption of science-based prevention: the role of coalition functioning. Prev Sci 16(8):1136–1146, 2015

Solantaus T, Toikka S, Alasuutari M, et al: Safety, feasibility and family experiences of preventive interventions for children and families with parental depression. International Journal of Mental Health Promotion 11(4):15–24, 2009

Spence SH, Shortt AL: Research review: Can we justify the widespread dissemination of universal, school-based interventions for the prevention of depression among children and adolescents? J Child Psychol Psychiatry 48(6):526–542, 2007

Stiles J, Jernigan TL: The basics of brain development. Neuropsychol Rev 20(4):327–348, 2010

Stockman J: Lifetime prevalence of mental disorders in U.S. adolescents: results from the National Comorbidity Survey Replication—Adolescent Supplement (NCS-A). Yearbook of Pediatrics 2012:385–387, 2012

Substance Abuse and Mental Health Services Administration: Key substance use and mental health indicators in the United States: results from the 2015 National Survey on Drug Use and Health. Center for Behavioral Health Statistics and Quality. 2016. Available at: www.samhsa.gov/data/sites/default/files/NSDUH-FFR1-2015/NSDUH-FFR1-2015/NSDUH-FFR1-2015. Accessed February 20, 2020.

U.S. Preventive Services Task Force; Curry SJ, Krist AH, et al: Interventions to prevent perinatal depression. JAMA 321(6):580–587, 2019

van Zoonen K, Buntrock C, Ebert DD, et al: Preventing the onset of major depressive disorder: a meta-analytic review of psychological interventions. Int J Epidemiol 43(2):318–329, 2014 van't Veer-Tazelaar PJ, van Marwijk HWJ, van Oppen P, et al: Stepped-care prevention of anxiety and depression in late life. Arch Gen Psychiatry 66(3):297–304, 2009

Weir K: The beginnings of mental illness. American Psychological Association, 2012. Available at: www.apa.org/monitor/2012/02/mental-illness. Accessed February 20, 2020.

Weissman MM, Pilowsky DJ, Wickramaratne PJ, et al: Remissions in maternal depression and child psychopathology: a STAR*D-Child report. JAMA 295(12):1389–1398, 2006

West CP, Dyrbye LN, Shanafelt TD: Physician burnout: contributors, consequences and solutions. J Intern Med 283(6):516–529, 2018

Wickramaratne P, Gameroff MJ, Pilowsky DJ, et al: Children of depressed mothers 1 year after remission of maternal depression: findings from the STAR*D-Child study. Am J Psychiatry 168(6):593–602, 2011

World Health Organization: Prevention and promotion in mental health. 2002. Available at: www.who.int/mental_health/media/en/545.pdf. Accessed February 20, 2020.

9

Peer and Recovery Support Services

Keris Jän Myrick, M.B.A., M.S.
Allen S. Daniels, Ed.D.

Background and Overview

Peer support services have an established role in behavioral health systems of care. There is a rich history that includes long-standing engagements of patients helping others with similar conditions in mental asylums and institutions dating as far back as 1795 (Davidson et al. 2018). The earliest known peer advocacy and support organization, started by John Perceval in England around 1845, was known as the Alleged Lunatics' Friend Society (Podvoll 2003). A variety of organizations and individuals since that time have attempted to enlist those who have experienced disruption of their mental health in the support of others who are struggling. More recent examples include the twentieth-century work of Abraham Low, who founded the Association of Nervous and Former Mental Patients (due to issues related to stigma of their members, the organization was later renamed Recovery, Inc., and then, more recently, Recovery International) (https://recoveryinternational.org/about/#History), and Harry Stack Sullivan, who recognized and deployed the role and mutual support of peers in therapeutic communities (Davidson 2013). Twelve-step programs date back to 1934 with the origin of Alcoholics Anonymous, which focused on alcohol recovery. It has since spawned a number of other programs of peer support for a variety of other emotional health conditions with compulsive elements.

The contemporary roots for peer support services have many key milestones, including recognition in national mental health policy reports, such as those of the President's Commission on Mental Health (1978), the Surgeon General (U.S. Department of Health and Human Services 1999), and the President's New Freedom Commission on Mental Health (2003). The combined findings of these reports indicate that there is a clear consensus that a person-centered behavioral health system must recognize the value that an individual with lived experience managing an illness brings to helping others to find hope and become engaged and activated in their own recovery.

The Substance Abuse and Mental Health Services Administration (SAMHSA) has described *peer support services* as direct services provided by individuals with mental illness and/or substance use disorder who have progressed in their recovery from illness and disability and in the management of their mental health challenges (Chinman et al. 2014). SAMHSA recognizes that with this experience, these individuals can help other people with a similar condition in their journeys toward long-term recovery. Service goals are commonly focused on aiding in the development of problem-solving and coping skills in the self-management of an individual's mental illness. This is achieved as the peer support specialists (PSSs) draw on their own life experiences to share the lessons they have learned and to promote engagement in treatment. This process fosters hope and the belief that recovery is possible. PSSs also help clients to develop the necessary community supports to establish a satisfying and fulfilling life. These services may be provided in a range of settings, including outpatient and inpatient facilities, community-based systems of care coordination and supports, and consumer-run organizations. Although SAMHSA has described these services for individuals with serious mental illness, a number of state Medicaid programs and commercial payers have expanded the scope for these services well beyond that range of individuals. Peer support services have been employed for youth with behavioral health issues, as well as transitional-age adults, parents and family caregivers, and adults. The scope of services in behavioral health includes both mental health and substance use conditions.

Peer support staff undergo specific training and must obtain certification in most states to qualify for this work. The training enables them to provide effective outreach and use their experience to promote engagement and activation in recovery and to sustain community tenure. Davidson and colleagues (2018) cite these roles in describing the evidence base for these services:

When reviewing this evidence, it is important to recognize that neither peer nor non-peer non-clinical staff "treat" mental illness, that is not their role. Peer-support staff complement clinical care; their role is to instill hope, engage patients in self-care and health services, help them navigate complex and fragmented systems, and promote their pursuit of a meaningful life. When assessed on their ability to do these jobs for which they have been trained, peer-support staff clearly demonstrate effectiveness. (p. 2)

Vignette: When Peer Support Services Work Well

Mary is a 30-year-old woman diagnosed with schizophrenia who reported to her psychiatrist that she experiences ongoing feelings of loneliness. Her inability to trust people makes social interactions stressful, and her fear of rejection causes her to isolate. She often hears voices and responds to them out loud, which she later realizes seems strange to others around her. She also feels that the people she does know, including her family, mostly try to avoid her. All this makes her feel depressed and anxious, increasing her hallucinations and isolation. All she has are the voices to keep her company.

She feels pretty comfortable with her psychiatrist, Dr. Crane, who inquires about her goals related to relationships and social activities. Mary expresses her desire to be more connected to people who will understand and accept her, but she also shares her fear of socializing and states, "I tried before and I only get hurt, so I think that would happen again." Because of Mary's fear of rejection, Dr. Crane recommends that she connect with one of the mental health center's PSSs, who meet one on one with individuals and organize groups and events that help people build social capital. Dr. Crane explains to Mary that PSSs are individuals living with mental illness, like hers, who have faced similar challenges and have been trained to use their experience to help others. Dr. Crane calls Jill, a PSS, to meet with her and Mary prior to the end of their session. She documents the referral and the "warm handoff" to the PSS.

The following week, during the mental health center's team meeting (which includes social work/service coordinators, PSSs, a nurse practitioner, and a substance use specialist), Dr. Crane provides an update on her visit with Mary and inquires about Jill's interaction with her. Jill reports meeting with Mary for about 30 minutes for them to get to know each other. She notes that Mary's strengths include being inquisitive and motivated to make things better for herself. Mary asked about Jill's recovery journey and how she got her job. As they shared their personal stories, Mary also revealed that she wants to go back to work, but she is afraid that she would be too nervous around others. After they explored several options, Mary agreed to attend the Walking Warriors support group. She liked the idea of increasing her activity level and maybe losing some weight. She hoped that she could learn how to be more comfortable in public by being with a group of people like her. Jill said that Mary came to her first Walking Warriors group but started to leave after a few moments. Jill was able to get Mary to stay and talk with her while the group went to the park. Mary attended the group a second time, and with Jill by her side, she was able to walk in the park with the group. Afterward, she said she would like to come back again.

The social worker and Dr. Belosi, another psychiatrist, note that they had tried to refer Mary to these groups previously but she had refused to go. Dr. Crane suggests that making the warm hand-off to Jill may have made the difference in increasing Mary's courage and willingness to go to the group, because she had someone to support her. Dr. Belosi asks whether there have been any recent struggles with Mary's medications, which had been an issue discussed previously in team meetings. Jill reported that Mary had mentioned some discomfort with side effects ("being really tired") but had been reluctant to bring it up in her last med check, fearing she would have to change her medication. Mary had said, "I am tired of feeling like a guinea pig." Jill had shared her own struggles with medication changes with Mary and offered to go with her to her next appointment with Dr. Crane to help her discuss her feelings and provide extra support. Mary agreed to let Jill help her create a list of questions she could ask Dr. Crane in preparation for her next appointment and was happy that Jill would be there with her.

In this vignette it is clear that this team has a well-developed role for the PSS and that team members are knowledgeable about the ways they can work together to achieve the best outcomes for their clients. Although the psychiatrist has a good relationship with her patient, she understands that there may be some barriers to communication with her, and that the PSS can offer many things that she cannot. There is a sense of mutual respect and shared responsibility in the team's interaction, and the team members have created a forum for the easy exchange of information about their clients. The team responds to the client's concerns in a multifaceted manner, recognizing that one-dimensional approaches have limited chances for success. Meeting with the client concurrently provides valuable collateral information and eases the client's reluctance to say all the things she is concerned about. Obviously, not all treatment teams function this well, or recognize all of the various ways that PSSs can contribute. This chapter further delineates the potential of peer support and considers how this workforce can contribute to systems seeking value in psychiatric care.

Differentiating Mutual Peer Support and Professional Peer Support Services

An important distinction exists between mutual peer support and professional peer support services. Although both activities can significantly contribute to improved well-being and recovery, their structure and intentions are different. Peer support is a *mutual* support process between two or more peers. This might include a group of peers who are meeting in mutual support groups with shared goals of improving their well-being and developing recovery goals. This type of support occurs in Alcoholics Anonymous for individuals with substance use issues, or in Al-Anon or Alateen for their families. Professional peer support services, on the other hand, are activities in which one individual with lived experience of a behavioral health condition is trained and paid to provide services to another person who is struggling with a mental health and/or substance use condition. The professional PSS is able to use that experience to inform a process of support with a set of client-defined goals that address the person's recovery journey.

Professional peer support services have been variously defined in the literature. Myrick and del Vecchio (2016) cite SAMHSA's definition of a peer provider as an individual using their lived experience in recovery plus skills learned in formal training to deliver services that promote mind-body recovery and resilience. They also note that several studies have identified core principles and values of peer support: being noncoercive, nonjudgmental, empathic, and respectful, and promoting honest and direct communication, mutual responsibility, power sharing, and reciprocity, all of which are required for the process. A national consensus panel has defined a set of core pillars of peer support and key tenants of workforce development (Daniels et al. 2012), including how U.S. states and others can promote the PSS workforce. These pillars support the need for the peer workforce to do the following:

- Receive necessary education.
- Achieve certification.
- Obtain employment as a PSS.
- Maintain professionalism.
- Promote community advocacy.

Differentiating Peer Support Services From Clinical Roles

An important distinction to make is between peer support services and more conventional clinical services. While the behavioral health workforce is defined by the scope of services in which each profession engages, professional peer support services are somewhat distinct in their roles and functions as part of the health care team. As described by Hendry and colleagues (2015), peer specialists provide the following: 1) *emotional support* that fosters hope and empowerment; 2) *informational support* that promotes informed decision making; 3) *instrumental support* that provides tangible and concrete supports to help others complete necessary tasks to attain tangible goals; and 4) *affiliation support* that helps others improve interpersonal skills and social integration. Some of the distinctions between peer professionals and clinicians are described in Table 9–1.

The clinician's role has evolved in a more collaborative, less prescriptive direction in recent years, as a recovery-oriented, person-centered perspective has become more prominent. This change has allowed clinicians and PSSs to work together in a more complementary fashion. Understanding the role of peer and recovery support services as part of a behavioral or integrated health treatment team is important for promoting best practices and improving health outcomes.

Among the key issues that face the peer support workforce are those of professionalism, licensure, and certifications. Differentiating peer support from clinical services has led some in the workforce to question whether peer support services are professional or paraprofessional services. Because peer support workers generally receive training that is not associated with an academic degree and they are certified rather than licensed, there is continuing controversy related to this issue. A number of national organizations have attempted to elevate the professionalism of the workforce through the development of occupational associations and certifications. Examples include the International Association of Peer Supporters and Mental Health America's National Certified Peer Specialist certification.

Differentiating Peer Support Services From Other Community-Based Services

Health care systems are increasingly recognizing the value of a workforce that can extend care and coordination of services beyond a treatment facility and into the community. In mental health, PSSs have been deployed to foster improved transitions between hospital and community-based care, and as ongoing support resources to improve health care engagement, foster community engagement and tenure, and promote hope and the belief of recovery. Peer recovery support services (PRSSs), a role commonly referred to as *recovery coach* (see section "Peer Recovery Support in Addictions" later in this chapter), have also been developed and deployed in substance use care. Recovery coaches, similar to PSSs, are trained and use their lived experience to support those with substance use disorders in their recovery. They are distinct from mutual peer supports, such as sponsors, who have no formal training, receive no supervision, and do not provide clinical services.

TABLE 9–1. Distinctions between peer professionals and clinicians

What a peer supporter or recovery coach is/does	*What a clinician is/does*
Is a person in recovery	Is a clinical professional
Shares lived experience	Gives professional advice
Is a role model	Is an expert or authority
Sees the person as a whole person in the context of the person's roles, family, community	Is expected to diagnose and treat the person
Motivates through hope and inspiration	Motivates through persuasion and rationality
Supports many pathways to recovery	Prescribes specific pathways to recovery
Functions as an advocate for the person in recovery, both within and outside of the program	Is expected to treat more than advocate for the person
Teaches the person how to accomplish daily tasks	Focuses on reducing the symptoms of illness
Teaches how to acquire needed resources, including money	Acquires resources and money for the person
Helps the person find basic necessities	Assists in the acquisition of basic needs
Uses language based on common experiences	Uses clinical language
Helps the person find professional services from lawyers, doctors, psychologists, financial advisers	Provides professional services
Shares knowledge of local resources	Provides case management services
Encourages, supports, praises	Diagnoses, assesses, treats
Helps to set personal goals	Suggests tasks and behaviors
A role model for positive recovery behaviors	Advises the person on how to achieve recovery

Source. Adapted from Hendry et al. 2015.

There has been a historical lack of integration among PSSs in mental health and PRSSs in substance use care, which reflects the division in the treatment system in general. Better integration of these two areas of behavioral health and consolidation of training programs will likely serve the needs of the population more effectively.

Health systems are increasingly utilizing community health workers (CHWs), sometimes referred to as *promotores* in Spanish-speaking communities, to provide community-based outreach and education for individuals with chronic health conditions. CHWs and promotores (hereafter, both are referred to simply as CHWs) frequently share a community and sociocultural peer status with those they serve and have been described as cultural peers (Daniels et al. 2017). These workers are used mostly in primary care settings, and in most cases they do not have lived experience to share with the people they are serving. Principal roles for this workforce include health promotion through liaison activities with health care and community agencies. Outreach, education, and improved education for community members on behalf of health care organizations are also provided, as well as linguistically and culturally appropriate supports for outreach and engagement services. To date, there has been limited consideration of how to use PSSs and CHWs in a complementary manner for integration of physical and behavioral care; this is due in part to the overall fragmentation between physical and behavioral health systems of care. In addition, their roles have been somewhat distinct: CHWs focus more on outreach and engagement, whereas PSSs place more emphasis on recovery and resiliency.

Differentiating the scope of services and peer status between PSSs and CHWs is important in understanding how best to use these workers. The key differences lie in the level of their peer status (mutuality with those they serve) that impacts their work roles. CHWs are most often engaged in patient education and community outreach, which supports prevention, and they usually share racial, ethnic, and culturally similar attributes with those they serve. PSSs function in roles that are more often based in shared health conditions and common life situations that support activation for health improvement, shared decision making, and adherence to a care plan. These differences are depicted in Figure 9–1, which illustrates the overlapping roles for CHWs and PSSs. In this figure, the top row describes the activities of both groups and the bottom row represents shared characteristics (mutuality) with community members. The diagonal indicates the proportional engagement of CHWs (above the line) and PSSs (below the line) in the characteristics listed in the rows above and below (Daniels et al. 2017). PSSs are noted for their attributes of sharing common health conditions and similar life situations (as seen in the figure's lower rightmost cell), and their primary role is promoting self-care, shared decision making, and activation to support wellness and health improvement (upper rightmost cell). PSSs also use their peer status (bottom right) to promote support and activation through shared health conditions and similar life situations (upper right). Conversely, CHWs are noted for shared attributes of racial, ethnic, and cultural similarities, and their primary role involves education and connection to treatment services and prevention to avoid illness, as seen in the left upper and lower cells.

Primary roles of CHW and PSS	Education and connection to treatment services	Prevention to avoid illness	Addressing hopelessness and trauma of illness conditions	Activation to support wellness and health improvement	Promoting self-care, shared decision making, and care plan adherence
Community Health Worker (CHW)	CHW—primary roles and peer status high → low				
Peer Support Specialist (PSS)				PSS—primary roles and peer status low → high	
Peer status CHW and PSS	Racial and ethnic similarities	Cultural similarities	Living in the same community	Common life situations	Common health conditions

FIGURE 9–1. Primary roles and status of community health workers and peer support specialists.

Peer Support Services Across the Life Cycle

Peer support services in mental health exist across all phases of the life cycle—for youth, transitional-age adults (young adults), adults, and older adults. However, there has been little cross-phase integration of the workforce. Each of these phases seems to have a different scope of services and evolving standards for the peer specialists. Peer support services for adults are arguably the most developed of these subspecialties.

Peer Support Services for Youth

Youth peer support is an emerging service providing support services for youth and young adults who are living with emotional and behavioral health conditions. For the most part, youth peer support services have focused on self-empowerment and activation for improved health outcomes, as well as recovery management. Research supports that half of all behavioral health conditions start by age 14, and roughly three-quarters are developed by the mid-twenties (Kessler et al. 2005). Evidence-based services and supports can be protective and are vital for adolescents and young adults (Kessler et al. 2005). Peer support services for youth provide education, emotional support and guidance, advocacy, and empowerment for this population. These peer support services are generally delivered within youth serving organizations, which provide a structure for the delivery and funding of these services. Because less formal training and fewer certification standards are required for youth-focused peer support, organizational delivery systems often provide on-the-job training and supervision.

Notable outcomes of youth support services include a range of findings that indicate better engagement with peers, who have increased credibility and understanding relative to clinicians (Gopalan et al. 2017; Tindall and Black 2019). Additionally, these peers can be helpful in supporting the navigation through complex health care and social systems, promoting successful engagement and transitions (Clark and Unruh 2009). For young adults, developmentally similar peers can also serve as effective role models, and can foster encouragement, hope, and empowerment (Rickwood et al. 2007).

Parent, Family, and Caregiver Support Services

Parent, family, and caregiver support services commonly focus on the interactions between parents, concentrating on better understanding of caring for family members facing behavioral health challenges and the systems of care that provide the necessary services. Parent, family, and caregiver support services are provided by a peer who is a family member with similar lived experiences caring for a loved one experiencing social, emotional, and behavioral health challenges. Peers in this workforce are trained to support others in navigating situations similar to what they have experienced. This peer workforce provides services in a variety of settings and participates in care teams for this population. Primary family peer support roles include advocacy, education and training, information and referral, aiding in systems navigation, and strengthening parenting skills and competencies.

Research outcomes support the effectiveness of these practices in a number of areas. These peer support services demonstrate improved parent and child understanding of the challenges and resources associated with mental, emotional, and behavioral conditions (Robbins et al. 2008). They also support improved engagement with services (Koroloff et al. 1996) and better adherence to treatment and care transitions (Davis-Groves et al. 2011).

Parent, family, and caregiver support service providers receive specialized training, and certification for the provision of these services is available. Qualifications for this workforce vary by state, and there is limited standardization nationally. However, a national certification has now been established by the National Federation of Families for Children's Mental Health (2017). Other major national organizations providing support services for families with mental health challenges include the National Alliance on Mental Illness, Mental Health America, and the Depression and Bipolar Support Alliance. Support services available from these organizations are provided primarily by volunteers.

Peer Support Services for Adults and Older Adults

Peer support services for adults and older adults with mental health conditions are provided in a variety of settings including consumer-run organizations, community behavioral health organizations, hospitals, and managed care organizations. PSSs in these services are active in crisis and respite services, assistance in level of care transitions, and ongoing community engagement and supports (U.S. Department of Health and Human Services 2015). Peer services in integrated care settings are also evolving. These services can be provided in either individual or group arrangements and can be based in either community or institutional settings. In many states, Assertive Community Treatment teams are required to employ peer specialists.

Training and certification for PSSs who work with adults and older adults are similar across different states, and universal practice standards are emerging. A national advanced certification for PSSs has been established by Mental Health America. This is intended as an additional certification beyond what is available at the state level. Peer support services for older adults is an emerging practice for this population. A certification for this workforce with older adults has been established by the Pennsylvania Department of Aging and the Center for Mental Health Policy and Services Research at the University of Pennsylvania.

Peer Recovery Support in Addictions

There has been a robust history of mutual peer support and peer providers to help people with addictions. Alcoholics Anonymous (AA) was founded in 1935 and provided both a philosophy of recovery and a practical methodology for how to recover. AA was built on the principles of mutual support, in which one recovering alcoholic helps another. In addition to group support in AA, a designated sponsor serves as an individual to provide support and mentoring within the structure of the overall program.

The foundations of PRSSs and the use of recovery coaches have developed from the AA 12-step principles and the history of mutual aid recovery to support (or in conjunction with) treatment (Humphreys 2004). Recovery coaches are trained in much the same way as PSSs are in mental health settings. The role of PRSSs with lived experiences of substance use recovery has been prevalent within the evolution of treatment programs and centers. Within these centers it is not uncommon to have both voluntary mutual support programs such as AA and peer recovery coaches who are employed staff and deliver recovery coaching and support for those they serve. It is important to differentiate between those individuals with a self-disclosed substance use history who are working in treatment centers in defined clinical roles, and those who are providing voluntary peer support through 12-step or other organized mutual support networks.

PRSSs have been defined by Reif and colleagues (2014) as a set of peer-based activities that support individuals who are seeking to recover from substance use or co-occurring substance use and mental health disorders. For the most part, the roles of the recovery coach are similar to those of the PSS in mental health, with a specific focus on substance use recovery. Services include peer support for emotional, informational, and instrumental assistance for specific needs; help with social skill building; and support for social connectedness and inclusion. Recovery coaches help to guide the recovery process while supporting an individual's goals and decisions; these efforts may occur in conjunction with or separate from participation in an AA program.

Common PRSS goals include self-empowerment, abstinence or decreased use, and improved purpose and self-esteem. Additionally, PRSSs are active in providing support to resolve or improve the social determinants of health, including social connectedness, housing, education, employment, and decreased criminal justice involvement, all of which can be factors in meeting recovery goals. These services are offered in a variety of settings and may occur before, during, and after treatment.

SAMHSA has also fostered the role of PRSSs through grant funding and program support for Recovery Community Services Programs and Recovery-Oriented Systems of Care. According to SAMHSA, the role of a PRSS is to help support an individual's capacity to assess internal and external recovery capital, help the individual make informed recovery-based choices and decisions, and assist the person in setting and achieving recovery goals. A mutual and trusting relationship between a recovery coach and a peer is essential. The recovery coach does not give advice or diagnose; rather, a recovery coach serves as a recovery role model by offering encouragement and hope, helping others to explore a range of recovery options, and helping to set recovery goals and the strategies to achieve them (Substance Abuse and Mental Health Services Administration 2009). An important distinction between the recovery coach role and that of a sponsor in AA is the one-directional support that is provided by the recovery coach. In AA all support is mutual and provided in unpaid roles.

The effectiveness of PRSSs has been rated as moderate (Reif et al. 2014). Studies have demonstrated increased treatment participation and retention, reduced relapse rates, improved social supports, and higher levels of treatment satisfaction. Methodological challenges to the research are also noted; these include the lack of definitive or consistent outcomes, the inability to distinguish service roles, and a lack of consistent or definitive comparison groups. Additional research is needed to better distinguish which aspects of PRSSs are key to improving health outcomes.

Evidence Base for Peer Support Services

In 2007 the Centers for Medicare and Medicaid Services (CMS) identified peer support services as billable under approved state plans and described them as evidence based. A 2014 review (Chinman et al. 2014) of the evidence for peer support services described the strength of the combined findings as moderate. While focusing on notable outcomes, this review also found that the evidence related to these services was equivocal because some of the studies had methodological shortcomings and used different outcome measures. The review found that service effectiveness varied by the type of service provided. It examined outcomes in the following areas: 1) impact of peer support added to traditional services, 2) peers assuming regular provider positions, and 3) peers delivering structured curricula. The review included over 20 randomized controlled trials as well as some less rigorous experimental and correlational designs. Chinman and colleagues (2014) noted that across the different types of peer support services that were studied, outcome improvements were demonstrated for 1) reduced inpatient service use, 2) improved relationships with providers, 3) better levels of engagement in care, 4) higher levels of empowerment, 5) higher levels of activation, and 6) higher levels of hopefulness for recovery.

Davidson and colleagues (2018) note that when people in recovery are working in peer support roles, they are successful at engaging people in caring relationships, which also improves relationships between those served and other clinical providers, and allows engagement in less costly levels of care. Decreased substance use and fewer unmet needs are also associated with effective peer support services. Increased hope and decreased demoralization promote empowerment and self-efficacy. These qualities lead to improved social functioning and activation of self-care (Repper and Carter 2011). Improved quality and satisfaction with life are also promoted by peer support services.

In a review of the peer support services literature, Repper and Carter (2011) found that the strength of the evidence base for peer support services is at a level similar to that described by Chinman and colleagues (2014). However, they also note that PSSs are more successful than other professional staff in creating hope for the possibility of recovery, increasing engagement and empowerment, and promoting self-esteem and autonomy. PSSs also improve the development of social integration and the formation of social networks. These are the milestones that have been realized by the PSSs and enable them to demonstrate that these accomplishments are possible.

As the role of peer support services expands across behavioral health systems of care, it is vital that ongoing investigation into their effectiveness and outcomes keeps pace. The following are needed: greater attention to the fidelity measures (Chinman et al. 2016) that define the roles and scope of services provided by PSSs, methodological design and rigor for service effectiveness, and funding to support this work. Peer support services have become a standard component of recovery-based behavioral health care.

Understanding their contributions to effective outcomes must be a priority for the field.

Training and Certification of the Peer Workforce

Training and certification standards currently vary across states. This is due, in part, to the 2007 CMS guidance letter that established peer support services as reimbursable under state Medicaid plans (Centers for Medicare and Medicaid Services 2007). CMS guidelines stipulate three key minimum requirements for states to implement peer support service programs: training and credentialing, supervision, and care coordination. Nevertheless, states have taken different approaches to applying Medicaid coverage to peer support services, and as a result, implementation of training and certification programs has been variable from state to state.

The certified peer specialist workforce is relatively recent, with the first state programs being established in 2001. As of 2016, forty-one states and the District of Columbia had developed training and certification, and more states are in the process of developing these (Kaufman et al. 2016). As of 2014, the required training hours for state programs generally ranged between 40 and 80 hours (U.S. Department of Health and Human Services 2015), and the majority of states also require passing a certification exam. Most states also have established requirements for continuing education, requiring between 10 and 40 hours in 2-year cycles. Core competency areas generally include advocacy, professional responsibility, mentoring, recovery supports, and cultural competency. However, these requirements and competencies lack consistency and also differ across the states.

Hendry and colleagues (2015) described the following 21 common elements in training programs for peer specialists:

- History of the peer movement
- Personal recovery insight (awareness and knowledge)
- Five stages of recovery
- Peer support roles
- Creating recovery environments
- Stages and dynamics of change
- Effective goal setting for change
- Facilitating groups that support recovery
- Effective listening skills
- Motivational interviewing

- Facing personal fears
- Combating negative self-talk
- Problem solving
- Ethics and boundaries for peer specialists
- Workplace power, conflict, and integrity
- Creating the life one desires
- Wellness Recovery Action Plans (WRAP)
- Understanding trauma's impact
- Shared responsibility
- Seeing crisis as an opportunity
- Personal sharing and disclosure

Notably absent from this list is attention to integration of the PSS into behavioral health and primary care treatment teams. This collaboration has been lacking in most training curricula for PSSs as well as in the training of psychiatrists and other professionals. Unfortunately, this lack of integration often leaves the PSS feeling marginalized and isolated, while other clinicians are uncertain of the PSS's role. Integration and the appropriate assumption of the role of a full-fledged team member would likely be greatly expedited if this were better addressed in training.

A national advanced certification program for PSSs has been established by Mental Health America (www.mentalhealthamerica.net/national-certified-peer-specialist-ncps-certification-get-certified). Candidates are required to have a state certification with a minimum of 40 training hours; 3,000 hours of supervised experience providing direct peer support; one professional and one supervisory letter of support; and National Certified Peer Support certification training. Candidates also must pass a 3-hour, 125-question exam, and maintain 20 hours of continuing education every 2 years.

The peer support workforce also includes service providers for substance use (recovery coaches), youth and transitional age peer support, and parent and family peer supporters. The training and certification of these peer support providers vary by their scopes of services. The National Federation of Families for Children's Mental Health offers a certification program for their workforce (www.ffcmh.org/certification). The core competencies include ethics, confidentiality, effecting change, educational information, communication, parenting for resiliency, empowerment, wellness and natural supports, and resource information. Certification requires completion of an eligibility application and passing of a national exam.

As training and certification standards evolve across the different peer support workforce specialties, there appears to be little standardization. Better definitions of the scope of practice for these services and improving the development and expectations for the use of core competencies across the different peer workforces will promote clearer delineations of the work that peers do and ways to measure their outcomes. This standardization will also promote improved portability across the states for the workforce. There are also opportunities for the development of specialty training and certifications as peer specialists increasingly work with unique populations, such as the military or gender-specific populations, and in primary health care settings.

Employment and Pay Scales

The U.S. Bureau of Labor Statistics maintains the Standard Occupational Classification system of more than 800 job classifications. Included in this system are descriptions of the workforce distribution and data on mean annual wages by classification and geographic region. PSSs do not have an established classification. Rather, some aspects of peer support are included in the classification for community health workers (U.S. Bureau of Labor Statistics 2018). The peer support services workforce would greatly benefit from being recognized in the routine data collected by this governmental group.

Although little data have been accumulated for the unique PSS workforce, a 2015 study (Daniels et al. 2016) surveyed the peer support workforce regarding compensation. Two parallel surveys were used to question both peer specialists and the organizations that employ them. Over 1,600 peer specialists and over 270 organizations responded to the survey. The findings of the study indicate that peer specialists are employed in various settings. The majority of respondents (72%) indicated that they were employed full time. Wages differed among the organizations that employ peers, with the lowest rates paid by consumer and peer-run organizations and the highest by health plans and managed care organizations. The average wage rate for full-time employed peer specialists was $16.73/hour; however, the range of reported hourly wages varied from a low of $7.00/hour to a high of $31.30/hour. These rates were generally above state minimum wage rates but well below those of clinical professionals. Many of the study participants at the lower end of this range noted that they were paid at a rate that was significantly below others in the facilities where they worked, including staff who do not have direct client contact or responsibilities. This compensation also varied by tenure in the position; employment location, including both type of organization and geography; and number of hours worked per week. Additionally, female peer specialists received a disproportionate rate of $2.06/hour less than their male counterparts. The reason for this discrepancy is unclear, other than perhaps common trends across the general workforce population.

A geographic analysis of peer wages was conducted using the 10 U.S. Department of Health and Human Services regions. There were distinct regional differences in wages, with the highest rate of $17.37/hour in Region 1 (Northeast) and the lowest of $13.44/hour in Region 7 (Midwest). Discrepancies in wages by gender were seen in all regions favoring male peer specialists except in Region 2 (New York and New Jersey). The highest overall gender-based wage was for males in Region 1, who were paid an average of $18.30/hour, and the lowest rate was for females in Region 7 at $12.73. Separate wage information is not available for recovery coaches in substance use care or for youth and parent/family peer specialists; however, these populations were not excluded from the peer wage study.

Financing and Reimbursement

Various contracting and reimbursement strategies are used across states to fund peer support services. The greatest impact on reimbursing for these services occurred when CMS deemed peer support services to be reimbursable under State Medicaid plans in 2007 (Centers for Medicare and Medicaid Services 2007). This change has affected the development and evolution of training, certification, supervision, and reimbursement for these services. In states that have built peer support services into their Medicaid plans, reimbursement is available, but rates vary among states. States that have adopted managed care plans for their covered Medicaid population usually provide reimbursement that is embedded in this coverage. Other states have also adopted programmatic reimbursements that utilize grants and other administrative funding streams. Some states continue to pay for peer support services through administrative grants and contracts. Peer support services are also beginning to be included in funding for primary care integration and some specialty care services for both acute and chronic conditions.

Peer support services that are deployed and reimbursed through managed care plans have in many cases adopted guidelines that are similar to those of other covered health services. For example, a standard in health plan management is the concept of medical necessity and level of care criteria that governs the quantity and type of services that are best suited to an individual's condition. The development of this type of criteria for peer support services is an important step in role definition and implementation in health systems. One managed care plan has developed level of care criteria for the determination and review of peer support services (Daniels et al. 2013). These criteria provide direction for the necessity and duration of peer services across different levels of care. These types of guidelines also help standardize the services provided and the approaches to reviewing their status for reimbursement. As managed care and other payer systems increase reimbursement for peer services beyond just Medicaid, these coverage criteria help establish peer services as a part of the continuum of available health services.

Future Opportunities

The future for peer-delivered services appears robust, but not without challenges. There is a growing recognition that enabling shared experiences among those with similar health conditions can foster better engagement and activation for improved health outcomes. However, widespread adoption and funding for these services remain limited. Gaps in the research base exist, yet these are rapidly being addressed and the quality of studies is improving. The evolving maturity in the preparation of the workforce's training and certification leads to better standards of care and improves the quality of effectiveness research studies. To fully realize these opportunities, better integration of the workforce into routine care is necessary. This requires psychiatrists and other behavioral health clinicians to accept these roles and this workforce into standard practice.

Opportunities for career advancement for peer support specialists need to expand beyond the basic training and certification. Advanced training and new career opportunities need to be developed. At this time, requirements for supervision of the peer workforce generally stipulate the involvement of clinical professionals. New approaches to supervision, which include advanced peer specialists in these roles, need to be enhanced, and appropriate training must be developed to support them. Advocacy for the inclusion of peer specialists in all physical, behavioral health, and integrated health service programs will also create new opportunities and new challenges.

As the scope of health services continues to become better integrated across physical and behavioral health care, there is an emerging role for peer support services and other resources that promote engagement and recovery activation for improved self and wellness care. A challenge for these services will be to assimilate the mental health perspective into the cultures of substance use treatment and physical health services, including integration with community health workers. Greater attention also needs to be focused on the role that peer support services can have in other specialized health services, such as physical therapy, cardiac rehabilitation, and oncology.

Technology also has an emerging role in peer support services. Online peer support groups are becoming common, and new technology is emerging to provide platforms for peer support. Other forms of health technology, such as virtual reality programs, might be developed for the delivery of innovative peer support services (see Chapter 10, "Applications of Technology"). As the roles for peer support services in systems of care increase, there will be additional opportunities for technical tools to support care coordination and integrated care teams.

Conclusion

This chapter has considered the role of peer support and particularly that of the trained peer support specialist (PSS). A review of the literature indicates the many ways in which the PSS enhances the treatment services that are available and improves the overall quality of care for people attempting recovery. Working with PSSs, the psychiatrist can be more effective in the development of treatment plans and have greater confidence regarding adherence to the plans established with clients. Establishing a positive working relationship with PSSs enables them to be a tremendous resource for the psychiatrist as well as the treatment team. Accomplishing this requires attention to the integration process, creating a welcoming environment, and the demonstration of mutual respect.

Under fee-for-service financing, it has been difficult to obtain adequate funding for PSS services. Although this has gradually started to change, inclusion of PSSs is much more common and viable in settings in which all-inclusive rates (i.e., per diems) are in place. Expansion into new areas of practice will be facilitated by alternative financing methods, which are being developed. In any case, PSSs are an important human resource relative to clinical professionals. As such, they bring significant added quality to a person's clinical experience and have a positive impact on the value equation. With flexible funding in place, it is hard to imagine that payer and provider organizations could afford to neglect this resource.

The presence and scope of peer support services in behavioral health care are rapidly expanding and evolving. By partnering with and referring clients to peer supports, psychiatrists can take advantage of the positive outcomes that peers can facilitate in behavioral health. The psychiatrist is well positioned to have a working understanding of how this workforce is best deployed and the key opportunities for inclusion of peer supports in the recovery process and in systems of care. As the mental health workforce evolves, there will be many new approaches to providing optimal care to a population with growing needs. The importance of PSSs in that workforce should continue to grow, and these specialists will undoubtedly add value to services delivered.

References

Centers for Medicare and Medicaid Services: State Medicaid Director letter—peer support services, SMDL #07-011. Department of Health and Human Services, August 15, 2007. Available at: www.cms.hhs.gov/SMDL/downloads/SMD081507A.pdf. Accessed July 22, 2019.

Chinman M, George P, Dougherty R, et al: Peer support services for individuals with serious mental illness: assessing the evidence. Psychiatr Serv 65(4):429–441, 2014

Chinman M, McCarthy S, Mitchell-Miland C, et al: Early stages of development of a peer specialist fidelity measure. Psychiatr Rehabil J 39(3):256–265, 2016

Clark HB, Unruh DK: Understanding and addressing the needs of transition-age youth and young adults and their families, in Transition of Youth and Young Adults With Emotional or Behavioral Difficulties: An Evidence-Supported Handbook. Edited by Clark HB, Unruh DK. Baltimore, MD, Paul H Brookes Publishing, 2009, pp 3–24

Daniels AS, Bergeson S, Fricks L, et al: Pillars of peer support: advancing the role of peer support services in promoting recovery. Journal of Mental Health Training, Education and Practice 7(2):60–69, 2012

Daniels AS, Cate R, Bergeson S, et al: Level-of-care criteria for peer support services: a best practice guide. Psychiatr Serv 64(12):1190–1192, 2013

Daniels AS, Ashenden P, Goodale L, et al: National survey of compensation among peer support specialists. The College for Behavioral Health Leadership, January 2016. Available at: www.leaders4health.org/images/uploads/files/PSS_Compensation_Report.pdf. Accessed February 23, 2020.

Daniels AS, Bergeson S, Myrick K: Defining peer roles and status among community health workers and peer support specialists in integrated systems of care. Psychiatr Serv 68(12):1296–1298, 2017

Davidson L: Harnessing the power of peer support, in Pillars of Peer Support Summit IV: Establishing Standards of Excellence. Edited by Daniels AS, Tunner TP, Bergeson S, et al. January 2013. Available at: www.pillarsofpeersupport.org/POPS2012.pdf. Accessed February 23, 2020.

Davidson L, Bellamy C, Chinman M, et al: Revisiting the rationale and evidence for peer support. Psychiatric Times, June 29, 2018. Available at: www.psychiatrictimes.com/special-reports/revisiting-rationale-and-evidence-peer-support. Accessed February 23, 2020.

Davis-Groves SA, Byers S, Johnson K, et al: Implementation of the parent support and training practice protocol with community mental health teams in Kansas. 2011. Available at: https://childrenandfamilies.ku.edu/sites/childrenandfamilies.ku.edu/files/docs/FY11%20PST%20Report%20FINAL.pdf. Accessed February 23, 2020.

Gopalan G, Lee SJ, Harris R, et al: Utilization of peers in services for youth with emotional and behavioral challenges: a scoping review. J Adolesc 55:88–115, 2017

Hendry P, Hill T, Rosenthal H: Peer Services Toolkit: a guide to advancing and implementing peer-run behavioral health services. College for Behavioral Health Leadership and Optum, April 30, 2015. Available at: https://mhanational.org/sites/default/files/Peer_Services_Toolkit%204-2015.pdf. Accessed February 23, 2020.

Humphreys K: Circles of Recovery: Self-Help Organizations for Addictions. Cambridge, UK, Cambridge University Press, 2004

Kaufman L, Brooks W, Bellinger J, et al: Peer specialist training and certification programs: a national overview—2016 update. 2016. Available at: http://sites.utexas.edu/mental-health-institute/files/2017/01/Peer-Specialist-Training-and-Certification-Programs-A-National-Overview-2016-Update-1.5.17.pdf. Accessed February 23, 2020.

Kessler RC, Chiu WT, Demler O, et al: Prevalence, severity, and comorbidity of twelve-month DSM-IV disorders in the National Comorbidity Survey Replication (NCS-R). Arch Gen Psychiatry 62(6):617–627, 2005

Koroloff NM, Friesen BJ, Reilly L, et al: The role of family members in systems of care, in Children's Mental Health: Creating Systems of Care in a Changing Society. Edited by Stroul BA. Baltimore, MD, Paul H Brookes Publishing, 1996, pp 1–25

Myrick K, del Vecchio P: Peer support services in the behavioral healthcare workforce: state of the field. Psychiatr Rehabil J 39(3):197–203, 2016

National Federation of Families for Children's Mental Health: National certification for parent family peers. 2017. Available at: www.ffcmh.org/certification. Accessed February 23, 2020.

Podvoll E: Recovering Sanity: A Compassionate Approach to Understanding and Treating Psychosis. Boston, MA, Shambhala Publishing, 2003, pp 55–68

President's Commission on Mental Health: Report to the President from the Commission on Mental Health 1978. 1978. Available at: https://archive.org/details/reporttopresiden00unit_5. Accessed February 23, 2020.

President's New Freedom Commission on Mental Health: Achieving the promise: transforming mental health care in America. 2003. Available at: http://govinfo.library.unt.edu/mentalhealthcommission/reports/reports.htm. Accessed February 23, 2020.

Reif S, Braude L, Lyman D, et al: Peer recovery support for individuals with substance use disorders: assessing the evidence. Psychiatr Serv 65(7):853–861, 2014

Repper J, Carter T: A review of literature on peer support in health services. J Ment Health 20(4):392–411, 2011

Rickwood DJ, Deane FP, Wilson CJ: When and how do young people seek professional help for mental health problems? Med J Aust 187(7 Suppl):S35–S39, 2007

Robbins V, Johnston J, Barnett H, et al: Parent to parent: a synthesis of the emerging literature. July 2008. Available at: http://cfs.cbcs.usf.edu/_docs/publications/parent_to_parent.pdf. Accessed February 23, 2020.

Substance Abuse and Mental Health Services Administration: What are peer recovery support services? (HHS Publ No SMA-09-4454). 2009. Available at: https://store.samhsa.gov/system/files/sma09-4454.pdf. Accessed February 23, 2020.

Tindall J, Black D: Peer Programs: An In-Depth Look at Peer Programs Planning, Implementation, and Administration, 2nd Edition. New York, Routledge, Taylor & Francis, 2019, pp 27–35

U.S. Bureau of Labor Statistics: Occupational employment statistics. May 2018. Available at: www.bls.gov/oes/current/oes211094.htm. Accessed February 23, 2020.

U.S. Department of Health and Human Services: Mental health: a report of the Surgeon General. 1999. Available at: www.loc.gov/item/2002495357. Accessed February 23, 2020.

U.S. Department of Health and Human Services: An assessment of innovative models of peer support services in behavioral health to reduce preventable acute hospitalization and readmission. Office of the Assistant Secretary for Planning and Evaluation, December 1, 2015. Available at: https://aspe.hhs.gov/report/assessment-innovative-models-peer-support-services-behavioral-health-reduce-preventable-acute-hospitalization-and-readmissions. Accessed February 23, 2020.

10

Applications of Technology

Sy Atezaz Saeed, M.D., M.S.
Nubia Lluberes, M.D., CCHP-MH, FAPA
Victor J.A. Buwalda, M.D., Ph.D.

Over the past few decades, the treatment of psychiatric disorders has advanced at a rapid pace. There is clear evidence for the effectiveness of many methods for the care of these disorders. Health care delivery systems are making efforts to provide enhanced outcomes at lower costs. Technology continues to play a key role toward meeting such goals. In this chapter we provide examples of how the use of new technology in routine clinical practice is transforming health care and maximizing the policies and practices that support value in the delivery of individual and population health care.

Many people with mental health and substance use disorders do not have access to psychiatric services, yet most have access to a mobile phone. Rapid growth in health technologies within our society presents opportunities to leverage these technologies for advancing mental health care by enhancing access, quality, and experience for both consumers and providers. Technology holds the potential to become one of the main drivers of change in mental health care delivery systems. *Value* is defined as care effectiveness or quality outcomes in relationship to cost of care. It is the balance between the health outcomes that patients want and the cost required to achieve them. Technology offers the promise to enhance outcomes at the same or reduced costs, resulting in better value.

Use of communication technologies (e.g., Internet, e-mail, video conferencing, telephone) to prevent and/or treat mental and substance use disorders has been recognized by the Center for Substance Abuse Treatment (2009) as important in helping to meet unaddressed treatment needs. Indeed, the use of new technology in routine clinical practice settings is already transforming health care and maximizing the policies and practices that support value in the delivery of individual and population health. Technological advances and their incorporation into routine health care continue to improve outcomes, lower costs, and significantly contribute to both consumer and provider satisfaction. In this chapter we consider the impact of these technologies on various stakeholder groups: purchasers, payers, providers, products, and patients.

Digital Health Technology

Since the introduction of the Internet, technology continues to influence daily lives. The penetration of the Internet has increased dramatically over the last decade. People are more familiar with health care–related technological advances as they surf the Web using a tablet or smartphone. Worldwide, the use of digital health technology (DHT) is rapidly expanding. According to findings from Accenture's (2018) survey in seven countries (Australia, Finland, Norway, Singapore, Spain, United Kingdom, and United States), health care consumers are increasingly using technology to manage their health. Of the responders, the number who had smartphones increased from 36% in 2016 to 46% in 2018. People who use social media to manage their health care increased from 23% in 2016 to 35% in 2018. The number of users of wearable technology (smart electronic devices that can be worn on the body as implants or accessories) increased from 26% in 2016 to 33% in 2018. The use of health apps also continued to rise sharply. Interestingly, consumers are so familiar with their wearables and new DHT that they are willing to share their health care data with doctors (90%), nurses and other health care professionals (88%), friends or family (76%), health insurance plan (72%), and even employer (38%) or government agency (41%). Also, health consumers see wearables as beneficial for their health tracking, such as monitoring glucose, heart rate, physical activity, sleep, or weight. The percentage of health care consumers using virtual care services rose from 21% in 2017 to 25% in 2018. The commonly reported advantages of virtual care include reducing costs, accommodating patients' schedules, and providing timely care for patients (Accenture 2018).

Benefits of DHTs for health care professionals include minimizing avoidable or unnecessary service use, improving outcomes, promoting patients' independence, and focusing more on prevention. There is emerging evidence that the use of health technology can reduce paperwork, increase face-to-face time with patients, and allow providers to see more patients per day. The benefits of DHTs for patients include sharing information on symptoms and medical condition, helping with health care provider communication, and accessing health records, including test results. Factors that increase the use of health apps include reliability and accuracy of data, ease of use, simplicity in design, and security of data.

Use of health technology in mental health ranges from simple to complex and has a wide range of applicability, from chronic care management to complex population health analyses. Mental health is likely to become an important partner in the new health care transformation in which the organization of health care is shifting toward a more patient-centered, outcome-based delivery model with an emphasis on value. Today, we face a paradigm shift in the doctor-patient relationship. Since the 1990s, there has been a gradual change from a paternalistic attitude to a more egalitarian relationship in which the doctor becomes more of a coach or partner with the patient (Buwalda et al. 2004). This evolution has created a more empowering environment for the people who use services. Empowerment has also been stimulated by the growth of Internet and other technological advances. In the past, patients almost exclusively relied on health care providers to receive information, diagnoses, and referral. It was difficult for patients to gather reliable information and to navigate health care and social services. Technology has enabled them to obtain information that can be trusted and utilized to share the ownership of their health care.

DHT in psychiatry encompasses a large list of uses with various types of technological modalities. They can be categorized according to the primary user (consumer vs. provider), the purpose (improving interaction, collecting data, delivering care, etc.), or the information that is being collected (subjective or objective). Next, we consider the spectrum of technological applications.

Telemedicine and Telepsychiatry

Telemedicine refers to all health services delivered through audiovisual media. It is the second fastest growing industry in the United States. Winfrey (2015) reported that in 2014 the industry revenue approached $585 million, with a projected revenue growth (2014–2015) of 49.4%. Winfrey also anticipated that the telehealth revenue would grow to $3.1 billion by 2020. According to the World Health Organization (WHO), telemedicine is "the delivery of health care services, where distance is a critical factor. The telemedicine approach uses information and communication technologies for the exchange of information for diagnosis, treatment and prevention of diseases and injuries, research and evaluation, and for the continuing education of health care providers. Some of the more established fields of telemedicine include, teleradiology, teledermatology, telepathology, and telepsychiatry" (World Health Organization 2009). It should be noted that this definition includes many communication modalities, such as phone, fax, e-mail, still imaging, and store-and-forward, most of which are typically not reimbursed by third-party payers for mental health in the United States. Live, interactive two-way audiovideo communication (videoconferencing) is the modality that is typically reimbursed for telepsychiatry.

Telepsychiatry has been referred to by various terms, including telebehavioral health, telemedicine, e-behavioral health, telemental health, e-care, and telecare. A significant body of literature supports the assertion that utilizing telepsychiatry to provide mental health care has the potential to mitigate the workforce shortage that directly affects access to care, especially in remote and underserved areas (Antonacci et al. 2008). Recruiting and retaining mental health professionals in rural areas has been a problem for many years. In 2010, a nationwide survey, published by the journal *Rural Remote Health*, showed that physician shortages were reported by 75.4% of the responding rural hospitals (MacDowell et al. 2010). Since then, many large cities have also witnessed the growth of telepsychiatry services for underserved portions of the urban population.

Telepsychiatry has also been favored in the correctional system of care because of its ability to reduce transportation and staffing costs while increasing access to effective mental health care. It often appeals to professionals who otherwise would not consider working in a correctional setting (Deslich et al. 2013). A randomized study in California compared 40 parolees who received treatment utilizing telepsychiatry with 64 parolees who received treatment in face-to-face sessions. The study showed comparable effects regarding psychological functioning and medication adherence, with a neutral to favorable perception of telepsychiatry, except for a decline in the therapeutic alliance in the telepsychiatry group (Farabee et al. 2016).

Utilizing remote video connection for educational and consultation efforts among practitioners and providers has been successfully attempted and may continue to grow. One novel use of this remote video connection is being developed by a major metropolitan sheriff's department to connect officers of the Crisis Intervention Response Team with medical professionals for guidance and triage of cases encountered. This approach aids in diverting patients with mental illness from jails and prisons and providing treatment in a timely manner (Blakinger 2017).

In addition to the direct benefits of telepsychiatry to patients and providers, other, more indirect benefits have been identified. The reduction of time and expenses associated with travel may improve consumer compliance. Coordination of care, the education of mental health professionals, and improved recruitment and retainment of medical professionals are other benefits of this approach. There is also the potential for reduction in the impact of stigma associated with receiving mental health services that sometimes deters patients from seeking care (Farrell and Mckinnon 2003).

Some of the barriers for the utilization of telemedicine include infrastructure limitations (e.g., lack of access to Internet, poor connection quality), cost (e.g., equipment, installation, staff allocation cost), legal limitations (which vary by jurisdiction), and cultural acceptance (or lack thereof). The American Psychiatric Association (APA) and American Telemedicine Association (2018) collaborated in the creation of a document that summarizes the best practices and resources for implementation of telepsychiatry. The document specifically covers legal and regulatory issues related to these practices, emphasizing that "[p]roviders of telemental health *shall* comply with state licensure laws, which typically entail holding an active professional license issued by the state in which the patient is physically located during a telemental health session, and *shall* have appropriate malpractice coverage" (p. 2). The Interstate Medical Licensure Compact is an agreement between 29 states, the District of Columbia, and the Territory of Guam, where physicians are licensed by 43 different medical and osteopathic boards. Under this agreement licensed physicians can qualify to practice medicine across state lines within the compact if they meet the agreed-on eligibility requirements. Approximately 80% of physicians meet the criteria for licensure through this compact (Interstate Medical Licensure Compact Commission 2020). WHO provides free access to the *Directory of eHealth Policies* (www.who.int/goe/policies/countries/en), a compilation of policies gathered by WHO representatives at the regional and national levels via Ministries of Health and other governing institutions in the participating countries.

In the United States, significant variability exists across states regarding telehealth standards for physicians. These standards change rapidly, so it is imperative for telehealth providers to stay up to date. For example, in 2016 Georgia and Texas required an in-person follow-up after a telemedicine encounter, but in 2017 Texas enacted a new set of rules and no longer requires face-to-face consultation following the telemedicine encounter (Texas Medical Association 2019). Reimbursement also varies from state to state.

In the vast majority of jurisdictions, fax, telephone, and e-mail communications are not covered. Some jurisdictions allow for reimbursement of synchronous (real-time) communications and specific types of asynchronous communications (stored medical information), whereas other jurisdictions allow only synchronous encounters.

Not all telepsychiatry software programs are the same. The majority of platforms rely on computer-based video conferencing, and only a handful of them allow for both the consumer and the provider to connect via cell-phone videoconferencing. Some platforms include capabilities for documentation or are part of an electronic medical record (EMR), whereas others are standalone performers with or without good interoperability (ability to communicate with the EMR). The creation of the Fast Healthcare Interoperability Resources (FHIR) by a nonprofit organization called Health Level Seven International (HL7) is an effort to improve the interaction among different apps, platforms, and EMRs (www.hl7.org). Newer telepsychiatry platforms with advanced forms of complementary technology that integrate the videoconferencing component, medical records, mobile apps, and wearable technology are very promising. They may facilitate better care by simplifying the connection and information collection, potentially lowering the overall cost for the patient and the provider. Nevertheless, Yellowlees and colleagues (2018) emphasize that one of the key concepts in the implementation of telepsychiatry is that "choosing the best available technology is always going to involve aiming at a moving target" (p. 69).

Hilty and colleagues (2013) reviewed the published literature on effectiveness of telepsychiatry compared to face-to-face services. Their findings suggest that telepsychiatry is effective for diagnosis and assessment across many populations and disorders and it appears to be comparable to face-to-face care. Outcome studies with randomized controlled trials are scarce. Some of the pioneering large-scale studies show that outcomes in the groups receiving videoconferencing-based interventions are frequently equivalent, sometimes superior, but almost never inferior, to conventional treatment (Fortney and Pyne 2007). According to Urness and colleagues (2006), 96% of telepsychiatry clients studied felt satisfied with the session, and 93% felt that they could present the same information as in person; these results were similar to those for in-person clients. On the other hand, compared with in-person clients, telepsychiatry clients reported slightly lower levels of satisfaction in relation to feeling supported or encouraged.

One example of a successful telepsychiatry program is the North Carolina Statewide Telepsychiatry Program (NC-STeP), which has been providing expert psychiatric assessments and consultations through a network of 60-plus hospitals statewide. This program, developed by one of this chapter's authors (S.A.S.), addressed the lack of access to psychiatrists in many parts of North Carolina. Before the start of the program, this deficit resulted in long length of emergency department stays for patients with mental health crises. Those emergency departments now use telemedicine technologies to assess and treat patients in rural and underserved areas. NC-STeP's level of reach has enabled over 35,000 patient assessments. The emergency departments implementing these technologies have seen shorter lengths of stay, fewer involuntary commitments, less recidivism, and measurable cost savings. The $2 million per year investment from the state has generated $5–$6 million in cost savings per year by preventing unnecessary hospitalizations, improving emergency department throughput, and providing evidence-based treatment recommendations (North Carolina Department of Health and Human Services 2018; Saeed 2018a, 2018b).

Some ethical concerns may arise when using telepsychiatry to treat patients who have severe pathology or those who may be at an increased risk for poor outcomes. For this reason, the American Medical Association released ethical guidelines for physicians engaging in telemedicine. These guidelines include recommendations about disclosing any financial interests in the telemedicine application, protecting the patient's privacy and confidentiality, and recognizing the limitation of the technology. See "AMA Adopts Ethical Guidelines forTelemedicine Providers" 2016 for a summary of these recommendations.

The Telehealth Modernization Act of 2015 was introduced in the House of Representatives with the goal of promoting the provision of telehealth (includes all forms of remote care provision) by establishing a federal standard. Previously established federal regulations with telemedicine implications include the Health Insurance Portability and Accountability Act of 1996 (HIPAA) and the Children's Online Privacy Protection Act of 1998 (COPPA). HIPAA requires the use of equipment that allows for audit trails to facilitate confidentiality risk assessments, and COPPA imposes certain requirements on operators of websites or online services about collecting personal information online from a child under 13 years of age. Liability concerns vary depending on many factors. The use of telepsychiatry for education is considered to pose a lower risk, whereas its use for the treatment of substance use presents a higher risk. Ways of decreasing the liability risk include adhering to the standard of care of the profession, knowing and abiding by the laws of each jurisdiction, and seeking counsel when facing ethical conundrums.

Electronic Health Record Technology

Paper-based records are rapidly becoming obsolete in medical practice. The growth and development of *electronic health records* (EHRs), also referred to as *electronic medical records* (EMRs), have been fairly rapid, with ever-evolving capabilities to address the need for better record keeping, rapid access to information, statistical evaluations (analytics), and information sharing. Because of this constant evolution, the technological advancement of data collection and sharing can be challenging, in addition to being advantageous, for the provider of services. Although EHRs are a technological advancement meant to improve clinical and fiduciary processes as well as the collection of data, they have a downside too. In the last 10 years, the proliferation of EHRs has also been described as a possible cause of physician burnout. A study by Sinsky and colleagues (2016) showed that during the office day, nonpsychiatrist physicians spent 27.0% of their total time on direct clinical face time with patients and 49.2% of their time on EHR and desk work. Despite the concerns about disruption of the doctor-patient relationship and the workflow in the Sinsky et al. study, the research conducted by Entzeridou and colleagues (2018) indicates that 46% of the public and 91% of physicians who had experience with EHRs sensed that there was better coordination between hospitals and clinics with higher quality and reduced cost of health care.

Providers in solo practice face the challenge of selecting an EHR among a long list of possible candidates. This can be an overwhelming task. Overall cost and performance are essential concerns that are relatively easy to compare, but the list of specific details may be less clear in the initial stages of the selection process. EHR products offer a variety of services, including patient information collection, clinical note writing, provider-to-provider communication, ordering labs, e-prescribing, billing, integrated ambulatory services, patient portals, scheduling, and comprehensive practice management. Some platforms allow for some level of personalization to the specific needs of a small practice. Otherwise, it is up to the practitioner to make the most out of the product selected.

In larger practice settings, such as group practices, hospitals, and other institutional settings, selection of the EHR rarely relies on practitioners' preferences. An institution must balance the organization's needs against the sometimes exorbitant institutional costs. Implementation is a challenging process, both for those who are starting from ground zero and for those switching from one product to another. The path to stability, from the bidding process to the acceptance of the providers, can take years. To assist, the U.S. Department of Health and Human Services has made available a guide for EHR implementation called the *Health IT Playbook* (Office of the National Coordinator for Health Information Technology 2019). Despite the difficulties, the adoption of EHR platforms has been consistently incentivized. The Centers for Medicare and Medicaid Services (2019) established the Medicare and Medicaid EHR Incentive Programs in 2011 to encourage eligible professionals, hospitals, and Critical Access Hospitals (hospitals established by the federal government in rural areas) to adopt, implement, upgrade, and demonstrate meaningful use of certified EHR technology.

EHRs are not without risks. The confidentiality risks inherent to electronic data sharing can translate to poor patient outcomes and severe fines. HIPAA requires doctors, hospitals, and other health care providers to report any "breaches" of information. The law also requires the health care provider to notify the Secretary of Health and Human Services if a breach occurs and affects more than 500 residents of a state or jurisdiction. The health care provider must also notify prominent media outlets serving the state or jurisdiction (U.S. Department of Health and Human Services, Office for Civil Rights 2018). Accidental breaches related to cyber attacks, limited security capabilities, or malfunctioning technology are the responsibility of the health care provider and may require extra financial investment. Unethical breaches, even when related to lawful access to the platform (e.g., an employee with granted access who looks up lab results of a family member or a famous person), will require investment in ongoing training for personnel.

An important concern is how information collected in EHRs is stored. Choices are traditional server-based EHR storage or cloud-based storage. There is not much difference between cloud-based and server-based EHRs in terms of confidentiality or security risks. However, some believe that cloud-based EHRs are less liable to malware. Another risk that may be less well known to providers is exemplified in the case of eClinicalWorks, an EHR and patient portal vendor that was fined twice by the Office of Inspector General for the U.S. Department of Health and Human Services. Allegedly, eClinicalWorks misled providers who submitted false claims to the Medicare and Medicaid EHR incentive program, not knowing that the platform did not meet "meaningful use" certification requirements (Davis 2018).

Patients' experience appears to be positive in terms of access to their medical information with the development of EHR products with patient portals. These portals are patient-centered tools created with the goal of allowing patients to have access to their health information online and thus promoting an active role in the shared decision making. Evidence that patient portals improve health outcomes, cost, or utilization is insufficient (Goldzweig et al. 2013), but these portals may account for higher patient retention rates (Hogan et al. 2014). It is apparent that the future of EHR products will include the use of machine learning, predictive models, and improved analytics. The president of the large EHR vendor Epic opines, "On a deeper level, it also helps us form a more detailed understanding about how disease forms and what clinicians and patients can do to influence outcomes" (Siwicki 2018). Although this claim may appear lofty, it illustrates how some of the major EHR companies may be envisioning where EHRs are headed and how they may play a larger role in health care of the future.

Prescribing electronically, or e-prescribing, has been incentivized as a way of improving the workflow and limiting medication errors. The Centers for Medicaid and Medicare Services included e-prescribing in the Medicare Prescription Drug, Improvement, and Modernization Act of 2003. Currently, most EHR platforms include e-prescribing. Platforms that observe the Drug Enforcement Administration's (DEA's) regulations for electronic prescription of controlled substances can be used to prescribe Schedule III medications. The vendors may voluntarily acquire accreditation by the Electronic Healthcare Network Accreditation Commission to ensure they are in compliance with the DEA's recommendations (Electronic Healthcare Network Accreditation Commission 2015).

Mobile Applications

Mental health apps offer a unique opportunity to enhance access to mental health treatment. The number of mobile health (mHealth) apps focused on mental health continues to increase rapidly. These apps are also increasingly being prescribed to supplement psychiatric treatment and help patients self-manage their mental health conditions. In theory, apps can assist consumers in monitoring, managing, or understanding their conditions, as well as communicating with peers, providers, and other sources of support. The two major categories of health care apps are disease-specific apps and wellness management apps. According to "Patient Adoption of mHealth," a report from the IMS Institute for Healthcare Informatics (Aitken and Lyle 2015), only a small number of health care apps are responsible for 90% of consumer downloads. The most common mental health apps in disease-specific groups are concerned with autism, anxiety, depression, attention-deficit/hyperactivity disorder, and Alzheimer's disease. Together, they constitute almost one-third of these types of apps.

Some apps consist of "gamified software." This refers to applying game mechanics to nongame contexts in order to improve engagement. A gamified intervention may not operate as a full game experience but contains gaming elements, such as the scoring of points, in-game rewards, or engaging in quests (Fleming et al. 2017). Mental health–related gamified apps are available for therapy and risk assessment and for facilitating learning. Examples of therapeutic apps include SPARX and SuperBetter providing cognitive-behavioral therapy, and Freeze-Framer and Journey to the Wild

Divine providing biofeedback. One example of risk assessment is the work of Ormachea and colleagues. This group developed a mobile app to be used on a tablet for the evaluation of recidivism risk in criminal justice cases. The app compiles known psychological tests to measure executive function, risk-taking behavior, impulse control, reactive aggression, cognitive empathy, and planning abilities. The tests were gamified, and the battery was used in a population that had been evaluated using the Texas Risk Assessment System (TRAS). The researchers found that by combining these variables with the TRAS, they achieved a significant improvement in criminal recidivism risk prediction (Ormachea et al. 2017).

Despite the optimism about potential positive outcomes and opportunities from utilizing apps, there are multiple concerns. One of the earliest concerns arising in the initial years of app development was the possibility that economic and racial health disparity gaps would be widened if the health apps are only available to populations that are of a privileged class. Recently, however, more people have access to phones and portable computers than in the past. According to the Pew Research Center, an exponential increase in technology adoption by consumers was observed in surveys conducted from 2000 to 2016. In 2016, roughly 77% of Americans owned a smartphone and 73% had broadband service at home (Smith 2017).

Another difficulty is deciding which app would be more beneficial or a better fit for a particular individual. Today, there are more than 40,000 health care apps available. Billions of dollars are being devoted to the creation of apps, some of which are never downloaded. There is little evidence that these apps provide the results envisioned by the creators. Without data to support the effectiveness of the numerous health apps, the selection can be confusing for both consumers and providers. Lastly, the quality of the app, including its fidelity to the nascent federal laws and regulations, may be difficult to measure. The quality of an app is defined by variables such as the ease of use, completeness, and good functionalities, but only a few apps have been subject to formal research in these areas.

The American Psychiatric Association (APA) designed an evaluation model for apps in 2018 and relaunched an upgraded version in June 2019 (Henson et al. 2019). The APA notes that "the goal of a hierarchical rating system and rubric is simply to make APA members aware of very important information that should be considered when picking an app that is not exactly the same as the information used to judge a medication or therapy." Although the APA App Evaluation Model offers examples of how to use this model, it does not explicitly rate apps (American Psychiatric Association 2018). Given that apps are constantly updating and changing, such information would quickly be out of date. Also, determining the inherent usability is very subjective. The APA identified the following steps for evaluating an app, which are described in greater detail on the model's Web page (American Psychiatric Association 2018):

- Step 1: Gather background information.
- Step 2: Assess risk/privacy and security.
- Step 3: Evaluate any evidence for potential benefits.
- Step 4: Assess overall functionality and ease of use.
- Step 5: Consider capacity for data integration and interoperability to meet therapeutic goals.

When apps are being created, some federal laws may apply depending on the type of app. The Federal Trade Commission (FTC) has made an effort to provide guidance to developers. They have created the Mobile Health Apps Interactive Tool (Federal Trade Commission 2016), which allows anyone to identify which federal laws will apply to their specific product. Among the federal laws that must be followed by health apps are the following:

- *Health Insurance Portability and Accountability Act, or HIPAA:* The Office for Civil Rights within the U.S. Department of Health and Human Services enforces the HIPAA rules, which protect the privacy and security of certain health information and require certain entities to provide notifications of health information breaches.
- *Federal Food, Drug, and Cosmetic Act:* The U.S. Food and Drug Administration (FDA) enforces this act, which regulates the safety and effectiveness of medical devices, including certain mobile medical apps. The FDA focuses its regulatory oversight on a small subset of health apps that pose a higher risk if they do not work as intended.
- *Federal Trade Commission Act:* This act prohibits deceptive or unfair practices in commerce relating to privacy and data security, and those involving false or misleading claims about apps' safety or performance.
- *FTC's Health Breach Notification Rule:* This rule requires certain businesses to provide notifications following breaches of personal health record information.

In terms of outcomes, however promising, the health apps have yet to undergo randomized controlled trials before a definitive conclusion can be delineated (Federal Trade Commission 2016).

Use of Social Media

Social media platforms such as Facebook, YouTube, SnapChat, Twitter, and Instagram improve connectivity by sharing information in real time with other users. These platforms provide different possibilities in terms on how the information will be shared (e.g., word based: blogs, images, videos) and who will be the targeted audience (e.g., general public: Facebook; other professionals: LinkedIn; other physicians: Doximity). Some professionals have used these tools to maintain a presence for marketing purposes, sharing events, teaching, and connecting with colleagues. Celebrities and politicians have started to use social media to advocate and to share their mental health stories. More recently, providers, health care organizations, scientific journals, and consumers have started to use social media routinely. Physicians, in general, have several ways to use social media platforms in a professional context to improve patient care and physician wellness. Psychiatrists, in particular, have started to use social media to have a presence in the daily life of the community at large outside of the office walls. The most traditional use of social media in psychiatry has been to share ideas, news, or articles. This approach provides an opportunity for a blend of educational efforts and marketing of services, treatment options, and so forth, but raises concerns about privacy, confidentiality, and other ethical issues. When used appropriately, marketing via social media can be powerful and engaging, allowing people in the community to find the services that meet their specific needs in a timely manner.

Depending on which platform is being used, the type of marketing strategy will vary. For example, Facebook allows for the publication of advertisements. The ads can be set up to target a specific audience (by geographic location, age, income level, education level, and other factors). The payment required depends on the length of time the ad will be running and the level of dissemination intended. All ads are evaluated prior to publishing and will not run until approval is confirmed. To be approved, ads must contain a picture and a description with sufficient information and clarity. The platform will provide statistical information regarding the acceptance and success of the ad campaign. Twitter also allows for marketing opportunities in the form of written information without images; however, each post is limited to 280 characters or less. Many concerns arise in marketing health-related products or services, especially when the character limitation may restrict the amount of information that can be published. The FDA released guidance documents to assist in the understanding of the risk and benefits of these activities. (These guides were the product of a public hearing held by the FDA in 2009.) They are available online and include case examples and recommendations regarding responding to unsolicited off-label treatment information and misinformation published by third parties (U.S. Food and Drug Administration 2014).

In terms of collegial interaction, Facebook provides the opportunity for developing closed groups within which professionals can interact, allowing for networking and professional growth. A search of Facebook groups containing the word *psychiatry* shows more than 30 groups, including professional closed groups as well as some antipsychiatry groups. Psychiatry-related groups, such as Women's Psychiatry Group, Psychiatry Network, and Developmental Psychiatry and Psychology, have experienced incredible growth in recent years, with memberships of 4,000, 9,000, and 82,000, respectively. Although there is an impression of confidentiality when sharing information within closed or secret groups, the reality is that confidentiality is not guaranteed. Each group will run by the rules established by the group administrators according to the purpose of the group. These groups are recommended to have moderators (monitors) to maintain the fairness of the interactions and to approve or deny posts and to remove or block participants. Facebook also has behind-the-scenes moderators, looking for posts that may be against community standards. When a group is reported to Facebook, the content is reviewed and removed if it violates the company's terms and conditions, but there is no guarantee that it will be removed (Facebook 2018).

Medical professional associations have opened social media accounts for their members to interact under the institutional umbrella. APA has a presence on Facebook, Twitter, LinkedIn, and Instagram and thereby encourages all members to share information and start conversations, providing the opportunity for collaborations. A short video on how to get started is available on the APA member Web site.

Many physicians elect to separate their social media accounts into two different identities (one personal and one professional) in an effort to preserve their own privacy. DeCamp and colleagues (2013) argue that this separation may inadvertently be harmful for both the professional and the patient. They explain that the depersonalized online interaction may be less clinically effective or could even reduce trust in the patient-physician relationship.

Engaging patients is vital for all mental health professionals. Having an online presence can enable mental health professionals to correct misconceptions, spread new knowledge, and fight stigma (see Chapter 15, "Advocacy"). Due to the ability of Twitter to spread concise information very rapidly, it is often used for the purpose of advocacy. Many professionals use this platform, knowing that their tweets have the potential to get shared (retweeted) endlessly by their followers. Chretien and colleagues (2011) examined the tweets of self-identified physicians with 500 or more followers between May 1 and May 31, 2010 (a total of 5,156 tweets). Of those tweets, 2,543 (49%) were health or medical related, 1,082 (21%) were personal communications, 703 (14%) were retweets, and 2,965 (58%) contained links. Seventy-three tweets (1%) recommended a medical product or proprietary service, 634 (12%) were self-promotional, and 31 (1%) were related to medical education. One hundred forty-four tweets (3%) were categorized as unprofessional, 38 tweets (0.7%) represented potential patient privacy violations, 33 (0.6%) contained profanity, 14 (0.3%) included sexually explicit material, and 4 (0.1%) included discriminatory statements. Of the 27 users (10%) in the sample responsible for the potential privacy violations, 25 (92%) were identifiable by full listed name on the profile, profile photograph, or full listed name on a linked Web site. Fifty-five tweets (1%) were coded "other unprofessional," including 12 possible conflicts of interest.

Social media platforms are also being explored for the purpose of large-scale data collection. The "Social Media Collection Tools" Web page allows users to collect data for research purposes. The tools vary in quality, specific platform of study, and performance (Freelon 2020). One important concern when releasing research information via social media is the risk of manipulation of the content to produce misinformation. Merchant and Asch (2018) recommend specific countermeasures to protect the value of medical science. These include *provenance* (giving credit to the scientific source), *engagement* (organized scientific campaigns that include strong responses to misinformation), *transparency*, *narrative* (avoiding systematic data sharing that weakens emotional appeal), and *reputation* (finding new ways of building the right type of reputation in the world of social media, where peer review citations are no longer the metric used).

Self-promotion in social media serves to advertise services and to gain reputation. Research done using social media tools or published in social media will add to achieving those goals. Although the time investment appears to be subjectively perceived as more or less depending on generational differences, it is clear that the value of social media in formal research has gained acceptance. Some researchers are paying attention to the cultural evolution of digital media use (Acerbi 2016) and the biological underpinnings of the rewards perceived during social media use (Meshi et al. 2013). There is also the possibility of gaining better understanding of mental illness and substance use disorder by utilizing social media data (Hassanpour et al. 2019). Social media may also play a role in suicide prevention efforts. With this in mind, Facebook launched a campaign to use artificial intelligence software to identify people at risk and prioritize the contacts with moderators. Facebook is also dedicating more moderators to monitor suicide risk, training them to deal with the cases 24/7, and partnering with local resources to offer help in a timely manner (Constine 2017).

It is important for the mental health provider to understand the individual patient's exposure to and interest in social media. The use of social media and its impact on the emotional stability of individuals has also been a focus of attention. Block and colleagues (2014) found that there is a consistent pattern that links self-reported depression with increased media use, and Hassanpour and colleagues (2019) found an association between the use of social media and the risk for substance use disorder. The Facebook Intensity Scale, developed by Ellison and colleagues (2007), measures the platform's ability to add emotional connectedness related to the frequency and duration of use.

The possibility of consulting with other providers about patients and offering medical advice via social media is still very controversial. The general guidelines put forth by many professional groups always stress the importance of adhering to the privacy and confidentiality laws that govern our profession. Being cognizant of privacy settings, understanding risks for privacy breaches, and taking the time to evaluate potential ethical dilemmas are only some of the important tasks to keep in mind when interacting in social media platforms.

Virtual Reality Applications for Treatment

Interest in medical applications of virtual reality (VR) has grown considerably in recent years (Pensieri and Pennacchini 2014). In the reality-virtual continuum, "real" reality and VR lie at opposite ends of the continuum. *Real reality* is described as the direct perception of "real" objects without artificial alteration, whereas *virtual reality* is understood as an environment consisting of a mediated perception of solely virtual (digital) objects (Milgram and Kishino 1994). In between, there are *mixed realities* in which real-world and virtual-world objects are combined. Different terms are used to designate the space within the mixed reality boundaries, such as *augmented reality*, *augmented virtuality*, *trans-realities*, and *altered reality*, based on the ratio between real and virtual objects and the reality-to-fiction proportion of the virtual objects.

In essence, VR provides the participants with a three-dimensional computer-generated environment that is immersive, interactive, and multisensory. Earlier definitions of VR focused on the technology that supported it—for example, VR as three-dimensional realities implemented with stereo viewing goggles and reality gloves. Steuer (1992) broadened this definition and defined VR as a particular type of experience rather than as a collection of hardware. VR can be seen as a mediated perception of being present and immersed in an environment. Van Gisbergen (2016) explained VR as a specific combination of technologies that are expected to increase an experience and sense of realism. The combination consists of the following four dimensions: sensory, interactivity, control, and location. The *sensory* dimension relates to technologies used to create content. It is often stated that a mediated experience will feel more real if more senses are engaged. With technological advances, innovative sound and touch technologies have become more important. The *interaction* dimension refers to technologies used to navigate and explore through virtual environments, and they range from simple keyboard input technologies to more advanced headset, goggles, and glove technologies. *Control* technologies provide users with the potential to regulate real-time interaction with the virtual environment, such as the freedom to look around and the opportunity to manipulate and change the virtual world. More recently, control technologies also make it possible to share content and socially interact with others within a virtual environment. *Location* refers to technologies used to automatically locate and track the user in the physical and virtual world. These include technologies used in smartphones and wearables, as well as more sophisticated eye and full-body motion trackers.

VR is being increasingly used in treatment for mental health and substance use disorders. For example, VR can replicate the scenario in which addiction behavior is likely to occur, which can allow cognitive-behavioral therapists to tailor specific client-focused treatment plans. VR can add enhanced effectiveness by using cue-exposure techniques using multiple variables and inputs that enable personalized alcohol use assessment and treatment. VR has also been used in the treatment of anxiety disorders, eating disorders, and posttraumatic stress disorder. It is used to help autistic adults or children develop the skills that are important for independent living and functioning, such as how to pick up visual cues as one pays attention to another person speaking. It has been used in the treatment of phobias, such as the fear of heights (Schuemie et al. 2000). The most common and most successful treatment for acrophobia is in vivo graded exposure. A promising alternative to in vivo treatment in which the patient is exposed to real stimuli, VR can provide graded exposure to extinguish fearful responses in a safe environment. VR has also been used in the treatment of fear of public speaking and performance anxiety (Stupar-Rutenfrans et al. 2017).

VR also brings new possibilities in adjuvant treatment for patients with treatment-resistant schizophrenia (du Sert et al. 2018). Patients with treatment-resistant schizophrenia continue to suffer from persistent psychotic symptoms, notably auditory-verbal hallucinations (AVHs), which are highly disabling. Recently, a psychological therapy using computerized technology has shown large therapeutic effects on AVH severity by enabling patients to engage in a dialogue with a computerized representation of their voices. These very promising results have been extended by du Sert and colleagues (2018) using immersive VR. They found that VR therapy produced significant improvements in AVH severity, depressive symptoms, and quality of life that lasted for the 3-month follow-up period. The study results suggested that VR therapy might be efficacious in reducing AVH-related distress.

A systematic review of individuals with alcohol use disorder (AUD) showed that many experience relapses after treatment and that alcohol craving has been repeatedly implicated as the cause (Ghita and Gutierrez-Maldonado 2018). Cue exposure therapy, widely used for treatment of patients with AUD, has had inconsistent outcomes. According to the studies included in the review, VR can enhance effectiveness by using cue-exposure techniques with multiple variables and inputs that enable individualized alcohol use assessment and treatment. VR is seen as a promising tool for the assessment and treatment of craving among individuals with AUD.

All kinds of apps and VR applications can be downloaded on a smartphone. The smartphone can be used to download VR apps and experience the VR environments. A smartphone of high quality is required to personalize VR apps, allowing data collection on the effect of the VR app on patients' treatment outcomes. The penetration of smartphones in today's society is high, and therefore VR is available and affordable for most consumers. Ease and simplicity are keys to success. Because of rapid technological developments, VR is becoming more and more available and personalized.

"MyRecovery," a research tool for alcohol relapse prevention, offers a kind of a therapist-guided cue exposure therapy. In this VR app, the therapist gradually guides the patient in the detoxification program from a relaxed and safe environment to environments in which the patient will encounter some difficulties, which will require different levels of resistance to cues initiating craving for alcohol. One virtual world would be a messy apartment that will trigger craving, and another would be a bar environment where others are drinking and seduce the patient to drink. Through exposure to one of these worlds for some time per session, the patient can learn to cope with the triggers in a safe environment guided by the therapist. The aim is for patients to learn to reject alcohol at their most vulnerable moments and reduce their relapse frequency and thus reduce the likelihood for clinical detoxification admissions (Buwalda et al. 2019).

There are several concerns related to the use of VR. Little is known about the psychological impact of VR as it replaces real human social contacts with virtual social contacts. It could potentially increase loneliness, for example (Perry and Singh 2016; van Est et al. 2017). What is the likely impact on children who are exposed to a VR world that is violent, frightening, and unsafe? One concern is possible adverse reactions to VR content that may be upsetting. The Simulator Sickness Questionnaire (Kennedy et al. 1993) is the most widely used instrument to measure the severity of distress related to the simulated experience. It measures symptoms categorized in several domains, including nausea, oculomotor signs, disorientation, general autonomic activation, vertigo, difficulty concentrating, eyestrain, and dizziness. Another concern is the potential for people to get addicted to the use of VR, as demonstrated by the inclusion in DSM-5 (American Psychiatric Association 2013) of Internet gaming disorder as a condition for further study. VR is a form of information technology and therefore raises privacy issues. It involves collecting data about the user and linking these data to all kinds of other personal data from social networks (Scheerder et al. 2014; Zuckerberg 2014). People have little visibility and control of this interconnectedness (Lemley and Volokh 2017; O'Brolcháin et al. 2015; van Est et al. 2017). When organizations such as schools and hospitals decide to use VR because of its benefits for pupils or patients, attention to possible privacy violations via this "shortcut" is also important. Privacy must be safeguarded from access by other parties.

Measurement-Based Care

Measurement-based care involves using standardized rating scales for measuring symptoms and using the results to inform clinical decision making in individual patient care. Although many reliable and valid scales have been available for decades, they have not been widely embraced in routine clinical practice settings. Studies have documented that mental health professionals are more likely to detect lack of clinical response, or clinical deterioration, when they use these rating scales than by using clinical judgment alone. Using rating scales to monitor outcomes helps prompt clinicians to change treatment plans when indicated and hence enhance treatment outcomes. Studies of measurement-based care among both pharmacotherapy and psychotherapy patients have consistently documented that patients in measurement-based care have better outcomes than patients randomly assigned to usual care. Additionally, without the routine use of symptom rating scales, clinical practices cannot easily evaluate the effectiveness of their quality improvement initiatives or demonstrate to payers that their treatments are effective (Fortney et al. 2017).

The reasons for not using such rating scales have included lack of training or access, and concerns about the time it takes to administer the scales. There are now many user-friendly, structured, and brief scales that are easier to use in busy clinical settings. Many such scales are in the public domain and are free to use. Technology makes it more convenient to access, administer, and score these rating scales. For example, such scales can be used on handheld devices and within EHRs, potentially increasing the efficiency of routinely gathering symptom severity data from patients and informing the providers' clinical decisions during the clinical encounter.

Stakeholder Perspectives

The rapid expansion of technology is transforming behavioral health care and bringing "disruptive" innovation into health care delivery. Integrating technology-based tools in health care holds the promise to transform behavioral health care. A growing body of research demonstrates the acceptability, effectiveness, and cost-effectiveness of behavioral intervention technologies (Mohr et al. 2013). For this promise to be realized, however, it is important to understand stakeholders' perspectives on the use of technologies.

As one reviews the available literature on this area, it becomes obvious that the stakeholders' perspectives are not exactly aligned. Whereas the consumer may be looking for an easy-to-use, low-cost health app, the provider may be more concerned about connectivity to other work-related systems, confidentiality and privacy limitations, and reimbursement limitations. The results of a recent study indicated that while technology was expected to disrupt current health care models, there was a need for stakeholder collaboration, because no single group was considered to have sufficient expertise and resources to develop successful, effective behavioral health technologies on its own (Sucala et al. 2017). Similar studies can contribute to a better understanding of how technology is affecting behavioral health care from the standpoint of its stakeholders, which may lead to better and mutually satisfying research and care delivery.

Implementation

Implementation implies introducing an innovation in daily routines. This requires effective communication strategies and removal of obstacles to implementation (Davis and Tailor-Vaisey 1997). Implementation involves both an active execution and behavioral change (Swinkels and Buwalda 2011); it is a process with several steps: making a plan, executing it, and securing it. Swinkels and Buwalda (2011) also point out that implementation often requires a cultural change. It is therefore important to involve all personnel in this process. Grol and Wensing (2006) designed an implementation model that consists of six phases:

1. *Preparation:* Describe a proposal for change, which requires systematically planning the entire implementation.
2. *Diagnosis:* Evaluate actual care and establish concrete goals for improvement.

3. *Analysis:* Understand context, characteristics of the target group, and impeding and facilitating factors regarding the proposed change.
4. *Selection:* Implement the plan and disseminate knowledge, generate interest, and promote positive attitudes (the activation of the change).
5. *Testing:* Collect data from the implementation activities.
6. *Evaluation:* Review outcomes and adjust the plan accordingly.

During implementation, the plan-do-check-act cycle is continuously used as part of the continuous quality improvement process. The implementation also depends on the setting in which the innovation will be used; every setting may require a different approach (Grol and Wensing 2006).

Leadership challenges include understanding and overcoming various barriers to successful implementation. The barriers include legal issues, reimbursement, and infrastructure costs. For example, legal and regulatory ramifications include the following:

1. Subtitle D of the Health Information Technology for Economic and Clinical Health Act of 2009 addresses the privacy and security concerns associated with the electronic transmission of health information, in part through several provisions that strengthen the civil and criminal enforcement of HIPAA rules.
2. Some malpractice providers cover telepsychiatry as part of their standard coverage, whereas others may require additional coverage for providing telepsychiatry services.
3. Providers issuing a prescription for a controlled substance are required, by law (Ryan Haight Online Pharmacy Consumer Protection Act of 2008), to conduct an in-person medical evaluation at least once every 24 months.
4. A provider must be credentialed in the services that he or she provides, which in many cases necessitates credentialing in multiple systems. This requirement significantly increases the burden on providers for completing applications, waiting for the review process to complete before services can start, and paying associated dues.
5. Health care services are considered to be delivered in the state where the patient is located. Therefore, when telepsychiatry services are being provided across state lines, providers must comply with licensure laws, which typically entail holding an active professional license issued by the state in which the patient is physically located during a telemental health session. Providers also must conduct their own due diligence to determine the type of licensure required, and must ensure they are in compliance with state licensing board regulations.

Implementing innovation requires skills in change management. Making an innovation part of the routine workflow requires specific knowledge, skills, and attitude, and psychiatrists' training makes them well positioned for such change (Buwalda 2012). Their competencies include expertise in content area, in communication, in collaboration, and in advocacy (Saeed et al. 2018).

Recommendations

Sustained change in workplace behaviors requires a restructuring of the flow of daily work so that routine procedures make it natural for the clinician to give care in the new way. If the organization's goal is to promote the use of telepsychiatry, then telepsychiatry must be integrated with the current process of delivering patient care. For successful implementation, both providers and consumers must see technology as an approach or addition to treatment that is likely to increase the possibility of successful outcomes. Overcoming the barriers to implementation will require a combination of consumer, provider, and governmental advocacy.

There is a need for an organizational entity that can enhance the dissemination of telemental health systems so that cities and rural settings across all states can have the benefit of the network. Devices being used in mental health care must fulfill the requirements of good clinical practice and meet the national HIPAA security requirements. With the creation of hundreds of thousands of apps, we need a system that reviews them according to established criteria to bring more clarity in identifying appropriate apps that can be effectively used by health care professionals (Torous et al. 2018).

The biggest challenge is not the development and implementation of new technology but rather ensuring equality of access. Investing in a "connected network" that is available to everyone, with health care provided at the point of convenience, must be a priority. The purpose and fit of telecare services in the wider care system, not the technology itself, should drive the change. DHT should be used to ensure that those individuals who are uninsured or underinsured and have behavioral health diagnoses can access all services in the continuum of care. As technology continues to advance at a rapid pace, pragmatic and realistic models for academia-industry partnerships are needed. Exploring innovative models, such as integrated care clinics where psychiatrists are linked via videoconferencing to the primary care clinics, also requires attention.

Conclusion

Many studies support the feasibility and acceptability of digital health technology in the diagnosis and treatment of mental health and substance use disorders. Numerous studies also have shown the potential effectiveness of telepsychiatry, information technology–based clinical decision support, and telephone support interventions in both clinical and community settings. Technologies such as smartphones, tablets, health apps, and virtual reality make health care more accessible, user friendly, and cost efficient for consumers and strive to make the community healthier. Electronic health records have now incorporated enhancements for both the providers and the consumers. For the providers, such enhancements include practice management systems, clinical decision supports, e-prescribing, alerts/reminders, e-journals, and digital imaging. For the consumer, enhancements include access to their health records, access to health Web sites, e-visits, and virtual support communities. Telepsychiatry is now a viable and reasonable option for providing psychiatric care to those who are currently underserved or who lack access to services.

Using technological advances helps us in getting closer to the Quadruple Aims of improved outcomes, lower cost, user satisfaction, and provider satisfaction (see Chapter 1, "Defining and Measuring Value"). Technology can reduce ineffective use of health services, enable health care professionals to integrate different areas of health care, enhance the availability of mental health care specialists, add more efficient access for people with different cultural backgrounds, and facilitate better support of families and peers. Technology helps us deal more effectively with the current inefficiencies of our systems of care (Krausz et al. 2016). Digital health technology can enable or empower patients' self-management and make the doctor-patient relationship more efficient when patients can access health information, advice, and support, and this technology can transform patients from being passive recipients of care to being actively engaged in their own care (Deloitte 2013).

Finally, telepsychiatry is technology based and driven, yet it lengthens and strengthens the reach of the health care providers to patients they might not otherwise have an opportunity to engage. It is still about building relationships, bridging distances, and making health care convenient for people. *It is still about relationships, not technology!* As health care technology expands, the key stakeholders need to understand how to work with each other in terms of how to adopt new behavioral health technologies into practice, as well as how to secure funding to do that.

References

Accenture: Insight. Latest thinking. Meet today's healthcare team: patients+doctors+machines. Accenture 2018 consumer survey on digital health. 2018. Available at: www.accenture.com/us-en/insight-new-2018-consumer-survey-digital-health. Accessed February 23, 2020.

Acerbi A: A cultural evolution approach to digital media. Front Hum Neurosci 10:636, 2016

Aitken M, Lyle J: Patient adoption of mHealth: use, evidence and remaining barriers to mainstream acceptance. IMS Institute for Healthcare Informatics, September 2015. Available at: www.iqvia.com/-/media/iqvia/pdfs/institute-reports/patient-adoption-of-mhealth.pdf. Accessed February 23, 2020.

AMA adopts ethical guidelines for telemedicine providers. Foley's Health Care Law Today (blog) July 28, 2016. Available at: www.healthcarelawtoday.com/2016/07/28/ama-adopts-ethical-guidelines-for-telemedicine-providers. Accessed February 24, 2020.

American Psychiatric Association: Diagnostic and Statistical Manual of Mental Disorders, 5th Edition. Arlington, VA, American Psychiatric Association, 2013

American Psychiatric Association: App evaluation model. 2018. Available at: www.psychiatry.org/psychiatrists/practice/mental-health-apps/app-evaluation-model. Accessed February 23, 2020.

American Psychiatric Association, American Telemedicine Association: Best practices in videoconferencing-based telemental health. April 2018. Available at: www.psychiatry.org/psychiatrists/practice/telepsychiatry/blog/apa-and-ata-release-new-telemental-health-guide. Accessed February 23, 2020.

Antonacci DJ, Bloch RM, Saeed SA, et al: Empirical evidence on the use and effectiveness of telepsychiatry via videoconferencing: implications for forensic and correctional psychiatry. Behav Sci Law 26(3):253–269, 2008

Blakinger K: Harris Co. Sheriff's office tests telepsych program to help with mental health cases. The Houston Chronicle, December 18, 2017. Available at: www.chron.com/news/houston-texas/houston/article/Harris-Co-sheriff-s-office-tests-telepsych-12440282.php. Accessed February 23, 2020.

Block M, Stern DB, Raman K, et al: The relationship between self-report of depression and media usage. Front Hum Neurosci 8:712, 2014

Buwalda VJA: Implementation of outcome assessment and the role of the psychiatrist, in Outcome Assessment: A Guideline for the Psychiatrist. Utrecht, The Netherlands, Dutch Association of Psychiatry, 2012, pp 31–35

Buwalda VJA, Sleeboom-van Raaij CJ, van Tilburg W: Changes in training program for psychiatrists in the 21st century. Psychiatrie 46:621–626, 2004

Buwalda VJA, Obermair K, Weber J, et al: Virtual reality in alcohol use disorder treatment. Poster Annual Meeting, Maastricht, 2019

Center for Substance Abuse Treatment: Considerations for the provision of E-therapy (HHS Publ No SMA-09-4450). Rockville, MD, Center for Substance Abuse Treatment, Substance Abuse and Mental Health Services Administration, 2009

Centers for Medicare and Medicaid Services: Promoting interoperability programs. June 18, 2019. Available at: https://www.cms.gov/Regulations-and-Guidance/Legislation/ehrincentiveprograms/index.html. Accessed February 24, 2020.

Chretien K, Azar J, Kind T: Physicians on Twitter, research letter. JAMA 305(6):566–568, 2011

Constine J: Facebook rolls out AI to detect suicidal posts before they are reported. November 27, 2017. Available at: https://techcrunch.com/2017/11/27/facebook-ai-suicide-prevention/. Accessed February 23, 2020.

Davis D, Tailor-Vaisey A: Translating guidelines into practice: a systematic review of theoretic concepts, practical experiences, and research in the adoption of clinical guidelines. CMAJ 157(4):408–416, 1997

Davis J: eClinicalWorks fined $132,500 by HHS OIG for patient safety risk. HealthcareITNews.com, 2018. Available at: www.healthcareitnews.com/news/eclinicalworks-fined-132500-hhs-oig-patient-safety-risk. Accessed February 23, 2020.

DeCamp M, Koenig T, Chisolm M: Social media and physician's online identity crisis. JAMA 310(6):581–582, 2013

Deloitte: Connected health: how digital technology is transforming health and social care. Deloitte Centre for Health Solutions, 2013. Available at: www2.deloitte.com/content/dam/Deloitte/uk/Documents/life-sciences-health-care/deloitte-uk-connected-health.pdf. Accessed February 23, 2020.

Deslich SM, Thistlethwaite TM, Coustasse A: Telepsychiatry in correctional facilities: using technology to improve access and decrease costs of mental health care in underserved populations. Perm J 17(3):80–86, 2013

du Sert OP, Potvin S, Lipp O, et al: Virtual reality therapy for refractory auditory verbal hallucinations in schizophrenia: a pilot clinical trial. Schizophr Res 197:176–181, 2018

Electronic Healthcare Network Accreditation Commission: EHNAC approved as a certifier by DEA for e-prescribing of controlled substances. Press Release, January 27, 2015. Available at: www.ehnac.org/?press-release=ehnac-approved-as-certifier-by-dea-for-e-prescribing-of-controlled-substances. Accessed February 23, 2020.

Ellison N, Steinfield C, Lampe C: The benefits of Facebook friends: social capital and college students use of online social network sites. Journal of Computer Mediated Communication 12(4):1143–1168, 2007

Entzeridou E, Markopoulou E, Mollaki V: Public and physician's expectations and ethical concerns about electronic health record: benefits outweigh risks except for information security. Int J Med Inform 110:98–107, 2018

Facebook: Facebook help center, group management for admins. 2018. Available at: www.facebook.com/help/1686671141596230?Helpref=about_content. Accessed February 24, 2020.

Farabee D, Calhoun S, Veliz R: An experimental comparison of telepsychiatry and conventional psychiatry for parolees. Psychiatr Serv 67(5):562–565, 2016

Farrell SP, Mckinnon CR: Technology and rural mental health. Arch Psychiatr Nurs 17(1):20–26, 2003

Federal Trade Commission: Mobile health apps interactive tool. April 2016. Available at: www.ftc.gov/tips-advice/business-center/guidance/mobile-health-apps-interactive-tool. Accessed February 24, 2020.

Fleming T, Bavin L, Stasiak K, et al: Serious games and gamification for mental health: current status and promising directions. Front Psychiatry 7:215, 2017

Fortney J, Pyne J: A randomized trial of telemedicine-based Collaborative Care for Depression. J Gen Intern Med 22(8):1086–1093, 2007

Fortney JC, Unutzer J, Wrenn G, et al: A tipping point for measurement-based care. Psychiatr Serv 68(2):179–188, 2017

Freelon D: Social media data collection tools. Wikidot.com, 2020. Available at: http://socialmediadata.wikidot.com/. Accessed February 24, 2020.

Ghita A, Gutierrez-Maldonado J: Applications of virtual reality in individuals with alcohol misuse: systematic review. Addict Behav 81:1–11, 2018

Goldzweig CL, Orshansky G, Paige NM, et al: Electronic patient portals: evidence on health outcomes, satisfaction, efficiency, and attitudes: a systematic review. Ann Intern Med 159(10):677–687, 2013

Grol G, Wensing M: Implementatie: Effectieve Verbetering van de Patiëntenzorg. Maarssen, The Netherlands, Elsevier Gezondheidszorg, 2006

Hassanpour S, Tomita N, Delise T, et al: Identifying substance use risk based on deep neural networks and Instagram social media data. Neuropsychopharmacology 44(3):487–494, 2019

Henson P, David G, Albright K, et al: Deriving a practical framework for the evaluation of health apps. The Lancet Digital Health 1(2):E52–E54, 2019

Hilty D, Ferrer D, Parish MB, et al: The effectiveness of telemental health; a review. Telemed J E Health 19(6):444–454, 2013

Hogan TP, Nazi KM, Luger TM, et al. Technology-assisted patient access to clinical information: an evaluation framework for blue button. JMIR Res Protoc 3(1):e18, Mar 27, 2014

Interstate Medical Licensure Compact Commission: Interstate medical licensure compact: a faster way to medical licensure. 2020. Available at: https://imlcc.org. Accessed February 23, 2020

Kennedy RS, Lane NE, Berbaum KS, et al: Simulator Sickness Questionnaire: an enhanced method for quantifying simulator sickness. International Journal of Aviation Psychology 3(3):203–220, 1993

Krausz M, Ward J, Ramsey D: From telehealth to an interactive virtual clinic. e-Mental Health, 2016. Available at: http://med-fom-krauszresearch.sites.olt.ubc.ca/files/2015/12/Krausz-Ward-Ramsey-2016-From-telehealth-to-an-interactive-virtual-clinic.pdf. Accessed February 23, 2020.

Lemley MA, Volokh E: Law, virtual reality, and augmented reality. Stanford Public Law Working Paper No. 2933867: UCLA School of Law, Public Law research Paper no. 17–13, 2017

MacDowell M, Glasser M, Fitts M, et al: A national view of rural health workforce issues in the USA. Rural Remote Health 10(3):1531, 2010

Merchant R, Asch D: Protecting the value of medical science in the age of social media. JAMA 320(23):2415–2416, 2018
Meshi D, Morawetz C, Heekeren HR: Nucleus accumbens response to gains in reputation for the self relative to gains for others predicts social media use. Front Hum Neurosci 7:439, 2013
Milgram K, Kishino F: A taxonomy of mixed reality visual displays. IEICE Transactions on Information Systems 77(12):1321–1329, 1994
Mohr DC, Burns MN, Schueller SM, et al: Behavioral intervention technologies: evidence review and recommendations for future research in mental health. Gen Hosp Psychiatry 35(4):332–338, 2013
North Carolina Department of Health and Human Services: North Carolina telepsychiatry program. 2018 Profile. 2018. Available at: https://files.nc.gov/ncdhhs/2018%20NC%20DHHS%20ORH%20Telepsychiatry%20Program%20One%20Pager_0.pdf. Accessed February 24, 2020.
O'Brolcháin F, Jacquemard T, Monaghan D, et al: The convergence of virtual reality and social networks: threats to privacy and autonomy. Science and Engineering Ethics 22(1):1–29, 2015
Office of the National Coordinator for Health Information Technology: Health IT Playbook. 2019. Available at: www.healthit.gov/playbook/electronic-health-records. Accessed March 20, 2020.
Ormachea P, Lovins B, Eagleman D, et al: The role of tablet based psychological tasks in risk assessment. Criminal Justice and Behavior 44(8):993–1008, 2017
Pensieri C, Pennacchini M: Overview: virtual reality in medicine. Journal of Virtual Worlds Research 7(1):1–34, 2014
Perry BI, Singh S: A virtual reality: technology's impact on youth mental health. Indian Journal of Social Psychiatry 32(3):222–226, 2016
Saeed SA: Successfully navigating multiple electronic health records when using telepsychiatry: the NC-STeP experience. Psychiatr Serv 69(9):948–951, 2018a
Saeed SA: Tower of Babel problem in telehealth: addressing the health information exchange needs of the North Carolina Statewide Telepsychiatry Program (NC-STeP). Psychiatr Q 89(2):489–495, 2018b
Saeed SA, Silver S, Buwalda VJA, et al: Psychiatric management, administration, and leadership: a continuum or distinct concepts? Psychiatr Q 89(2):315–328, 2018
Scheerder J, Hoogerwerf R, de Wilde S: Horizonscan 2050: Anders Kijken naar de Toekomst. Den Haag, The Netherlands, Stichting Toekomst beeld der Techniek, 2014
Schuemie MJ, Bruynzeel M, Drost L, et al: Treatment of acrophobia in virtual reality: a pilot study, in Proceedings of the Euromedia 2000, Antwerp, Belgium, May 8–10. Edited by Broeckx F, Pauwels L. Ostend, Belgium, EUROSIS—ETI Publications, 2000, pp 8–10
Sinsky C, Colligan L, Li L, et al: Allocation of physician time in ambulatory practice: a time and motion study in 4 specialties. Ann Intern Med 165(11):753–760, 2016

Siwicki B: Next-gen EHRs: Epic, Allscripts, and others reveal future of electronic health records. Healthcare IT News, May 21, 2018. Available at: www.healthcareit-news.com/news/next-gen-ehrs-epic-allscripts-and-others-reveal-future-electronic-health-records?Mkt_tok=eyjpijoiwwpkallqbghprfjqwkdjncisinqioiirtdrim1njs3dmazu2vwxpy3nydvlevyt0qjrwzitinkx2exvyduy1btnmn2jtmuhqouowuw9rc2lrbstkag84rup1. Accessed February 23, 2020.

Smith A: Numbers, facts, and trends shaping your world. Pew Research Center, 2017. Available at: www.pewresearch.org/fact-tank/2017/01/12/evolution-of-technology. Accessed February 23, 2020.

Steuer J: Defining virtual reality: dimensions determining telepresence. Journal of Communication 42(2):73–93, 1992

Stupar-Rutenfrans S, Ketelaars LEH, van Gisbergen MS: Beat the fear of public speaking: mobile 360° video virtual reality exposure training in home environment reduces public speaking anxiety. Cyberpsychol Behav Soc Netw 20(10):624–633, 2017

Sucala M, Nilsen W, Muench F: Building partnerships: a pilot study of stakeholders attitudes on technology disruption in behavioral health delivery and research. Transl Behav Med 7(4):854–860, 2017

Swinkels JA, Buwalda VJA: Implementation, the art of temptation, in Routine Outcome Monitoring in the Mental Healthcare: A Guideline for the Usage and Implementation of Measurement Instruments. Edited by Buwalda VJA, Nughter MA, Swinkels JA, et al. Utrecht, The Netherlands, 2011, pp 33–50

Texas Medical Association: Texas Laws and Regulations Relating to Telemedicine. August 2019. Available at: https://www.texmed.org/Template.aspx?id=47554. Accessed June 19, 2020.

Torous JB, Chan SR, Gipson SYT, et al: A hierarchical framework for evaluation and informed decision making regarding smartphone apps for clinical care. Psychiatr Serv 69(5):498–500, 2018

Urness D, Wass M, Gordon A, et al: Client acceptability and quality of life—telepsychiatry compared to in-person consultation. J Telemed Telecare 12(5):251–254, 2006

U.S. Department of Health and Human Services, Office for Civil Rights: Privacy, Security, and Electronic Health Records. Washington D.C.: HHS.gov., 2018. Available at: www.hhs.gov/sites/default/files/ocr/privacy/hipaa/understanding/consumers/privacy-security-electronic-records.pdf. Accessed February 23, 2020.

U.S. Food and Drug Administration: Industry Internet/social media platforms: correcting independent third-party misinformation about prescription drugs and medical devices. June 2014. Available at: www.fda.gov/downloads/Drugs/guidancecomplianceregulatoryinformation/Guidances/UCM401079.pdf. Accessed February 23, 2020.

van Est QC, Gerritsen J, Kool L: Human Rights in the Robot Age: Challenges Arising From the Use of Robotics, Artificial Intelligence, and Virtual and Augmented Reality. Den Haag, The Netherlands, Rathenau Instituut, 2017

Van Gisbergen MS: Contextual connected media: how rearranging a media puzzle, brings virtual reality into being. Inaugural lecture, Breda University of Applied Sciences, 2016. Available at: https://pure.buas.nl/ws/portalfiles/portal/683141/Gisbergen_Contextual_Connected_Media_and_VR.pdf. Accessed February 23, 2020.

Winfrey G: The 5 fastest-growing industries in the U.S. March 2015. Available at: www.inc.com/graham-winfrey/the-5-fastest-growing-industries-in-the-us.html. Accessed February 23, 2020.

World Health Organization: Global observatory for eHealth: survey 2009 figures: telemedicine. 2009. Available at: www.who.int/goe/survey/2009/figures/en/index1.html. Accessed February 23, 2020.

Yellowlees P, Kaftarian E, Caudill RL, et al: The business of telepsychiatry, in Telepsychiatry and Health Technologies: A Guide for Mental Health Professionals. Arlington, VA, American Psychiatric Association Publishing, 2018, pp 59–95

Zuckerberg M: Post on Oculus acquisition: I'm excited to announce that we've agreed to acquire Oculus VR, the leader in VR technology. Genius, 2014. Available at: https://genius.com/Mark-zuckerberg-post-on-oculus-vr-acquisition-annotated. Accessed February 23, 2020.

Part III

Where We Want to Go

Professional Interventions

11

An Expanded Role for Psychiatry

Donovan Wong, M.D.
Wesley E. Sowers, M.D.

Psychiatrists have historically had a wide range of roles within mental health care systems. These roles have diminished over the course of time due to a variety of economic factors and the rising prominence of medication management in training and practice. Although medication management is an important aspect of psychiatric practice and will likely continue to be, many would argue that restoring a broader scope of practice would maximize the value of psychiatric care. As systems of care continue to evolve, there will need to be ongoing reassessment and redefining of the roles that psychiatrists can take on to improve the delivery of mental health care. This chapter looks at specific ways that psychiatrists' roles and scope of practice can be enhanced. Some of the issues to be considered regarding scope of practice include systems-based services, consultative and supervisory activities, psychiatrists' participation in pharmacological and nonpharmacological treatments, provision of some aspects of primary care, and educational activities. Because psychiatrists are a scarce and costly resource, it will be important to consider how an expansion of their activities would impact the value equation.

When psychiatrists are trained in all the diverse aspects of mental health treatment, they are clearly able to make more valuable contributions to treatment planning. Knowledge of issues such as entitlements, advocacy, recovery management, and education are essential for that process (Ranz et al. 2012). The continuing practice of various psychotherapies, involvement in consultative practices, the provision of some primary care and preventive interventions, and an adequate knowledge base regarding social interventions will also enhance this capacity. This expansion of activity may seem to be at odds with cost reduction strategies, because psychiatrists would then have less time for direct care and "billable" medication management, but this would be the case only in the context of current financing arrangements. Psychiatrists can be more effective members of a team treatment planning process if they have fluency with all of the tools at their disposal. Ultimately, determining the scope of practice that most wisely uses this human resource is a complicated, dynamic process. This chapter considers some potential activities that can help increase the effectiveness of psychiatrists, while optimizing patient care and job satisfaction for providers.

Systems-Based Practices

Much of the care currently provided by psychiatrists takes place in organizational settings rather than in private practices, which was more common in the past (Ranz et al. 2006). The Accreditation Council for Graduate Medical Education (ACGME) designates systems-based practice (SBP) as one of six core competencies required for psychiatric training programs.

As cited by Ranz and colleagues (2012), ACGME describes SBP as an "awareness of and responsiveness to the larger context and system of healthcare, as well as the ability to call effectively on other resources in the system to provide optimal healthcare." The study by Ranz and colleagues (2012) (members of the Mental Health Services Committee of the Group for Advancement of Psychiatry) determined that both trainees and faculty of training programs understood SBP concepts poorly, and that training programs struggled to define and measure this competency. Based on ACGME's six core expectations for SBP and ACGME's Psychiatry Residency Review Committee's additional eight core expectations for psychiatry, the research group developed an instrument used to survey psychiatric residents in 12 programs across the country regarding their experience with SBP competencies at various levels of their training. Through a factor analysis of the data obtained, the study identified four essential factors integral to SBP for psychiatrists. The activities defining these factors are observable and measurable. The resulting four-factor model for systems-based care describes four roles that psychiatrists should assume in organizational settings:

- Information integrator
- Team member

- Resource manager
- Patient care advocate

In the role of *information integrator*, the psychiatrist collects information from as many sources as possible to provide a comprehensive assessment and analysis of a patient's life circumstances and functioning, and identifies the interventions and professional resources needed to adequately meet the patient's needs. As a *team member* the psychiatrist works with other members of the treatment team to gather and organize this information and participates in its application to treatment planning. Communication and coordination with all parties involved in a person's care will be part of this role as well. As a *resource manager* the psychiatrist provides awareness of cost considerations in the selection of interventions, which is particularly relevant to value assessment. Insurance limitations, medication prices, level of care decisions, and outcome evidence will all be important considerations in developing the service plan. As *patient care advocate* the psychiatrist works with and facilitates the patient's interface with various systems. This role may involve obtaining entitlements and basic needs, maintaining housing, providing access to transportation, establishing eligibility for needed services, and many other actions to help further a patient's well-being in an environment that can be quite hostile toward those with few resources.

In these four roles, the psychiatrist assists in all aspects of a person's care and ensures that biopsychosocial needs are addressed. This integration maximizes the possibilities for good outcomes and reduces inefficiencies related to fragmentation and lack of coordination. In an earlier article, Ranz and Stueve (1998) examine the role of psychiatrists as program medical directors. Although not all psychiatrists will necessarily hold these positions, the results of this study suggest that for many occupying these roles, satisfaction and performance are enhanced, leading ultimately to better performance and longevity in organized systems of care. In the sections that follow, various clinical and administrative activities in which psychiatrists could be involved will be considered. Many of these activities will enhance the psychiatrist's ability to manage these four roles effectively and add value to behavioral health services.

Indirect Services: Supervision, Consultation, and Team Work

The inadequate supply of psychiatrists in the behavioral health workforce creates clear challenges in accessing psychiatric care. This access issue will continue to be a challenge, and likely worsen, as the psychiatric community ages and retires (Association of American Medical Colleges 2012; Health Resources and Services Administration/National Center for Health Workforce Analysis and Substance Abuse and Mental Health Services Administration/Office of Policy, Planning, and Innovation 2015; Lowes 2015). Confronting this workforce shortage requires consideration of alternatives to how patients traditionally access psychiatric care and how psychiatrists interact with other providers. Indirect consultation (including telepsychiatry), supervision, and teamwork are three somewhat overlapping ways to expand access to psychiatric care to a larger group of patients. Indirect consultation can also include curbside consultation, education, registry review, and e-consults. Psychiatrists' involvement in these activities will allow the health care systems to better confront the psychiatric shortage, and thereby potentially increase the overall quality of mental health treatment (i.e., decreased waiting times, more appropriate prescribing) and likely contribute to a healthier workplace.

Indirect consultation has the potential to greatly increase the number of patients who have access to psychiatric expertise. Because of prescriber scarcity, primary care providers already prescribe the majority of psychotropic medications (Mark et al. 2009). Collaborative care approaches are ways for psychiatrists to review cases and make recommendations to primary care providers, without necessarily seeing patients directly. In most cases, a consulting psychiatrist will typically discuss cases with a mental health coordinator on the primary care team who has assessed the patient. Following this discussion and a review of the patient's chart, the psychiatrist can make recommendations to the primary care provider and treatment team (Hegel et al. 2002). In most cases, the primary care provider remains responsible for ongoing medication management.

Collaborative care models have been gaining traction in recent years, but they are still not available in many health care systems. These models are typically used for patients with mild to moderate depressive or anxiety symptoms. Primary care providers learn from successive indirect consultations, allowing their own practice to become more sophisticated over time. A significant literature base shows that this approach achieves the Triple Aim of improving outcomes, lowering costs, and increasing patient satisfaction. This model can also improve system efficiency by ensuring that patients are treated in a timely manner at the appropriate intensity of care (American Psychiatric Association and Academy of Psychosomatic Medicine 2016).

Psychiatric supervision of advanced practice providers is another way to get psychiatric care to a broader patient population. Another obvious advantage of engaging advanced practice providers is cost reduction, because these providers cost nearly half as much as psychiatrists. The use of advanced practice providers is becoming more common. In 2013, there were 45,580 psychiatrists, 7,670 psychiatric nurse practitioners, and 1,280 physician assistants practicing in a prescribing capacity. As the number of advanced practice providers continues to grow (Health Resources and Services Administration/National Center for Health Workforce Analysis and Substance Abuse and Mental Health Services Administration/Office of Policy, Planning, and Innovation 2015), there will be more opportunities for systems and psychiatrists to work with these providers to increase access to psychiatric care. For the most part, advanced practice providers work very similarly to psychiatrists with respect to medication management, and often have some form of collaboration or supervision with a psychiatrist. In these professional relationships, psychiatrists have the opportunity to work in a mentoring capacity (National Council for Behavioral Health 2017). As in many other areas within the scope of practice, experience and training are important. This is not typically part of psychiatric residency training, so psychiatrists are not always confident in supervisory or consultative roles. Increased focus on preparing psychiatrists for this work will be helpful in enabling more of them to do so comfortably. Chapter 12 ("Psychiatric Workforce Development") considers workforce issues in greater detail.

Working in teams requires psychiatrists to interact in ways that include elements common to both indirect consultation and the supervision of advanced practice providers. As psychiatrists emerge from marginalized roles in fee-for-service payment systems, they can become a more integral part of treatment teams. Psychiatrists, due to their breadth of training, are uniquely positioned to provide leadership to mental health teams. An important aspect of teamwork is the better quality of care that can be delivered through collaborative processes and strong relationships with other professionals. Team members feel more effective when they are connected with their colleagues and take pride in the quality of care they provide (Herrman et al. 2002). Wise orchestration of the various elements of the team will allow systems to manage a larger number of clients effectively.

Pharmacological Practices

In recent years psychiatric practice has become increasingly focused on the prescription of medications and their management. Psychiatry training programs are 4 years long, 1 year more than most primary care training programs, which arguably have a more diverse and challenging array of health issues to address. The rationale for this extended training was initially to provide ample time to develop the skills necessary to provide various psychotherapeutic interventions. However, as various forces coalesced to reduce the scope of practice for psychiatry, many of these areas of competency were reduced in emphasis or dropped completely from training programs, and generally were replaced by more attention to biological aspects of care (Weisman 2011). As the array of pharmacological agents has expanded, and the mythology of medications' magic has grown through the efforts of pharmaceutical corporations, the use of medication in psychiatric care has markedly increased. The occurrence of ineffective polypharmacy, as well as the unwanted side effects associated with it, has increased proportionately. Research on the long-term impact of medication use has remained grossly inadequate (Sowers 2005). The full spectrum of this topic is considered in detail in Chapter 13 ("Pharmaceutical Management and Prescribing"), but this section focuses on novel aspects of psychiatrists' roles in prescribing—specifically, medication dosage reduction, or the concept of "deprescribing," and medication discontinuation (InformedHealth.org 2017; Moncrieff and Kirsch 2005; Pigott et al. 2010; Rimmer 2018).

Most of the attention in the pharmacological curricula in psychiatry is centered on the properties and indications for prescribing a relatively limited list of medications. Much less attention is given to the art or dynamics of prescribing, which may be equally important in terms of outcomes achieved (Weisman 2011). Many of the psychiatric medications commonly prescribed have outcomes that are only marginally better than the use of the placebos to which they are compared. This is most dramatically evident in the treatment of depression. Clinicians and laypeople alike are often surprised to learn that placebo treatments are almost as effective as antidepressants, achieving remission up to 40% of the time. The use of an antidepressant improves rates to about 60% at best, but this additional impact is noted primarily in persons with severe depression, who account for only a small percentage of those who are treated with these medications.

There has been some controversy regarding whether taking antidepressants offers any advantage over placebo in the long run (InformedHealth.org 2017; Moncrieff and Kirsch 2005; Pigott et al. 2010; Rimmer 2018). The advantages appear to be equivocal for many anxiety medications as well (Piercy et al. 1996). Anxiety and depression account for a large proportion of people engaged in mental health treatment, and these medications are prescribed quite extensively by primary care physicians as well as psychiatrists. Because relatively little information is available on the long-term effectiveness of these medications, it is unclear whether their positive effects have a lasting impact (Pigott et al. 2010). Confounding the picture further is the fact that depression is known to have a cyclic course, even in the absence of treatment.

The picture is less obscure for some other patients. Severe mental illnesses such as schizophrenia and bipolar disorder have much better outcomes when medication is used. Nevertheless, the numbers and types of medications used are often observed to be disproportional to their effectiveness and cost. Many critics believe that overtreatment with medication is the result of a number of forces impacting training and clinical structures, with an ultimate result being short visits where there is little time for diagnostic clarity or interventions other than medication manipulation (Smith 2012). Client pressures and the expectations of other clinicians, along with liability concerns, have created a milieu in which medications are often added to treatment regimens and less often discontinued from them, resulting in people taking multiple medications.

Although information regarding the effectiveness of medication is generally available to both the public and professionals, it is not promoted or emphasized. Pharmaceutical companies clearly have little interest in disseminating information that would reduce the use of their products and subsequently their profits, but it is less clear why it is not emphasized more in medical training or prescribing guidelines. Many ascribe this to an acquiescence of training curricula to biological reductionism and the narrowed scope of psychiatric expertise. As discussed in other sections of this chapter, training and continued practice of psychotherapeutic interventions contribute to a psychiatrist's holistic understanding of individual clients (Sowers and Thompson 2007). This is especially significant in prescribing. An important aspect of psychiatric care is understanding how an individual client will view the use of medication and developing strategies to ensure maximum benefit and minimize the potential detrimental effects of medications (Sowers and Golden 1999). In many cases, prescribing will include helping clients to reduce the number of medications they are taking, or their dosages, and to safely discontinue pharmacological treatment.

Several studies have indicated that many people who have had mental illness and have accomplished some degree of recovery following treatment, can eventually reduce their use of medication or can discontinue it entirely without a significant impact on various outcome measures (Harding et al. 1987; Steingard 2018). The reduction of medication use will in many cases improve overall health status and disability burdens by eliminating medication-associated side effects and risk factors. Issues related to the side effects associated with medications are especially prominent in the use of antipsychotics and mood stabilizers (Correll et al. 2015). Although wise or "conservative" prescribing can avoid or minimize side effects and risk factors at the outset, prescribers will often be confronted with clients who are new to them and who have previously been prescribed several medications of dubious effectiveness or that pose a significant threat to their function or well-being. It is frequently challenging to work with clients around the alteration of their medication regimen. Some people using medications may be wary of discontinuing medications, even those that are unlikely to be contributing to their stabilization, whereas other people will wish to discontinue medications that are very likely responsible for a reduction of their symptoms.

Prescribers need to have a sound understanding of the impact of substance use on psychiatric symptoms and clients' attitudes and beliefs regarding medication. This issue is considered in greater detail in Chapter 17 ("Addiction Treatment and Harm Reduction"), but a brief consideration of the impact of substance use on dosage reduction and medication discontinuation is warranted here. Because the effects of substance use often produce or mimic psychiatric symptoms, in both peri-intoxication phases and longer-term manifestations, it is not unusual for other psychiatric diagnoses to be dispensed prematurely and inaccurately. As a result, patients receive medication prescriptions that are ineffective or inappropriate. Even when medication is appropriately prescribed for the alleviation of specific target symptoms that are substance related, it often is not discontinued after clients are stabilized and substance use effects are unlikely to persist. In addition, clients' attitudes are often influenced by long-standing substance use. Coping skills may be poorly developed, tolerance for discomfort is generally low, and an external locus of control often results in patients' belief that medications are "substances" that can fix all of their discomfort (Sowers and Golden 1999). All of these factors may result in the overprescription of medication.

It is no small task to integrate the psychodynamics of each individual into a formulation of a strategy to minimize medication use while optimizing health outcomes. In developing these strategies, prescribers must recognize client beliefs and desires, estimate the likely impact of a medication on symptom reduction and long-term health, ensure that clients have adequate information to make informed decisions, and take into account cost relative to benefits (Deegan and Drake 2006). Psychiatric training must enable trainees to develop the skills to accomplish this task so that they will have the expertise to provide consultation and supervision in these processes. As the most highly trained prescribers, psychiatrists will be asked to work closely with clients who will benefit from medication reduction. Assumption of this role will contribute to cost reduction, better outcomes, and presumably greater client and clinician satisfaction.

Therapeutic Treatments

Group Treatments

Group treatments for individuals with psychiatric and substance use disorders have been effective methods for helping people recover from their behavioral health disabilities. Although psychiatrists once had a significant involvement in group treatments, this has not been the case in recent years, and most psychiatric training programs provide limited exposure to group treatment models. There are several reasons that these skills have receded in practice and in the curricula of residency training programs, as discussed elsewhere in this chapter (see section "Pharmacological Practices"). Economic forces that have been responsible for biological reductionism in psychiatry have played a significant role in limiting psychiatric involvement in group activities as well. In this section we consider whether involvement in group treatment by psychiatrists can improve the quality of care and do so with greater efficiency.

Group activities have long been part of milieu treatment of people with severe mental illnesses who were admitted to the state asylums of the late nineteenth century. In the early days of state asylums, "moral treatment," as espoused in the United States by Benjamin Rush and Dorothea Dix, consisted of a variety of activities to encourage patients to socialize with each other while engaging in productive activities. In later years, groups were commonly used to treat combatants suffering from "shell shock" after being exposed to trauma in World War II. Groups were originally introduced as an attempt to meet the demands for help that could not be met through individual therapy (see Barlow et al. 2014; Panman and Panman 2001). Through this experience, many clinicians felt that the interaction between patients in groups was, in many ways, superior to what could be accomplished with individual work. As a result, after the war, the use of groups proliferated in hospital settings and eventually in community service settings (Karterud 1993). At the same time, clinicians began to experiment with different types of groups and with a variety of formats and objectives. Irvin Yalom, a psychiatrist well known for the extensive use of group therapy in his practice, wrote about the benefits of group treatments for participants (Yalom 1970). He identified 10 factors potentially contributing to healing in groups:

1. Imparting of information (psychoeducation)
2. Installation of hope (overcoming helplessness)
3. Universality (understanding that other people are like you)
4. Altruism (pleasure derived from helping others)
5. Recapitulation of family experience (understanding significant relationships)
6. Socialization (reduction of isolation)
7. Imitative behavior (identifying effective behaviors)
8. Interpersonal learning (adopting successful methods of social interaction)

9. Cohesiveness (affiliation)
10. Catharsis (unburdening oneself)

Most group experiences expose participants to several of these healing factors, regardless of their specific format or focus (Yalom 1970). Groups have been used for treatment of a variety of disorders and disabilities. The outcomes related to group treatment have been studied extensively and indicate that most group treatments are quite effective. Although the value of group treatment is well established, little has been written or studied regarding the impact of psychiatric participation in group processes (Gise and Crocker 2012). Why, then, should group treatments have a place on the psychiatrist's palette?

The Case for Psychiatrist-Facilitated Groups

There are several ways in which group experience may contribute to the relationship and understanding between psychiatrists and their clients as well as their relationships with other members of the treatment team. Setting aside obstacles to psychiatrists doing group work, groups provide an opportunity to observe clients' social interactions in a more natural circumstance. As a member of the group, the psychiatrist is less stigmatized or alien, and the perceived power differential is significantly diminished. A more honest portrait of the client can be obtained, partly because group members will often confront erroneous or inappropriate statements made by other members. The group format allows clients to be seen more frequently and for more extended periods of time. These factors all contribute to the construction of trust, authenticity, and mutuality. Clients may initially object to the suggestion of group work, because of their own inhibitions and a variety of other factors, but generally, if they can be persuaded to join a group for some period of time, they find the experience quite enjoyable (Gise and Crocker 2012).

There are other advantages for psychiatrists who are also prescribing medication for group participants. The factors that help build trust with clients also help to inform the prescribing process and, in many cases, expedite it, however it is designed. The formation of a trusting, collaborative relationship increases the likelihood that clients will adhere to their medication regimens (Colom et al. 2003). Psychiatrists can prescribe more wisely having had an opportunity to evaluate the authenticity of reported symptoms and to obtain a more dynamic view of the client's mental status. Regardless of the group format, even when the group is not specifically medication related, there can be opportunities to insert psychoeducational elements to inform clients about medications, common side effects, health maintenance, and numerous other topics that would not be possible to cover in brief individual visits. Group interaction may more effectively counteract denial and provide additional information and encouragement from peers who support the wise use of medication (Gise and Crocker 2012).

Psychiatrists working in the context of a treatment team will find that the information obtained from their observations in group interactions can be very helpful to other members of the team. In more traditional individual interactions, the psychiatrist usually has a very brief, limited "snapshot" of a client's behavior and interaction with others. The group experience provides a more dynamic "motion picture" of the client's demeanor and interactions in a community. This insight creates added value to the psychiatrist's contribution to the team and the treatment planning process. These contributions enhance the psychiatrist's relationship to treatment team members in much the same way that self-disclosure and coaching operate with clients in group treatments. In most group formats, psychiatrists will facilitate the group with another clinician. This interaction is also helpful in evaluating behaviors and fortifying the relationship between the psychiatrist and other clinicians (Karterud 1993).

Design of the Group

Although the main purpose of this chapter is not to impart clinical information, it may be helpful to consider different ways in which groups can be structured to meet specific needs or circumstances. The group's design will often depend on setting and circumstance, as well as limitations encountered, but in most cases a satisfactory design can be arranged. Some aspects of group design are considered below (Gise and Crocker 2012; Karterud 1993).

Membership: The size of groups is variable, but most have 8–12 participants. Larger groups may be appropriate for educational formats, and smaller groups usually work best for process-oriented meetings. Homogeneous groups have members selected on the basis of some common characteristic or challenge (e.g., substance use or psychosis), whereas heterogeneous groups have members with a wide array of behavioral health challenges. Membership may be open (participation in flux, with a different constellation of members each meeting) or closed (membership is fixed or is only occasionally altered).

Duration: Group sessions generally last 60–90 minutes, although in some cases this may be too long to hold the attention of some members (i.e., those with various cognitive impairments). Open groups may be ongoing with no defined endpoint, whereas closed groups usually are planned with a specified time period or number of sessions. Educational groups may have a set curriculum, whereas process groups have a more open agenda, which may continue indefinitely.

Format: A variety of formats may be used depending on the main objective of the group. Most groups involving psychiatrists will need to incorporate medication management in some way. Some groups will make this the main focus, with prescribing taking place within the group context. Although this approach may provide some efficiency, it leaves little time for other group processes. If the objective is to incorporate some of the group therapeutic factors discussed earlier, leaders may choose an educational process or a supportive format, with prescribing taking place in brief individual meetings after the main group experience. Groups may also be organized around specific activities to facilitate interaction and relaxation, which may work well when working with clients who have difficulty expressing themselves.

Not all psychiatrists will be well suited for group work, but many will discover their ability to be effective group facilitators when they are adequately trained. As with other aspects of practice considered in this chapter, most training programs do not offer sufficient exposure to group work to enable graduates to feel comfortable leading groups. Clearly, greater exposure and better preparation would be critical for psychiatrists to have greater participation in this effective treatment modality.

Family Treatment

The value of family engagement and education, like that of group treatments, is well established. Family therapy evolved from psychoanalytic roots in the 1950s and 1960s. During that time, several theorists, many of whom were psychiatrists, independently developed family models before developing professional recognition and interaction in the years that followed. John Bell, Nathan Ackerman, Murray Bowen, and Carl Whitaker were among the seminal thinkers around the family's impact on the behavior of children and other family members. In the latter part of the twentieth century, these theorists and others began to examine how families are structured and interact, and began to develop interventions to alter families' function. The American Family Therapy Academy was established in 1977, and since then practitioners have become increasingly eclectic in their approaches rather than adhering to a particular school of thought (Broderick and Schrader 1991).

The initial development of psychoeducation for families with a member who has severe mental illness took place in the United States and the United Kingdom in the last three decades of the twentieth century. Ian Falloon in the United Kingdom and Carol Anderson in the United States developed education models for single families, and William McFarlane expanded Anderson's ideas to create the multifamily psychoeducation model (Deakins and McFarlane 2012). These treatment programs attempt to help families identify strategies to contribute to the recovery of their family member with severe mental illness. They do so by providing education about the illness, helping families to network and connect to resources, and teaching them to implement skills needed to provide support to their family member. These programs generally encourage involvement of the families over several months, with McFarlane's groups running for 18–24 months. Participating family members not only are able to provide better support for their loved one but also find that this involvement is supportive for themselves. There is extensive evidence for the effectiveness of these interventions (Falloon 2003; Hogarty et al. 1991; McFarlane 2002).

The rationale for including family interaction and education in psychiatrists' repertoire is much like the reasons given for psychiatrists' participation in group activities. Observation of a person in the context of his or her family constellation provides a clearer portrait of the individual's function and enhances the psychiatrist's ability to prescribe and contribute to the treatment planning process. In the role of prescriber, the psychiatrist needs to enlist the support of family members who will be involved in the care of their loved one and put them in the best position to provide it. That will be accomplished when family members understand the source of the symptoms they have witnessed and how prescribed medications may help. Psychiatrists are best suited to provide this information, and often they are the clinician on the team that family members are most eager to hear from. In the opening session of McFarlane's multifamily group model (Deakins and McFarlane 2012), the participants are given information about the biological basis of severe mental illness. Psychiatrists are chosen to provide this information when possible.

As with other elements that have been reduced or eliminated from the psychiatric scope of practice, there are several obstacles to the inclusion of family work. One major barrier lies with adult psychiatric training curricula. There are generally few clinical opportunities for family involvement and few positive mentors and supervisors to encourage it. As a result, many psychiatrists do not feel comfortable providing family treatment (Berman et al. 2008). Community behavioral health agencies are often not supportive of psychiatric involvement in family work, in part because of negative financial incentives. Despite the solid evidence of the effectiveness of family engagement and education, which ultimately reduces the cost of care through the decreased use of intensive services, short-term, agency-specific incentives often prevail, and the work of family education is frequently abdicated to NAMI (National Alliance on Mental Illness) or other mental health professionals (e.g., social workers, nurses, drug and alcohol counselors) (President's New Freedom Commission 2003). Enhancing psychiatrists' involvement in family interactions will only be accomplished through exposure and training. Reform of training curricula and on-the-job experience will increase the level of interest among psychiatrists and bolster their confidence for providing family treatment (Weisman 2011). Along with other elements of an expansion of the scope of practice, these skills will ultimately contribute to psychiatrists' versatility and overall quality of care, while making their experiences more fulfilling.

Individual Psychotherapy

As the scope of practice for psychiatrists has been reduced over time, there has been a corresponding decrease in their expertise and involvement in psychotherapy (Shorter 1997). Shortened visits, increased medication options, and the growing focus on biological treatments are major factors that have contributed to this change (Harris 2011; Mojtabai and Olfson 2008; Olfson et al. 2002). The decreased role in psychotherapy and increased focus on medication management have led to several unintended consequences (Carlat 2010; Mellman 2006; Pasnau 2000). Psychiatrists often feel marginalized as peripheral medication managers with little time to develop relationships with their clients (Fava et al. 2008). Many would argue that this lowers the overall quality of the treatment psychiatrists provide as they have a more limited view of their patients' behavioral dynamics.

Psychiatrists can do therapy as a part of their private practice with little difficulty. It may be more challenging in organizational settings. Psychotherapy cannot be offered to every client a psychiatrist sees, but it may be practical to carry a few cases to keep skills sharp. Thinking about psychological underpinnings of dysfunction even informs the prescribing process, as discussed earlier in this chapter. When limited to providing medication evaluations and treatment, psychiatrists are more likely to engage in counterproductive polypharmacy. "If your only tool is a hammer, everything will begin to look like a nail" is a well-known aphorism. Similarly, a limited focus on medication can lead psychiatrists to begin to see medication as the main solution to every problem. A broader scope of practice that includes psychotherapy would likely reduce the overuse of medications.

Having skill and expertise in therapy, along with medical knowledge, puts psychiatrists in a unique position to be able to have input into all parts of mental health treatment and be a more integral part of the treatment team. Psychiatric leadership is often provided informally at the outset, but as psychiatrists demonstrate both their wisdom and humility, this role often becomes more firmly established.

Psychiatrists' reduced involvement in psychotherapies is due in part to pressures to maximize billing with increased but shorter medication-focused visits. However, the resulting decrease in quality may offset any advantages derived from decreased cost (Carlat 2010). With the pendulum having swung to one extreme end with shorter medication management visits as the norm, it should now move back toward a more quality-focused approach. For most psychiatrists, psychotherapy would likely occupy a small portion of their time. Ideally, psychiatrists would do enough psychotherapy to maintain their skill set. Studies to determine the optimal amounts of time needed to maintain psychotherapy skills would be helpful, but any ongoing involvement would improve psychiatrists' capacity to contribute advantageously in organizational settings. Training curricula for psychiatrists should expand their attention to psychotherapeutic skills during the formal training period. If these fundamental skills are not established during the training period, it is less likely that they will be established as a psychiatrist's career progresses (DeMello and Deshpande 2011).

Provision of Primary Care

It has become clear that people with severe mental illness have a dramatically lower life expectancy than the general population. Psychiatrists have not traditionally been very attentive to or involved with physical health issues, despite the significant interaction of physical and mental health. The growing emphasis on integrated care for physical and mental health, and access to primary care for all members of the population, supports the need for psychiatrists to incorporate elements of primary health care into their practices. The level of involvement in the provision of primary care will vary according to circumstances, but attention to wellness and preventive activities will be a valuable addition to any psychiatric practice, decreasing days lost to both physical and mental disability.

Vanderlip and colleagues (2016) proposed five distinct domains that should be considered to determine the appropriate involvement by a psychiatrist in the provision of primary care: 1) the nature and severity of the problem, 2) the patient's access to existing primary care services, 3) the psychiatrist's general medical training and comfort, 4) the capacity of the provider's environment for management and follow-up, and 5) the patient's preference. Psychiatrists without special training in the provision of physical health care will obviously be less competent in the management of more complex, interacting, and severe physical health conditions. They could, however, easily manage simpler medical conditions such as hypertension or hyperlipidemia. It will make sense for psychiatrists to have greater involvement when clients' access to primary care is limited for any one of a variety of reasons. Patients' reluctance to visit a primary care provider may be a significant impediment to access for many clients. The management of medical conditions by psychiatrists will always need to be considered in the context of their training and competence as well as the capacity of the system in which they work to support primary care activities.

Considering these factors and several others, Sowers and colleagues (2016) describe three levels of complexity for the provision of primary care by psychiatrists. Level 1, universal basic psychiatric primary care, describes what all psychiatrists should be capable of incorporating into their practice: assessment of basic medical needs, health promotion, and health monitoring. It also includes communication with an outside primary care provider. Level 2 is enhanced psychiatric primary care. Psychiatrists should be able to provide this level of care when the client's access to primary care is impeded in some way. In addition to the activities described for Level 1, laboratory testing, limited physical examination, and the diagnosis and management of simple medical issues may be required. Continuing medical education related to these activities would be recommended for psychiatrists providing this level of primary care. Level 3 is fully integrated primary care and psychiatric management. The ability to obtain comprehensive care from one provider will be especially advantageous for some clients. Obviously, psychiatrists who are dually trained in primary care would be most capable of providing this level of care. Sowers and colleagues (2016) describe client characteristics and environmental circumstances for each level.

There have been many obstacles to the provision of primary care by psychiatrists. Perhaps foremost among these has been residents' inadequate preparation in training programs, which generally focus on tertiary care rather than placing residents in primary care settings to complete their physical health requirements. As a result, many psychiatrists are reluctant to provide this care and do not consider it part of their role. They express concerns that practicing primary care would expose them to increased liability risks or that this activity would harm the therapeutic relationship. Time constraints and lack of appropriate infrastructure to support some primary care functions also discourage its incorporation (Mojtabai and Olfson 2018). Last, but by no means least, the majority of current funding arrangements provide little or no incentives to psychiatrists to provide primary care or make it financially viable.

Clearly, these obstacles need to be overcome to move toward inclusion of primary care activities in psychiatric practice. The advantages of such inclusion are many, particularly for clients with severe mental illness. Greater attention to primary care needs will reduce morbidity and extend life expectancy, and therefore reduce the costs of tertiary care resulting from inadequate attention to health needs. Like other aspects of clinical practice that have been considered in this chapter, primary care must be included in the reformation of training programs, and health promotion and basic attention to the health status of clients need to be incorporated into standards of care for psychiatrists.

Education

Psychiatrists are likely to be the most highly trained professionals in behavioral health settings. Although their expertise and knowledge level will not necessarily surpass those of all other professionals in all clinical and administrative matters relevant to behavioral health care, psychiatrists do have some unique areas of expertise. In efforts to expand their scope of practice, psychiatrists may provide continuing professional education, community education, and patient education, as well as medical education and residency training. Most psychiatrists will find these educational opportunities attractive.

Some of the topics that psychiatrists are uniquely equipped to teach include the neurophysiology of psychiatric illness, the interface of mental and physical health, the effects of substance misuse on mental and physical health, the value of pharmacological interventions, and the physiology of stress reactions. There are many other areas in which psychiatrists have expertise that would allow them to make valuable contributions to educational programs. Despite this knowledge base, not all psychiatrists will be good teachers if they are not adequately prepared to take on these activities (Vassilas et al. 2003). As with other elements of the psychiatrist's role described in this chapter, adequate exposure in training, and ongoing inclusion in their practice activities, will enable them to be effective and confident in making these contributions.

At the most basic level, psychiatrists should be involved in the education of their clients. This is particularly relevant as the penetration of patient-centered, recovery-oriented care continues to advance. Providing relevant information to patients that enables them to make informed decisions about their care is an important element of this paradigm. Collaborative decision making enhances the investment of clients in the treatment plan and their likelihood of adhering to it. The education of family members and other involved supports will likewise be an advantageous investment of time by enabling these supports to be more effective and understanding as they attempt to help loved ones cope with their illness. Psychiatrists can also be useful to local advocacy and support groups, or any community organization that is concerned about the mental health of its community (Bird et al. 1983; Mushkin 2008). These educational activities will be important for combating stigma associated with people with mental health and substance use issues (Einat and George 2008).

Most psychiatrists, apart from those working in small private practices, will have significant interaction with allied behavioral health professionals. There is currently a broad spectrum of professionals, ranging from peer professionals and rehabilitation specialists to advance practice nurses and psychologists, who may be part of behavioral health teams. Exposure to aspects of psychiatric care in their training will vary considerably based on their discipline and training program (Leigh et al. 2008). These professionals are often eager to know more about diagnosis, medication, management of difficult behaviors, and other aspects of psychiatric care that psychiatrists can provide. Other health and service professionals often wish to know more about behavioral health as they encounter clients who struggle with these issues (Bird et al. 1983; Einat and George 2008). Education provided by psychiatrists via formal or informal encounters will be valuable for the coordination and integration of services.

Most psychiatrists do not hold a voluntary or full-time faculty position associated with a psychiatric training program or a medical school. Those who do are privileged to have opportunities to share their knowledge and experience with the next generation of psychiatrists. Involvement in training is a source of great satisfaction for many psychiatrists, even when these opportunities are a small part of their overall activity. Supervision and mentoring are often valued as much as more formal didactic involvement. These educational encounters with trainees often challenge more senior psychiatrists to keep their knowledge current by maintaining a personal program of self-education. This ongoing education, of course, is good for both trainer and trainees, and for the quality of care in general (Bromley and Braslow 2008). Extension of these opportunities to a greater number of psychiatrists would also benefit our systems of care.

Barriers to an Expanded Scope of Practice

One of the major factors to consider when thinking of scope of practice and how it affects value is the availability of psychiatrists. As noted earlier, there is a shortage of psychiatrists, and this will continue to be a challenge as psychiatrists age and retire (Association of American Medical Colleges 2012; Health Resources and Services Administration 2015; Lowes 2015). For patients to have sufficient access to psychiatric care and expertise, there must be a rethinking of standard approaches to service organization and the use of psychiatric resources. Shorter and less frequent visits can no longer be the primary response to growing demand. Alternatives to the traditional format of direct interaction between patient and psychiatrist must be implemented.

Cost is another commonly cited obstacle to using psychiatrists for nonpharmacological treatment methods. Billing options vary a great deal from insurer to insurer, by locality, and from state to state. Regardless of these variations, fee-for-service payment models make it more difficult to use psychiatrists in many of the ways outlined in this chapter. Alternative financing arrangements will be necessary to allow the most advantageous use of psychiatric services. All-inclusive per diem rates (e.g., residential treatment programs) or other global funding arrangements (e.g., capitated rate for a defined population) will offer much more flexibility in using psychiatric resources efficiently (see Chapter 6, "Innovative Financing").

Research is needed to clearly establish the value of a broader spectrum of psychiatric practices. Administrators may be wary of engaging psychiatrists in a full range of activities until systems are designed to use them most effectively. Expanding the reach of the psychiatric workforce through the development of alternative prescribers, telepsychiatry, and expanded consultation opportunities should be a primary consideration in these studies. Although the rationale for using psychiatrists with greater flexibility according to their skills makes intuitive sense, developing an evidence base to support these concepts should help overcome resistance from those who are doubtful.

Conclusion

The scope of psychiatric practice has been increasingly constricted over the past several decades, and this has not served the interests of our health service systems, those of people who use them, or those who provide care. This chapter considered how the scope of psychiatric practice should be expanded and how a diverse constellation of psychiatrist skills and activities will be beneficial to those who receive care by enhancing their health outcomes and satisfaction with services. Most psychiatrists will welcome the inclusion of a broader array of skills in their practices, because these will enrich the variety and complexity of their activity. This expansion should ultimately reduce "burnout" and other manifestations of their dissatisfaction.

Other chapters in this book will explore additional roles or skills that should be included in the scope of psychiatric services (e.g., Chapter 15, "Advocacy"; Chapter 16, "Psychiatric Leadership"; Chapter 17, "Addiction Treatment and Harm Reduction"). Engaging psychiatrists in the activities described throughout this volume will enhance their ability to effectively plan care and supervise other clinicians—which are appropriate responsibilities for highly trained professionals. Clearly, to accomplish this vision, we require significant changes in how we train clinicians (Chapter 12, "Psychiatric Workforce Development") and how we finance services (Chapter 6, "Innovative Financing"). When such changes occur, the cost and quality of care and the satisfaction of all stakeholders will be improved.

Ultimately, these adjustments to job descriptions will attract more medical students to this specialty and also improve organizations' capacity to recruit and retain them. From a population health perspective, many patients will be denied access to psychiatric care unless there are changes to treatment as it is currently being delivered. Psychiatrists should have a role in leading this change, but for that to occur, they must have a clear understanding of the forces that govern the systems of care in which they work. Shaping job descriptions in ways that would increase psychiatrists' sense of competence and accomplishment will be critical for their career satisfaction, but it must also bring value to services to be viable.

References

American Psychiatric Association, Academy of Psychosomatic Medicine: Dissemination of integrated care within adult primary care settings: the collaborative care model. 2016. Available at: www.psychiatry.org/File%20Library/Psychiatrists/Practice/Professional-Topics/Integrated-Care/APA-APM-Dissemination-Integrated-Care-Report.pdf. Accessed February 27, 2020.

Association of American Medical Colleges: 2012 Physician specialty data book. Center for Workforce Studies. November 2012. Available at: www.aamc.org/system/files/2019-08/2012physicianspecialtydatabook.pdf. Accessed February 27, 2020.

Barlow SH, Fuhriman AJ, Burlingame GM: The history of group counseling and psychotherapy, in Handbook of Group Counseling and Psychotherapy. Edited by DeLucia-Waack JL, Gerrity DA, Kalodner CR, et al. Thousand Oaks, CA, Sage Publications, 2014, pp 3–24

Berman EM, Heru A, Grunebaum H, et al: Family oriented patient care through the residency training cycle. Acad Psychiatry 32(2):111–118, 2008

Bird J, Cohen-Cole SA, Boker J, et al: Teaching psychiatry to non-psychiatrists,: I: the application of educational methodology. General Hospital Psychiatry 5(4):247–253, 1983

Broderick C, Shrader S: History of professional marriage and family therapy, in Handbook of Family Therapy. Edited by Gurman AS, Kniskern DP. New York, Routledge, Taylor & Francis Group, 1991, pp 3–40

Bromley E, Braslow JT: Teaching critical thinking in psychiatric training: a role for the social sciences. Am J Psychiatry 1165(11):1396–1401, 2008

Carlat DJ: Unhinged: The Trouble With Psychiatry: A Doctor's Revelations About a Profession in Crisis. New York, Free Press, 2010, pp 1–53

Colom F, Vieta E, Reinares M, et al: Psychoeducation efficacy in bipolar disorders: beyond compliance enhancement. J Clin Psychiatry 64(9):1101–1105, 2003

Correll CU, Detraux J, DeLepeleire J, et al: Effects of antipsychotics, antidepressants and mood stabilizers on risk for physical diseases in people with schizophrenia, depression and bipolar disorder. World Psychiatry 14(2):119–136, 2015

Deakins S, McFarlane W: Integrated family psycho-education: helping families help their loved ones recover, in Handbook of Community Psychiatry. Edited by McQuistion H, Sowers W, Ranz J, et al. New York, Springer, 2012, pp 339–345

Deegan PE, Drake RE: Shared decision making and medication management in the recovery process. Psychiatr Serv 57(11):1636–1639, 2006

DeMello JP, Deshpande SP: Career satisfaction of psychiatrists. Psychiatr Serv 62(9):1013–1018, 2011

Einat H, George A: Positive attitude change toward psychiatry in pharmacy students following an active learning psycho-pharmacology course. Acad Psychiatry 32(6):515–517, 2008

Falloon I: Family interventions for mental disorders: efficacy and effectiveness. World Psychiatry 2(1):20–28, 2003

Fava GA, Park SK, Dubovsky S: The mental health clinic: a new model. World Psychiatry 7(3):177–181, 2008

Gise L, Crocker B: Psychiatrist led outpatient groups: putting our minds together, in Handbook of Community Psychiatry. Edited by McQuistion H, Sowers W, Ranz J, et al. New York, Springer, 2012, pp 233–247

Harding CM, Brooks GW, Ashikaga T, et al: The Vermont longitudinal study of persons with severe mental illness, II: Long-term outcome of subjects who retrospectively met DSM-III criteria for schizophrenia. Am J Psychiatry 144(6):727–735, 1987

Harris G: Talk doesn't pay, so psychiatry turns to drug therapy. New York Times, March 5, 2011. Available at: www.nytimes.com/2011/03/06/health/policy/06doctors.html. Accessed February 27, 2020.

Health Resources and Services Administration/National Center for Health Workforce Analysis; Substance Abuse and Mental Health Services Administration/Office of Policy, Planning, and Innovation: National Projections of Supply and Demand for Behavioral Health Practitioners: 2013–2025. 2015. Available at: https://bhw.hrsa.gov/sites/default/files/bhw/health-workforce-analysis/research/projections/behavioral-health2013-2025.pdf. Accessed February 27, 2020.

Hegel MT, Imming J, Cyr-Provost M, et al: Role of behavioral health professionals in a collaborative stepped care treatment model for depression in primary care: Project IMPACT. Fam Syst Health 20(1):265–277, 2002

Herrman H, Trauer T, Warnock J, et al: The roles and relationships of psychiatrists and other service providers in mental health services. Aust NZ J Psychiatry 36(1):75–80, 2002

Hogarty GE, Anderson CM, Reiss DJ, et al: Family psychoeducation, social skills training, and maintenance chemotherapy in the aftercare treatment of schizophrenia: two-year effects of a controlled study on relapse and adjustment. Arch Gen Psychiatry 48(4):340–347, 1991

InformedHealth.org: Depression: how effective are antidepressants? Institute for Quality and Efficiency in Health Care, January 12, 2017. Available at: www.ncbi.nlm.nih.gov/books/NBK361016/. Accessed February 27, 2020.

Karterud SW: Community meetings in the therapeutic community, in Comprehensive Group Therapy, 3rd Edition. Edited by Kaplan HI, Sadock BJ. Baltimore, MD, Williams & Wilkins, 1993, pp 598–606

Leigh H, Mallios R, Stewart S: Teaching psychiatry in primary care residencies: do training directors of primary care and psychiatry see eye to eye? Acad Psychiatry 32(6):504–509, 2008

Lowes R: Psychiatry facing severe manpower crisis. Medscape, July 30, 2015. Available at: www.medscape.com/viewarticle/848884. Accessed February 27, 2020.

Mark TL, Levit KR, Buck JA: Datapoints: psychotropic drug prescriptions by medical specialty. Psychiatr Serv 60(9):1167, 2009

McFarlane W: Multiple Family Groups in the Treatment of Severe Psychiatric Disorders. New York, Guilford, 2002, pp 18–65

Mellman LA: How endangered is dynamic psychiatry in residency training? J Am Acad Psychoanal Dyn Psychiatry 34(1):127–133, 2006

Mojtabai R, Olfson M: National trends in psychotherapy by office-based psychiatrists. Arch Gen Psychiatry 65(8):962–970, 2008

Mojtabai R, Olfson M: Management of common medical conditions by office-based psychiatrists. Psychiat Serv 69(4):410–423, 2018

Moncrieff J, Kirsch I: Efficacy of antidepressants in adults. BMJ 331(7509):155–157, 2005

Mushkin PR: The teaching of psychiatry to non-psychiatrists: the patient as person. Acad Psychiatry 32(6):460–462, 2008

National Council for Behavioral Health: The psychiatric shortage: causes and solutions. March 28, 2017. Available at: www.thenationalcouncil.org/wp-content/uploads/2017/03/Psychiatric-Shortage_National-Council-.pdf. Accessed February 27, 2020.

Olfson M, Marcus SC, Druss B, et al: National trends in the outpatient treatment of depression. JAMA 287(2):203–209, 2002

Panman R, Panman S: Group counseling and therapy, in The Counseling Sourcebook: A Practical Reference on Contemporary Issues. Edited by Ronch JL, Van Ornum W, Stilwell NC. New York, Crossroad Publishing, 2001, pp 232–241

Pasnau RO: Can the patient-physician relationship survive in the era of managed care? J Psychiatr Pract 6(2):91–96, 2000
Piercy MA, Sramek JJ, Kurtz NM, et al: Placebo response in anxiety disorders. Ann Pharmacother 30(9):1013–1019, 1996
Pigott HE, Leventhal AM, Alter GS, et al: Efficacy and effectiveness of antidepressants: current status of research. Psychother Psychosom 79(5):267–279, 2010
President's New Freedom Commission: Achieving the promise: transforming mental health care in America. July 22, 2003, pp 27–46. Available at: https://govinfo.library.unt.edu/mentalhealthcommission/reports/FinalReport/downloads/FinalReport.pdf. Accessed February 27, 2020.
Ranz J, Stueve A: The role of the psychiatrist as program medical director. Psychiatr Serv 49(9):1203–1207, 1998
Ranz J, Weinberg M, Arbuckle M, et al: A four factor model of systems-based practices in psychiatry. Acad Psychiatry 36(6):473–478, 2012
Ranz JM, Vergare MJ, Wilk JE, et al: The tipping point from private practice to publicly funded settings for early and midcareer psychiatrists. Psychiatr Serv 57(11):1640–1643, 2006
Rimmer A: Large meta-analysis ends doubts about efficacy of antidepressants. BMJ Clinical Research 360:k847, 2018
Shorter E: A History of Psychiatry: From the Era of the Asylum to the Age of Prozac. New York, Wiley, 1997
Smith BL: Inappropriate prescribing. Monitor on Psychology, 2012. Available at: www.apa.org/monitor/2012/06/prescribing. Accessed February 27, 2020.
Sowers W: Reducing reductionism: reclaiming psychiatry. Psychiatr Serv 56(6):637, 2005
Sowers WE, Golden S: Psychotropic medication management in persons with co-occurring psychiatric and substance use disorders. J Psychoactive Drugs 31(1):59–70, 1999
Sowers WE, Thompson KS (eds): Keystones for collaboration and leadership: issues and recommendations for the transformation of community psychiatry. The American Association of Community Psychiatrists, Pennsylvania Psychiatric Leadership Council, Allegheny County Office of Behavioral Health, Coalition of Psychiatrists for Recovery, 2007. Available at: www.bgrosjean.com/files/TransformationofPsychiatryReport.pdf. Accessed February 27, 2020.
Sowers W, Arbuckle M, Shoyinka S: Recommendations for primary care provided by psychiatrists. Community Ment Health J 52(4):379–386, 2016
Steingard S: Five year outcomes of tapering antipsychotic drug doses in a community mental health center. Community Mental Health J 54(8):1097–1100, 2018
Stone WN: Group psychotherapy, in Psychiatry, 3rd Edition, Vol 2. Edited by Tasman J, Lieberman M, First M, et al. New York, Wiley, 2008, pp 1904–1919
Vanderlip ER, Raney LE, Druss BG: A framework for extending psychiatrists' roles in treating general health conditions. Am J Psychiatry 173(7):658–663, 2016
Vassilas CA, Brown N, Wall D: Teaching the teachers in psychiatry. Advances in Psychiatric Treatment 9(4):308–315, 2003

Weisman S: Are we training psychiatrists to provide only medication management? Psychiatric Times, January 28, 2011. Available at: www.psychiatrictimes.com/schizophrenia/are-we-training-psychiatrists-provide-only-medication-management. Accessed February 27, 2020.

Yalom ID: The therapeutic factors in group psychotherapy, in Theory and Practice of Group Psychotherapy, 3rd Edition. New York, Basic Books, 1970, pp 1–20

12

Psychiatric Workforce Development

Patrick Runnels, M.D., M.B.A.

Available data on workforce trends over the past 20 years point to a severe and worsening problem with access to psychiatric care. In one study, the Health Resources and Services Administration (HRSA) anticipated that the psychiatrist shortfall in 2025 would range from 6,080 to 15,400 (Health Resources and Services Administration 2016). A different HRSA study suggested that the shortfall in 2006 was already at least 24,000 and perhaps as high as 45,000 (Konrad et al. 2009). Whichever benchmark data you look at, the psychiatrist deficit is expected to *grow* by more than ten thousand over the next decade.

During the decade from 2003 to 2013, the number of psychiatrists per capita in the United States declined by 10%. More than 50% of the counties in the United States had no psychiatric provider in 2013 (Bishop et al. 2016), and more than 75% had a severe shortage and 96% had unmet "prescriber" need in an earlier study (Thomas et al. 2009). Additionally, more than 50% of psychiatrists are above age 55, making psychiatry the second-oldest physician discipline, trailing only physical medicine and rehabilitation (American Medical

Association 2015). Furthermore, from 1978 to 2012, the number of matched residency slots increased a paltry 141 slots (13%) from 939 to 1,080 (National Residency Matching Program 2017). Because graduation from psychiatric residency programs has held relatively steady for the past 35 years, the anticipated wave of retirement over the next 10 years is expected to further exacerbate the supply problem, even though available residency slots ballooned from 2013 through 2017 (increasing 28% from 1,080 to 1,491 slots).

Aggravating this supply problem, several factors have led to an increase in demand for psychiatry. The Patient Protection and Affordable Care Act of 2010 significantly expanded access to private insurance shortly after its implementation, and more than 15 million additional individuals were enrolled in the Medicaid expansions starting in 2014 (Centers for Medicare and Medicaid Services, Centers for Medicaid and CHIP Services 2018). Meanwhile, the demand to reduce health care costs—17.9% of gross domestic product as of 2017 (Centers for Medicare and Medicaid Services 2018)—has led to a focus on interventions that can prevent costly procedures and hospitalizations. Evidence confirming the value of psychiatric interventions in significantly reducing health care spending overall has proliferated over the past two decades (Grypma et al. 2006; Katon et al. 2006; Simon et al. 2007; Unützer et al. 2008), and health care organizations have caught on: psychiatry is now the second most in-demand specialty, and salaries for psychiatric providers have outpaced nearly every other specialty over the past several years (Merritt Hawkins 2018).

Taken together, these findings bring into sharp focus the need to address the psychiatric workforce shortage. A large emphasis has been placed on changing how and to whom psychiatrists provide care, most notably with the advent of models for integrated behavioral and physical health care and telepsychiatry. However, even the most efficient use of new models will not fully bridge the gap between supply and demand. Although advanced practice registered nurses (APRNs) are the most visible health care professionals to step in and fill the void, others have started to fill the gap as well, including physician assistants and pharmacists.

Psychiatric physicians often have a limited understanding of the background and scope of practice of other professional groups that are functioning in the prescribing role. In this chapter, we first consider factors related to scope of practice and the tension between different disciplines occupying the prescribing role. We then review the training and roles of several professionals: psychiatric APRNs, physician assistants (PAs), and pharmacists. We additionally briefly explore psychologist prescribing statutes and data for states where psychologists can obtain prescriptive authority. Finally, we consider how different professionals can function more effectively as a team and how psychiatric training and practice must change in order to accommodate this new environment.

Scope of Practice

Scope of practice refers to the range of actions and interventions that a health care professional is allowed to undertake, as well as the parameters under which the professional can practice as dictated by the terms of professional licensure. Scope of practice is determined primarily at the state level. Physicians have the broadest and least restrictive scope of practice of any health care professional, enjoying broad latitude to deliver care independently across most medical fields. Credentialing committees serve as the main limiting force on physician practice.

Licensure requirements for all other health care professions come with increased practice limitations. In this chapter, we concern ourselves primarily with scope of practice as it relates to APRNs, PAs, and pharmacists. Some limitations are secondary to depth of training; for example, primary care would be out of scope for psychiatric APRNs who receive no training in primary care. Other limitations are based on state regulations, which place restrictions on prescribing medications, procedures, and hospital admission privileges. Finally, autonomy and independence of other professionals are often limited, primarily through the requirement of collaborative agreements with physicians. These collaborative agreements serve as limiting agents themselves—that is, a professional cannot practice at all without having one in place—and can also endow supervising physicians with additional latitude to limit others' scope of practice as they see fit. Importantly, while physician practice is nearly uniform across the country, scope of practice for other professionals can vary considerably from state to state. Furthermore, within states, rules governing scope of practice are constantly evolving. Given the increasing ubiquity of interprofessional practice, it is recommended that physicians acquaint themselves with their state's rules and regulations for any and all professional groups with whom they actively collaborate. State medical, nursing, and pharmacy associations are typically excellent resources for gathering this information.

Controversy

Expansions in the scope of practice for other professions have been driven primarily by physician workforce shortages and restricted access to care. Efforts to increase or enhance scope for an expanding group of providers have been met with some alarm by psychiatrists. Physician advocacy groups often lobby against easing regulations on practice out of concern for diminished standards of care, whereas the other professions lobby for easing restrictions, arguing that such concerns are unfounded and unnecessarily interfere with expanding access to isolated and underserved populations. This debate is not trivial and has important ramifications. As a society, we are in the process of determining exactly what—if any—risk comes with various degrees of expanding scope for different professions so that we can establish the right balance of quality and access.

Economic Considerations and Disruptive Innovation

Of course, economic interests are also powerful motivating factors. Psychiatrists (like all other physicians) enjoy the privileged position of a tightly capped labor market that never fully meets demand. This limitation in the supply of practitioners enhances relative market power, impacting both remuneration and practice conditions. Depending on one's view, either this is necessary to ensure that the quality of care delivered meets a minimum standard, or physicians are capturing *monopoly rents*—that is, increased price that does not provide extra value but that can be charged in the absence of competition. Indeed, the possibility that consumers might believe physicians are charging monopoly rents has accentuated competition from professionals who perceive that they are trying to deliver the same value proposition to the same market segment.

However, the economic forces that have led to these sometimes heated and acrimonious debates have rarely been fully expounded on. For many decades, physicians held near monopoly power over the health care workforce supply. The impact of this position was less concerning through the mid-1960s because available health care interventions offered far less value to consumers while insurance was considerably less ubiquitous. However, the establishment of Medicare and Medicaid dramatically and rapidly increased the number of insured individuals. Over the next several decades, expanded insurance coverage paired with unparalleled innovation in practice and technology (computed tomography, magnetic resonance imaging, myriad surgical innovations, pharmaceutical breakthroughs) led to increased demand. That increase in demand fueled the spike in health care costs that is currently plaguing our country. Not only has health care become uncomfortably expensive, but workforce development has not kept up with demand: the ratio of psychiatrists per capita has actually diminished over the last 20 years (Bishop et al. 2016).

This market vacuum is inconsistent with sound economics. Eventually, the pressure to expand access and meet demand was bound to overcome physician resistance to new market entrants and soften public (and physician) concern about quality. Initially, expansion of scope to other professions appealed to only a smaller segment of health care consumers who were willing to trade the potential reduced quality of providers whose training was both less robust and unproven for increased access and lower price. Over time, however, the alternative training programs have adapted to improve the quality of their graduates, thereby increasing the appeal of their services. Although this topic has not been extensively studied, health care consumers in the United States appear to be increasingly comfortable with care delivered by APRNs and PAs (Dill et al. 2013), particularly when limited access to physicians is raised as a concern. Meanwhile, health care systems are eager to expand access to medication management at a lower price. An innovation in efficiency that seeks to upset a market dominated by a limited number of high-value, high-cost alternatives is termed a *disruptive innovation*. The expansion of scope to professionals with less training (and therefore cheaper to produce and pay) performing many of the same duties traditionally performed by physicians meets that definition precisely. At least in some market segments, these other professionals have become a reasonable, lower-cost substitute for the more expensive service provided by physicians (Hwang and Christensen 2008).

To be sure, this innovation has caused modest disruption to some market segments that are more price sensitive (e.g., some community mental health centers operating on very thin margins with challenging reimbursement rates). However, because access to psychiatry remains relatively poor, the increase in alternatives to psychiatrists has not had a negative impact on psychiatrists' salaries overall. To the contrary, salaries for both psychiatrists and psychiatric APRNs have continued to increase together. Furthermore, even this continued, robust addition of other professions is unlikely to fully meet demand, so other types of innovations will also be necessary to solve the access problem (e.g., integrated care, telepsychiatry, or even artificial intelligence, which is likely in the near future to streamline triage and data gathering, thereby improving efficiency).

Nevertheless, the concern generated by expansion of scope to other professions has been enough for psychiatrists to consider the following question: If much of what was traditionally performed by psychiatrists can be performed by those with less training and at lower cost, what is the value proposition of psychiatrists in the mental health landscape of the future? A more diverse role for psychiatrists was considered in the previous chapter (Chapter 11, "An Expanded Role for Psychiatry"), but in an environment in which demand is likely to outstrip need for the foreseeable future, this becomes a question not simply of who gets assigned what tasks, but also of how different professions can collaborate together most effectively to serve the population at large. This issue, in turn, requires us as psychiatrists to become considerably more familiar and comfortable with the range of professionals with whom we now share space, in addition to expanding the range of their own skills and knowledge.

Psychiatric Advanced Practice Registered Nurses

History

The first advanced practice nursing program for any discipline was the psychiatric advance practice program developed in 1954 and initiated a year later by Hildegard Peplau out of Rutgers University with a grant from the National Institute of Mental Health. The original role was called the clinical nurse specialist (CNS) and focused on managing the therapeutic milieu in addition to psychotherapeutic interventions. Perhaps more importantly, the core thrust of the role was to enhance the application of nursing theory and science to the practice of psychiatric nursing—to help psychiatric nurses practice more effectively through teaching, organizational analysis, consultation, and leadership (Drew 2014).

Just 10 years later, more than 30 programs had been established across the country. The CNS remained the sole APRN role until the development of the nurse practitioner (NP) role in the 1990s. Select prescriptive authority was granted to APRNs by some states as early as the 1980s, with all states providing at least limited prescribing privileges by 2007. In 1994, prescribing privileges had been attained by 20% of psychiatric APRNs; by 2007, the percentage had climbed to 68% (Drew 2014).

Broadly, the differences between the CNS and NP roles have been and continue to be small, but NP training has an enhanced focus on pharmacology, physical examination, and pathophysiology. In 2001, the American Nurse Credentialing Center developed a certification exam for NPs. In 2004, the National Panel for Psychiatric-Mental Health NP Competencies developed a standardized set of competencies for NP training programs, which helped to standardize training across the country. In a parallel development, APRN leadership across all disciplines developed a "National Consensus" model in 2008, which serves to standardize regulation of APRN practice at the state level across the country (Drew 2014).

Nursing Theory

APRNs do not view themselves as mid-level medical providers or as mere extenders of physician practice. Indeed, the terms *mid-level provider* and *physician extender* are offensive precisely because they minimize the value of nursing theory and perspective. Although APRNs must master the competencies of psychiatric diagnosis and treatment, this learning occurs alongside and in partnership with core nursing practice and theory, which are outlined below. Indeed, nursing theory, which is person-centric, offers an alternative approach to patient engagement and evaluation that can provide an important counterbalance to the predominant physician approach, which is traditionally disease-centric. Recovery-oriented, patient-centered care—which has become central to the practice of community psychiatry—has strong parallels with psychiatric nursing theory, and the synergy between these distinctive approaches can both be incredibly valuable and greatly enhance patient care.

Interpersonal Theory of Nursing

Hildegard Peplau, widely regarded as the "mother" of psychiatric nursing, pioneered the "interpersonal theory of nursing." Peplau postulated that unlike medicine—which seeks to identify specific disease elements, make diagnoses, and apply evidence-based treatment to cure or attenuate underlying disorders—nursing is an interpersonal process that seeks to relieve distress through the development of a relationship. That relationship proceeds sequentially through the development and understanding of an individual's "felt difficulties," the larger environment contributing to those difficulties, and the identification of common goals that are shared by both the nurse and the individual to help resolve the difficulties. In this paradigm, rather than seeking first to assess the individual's specific difficulties, the assessment phase seeks first to understand the whole person and their surrounding environment in order to get a full understanding of their difficulties and then to supplement that initial assessment with broader questioning (Varcarolis 2013).

Stuart Stress Adaptation Model

Gail Stuart is among the more influential modern psychiatric nursing theorists. In contrast to the health/illness model that dominates medicine, Stuart's Stress Adaptation Model is more consistent with the nurse's role. The model works on five assumptions: 1) that the individual is situated within a larger psychosocial context that must be fully understood; 2) that the nurse must deliver care that considers the entire biopsychosocial context of the individual's environment; 3) that an individual develops coping mechanisms to the stress that arises from their environments that exist on a range from highly adaptive to highly maladaptive; 4) that nursing interventions should be considered through the lens of primary, secondary, and tertiary prevention, and should exist in four phases—crisis, acute, maintenance, and health promotion; and 5) that the assumptions outlined above are grounded in the nursing process, separate and distinct from the medical model. Finally, according to the model, good mental health is measurable along six criteria: positive attitude toward self; growth, development, and self-actualization; integration, which is a balance between what is expressed and repressed; autonomy, including the acceptance of consequences for one's actions; reality perception; and environmental mastery (Stuart 2009).

Training

Pre–Master's Degree Work

The lowest level of nurse training and certification is the licensed practical nurse (LPN). LPN programs are typically 1- to 2-year certificate programs, with a focus on practical skills, compared with higher level analytic skills for any registered nursing degree, reflected by more difficult coursework. One can earn a degree in registered nursing by completing either a 2-year certificate program or a 4-year bachelor of science degree in nursing (BSN). Multiple pathways to attain a BSN degree are available for nurses with less than a BSN or with a bachelor's degree in another subject. The most common route is referred to as a conversion or bridging program, which allows a person to count associate degree coursework credit toward the BSN. The BSN is nondifferentiated by specialty; upon graduation, nurses can choose to focus their work in any specialty area and can shift to a different specialty at any point during their career.

Master of Science in Nursing

The master of science in nursing (MSN) degree refers to any graduate-level nursing program geared toward training APRNs. However, MSN programs are specific to different disciplines and have very different curricula. The following MSN degrees are offered: nurse practitioner, certified nurse specialist, certified registered nurse anesthetist, and certified nurse midwife. Nurse practitioner degrees are offered in multiple subspecialties: acute care, adult gerontology, emergency, family, neonatal, pediatric, psychiatric-mental health, and women's health. Psychiatric-mental health nurse practitioner (PMH-NP) programs train individuals to practice psychiatry. The American Psychiatric Nurses Association (2020) currently lists 133 individual PMH-NP degree programs across all 50 states. Successful completion of a PMH-NP program confers eligibility to sit for the Psychiatric NP certification exam, a prerequisite for obtaining licensure.

A BSN or an equivalent is required for admission to an MSN program. Previously, a minimum number of clinical years of practice was also required; although some programs still require at least a few years of practice, many programs have no clinical experience requirement. PMH-NP programs require 18–24 months of education, divided into classroom/didactic work and clinical placements. Coursework totals approximately 45 credit hours; this includes a minimum of 500 hours of clinical practicum over the course of the 2 years. Coursework in most programs is a mix of in-person and online participation, with some programs delivered entirely online, allowing NP students in one state to participate in programs in other states. Coursework for the PMH-NP degree includes, among other courses, overviews of psychiatric diagnoses, pharmacology, and other treatment interventions, along with application of nursing theory to mental health settings.

The clinical practicum experience is considerably more heterogeneous for students in a given graduate nursing program than for students in medical school, because students in most nursing programs are responsible for identifying and arranging their own clinical placements, which are usually not directly affiliated with the nursing school. Prior to each semester, students—with guidance from faculty and school alumni—reach out to potential preceptors, who must agree to supervise the student during an experience that meets the rotation requirements. This process, while flexible, risks exposing students to rotations that are highly observational, minimally engaging, and light on personalized supervision. The school does not typically pay preceptors for their time, but some clinical placements charge PMH-NP students a fee to cover supervisory costs.

The rotations are organized around the practice domains of individual psychotherapy, family and group psychotherapy, and medication management, rather than being organized around practice setting (e.g., consultation-liaison or inpatient psychiatry). PMH-NP students do not necessarily have robust experiences across all practice settings, so a PMH-NP may graduate with no experience in some settings. This does not preclude the PMH-NP from getting work in those settings (although most PMH-NP students focus their clinical experiences in settings where they intend to practice after graduating), so a core value of PMH-NP culture and training is *self-directed learning* across their careers (O'Shea 2003). In any new practice setting, PMH-NPs are expected to identify their limitations and identify collaborative partners to provide mentorship to shore up any deficits.

Doctor of Nursing Practice Degree

The doctor of nursing practice (DNP) degree involves an additional 30+ credit hours on top of the MSN degree. To attain a DNP degree, graduates typically must have completed 1,000 post-BSN hours of clinical practicum, which includes hours accumulated toward their MSN degrees. Most DNP degree students are already employed in a clinical setting, and those clinical hours can be counted toward this total. Unlike MSN programs, DNP programs are not specific to a particular discipline; psychiatric APRNs, nurse midwives, and others learn side by side. Meanwhile, coursework focuses on leadership, program development, and policy rather than further clinical study and preparation. All

DNP programs expect students to create a scholarly project that focuses on improving practice above the level of the individual provider.

The field of nursing has been debating for years whether to require all APRNs to attain a DNP degree to be eligible for the American Nurses Credentialing Center board exam, and some programs have rolled the training into one combined program. At present, however, attainment of the DNP degree is not required for a nurse to practice as an APRN in any state.

Residency and Fellowship

NP residencies and fellowships are post–master's degree clinical training programs, typically run by health care provider entities rather than academic institutions. They are focused entirely on providing enhanced clinical support and mentorship during the first year(s) of practice, with the goal of improving the clinical quality and skill level of participants. Residents and fellows typically earn a salary, which might be lower than the full salary they would otherwise earn. The terms *residency* and *fellowship* are used somewhat interchangeably, although typically *residency* refers to a general program and *fellowship* denotes a subspecialty training experience. These programs are *not* required for NPs to practice, and no formal accreditation process is required at this time. An accreditation process is in development, and implementation will likely accelerate the interest in postgraduate NP training (National Nurse Practitioner Residency and Fellowship Training Consortium 2019).

As the clinical experience prerequisite for admission to MSN programs has been eliminated and the experience level of PMH-NP graduates has dropped, the demand for such programs by recent MSN graduates has increased. At present, only a handful of psychiatry residency or fellowship programs for APRNs have been formalized (GraduateNursingEDU.org 2020). A larger number of organizations provide informal, structured mentorship programs during the first year of practice.

Scope of Practice and Collaboration

The American Nursing Association defines *scope of practice* as the "services that a qualified health professional is deemed competent to perform, and permitted to undertake—in keeping with the terms of their professional license" (American Nurses Association 2020). All APRNs are limited in scope based on their area of training and certification. Psychiatric APRN scope of practice extends to all areas of psychiatry but not, for instance, to primary care. Likewise, for example, the scope for clinical nurse midwives is limited to practice related to women's health and does not include critical care.

APRNs are trained to be acutely aware of their scope limitations and are responsible for making sure that the care they deliver is squarely in line with both their certification and training. Relatively minor violations of scope boundaries can be met with swift and severe sanctions by state nursing boards, even in the absence of a bad outcome. Further complicating matters, within a given specialty, gray areas exist. For instance, the ability of psychiatric APRNs to prescribe metformin to treat metabolic syndrome is under debate. APRNs are trained to interpret scope of practice conservatively until clear guidance is issued by state nursing boards or national accreditation bodies.

In addition to scope differences across APRN disciplines, scope within an APRN discipline varies dramatically across states, largely related to restrictions on prescriptive authority (American Association of Nurse Practitioners 2020). Presently, APRNs in 22 states have authority to prescribe independently within their scope of practice but outside a formal collaborative relationship with a physician; those in 16 states have the ability to prescribe largely autonomously through a formal collaborative relationship with a physician; and those in 12 states have significant restrictions on their ability to prescribe. The exact nature of collaborative relationships varies significantly, and these relationships are typically vaguely defined by state laws, rules, and regulations. APRNs and physicians are both well advised to fully understand rules related to APRN scope of practice in the state or states in which they practice (Minarik et al. 2001).

Independent prescriptive authority is a core area of advocacy for nursing groups, while being strongly opposed by most physician advocacy groups (Villegas and Allen 2012). Notably, the trend over the past decade has leaned heavily toward prescriptive independence and autonomy. Other scope restrictions apply to admitting privileges and test result interpretation. No research as to the impact on outcomes, practice patterns, and provider distribution in psychiatry has been undertaken as of the publication of this book, although several studies of other fields have demonstrated that prescribing patterns, patient satisfaction, and patient outcomes are comparable for APRNs and physicians (Jiao et al. 2018; Johantgen et al. 2012; Maul et al. 2015; Virani et al. 2016).

Workforce Data

As of 2017, the total number of psychiatric APRNs was 17,387 (Delaney and Vanderhoef 2019). At that time, annual rates of certification were around 1,100 psychiatric NPs per year, putting the country on track to have more than 17,000 psychiatric APRNs by 2025 (Drew 2014).

Physician Assistants

History

In response to shortages in physicians, particularly in rural areas and the military, the first physician assistant (PA) training program was established at Duke University in 1965 by Dr. Eugene Stead, enrolling four former navy corpsmen (Physician Assistant History Society 2020). By 1980, the number of training programs had climbed to 42, and over 9,400 PAs had been certified by the National Commission on Certification of Physician's Assistants (Physician Assistant History Society 2020). By the end of the 1980s, all but two states had rules and regulations that allowed for PAs to practice at the direction of a supervising physician (Mississippi would be the last in 2000) (Physician Assistant History Society 2020).

For several decades, PA training programs were not standardized. Some programs focused on training surgical assistants, others on primary care; some programs led to associate's degrees, others to bachelor's degrees (Physician Assistant History Society 2020). In 1990, accreditation standards for all types of training programs were consolidated to ensure uniformity of training for all PAs (Accreditation Review Commission on Education for the Physician Assistant 2020c). Though not clearly documented, the conversion to master's level programs—which is now the standard for the vast majority of programs—began in the 1990s (Physician Assistant History Society 2020). By 2000, more than 42% of PA programs were master's level (Larson and Hart 2007); today, nearly all programs are. By 2020, all PA training programs will be required to offer a formal graduate degree and all enrollees will be required to have a bachelor's degree. As of 2018, a total of 239 accredited PA training programs had been established, up from less than 150 programs just 8 years earlier (Accreditation Review Commission on Education for the Physician Assistant 2020a).

Training

Master's Degree

Parallel to physicians, all PAs, regardless of the discipline and the setting in which they practice after graduation, go through the same basic training program (in contrast to APRNs, whose training programs are specialized by discipline). To be admitted to graduate programs, individuals must have completed a bachelor's degree with certain prerequisite courses in the sciences. PA master's training programs are around 2 years in length and are accredited solely by the Accreditation Review Commission on Education for the Physician Assistant, which is overseen by a conglomerate of advocacy organizations led by physicians and PAs. Curricula are modeled on physician education.

The first year focuses on basic physiology and pathophysiology, which typically includes 400 hours in basic sciences, 175 hours in behavioral sciences, and 580 hours in clinical medicine. The second year consists primarily of clinical rotations in outpatient, emergency, inpatient, and long-term care settings across a variety of disciplines that include all medical disciplines (surgery, medicine, primary care, obstetrics and gynecology, behavioral health, pediatrics, emergency medicine). By the end of the program, students should have completed approximately 2,000 hours of supervised clinical practice (American Academy of Physician Assistants 2014).

PA students focusing on behavioral health and psychiatry have a didactic course in behavioral health during the first year of training, and then a clinical rotation, typically 4 weeks, during their second year of training (Case Western Reserve University School of Medicine 2020). In addition, students may choose elective work in psychiatry. Rotations are established with a broad set of competencies that students are expected to develop during the rotation, including diagnosis, clinical treatment, and interviewing. Schools leverage several different settings for each class, and students typically complete the clinical rotation in one setting. The result is a heterogenous set of experiences, in which some are more hands-on and others more observational (not so different from psychiatry rotations for medical students). After graduation, PAs must pass the Physician Assistant National Certifying Exam; they then must complete 100 hours of continuing education and take a recertification exam every 10 years.

Postgraduate Training

After obtaining a master's degree, PAs have available to them a variety of formal postgraduate training programs, akin to residency and fellowship programs, typically sponsored by health care systems. Some formal programs for psychiatry postgraduate training have been established (Association of Postgraduate Physician Assistant Programs 2020). These 1-year programs typically provide supervised clinical rotations aimed at establishing basic competency across a broad range of clinical settings in psychiatry. Didactics and supervision are typically included. No formal accreditation process has been adopted (Accreditation Review Commission on Education for the Physician Assistant 2020b).

Scope of Practice and Collaboration

The scope of practice for PAs is, by and large, more streamlined and homogeneous than the scope for APRNs. Scope of practice does vary state by state, with some states codifying supervision requirements, prescriptive authority, and scope of practice at the level of the state medical board, and other states delegating the decisions on each of those three areas to practices themselves. Currently, no states allow for independent practice by PAs: all states require a collaborative agreement between a PA and a physician who is responsible for overseeing the PA's practice. Because PA programs include training in all major medical disciplines, PA scope of practice includes all areas of medicine; interdisciplinary restrictions, such as on prescribing medications, are at the discretion of the practice in which a PA is working (Scope of Practice Policy 2020).

PA practice itself is heavily rooted in the concept of *collaborative team practice*, in which effective teams "utilize the skills and abilities of each team member most fully" (American Academy of Physician Assistants 2017a). PAs view their roles as more collaborative than subordinate, and although scope of practice and team roles are delegated by a physician, PAs can fulfill any role that the physician deems them capable of with the highest amount of autonomy possible, commensurate with their individual skill sets. More recently, PA advocacy groups have promoted *optimal team practice*, which seeks to eliminate the need for collaborative agreements with physicians while maintaining the legal expectation that PAs continue to practice in physician-led teams (though without delineated guidelines for how this would be monitored). This approach to practice would remove specific practice regulations from state laws (i.e., formulary, procedures, degree of autonomy), and the regulations would be shifted to the physician level entirely without state oversight otherwise. This policy position by PAs, advocating for the elimination of formal collaborative agreements altogether, should not be confused with the more general term *collaborative team practice* (American Academy of Physician Assistants 2017b).

Workforce Data

As of 2017, a total of 95,408 PAs were certified, of whom 1,347 were identified as practicing in psychiatry, representing about 1.4% of the PA workforce nationally. Although this represents an average of about 26 psychiatric PAs per state, the distribution around the country is variable (National Commission on Certification of Physician Assistants 2018).

Clinical Pharmacists

History

Over the past decade, pharmacists have gained scope of practice permitting them to modify prescribed medications in collaboration with physicians, consistent with their clinical focus on patient wellness and chronic disease management. Historically, bachelor's degrees were the terminal degree for pharmacists. After the first doctorate in pharmacy (PharmD) was introduced in 1950 at the University of Southern California, the predominant degree remained the bachelor's for several more decades. Not until 1992 did the American Association of Colleges of Pharmacy (AACP) vote to recommend that the PharmD should be the only accredited degree for pharmacists, and in 2000 the American Council on Pharmaceutical Education (renamed the Accreditation Council for Pharmacy Education in 2003) formally stopped accrediting bachelor's programs in pharmacy (Carter 2016).

This evolution in training was driven by a change in identity. Historically, pharmacists identified as dispensing agents. The advent of doctoral programs gave birth to the concept of pharmacists as clinicians. By 1975, the AACP had commissioned a report, *Pharmacists of the Future*, that explicitly identified pharmacists as clinicians and made recommendations for clinical training to be standardized into curricula. Over the following decades, this training has laid the foundation for the clinical identity of pharmacists today.

Starting in the 1980s, a significant number of hospital-based postgraduate training residencies emerged, offering opportunities for clinical pharmacists to further enhance their clinical skills. Over time, these residencies have evolved to include subspecialty training in the form of a second-year postgraduate residency, and pharmacists can now gain additional certification in a range of subspecialties.

Training

Doctoral Training

Traditional PharmD programs are 4-year doctoral programs. Most require a bachelor's degree for admission, although a handful of programs offer the bachelor's degree and PharmD in one 6-year program. A PharmD program includes coursework on pharmacotherapeutics and other aspects of managing a pharmacy; coursework covering a range of chronic diseases; and a year of clinical experience, referred to as the Advanced Pharmacy Practice Experiences. Although these programs include psychopharmacology in the coursework, they have no specific requirements related to psychiatry or mental health clinical experiences. After graduation, pharmacists take a board certification exam, which is required for licensure (University of Southern California School of Pharmacy 2020).

Residency and Subspecialty Certification

Although the pharmacy profession has debated making residencies a requirement for licensure, postgraduate residencies are currently elective experiences. Residencies—categorized as either hospital based or clinic based—typically take 1 year but can be extended an additional year for further subspecialization. Around 15,000 pharmacists graduate annually; in 2017 about one-third applied for approximately 4,200 total residency slots (American Association of Colleges of Pharmacy 2020; Moreau et al. 2017). Subspecialty accreditation can be attained either by completing a documented number of clinical hours in a subspecialty area or by completing a residency program focusing on that subspecialty area. The College of Psychiatric and Neurologic Pharmacists currently lists more than 50 accredited PGY-2 psychiatric pharmacy residencies around the country, and subspecialty certification in psychiatry is available (College of Psychiatric and Neurologic Pharmacists 2020).

Clinical Pharmacy Practice and Scope

Clinical pharmacists are trained to assess and monitor health problems; determine appropriateness of medication regimens with regard to effectiveness, side effects, and cost; consult with prescribing clinicians to select or optimize medications; provide consultations directly to patients to assess barriers to adherence; and provide patient education (American College of Clinical Pharmacy 2014). Medication therapy management (MTM) refers to a service, created by the Centers for Medicare and Medicaid Services in 2003 and traditionally performed by clinical pharmacists, that optimizes therapeutic outcomes through improved medication use and reduces risk of adverse events, including adverse drug interactions (Ramalho de Oliveira et al. 2010).

In addition to MTM, nearly all states have rules and regulations that allow pharmacists to initiate, modify, or discontinue medication treatment through collaborative prescribing agreements (CPAs) (Adams and Weaver 2016). CPAs typically allow a physician to determine which medications can be prescribed, what health conditions can be treated, and in what circumstances a pharmacist can initiate, modify, or discontinue treatment (National Alliance of State Pharmacy Associations 2017). CPA regulations are not bound to specific areas but rather defer to the physician nearly all authority for what a pharmacist can and cannot do autonomously. As such, the decision to be more or less restrictive is entirely up to the individual physician. A handful of states allow pharmacists to independently prescribe a specified set of medications outside of CPAs as set forth by the state medical and/or pharmacy boards.

Although pharmacists are reimbursed for performing MTM through the Medicare Part D benefit, pharmacists are not formally recognized as health care providers under the Social Security Act, and therefore they are not able to independently bill for services. The lack of a sustainable financial model has significantly curtailed development and expansion of clinical pharmacy services. Formally recognizing pharmacists as health care providers would likely change that dynamic.

Workforce Data

As of 2012, the Health Resources and Services Administration estimated the total number of pharmacists to be 264,100, about equal in their estimation to the total demand. At the time, they predicted that the supply of pharmacists would outstrip the growth in demand. However, this was based on modeling of pharmacy practice in 2012 and does not include the potential growth of clinical pharmacy (National Center for Health Workforce Analysis 2020). As of 2020, more than 1,200 pharmacists have been certified as psychiatric pharmacists by the Board of Pharmacy Specialties (Board of Pharmacy Specialties 2020), although this number does not necessarily correlate with pharmacists prescribing psychiatric medications or prescribing any medications in a mental health setting. The number of pharmacists participating in CPAs and prescribing medications of any type, much less psychotropic medications, is unknown because states do not track CPA agreements in the same way that they track collaborative agreements for other professions. However, clinical pharmacy practice does not require residency or specialty certification, so technically nearly all pharmacists are eligible to participate in clinical care and CPAs, contingent on the credentialing and privileging processes of the employer.

Prescriptive Authority for Psychologists

Although psychiatrists and psychologists have been practicing collaboratively together for decades, that working relationship has several well-documented areas of role conflict, including service-line leadership, hospital admitting privileges, and even the issue of whether a psychologist should be classified as a physician. The nature of these role disputes could fill a book and are beyond the scope of this chapter. Importantly, many of these disputes would likely be minimized with stronger models of interprofessional collaboration and training, outlined in later sections of this chapter. However, psychologist prescribing in particular overlaps greatly with the other professional roles outlined in this chapter, and a handful of states have laws permitting psychologist prescribing. Here, we provide a brief outline of the current state of psychologist prescribing in the United States.

Laws giving prescriptive authority to psychologists (a movement often referred to as RxP) have been passed in five states. New Mexico and Louisiana enacted their laws in 2002 and 2004, respectively. In New Mexico, 52 psychologists are currently listed as having active, full prescriptive authority, whereas an additional 13 are listed as having "initial conditional authority," compared with 251 active practicing psychiatrists (Association of American Medical Colleges 2017b). In Louisiana, 84 psychologists are currently listed as having active prescriptive authority and are currently practicing in Louisiana, compared with 423 active practicing psychiatrists (Association of American Medical Colleges 2017a). Meanwhile, since 2016, Idaho, Iowa, and Illinois have all passed laws permitting psychologist prescribing, but no formal workforce has completed training as of yet (Bethune 2017).

Prerequisite training requirements for prescriptive authority by psychologists vary significantly, with some states requiring a specific number of hours of coursework, and others requiring a full degree (the Idaho program mandates a full master's degree that is the equivalent of an MSN for APRNs). Once an individual meets educational requirements, these programs typically mandate a period of physician supervision (though not necessarily by a psychiatrist), with some degree of enhanced autonomy or full independence after that period. Formularies are typically restricted to psychotropic medications. Oversight of most programs is vested at least partially within state medical boards. Evidence in the literature about the effectiveness and safety of psychologist prescribing is absent (Lavoie and Barone 2006), in contrast with evidence for APRN prescribing practices (Gielen et al. 2014).

Collaborative Practice

Most mental health clinicians can identify various common problems associated with poor collaborative practice. These include, among others, failure of clear communication between psychiatric providers and pharmacists; misunderstanding of scope of practice around medication prescription; and detached, anemic mentorship in collaborative practice arrangements. Despite the common problems, optimal collaborative practice models for this panoply of psychiatric professionals have not been well defined; indeed, an exhaustive literature search uncovered no studies explicitly designed to determine optimal collaborative arrangements between any two psychiatric professions. Although collaborative agreements have existed for decades, most are shockingly vague, rarely addressing more than proximity of practice, availability of mentorship, and hours of supervision. CPAs between pharmacists and physicians can be quite specific but are also highly individualized and variable. Guidance or standards for collaborative relationships are not delineated, which makes sense when one considers that expansion of scope was not designed as a team-based activity, but rather as an effort to expand access to traditional care by new providers. Collaborative agreements were implemented to hedge against risk rather than to promote collaborative practice. Nevertheless, interprofessional teams have become ubiquitous in all mental health settings outside private practice, and creating high-functioning collaborative units will be necessary moving forward.

Broad studies examining interprofessional collaboration among health care teams appear to converge on transformation of practice along two intertwined domains: a shift away from subordination and toward complementarity, and the need to shift from cost containment to a focus on the unmet needs of patients. Physicians and other professionals easily assume a team dynamic built around hierarchical, rigid, preset roles. This dynamic tends to stifle collaboration by shoehorning nonphysician professionals into practicing well beneath the scope of their practice. This, in turn, limits contributions from everyone involved and is often poorly suited to managing the individual needs of specific patients (not to mention being professionally unfulfilling for everyone besides physicians). Complementarity, on the other hand, offers an alternative by which teams focus foremost on patient needs, with all team members occupying roles that embrace their full scope of practice, and developing care pathways that take patient needs into account first (Supper et al. 2015).

Actualizing this shift in practice is facilitated most effectively when individual practitioners display three characteristics: a shared interest in collaboration, a sense that effective collaboration can improve care, and an interest in expanding into new professional domains. Meanwhile, several barriers can impede good interprofessional collaborative care:

- Poor awareness of different professionals' roles and competencies *or* disagreement about roles

- Poor systems and mechanisms for sharing information
- Misconceptions about confidentiality and individual responsibility for outcomes
- Absent or impoverished team building and intraprofessional training
- Billing and funding models that lead to assignation of credit to individual providers rather than to teams

To ensure good collaborative practice, teams must devote adequate time during the early stage of collaboration to communication, training, building shared views and values, and overcoming prejudices and fears. Teams should have shared space, shared goals, and time devoted specifically to team-based collaboration and determining how to elaborate roles and responsibilities for all team members (Interprofessional Education Collaborative 2011). Effective leadership to ensure cohesive team functioning toward a common goal is necessary, but equally important is the belief that input from all team members will be adopted into team practice. Focusing on how best to meet patient needs can facilitate a sense of ownership and buy-in from all team members.

The Future of Interprofessional Collaboration in Psychiatry

From studies of interprofessional collaboration in primary care paired with the real-world experiments that have been taking place for years in mental health settings, a picture of interprofessional collaborative practice in psychiatry is emerging. Clinical professions will be emphasizing practice at the "top" of their scope. For APRNs and PAs, this will mean taking increasing responsibility for treating patients with moderate illness severity (with more mild illness being managed primarily in collaborative care models, as outlined elsewhere in this book; see Chapter 7, "Integration of Services"). Clinical pharmacists will increase their focus on medication adherence and interactions, management of side effects, and providing input on patients with multiple chronic illnesses and complicated medication regimens. To facilitate this transformation, interprofessional training hubs are likely to develop, focusing on residencies and fellowships for each profession.

Psychiatrists will likely focus their clinical time on the most difficult or complicated patients and situations. Sometimes they will be providing mentorship to a collaborative partner, but at other times they will be managing the case themselves. Some practices have established models in which psychiatrists perform diagnostic assessments, then have APRNs manage treatment initiation and follow-up. Other practices have psychiatrists and APRNs or PAs working equivalently, side by side, with some fluidity of caseload, whereby psychiatrists take on cases that are found to be more difficult, or alternatively, provide one-time consultations or in-depth supervision and mentorship around difficult cases.

Expectations around the level of value provided by psychiatrists will continue to expand. Psychiatrists will need to demonstrate comfort with addiction management, the interface between chronic physical and mental illnesses, and other more complicated diagnoses that test the capabilities of all but the most seasoned and capable advanced practice clinicians. Workflow design will increasingly rely on a range of other professions, including nurses and medical assistants. Psychiatrists will need to demonstrate comfort and capability with interprofessional collaboration and team-based work, as well as the range of clinical interventions outlined in Chapter 11, "An Expanded Role for Psychiatry."

Psychiatrist leadership, whether exercised informally or formally, will be important. The value of that leadership will likely be measured by how much psychiatrists enhance the performance of the team rather than more concrete administrative goals such as recruitment and performance measurement. Physician leadership today is exercised primarily through hierarchy. That will not suffice in the future. Advanced practice clinicians will demand that physicians add value to their practices, and will look for physician leaders who trust and empower them. Meanwhile, the value that psychiatrists can and ought to be delivering is not promoted well by current payment models. Payment models of the future will increasingly focus on outcomes and value, but those payment models are still emerging (see Chapter 6, "Innovative Financing"). Psychiatrists must invest time pushing for payment model change at the local level, as well as by engaging insurers. Psychiatrists can also become involved at the state and national levels through policy and legislative advocacy. These activities are considered in greater detail in Chapter 15 ("Advocacy").

Training Implications

Currently, most psychiatric residencies do not contain formalized interprofessional education (IPE), and we found no papers outlining such experiences in the literature. Although PA students sometimes share didactics with medical students, didactic training across professions is otherwise rarely shared. Clinical rotations for APRNs and PAs typically include exposure to other professions, but rarely do such rotations emphasize deliberate interprofessional work. Clinical pharmacy rotations and pharmacy residencies are a clear exception, because they have a strong intentional focus on communication with physician counterparts; however, evidence that psychiatrists specifically had opportunities during their training experiences to work intentionally with clinical pharmacists was absent.

Taking into consideration the evolving trends in scope of practice, interprofessional collaboration will be the rule rather than the exception in most psychiatric practice environments, particularly in academic training environments. As such, it is imperative that psychiatric providers of all professions, and psychiatrists more specifically, have robust IPE experiences during their training. Notably, the Association of American Medical Colleges identified IPE as one of two horizon issues for action back in 2008, whereas the Accreditation Council for Graduate Medical Education already includes core competencies related to the expectation that residents are able to work effectively on interprofessional health care teams (Interprofessional Education Collaborative 2011). Nevertheless, concrete and robust IPE is largely absent. Although training directors must get more support for building formal IPE programs, they first must be provided with templates of effective and achievable high-quality IPE programs.

Across the literature, interprofessional training simulations have emerged as a particularly effective mechanism for promoting effective interprofessional practice. Specifically, interprofessional training simulations have been shown to do the following:

- Enhance knowledge related to other professions.
- Nurture positive attitudes about working with other professions.
- Engender confidence working in interprofessional teams.
- Impart a sense of well-being across interprofessional teams.

Furthermore, and importantly, simulation training appears to alter individual clinician workflow and improve clinician self-efficacy. The preponderance of evidence suggests that formalized IPE (whether by simulation or in live settings) should be incorporated into residency programs and that increased exposure through training not only would improve team-based care, but also might reduce individual stress and improve attitudes about clinical work in general (Kowalski et al. 2018; Marcussen et al. 2019; Piette et al. 2018; Yang et al. 2017).

Building IPE into the classroom can also be of benefit. A broad IPE experience at the University of Toledo demonstrated high levels of learner satisfaction and improvement in the perception of other professions (Peeters et al. 2017), whereas several studies reveal that a range of IPE programs positively impact attitudes about collaborative practice and improve skills in negotiating interprofessional practice (Fox et al. 2018; Imafuku et al. 2018; Lairamore et al. 2018). Specific to mental health, the Public and Community Psychiatry Fellowship at Case Western Reserve University has been collaboratively training psychiatrists and nurse practitioners together since 2012, and surveys of their fellowship graduates indicated that the experience of learning together as peers improved confidence, increased positive attitudes, and reduced apprehension about interprofessional collaboration (Runnels and Ruggiero 2015).

Introducing IPE, then, should include the following elements: simulated interprofessional practice, real opportunities for interprofessional practice, opportunities to discuss interprofessional practice, and shared didactics. All experiences should occur across multiple professions, ideally inclusive of physicians, APRNs, registered nurses, PAs, pharmacists, psychologists, and social workers. Programs would benefit from introducing elements from any of these domains, but leadership should set the goal of establishing experiences in all of them. To achieve that goal, academic leaders from each profession must work together, and should create interprofessional committees for establishing and monitoring the quality of these experiences. For residencies that do not have academic training programs for a given profession, departments of psychiatry should provide academic appointments to clinicians representing each missing profession to help develop the curriculum. Quality should be measured through surveying participant experiences, including pre- and posttest attitudes about interprofessional practice, as well as about each profession's role in team-based settings.

Conclusion

The relative shortage of psychiatrists, which has gotten more acute over the past decade, has led to the delegation of diagnostic and prescribing responsibilities to several other professions. As with any new medical advance, the adoption of new providers should be approached with reasonable caution. Debates about scope are an appropriate piece of that process. Yet, psychiatrists cannot carry the burden for managing psychiatric illnesses on their own, and the expansion of scope to other fields, uncomfortable as it may be, is both necessary and humane.

In the larger context of health care reform, the very nature of how the system approaches mental illness is set to change over the next few years. Indeed, the intent of the Affordable Care Act was not only to expand traditional coverage, but to move our health care delivery system toward being more accountable for long-term outcomes and to carry the burden of cost more directly. The first 10 years of the ACA have been about pushing systems to lay the foundation necessary to make that change—through the implementation of electronic medical records, the reduction of fragmentation through provider consolidation and system alignment, and an expanded ability to gather and measure data. The next 10 years will focus on leveraging these new capabilities to provide more value at lower cost. The era of fee-for-service care that favors the delivery of high-cost procedures will give way to an era in which the services that produce the best outcomes at the lowest cost are prioritized. Systems have started to understand that behavioral health will be central to realizing that value. If psychiatry is to be at the center of reform efforts, psychiatrists will need to reimagine their value proposition, which will almost certainly include moving toward a population-based model of practice and away from the highly individualized approach that has dominated practice until now. Such an environment will call on psychiatrists to get comfortable working in teams and develop the skills necessary to lead—either formally or informally—those teams. As the number of providers with different professional backgrounds continues to grow, psychiatrists must get enhanced and intentional training in interprofessional collaboration. Indeed, leading the development of interprofessional practice represents a major area where psychiatrists can demonstrate their own value proposition.

References

Accreditation Review Commission on Education for the Physician Assistant: Accredited programs. 2020a. Available at: www.arc-pa.org/accreditation/accredited-programs. Accessed February 28, 2020.

Accreditation Review Commission on Education for the Physician Assistant: Postgraduate programs. 2020b. Available at: www.arc-pa.org/accreditation/postgraduate-programs. Accessed February 28, 2020.

Accreditation Review Commission on Education for the Physician Assistant: Standards of accreditation. 2020c. Available at: www.arc-pa.org/accreditation/standards-of-accreditation. Accessed February 28, 2020.

Adams AJ, Weaver KK: The continuum of pharmacist prescriptive authority. Ann Pharmacother 50(9):778–784, 2016

American Academy of Physician Assistants: PAs: Assessing clinical competence: guide for regulators, hospitals, employers, and third-party payers. September 2014. Available at: www.aapa.org/wp-content/uploads/2017/02/PAs-Assessing_Clinical_Competence_ 2014.pdf. Accessed February 28, 2020.

American Academy of Physician Assistants: PAs and team practice. February 2017a. Available at: www.aapa.org/wp-content/uploads/2017/02/Issue-brief_Team-Practice_Update_0217.pdf. Accessed February 28, 2020.

American Academy of Physician Assistants: What is optimal team practice? May 2017b. Available at: www.aapa.org/advocacy-central/optimal-team-practice. Accessed February 28, 2020.

American Association of Colleges of Pharmacy: Academic pharmacy's vital statistics. 2020. Available at: www.aacp.org/article/academic-pharmacys-vital-statistics. Accessed February 28, 2020.

American Association of Nurse Practitioners: State practice environment. 2020. Available at: www.aanp.org/legislation-regulation/state-legislation/state-practice-environment. Accessed February 28, 2020.

American College of Clinical Pharmacy: Standards of practice for clinical pharmacists. March 2014. Available at: www.accp.com/about/clinicalpharmacists.aspx. Accessed February 28, 2020.

American Medical Association: AMA physician masterfile. 2015. Available at: www.aamc.org/data/workforce/reports/458494/1-4-chart.html. Accessed March 4, 2020.

American Nurses Association: Scope of practice. 2020. Available at: www.nursingworld.org/practice-policy/scope-of-practice. Accessed February 28, 2020.

American Psychiatric Nurses Association: Psychiatric-mental health nursing graduate programs by state. 2020. Available at: www.apna.org/i4a/pages/index.cfm?pageid=3311. Accessed February 28, 2020.

Association of American Medical Colleges: Louisiana physician workforce profile. 2017a. Available at: www.aamc.org/system/files/2019-08/louisiana2017.pdf. Accessed March 31, 2019.

Association of American Medical Colleges: New Mexico physician workforce profile. 2017b. Available at: www.aamc.org/system/files/2019-08/newmexico2017.pdf. Accessed March 31, 2019.

Association of Postgraduate Physician Assistant Programs: Postgraduate PA programs listings. 2020. Available at: https://appap.org/programs/pa-programs-listing. Accessed February 28, 2020.

Bethune S: And Idaho makes five. Monitor on Psychology 48(6):18, June 2017. Available at: www.apa.org/monitor/2017/06/idaho. Accessed July 29, 2020.

Bishop TF, Seirup JK, Pincus HA, et al: Population of U.S. practicing psychiatrists declined, 2003–13, which may help explain poor access to mental health care. Health Affairs 35(7):1271–1277, 2016

Board of Pharmacy Specialities: Psychiatric pharmacy, 2020. Available at: www.bpsweb.org/bps-specialties/psychiatric-pharmacy. Accessed July 29, 2020.

Carter BL: Evolution of clinical pharmacy in the U.S. and future directions for patient care. Drugs Aging 33(3):169–177, 2016

Case Western Reserve University School of Medicine: Physician assistant curriculum overview. 2020. Available at: https://case.edu/medicine/physician-assistant/education/curriculum-overview. Accessed February 28, 2020.

Centers for Medicare and Medicaid Services: National health expenditure 2017 highlights. 2018. Available at: www.cms.gov/Research-Statistics-Data-and-Systems/Statistics-Trends-and-Reports/NationalHealthExpendData/Downloads/highlights.pdf. Accessed February 28, 2020.

Centers for Medicare and Medicaid Services, Center for Medicaid and CHIP Services: Medicaid and CHIP enrollment data highlights. October 2018. Available at: www.medicaid.gov/medicaid/program-information/medicaid-and-chip-enrollment-data/report-highlights. Accessed February 28, 2020.

College of Psychiatric and Neurologic Pharmacists: Psychiatric pharmacy residency programs. 2020. Available at: https://cpnp.org/career/residencies. Accessed February 28, 2020.

Delaney KR, Vanderhoef D: The psychiatric mental health advanced practice registered nurse workforce: charting the future. J Am Psychiatr Nurses Assoc 25(1):11–18, 2019

Dill MJ, Pankow S, Erikson C, et al: Survey shows consumers open to a greater role for physician assistants and nurse practitioners. Health Aff 32(6):1135–1142, 2013

Drew BL: The evolution of the role of the psychiatric mental health advanced practice registered nurse in the United States. Arch Psychiatr Nurs 28(5):298–300, 2014

Fox L, Onders R, Hermansen-Kobulnicky CJ, et al: Teaching interprofessional teamwork skills to health professional students: a scoping review. J Interprof Care 32(2):127–135, 2018

Gielen SC, Dekker J, Francke AL, et al: The effects of nurse prescribing: a systematic review. Int J Nurs Stud 51(7):1048–1061, 2014

GraduateNursingEDU.org: Nurse practitioner fellowship and residency programs. 2020. Available at: www.graduatenursingedu.org/nurse-practitioner-residency-programs. Accessed February 28, 2020.

Grypma L, Haverkamp R, Little S, et al: Taking an evidence-based model of depression care from research to practice: making lemonade out of depression. Gen Hosp Psychiatry 28(2):101–107, 2006

Health Resources and Services Administration: National projections of supply and demand for selected behavioral health practitioners: 2013–2025. November 2016. Available at: https://bhw.hrsa.gov/sites/default/files/bhw/health-workforce-analysis/research/projections/behavioral-health2013-2025.pdf. Accessed March 4, 2020.

Hwang J, Christensen CM: Disruptive innovation in health care delivery: a framework for business-model innovation. Health Aff 27(5):1329–1335, 2008

Imafuku R, Kataoka R, Ogura H, et al: What did first-year students experience during their interprofessional education? A qualitative analysis of e-portfolios. J Interprof Care 32(3):358–366, 2018

Interprofessional Education Collaborative: Core competencies for interprofessional collaborative practice: report of an expert panel. May 2011. Available at: www.aacom.org/docs/default-source/insideome/ccrpt05-10-11.pdf?sfvrsn=77937f97_2. Accessed February 28, 2020.

Jiao S, Murimi IB, Stafford RS, et al: Quality of prescribing by physicians, nurse practitioners, and physician assistants in the United States. Pharmacotherapy 38(4):417–427, 2018

Johantgen M, Fountain L, Zangaro G, et al: Comparison of labor and delivery care provided by certified nurse-midwives and physicians: a systematic review, 1990 to 2008. Women's Health Issues 22(1):e73–e81, 2012

Katon W, Unützer J, Fan MY, et al: Cost-effectiveness and net benefit of enhanced treatment of depression for older adults with diabetes and depression. Diabetes Care 29(2):265–270, 2006

Konrad TR, Ellis AR, Thomas KC, et al: County-level estimates of need for mental health professionals in the United States. Psychiatr Serv 60(10):1307–1314, 2009

Kowalski C, Attoe C, Ekdawi I, et al: Interprofessional simulation training to promote working with families and networks in mental health services. Acad Psychiatry 42(5):605–612, 2018

Lairamore C, Morris D, Schichtl R, et al: Impact of team composition on student perceptions of interprofessional teamwork: a 6-year cohort study. J Interprof Care 32(2):143–150, 2018

Larson EH, Hart LG: Growth and change in the physician assistant workforce in the United States, 1967–2000. J Allied Health 36(3):121–130, 2007

Lavoie KL, Barone S: Prescription privileges for psychologists: a comprehensive review and critical analysis of current issues and controversies. CNS Drugs 20(1):51–66, 2006

Marcussen M, Norgaard B, Arnfred S: The effects of interprofessional education in mental health practice: findings from a systematic review. Acad Psychiatry 43(2):200–208, 2019

Maul TM, Zaidi A, Kowalski V, et al: Patient preference and perception of care provided by advance nurse practitioners and physicians in outpatient adult congenital clinics. Congenit Heart Dis 10(5):e225–e229, 2015

Merritt Hawkins: 2018 review of physician and advanced practitioner recruiting initiatives. 2018. Available at: www.merritthawkins.com/uploadedFiles/Merritt_Hawkins_2018_incentive_review.pdf. Accessed February 28, 2020.

Minarik PA, Zeh MA, Johnston L: Collaboration with psychiatrists in Connecticut. Clin Nurse Spec 15(3):105–107, 2001

Moreau C, Hale G, Joseph T: The match: facts and figures. Pharmacy Times, October 1, 2017. Available at: www.pharmacytimes.com/publications/career/2017/careersfall2017/the-match-facts-and-figures. Accessed February 28, 2020.

National Alliance of State Pharmacy Associations: Collaborative practice agreements: resources and more. June 8, 2017. Available at: https://naspa.us/resource/cpa. Accessed February 28, 2020.

National Center for Health Workforce Analysis: Health workforce projections: pharmacists. 2020. Available at: https://bhw.hrsa.gov/sites/default/files/bhw/nchwa/projections/pharmacists.pdf. Accessed February 28, 2020.

National Commission on Certification of Physician Assistants: 2017 Statistical profile of certified physician assistants. 2018. Available at: http://prodcmsstoragesa.blob.core.windows.net/uploads/files/2017StatisticalProfileofCertifiedPhysicianAssistants%206.27.pdf. Accessed February 28, 2020.

National Nurse Practitioner Residency and Fellowship Training Consortium: Accreditation fact sheet. January 7, 2019. Available at: www.nppostgradtraining.com/Portals/0/Documents/ACCREDITATION%20FACT%20SHEET%20FINAL%20 2018%20v2%20pdf.pdf?ver=2019-01-10-195319-437. Accessed February 28, 2020.

National Residency Matching Program: Results and data: 2017 main residency match. 2017. Available at: https://mk0nrmp3oyqui6wqfm.kinstacdn.com/wp-content/uploads/2017/06/Main-Match-Results-and-Data-2017.pdf. Accessed March 4, 2020.

O'Shea E: Self-directed learning in nurse education: a review of the literature. J Adv Nurs 43(1):62–70, 2003

Peeters MJ, Sexton M, Metz AE, et al: A team-based interprofessional education course for first-year health professions students. Curr Pharm Teach Learn 9(6):1099–1110, 2017

Physician Assistant History Society: Timeline. 2020. Available at: https://pahx.org/timeline. Accessed February 28, 2020.

Piette AE, Attoe C, Humphreys R, et al: Interprofessional simulation training for community mental health teams: findings from a mixed methods study. J Interprof Care August 24, 2018 [Epub ahead of print]

Ramalho de Oliveira D, Brummel AR, Miller DB: Medication therapy management: 10 years of experience in a large integrated health care system. J Manag Care Pharm 16(3):185–195, 2010

Runnels P, Ruggiero R: Collaborative training in fellowship: implications for psychiatric workforce development. Acad Psychiatry 39(6):695–698, 2015

Scope of Practice Policy: Physician assistants overview. 2020. Available at: http://scopeofpracticepolicy.org/practitioners/physician-assistants. Accessed February 28, 2020.

Simon GE, Katon WJ, Lin EH, et al: Cost-effectiveness of systematic depression treatment among people with diabetes mellitus. Arch Gen Psychiatry 64(1):65–72, 2007

Stuart GW: Principles and Practice of Psychiatric Nursing, 10th Edition. New York, Elsevier, 2009

Supper I, Catala O, Lustman M, et al: Interprofessional collaboration in primary health care: a review of facilitators and barriers perceived by involved actors. J Public Health 37(4):716–727, 2015

Thomas KC, Ellis AR, Konrad TR, et al: County-level estimates of mental health professional shortage in the United States. Psychiatr Serv 60(10):1323–1328, 2009

University of Southern California School of Pharmacy: PharmD curriculum. 2020. Available at: https://pharmacyschool.usc.edu/files/2018/06/Four-Year-PharmD-Course-Plan-Class-of-2022-V5-Grade-Type.pdf. Accessed February 28, 2020.

Unützer J, Katon WJ, Fan MY, et al: Long-term cost effects of collaborative care for late-life depression. Am J Manag Care 14(2):95–100, 2008

Varcarolis EM: Essentials of Psychiatric Mental Health Nursing: A Communication Approach to Evidence-Based Care, 2nd Edition. New York, Elsevier, 2013

Villegas WJ, Allen PE: Barriers to advanced practice nurse scope of practice: issue analysis. J Contin Educ Nurs 43(9):403–409, 2012

Virani SS, Akeroyd JM, Ramsey DJ, et al: Comparative effectiveness of outpatient cardiovascular disease and diabetes care delivery between advanced practice providers and physician providers in primary care: implications for care under the Affordable Care Act. Am Heart J 181:74–82, 2016

Yang LY, Yang YY, Huang CC, et al: Simulation-based inter-professional education to improve attitudes towards collaborative practice: a prospective comparative pilot study in a Chinese medical centre. BMJ Open 7(11):1–11, 2017

13

Pharmaceutical Management and Prescribing

David A. Stern, M.D.
Brian G. Mitchell, Pharm.D., BCPS, BCPP
Ali Abbas Asghar-Ali, M.D.

In this chapter we consider the development and marketing of medications and the effects that pharmaceutical industry behaviors have on the insurer and provider organizations that attempt to manage their expenses. This discussion provides a backdrop for consideration of prescribing practices that undermine high-value care and the practices that can enhance it. We begin with a brief vignette.

Vignette 1

It is 2014. A psychiatry resident begins her meeting with a patient who reports depressive symptoms that have not improved despite trials of several different selective serotonin reuptake inhibitors. As the resident considers the best pharmacotherapeutic recommendation for the patient, she remembers from a dinner presentation the night before about the benefits of a medication approved by the U.S. Food and Drug Administration (FDA) as an adjunct to treat major depressive disorder (MDD).[1] Although she has never prescribed the drug before, there seems to be good data about its efficacy, and it might help the seemingly refractory depressive illness. She discusses her recommendation with her attending physician, who asks how long the medication has been available and its FDA-approved indications. She responds that the medication first came to market in 2002, is now approved by the FDA as an adjunct for treating MDD, and has a favorable side-effect profile. With that information, the attending physician agrees with the resident's recommendation; the resident returns to the patient and reviews the recommendations.

Two weeks later the patient misses his follow-up appointment. The resident reaches the patient at his home; he tells her that the depression has worsened to the point that he cannot get out of bed. He explains he went to the pharmacy, and they said the price of her prescription would be over $1,000 per month. Apparently his health insurance had lapsed, and he could not afford the medication. "I had to choose between paying my rent or trying this new medication," said the patient. "Although I'm sick and tired of feeling this way, I know I'd feel much worse if I had no place to live."

In this vignette, we encounter a physician whose decision was influenced by pharmaceutical industry interests and lacked an adequate evidence base. Her approach was insufficiently oriented toward the patient's interest, was subtly directed by pharmaceutical research, and was indirectly supported by the health care infrastructure. This decision, multiplied, can cause great waves in our health care system, as billions of dollars are annually misspent on services that are unnecessary, inefficient, or harmful. Because physicians make recommendations to and at times make decisions for patients, much of the responsibility rests with prescribers.

The purpose of this vignette is not to blame the pharmaceutical industry or single out an individual medication; rather, it is to illustrate how our health care system does not facilitate high-value use of medications. Clearly, the interests of various stakeholders in this vignette were not aligned. The goals of this chapter are to help readers understand 1) pharmaceutical de-

---

[1]The medication in the introductory scenario is Abilify (aripiprazole). Introduced to the U.S. market in 2002, Abilify remained on patent until 2014; due to a pediatric extension, a generic did not become available until 2015. In 2007, Abilify gained FDA approval for adjunctive treatment of MDD, although the medication showed benefit over placebo in only one of two double-blind randomized placebo-controlled trials (Bristol-Myers Squibb 2007). The 2014 sales of Abilify—which was approved by the FDA for treatment of schizophrenia, bipolar disorder (depressive episode), and autism spectrum disorders, and as an adjunctive treatment for MDD—totaled $7.8 billion (IMS Institute for Healthcare Informatics 2015).

velopment and marketing and their impact on the health care system, 2) best practices in high-value pharmaceutical management, and 3) the perspectives of all stakeholders. This chapter crosses the chasm between systemic and professional interventions because they are so closely intertwined. The case will be made that the professional actions described here can have a significant impact on the value obtained from medication management and needed systemic changes.

Pharmaceutical Development, Marketing, and Pricing

The first step in moving toward value-based decision making in pharmaceutical management is to understand the relationship between our health care system and pharmaceuticals. This is no easy task, as physicians are not generally exposed to the complicated process of pharmaceutical development. We begin with the well-known fact that governmental agencies, academic institutions, private foundations, and industry fund the gamut of research, from the more basic testing procedures through clinical pharmaceutical trials. The goal of clinical pharmaceutical trials is to ascertain whether the drug being studied is safe and useful when administered to people.

When research funding comes through government grants, there is regulation and oversight from government as well as institutional review boards, which are peer-review bodies composed of interdisciplinary medical professionals whose responsibility is to protect the safety and welfare of subjects. Researchers spend countless hours on their work, which remains private until and unless they choose to publish it in manuscript form. Manuscripts submitted to scientific journals then undergo peer review, a process whereby manuscripts are reviewed by researchers with expertise in the topic of the submitted manuscript. Each reviewer can accept or reject the manuscript or request revisions.

Once a manuscript is accepted for publication and trial results become available, a pharmaceutical company may elect to develop a promising compound. After a drug is developed by the pharmaceutical industry, it must obtain approval for sale and marketing from the FDA. Phase III drug trials are then conducted by pharmaceutical companies. This level of trial requires that companies conduct randomized controlled, double-blinded, and multicenter investigations, in which the drug under consideration may be compared against placebo only, or with an existing, accepted standard treatment (Askin and Moore 2014). The pharmaceutical company then submits an application with all known information, positive and negative, to the FDA. If approved, a drug receives a patent as an intellectual property, usually with a new "brand" name; this protects competitors from developing a molecularly identical competing formulation for a certain amount of time, usually around 10 years. The implications of these patents will be considered below.

After the patent expires, other pharmaceutical companies can produce their own version of the same molecule, usually referred to as a generic medication. A generic medication is expected to be pharmaceutically equivalent, bioequivalent, and therapeutically equivalent to the reference listed drug (RLD) or brand-name product. To be considered *pharmaceutically equivalent*, the generic drug product must have the same active ingredient, dosage form, strength, and route of administration under the same conditions of use. *Bioequivalence* to the RLD means that the generic drug product must show no significant difference in the rate and extent of absorption of the active pharmaceutical ingredient. Consequently, *therapeutic equivalence* must also be met, which entails that the generic drug product be substitutable for the RLD, with the expectation that the generic product will have the same safety and efficacy as its RLD (U.S. Food and Drug Administration 2018a).

The benefits of medical research are multiple. For example, approximately 50% of the gains in longevity in the past century are estimated to be attributable to advances in medical research and progress in the development of unique, new medications (Cutler et al. 2006). Antibiotics and statins have saved millions of lives, and the development of chlorpromazine (Thorazine) and fluoxetine (Prozac) has undoubtedly relieved the suffering of millions more. These past successes contribute to the fanfare generated around the release of a new medication and often lead to the assumption that newer medications are better than older ones. Patients, seeing advertising, desperate for relief from suffering, and disappointed with previous treatments, may want a new medication.

One important issue that may not be obvious from the preceding description of pharmaceutical development, however, is the negative impact that pharmaceutical control of the development process can have. Two considerations are that 1) industry-funded trials, as opposed to publicly funded ones, can be prematurely terminated for financial rather than for scientific or ethical reasons (Lièvre et al. 2001) and 2) industry-sponsored trials are more often positive than government-funded trials. Bourgeois and colleagues (2010) found that industry-funded trials reported positive outcomes 85% of the time, compared with 50% for government-funded trials and 72% for trials funded by nonprofit or nonfederal organizations. In addition, among the nonprofit or nonfederal trials, those that had industry contributions (nearly half) were more likely than those without to report positive outcomes (85% vs. 61%). These differences were all statistically significant, according to the press release.

Additionally, trials comparing name-brand with generic medications are infrequent, and trials that are completed are slow to be published (Flacco et al. 2016). These issues present problems when trying to argue that generic medications are a valuable alternative to newer medications. More funding comparing a standard generic medication to newer brand-name medications would likely be high yield. One example of such a trial was the National Institute of Mental Health–funded Clinical Antipsychotic Trials of Intervention Effectiveness (CATIE). CATIE was a nationwide, public health–focused study that compared the effectiveness of the typical antipsychotic medication, perphenazine (Trilafon), first available in the 1950s, with newer, atypical antipsychotic medications (available since the 1990s) used to treat schizophrenia.

The National Institute of Mental Health (2005) noted that although research has shown that antipsychotic medication is better than no medication for the treatment of schizophrenia, there were no definitive data about whether atypical antipsychotic medications were more effective than the older "typical" antipsychotic medications. Nonetheless, newer medications were about 10 times more expensive than older medications. Additionally, none of the medications proved to be remarkably effective, as all were associated with high rates of discontinuation due to intolerable side effects or inadequate control of symptoms.

This outcome ran contrary to the common belief that newer medications are superior to typical antipsychotic medications. Much of that belief arises out of industry-sponsored research. In one paper about CATIE, Lieberman and Stroup (2011) stated that the trials "demonstrated the value and importance of independently sponsored and conducted comparative effectiveness trials to inform clinicians, consumers, and policy makers of the relative value of marketed treatments for medical disorders." These findings underscore the inherent conflict of interest in industry-sponsored research, and the disincentive that industry has to share outcomes unfavorable to its products.

The development of novel therapeutics is an expensive business: it costs more than a billion dollars to bring a medication to market, and only one-fifth of medications brought to market prove profitable (Askin and Moore 2014). In the United States, public funding in research and development plays a major role in identifying the biological targets of novel agents. However, the government does not receive the potential profits from these novel agents to fund more research. Rather, the government's work is typically purchased, modified, and patented by companies, which subsequently receive the profits of successful medications that originated with taxpayer money

(Zaitchik 2018). Research by Cleary and colleagues (2018) shows that National Institutes of Health (NIH) funding contributed to published research associated with each of the 210 new drugs approved by the FDA from 2010 to 2016. The role of NIH funding thus complements research and development of the pharmaceutical industry, which more recently shifted its focus to predominantly applied research. Additionally, pharmaceutical companies spend billions of dollars on marketing. According to the Pew Charitable Trust (2013), in 2012 the pharmaceutical industry spent more than $24 billion on marketing to physicians. Most of that is spent on pharmaceutical detailing—that is, educating a physician about a vendor's products in hopes that he or she will prescribe the company's products more often.

In the past 10 years or so, there has been growing interest in regulating real and perceived conflicts of interest between physicians and industry. For example, more and more academic medical centers have enacted policies restricting pharmaceutical representative sales visits to physicians. A study by Larkin and colleagues (2017) examined whether these restrictions (between 2006 and 2012 in the study) changed prescribing practices. The results showed a modest but significant lowering in prescriptions of name-brand medications, including medications for attention-deficit/hyperactivity disorder and depression.

An additional advance in the reduction of conflicts of interest is in the transparency of payments made by pharmaceutical and medical device companies to physicians. The Physician Payments Sunshine Act of 2010, included as Section 6002 in the Patient Protection and Affordable Care Act, requires pharmaceutical and medical device companies to disclose any payments or other transfers of value made to physicians or teaching hospitals. The information is readily accessible on a database on the Centers for Medicare and Medicaid Services (CMS) Web site (Tigas et al. 2018). Although it is easier to see potential conflicts as information becomes more transparent, there are still other avenues for biased influences. For example, the Accreditation Council for Continuing Medical Education continues to allow commercial support in the hundreds of millions of dollars allocated for continuing education (Steinbrook 2011).

Most physicians do not know the cost of the medications they prescribe. Allan and colleagues (2007) found physicians' awareness of medication cost to be poor. In their study, physicians' median estimate for the cost of a medication was 243% off the true cost. Additionally, physicians were more likely to underestimate the cost of expensive drugs and overestimate the cost of inexpensive drugs. It is widely acknowledged that the complexity of medical charges and reimbursements across insurance plans and the variability in markups by retail pharmacies make it impossible for any physician to know the exact cost of any specific service or product for a given patient. Price transparency has come a long way, and medication costs are now easier to discern. Still, the cost of a medication can vary in unforeseen ways, based on coverage, formulary, and pharmacy selection. Individuals who attempt to purchase generic medications without using insurance can face wide-ranging price differences. For example, one study noted a price differential of more than 10 times for the same medication (Barkil-Oteo et al. 2014).

In the realm of health care costs, the rising cost of medications has been of significant concern. In an Issue Brief in 2017, Sarnak and colleagues reported that in 1980 the U.S. expenditure on prescription medications was $53 per capita and similar to the nine other comparable countries. In 2016, the cost for pharmaceuticals had risen to $1,011.40 per capita in the United States, with the next highest per capita cost being in Switzerland at $783.30. In a review in 2016, Kesselheim and colleagues addressed the increasing cost of prescription medications in the United States. The main reason they identified for the increased spending on medications was the high price of branded medications. They noted that although brand-name medications (those usually sold by the original sponsor of the application for approval and patent protected) constitute only 10% of dispensed prescription medications, they constitute 72% of medication spending. Based on these authors' findings, the main causes for the faster rate of increase in the cost of prescription medications in the United States than in other countries are the absence of price controls and the fact that manufacturers are allowed to set their own prices for their products. In contrast to the United States, most industrialized countries with national health insurance systems first review a new medication and decide whether they want to offer it; then they negotiate a price with the manufacturer that they are willing to pay. In the United States only the Veterans Health Administration receives rebates from pharmaceutical manufacturers and can create a formulary in which it can exclude medications. This allows it to have lower prices than Medicare (which cannot negotiate prices) and Medicaid (which cannot restrict its formulary).

Formulary Management

A formulary is a continually updated list of medications and related information, representing the clinical judgment of pharmacists, physicians, and other experts in the diagnosis and treatment of disease and promotion of health. A formulary includes, but is not limited to, a list of medications and medication-associated products or devices, medication-use policies, important ancillary drug information, decision-support tools, and organizational guidelines (American Society of Health System Pharmacists 2008b). The multiplicity of medications available, the complexities surrounding their safe and effective use, and differences in their relative value make it necessary for health systems to have medication-use policies that promote rational, evidence-based, clinically appropriate, safe, and cost-effective medication therapy. The formulary system is the ongoing process through which health care organizations establish policies on the use of drugs, therapies, and drug-related products, and identify those that are the most medically appropriate and cost effective to best serve the health interests of a given patient population (American Society of Health System Pharmacists 2008b).

Pharmacy benefits managers (PBMs) are third-party administrators of prescription drug programs for a number of institutions, including commercial health plans, state and federal employee health plans, and Medicare Part D. PBMs were created to curb prescription drug costs that were rising at a rate that far exceeded inflation. PBMs largely offer services that range from tiered formularies to prior authorization requirements, intended to institute limits on the use of more expensive medications by their beneficiaries. These approaches reduce medication costs and increase generic drug use while decreasing overall drug use (Shrank et al. 2009). PBMs obtain discounts on drugs for health plans and beneficiaries through negotiation and administration of drug manufacturer rebates and discounts from retailers. Because PBMs have direct access to manufacturers and pharmacies, they can negotiate discounts from wholesalers and purchase discounts from drug developers (Beaton 2017a). PBMs use a variety of solutions that help payers implement generic utilization into health plans, including cost sharing on generic drugs (e.g., deductibles, coinsurance, copays), promotion of generic incentive programs (e.g., promotion of a three-tier copay structure), and the use of home delivery and mail-order pharmacies (Beaton 2017a).

The use of value-based pharmaceutical contracts is one way in which payers manage prescription drug benefits to fit their business needs and improve patient outcomes (Beaton 2017b). The three types of value-based pharmaceutical contracts are indication-based management contracts, outcomes-based contracts, and cost-cap contracts. Indication-based management contracts determine the value of the drug based on the relative cost of a patient's health condition. Indication-based management helps ensure that the right patient gets the right drug for the right condition. This can increase competition among products that are safe and effective for patients with a common condition, helping to lower costs (Beaton 2017b). A recent example of value-based pharmaceutical contracting occurring on a major scale is the announcement by CMS that it will offer Medicare Part D plan sponsors the opportunity to choose indication-based formulary design beginning in contract year 2020 (Centers for Medicare and Medicaid Services 2018). Outcomes-based contracts are based on a value-based contract design that ties drug reimbursement rates to actual health outcomes. In an outcomes-based contract, a manufacturer may be required to show, for example, that a medication would lower hemoglobin A_{1c} levels for people with diabetes by a certain percentage that is in line with the standards set for FDA approvals. In an outcome-based value contract, if the patient receiving the medication does not reach the goals outlined in the FDA approval process, a manufacturer could pay incremental rebates back to the purchasers (i.e., insurers and health care systems) to meet outcome-based value. Payers may also find that cost-cap contracts best fit their value-based care goals if they are looking to treat a large beneficiary population through novel therapy-class medications (Beaton 2017b). In a cost-cap contract, a PBM would negotiate formulary placement and a maximum cost of the drug per member per month. The cost-cap arrangement is likely to be useful when a new medication comes to market and is set at a much higher price than other drugs in the same drug class.

Negotiating Minimum Pricing

There are three main avenues for purchasing pharmaceuticals at discounted rates: group purchasing organization (GPO) contracts, facility contracts, and wholesaler own-use contracts. GPOs use the aggregate purchasing power of many facilities in negotiating pricing agreements with manufacturers. Although some GPOs focus exclusively on drugs, the majority of GPOs offer contracts for medical and surgical supplies, as well as food and other support products and services, in addition to pharmaceuticals. GPO contracts address the unit cost of the pharmaceutical, the allowable distribution methods for the pharmaceutical, payment terms, returns policies, and supplier performance requirements (American Society of Health System Pharmacists 2008a). Market-share agreements are typically used when two or more products can be used to treat the same disease, and no generic equivalent exists. The incentive, such as a rebate, a lock-in of a current discount, or achievement of a higher discount, is contingent on attaining a given market share for a particular product in the institution's market basket. To achieve the greatest financial advantage from the contract (lowest net drug cost), the pharmacy must work with the medical staff. This process requires a careful evaluation of comparative efficacy and safety of the product and its alternatives (American Society of Health System Pharmacists 2008a). GPOs are evolving and adding other services, especially market research, data collection, and data analysis, to help inform their members about products and services that offer the best value (Drug Topics 2016).

The alternative to GPO contracting is individual facility contracting. In some cases, individual facilities, especially large facilities or integrated delivery networks, can contract equal or better pricing than GPOs can provide. Opportunities for better pricing through individual contracting may exist for specialized health systems that purchase a large volume of a selected drug and are able to commit to maintaining a market share for the drug (American Society of Health System Pharmacists 2008a). However, continual use of individual facility contracts that encroach on GPO contracts can erode the GPO's ability to consistently contract aggressively for its members. Because of larger GPO volume, manufacturers often will not offer the same pricing or other terms to individual facilities as they offer to GPOs. Finally, the amount of time required to negotiate, write, and maintain an individual contract should be weighed against the incremental value gained over what a GPO contract would offer.

Wholesalers are also able to take advantage of special pricing on certain branded and generic drugs and offer those products to their customers in the wholesaler's proprietary contract portfolio. This practice creates allowance for the wholesalers that can be used to fund distribution discounts. Wholesalers also take advantage of cash discounts and quick-payment terms from manufacturers to increase their margin and to offer discounts to customers (American Society of Health System Pharmacists 2008a).

Drug Shortages and Value

Prescription drug shortages have become common occurrences in the U.S. health care system. As these shortages have become more frequent and more serious, life-threatening shortages are a constant fear (Teagarden and Epstein 2013). Drug shortages gravely impact value through increased labor costs, the gray market, greater numbers of medical errors, and delays in treatment. The gray market in this sense can be defined as the sale of a pharmaceutical agent through unauthorized distribution channels or unintended by the original manufacturer. In these unauthorized distribution channels, pharmaceutical agents are being purchased and sold multiple times, each time with a markup in price. The questionable business practices of the distributors and pharmacies engaging in gray market sales result in higher healthcare costs and potential risk to patients. The FDA states that quality and manufacturing issues, delays in manufacturing and obtaining raw materials, and discontinuation of drugs are the main contributors to drug shortages (U.S. Food and Drug Administration 2018a). The hours spent managing shortages have greatly expanded in recent years (Morrison and Molina 2011).

A nationwide survey of 353 hospital pharmacy directors conducted by the American Society of Health System Pharmacists revealed that the time pharmacists spend managing drug shortages has tripled between 2004 and 2011 (from 3 to 9 hours/week), creating an annual labor cost of $216 million for all health systems nationwide. This survey also revealed that 32% of hospitals have reallocated existing staff to allow time for managing drug shortages (Morrison and Molina 2011).

Findings from different organizations suggest that drug shortages could cost U.S. hospitals at least $415 million annually through the purchase of more expensive drug substitutes and additional labor costs. Drug shortages force hospitals to buy from gray-market drug distributors that charge as much as 335% more than the normal market price (Morrison and Molina 2011). The FDA has allowed unapproved drugs to be imported from Europe to fill the gap, but drugs from these sources are highly expensive as well as potentially unsafe. Sourcing alternative drugs from the gray market compromises patient safety. The guidelines for handling and manufacturing these drugs are often lax, putting drugs at risk of being stolen and then sold back to pharmacies. They might be either adulterated or have quality issues as a result of sustaining heat and not being stored properly during the theft (Morrison and Molina 2011). Unfortunately, gray-market pharmaceutical distribution, driven by wholesaler stockpiling to raise prices, is separate from manufacturer-driven shortages and falls outside the FDA's regulatory purview and institutional mitigation strategies (Shaban et al. 2018). Gray-market pharmaceutical purchasing within the U.S. Department of Veterans Affairs (VA) is complicated by regulatory barriers found within the Trade Agreements Act of 1979 and the Federal Acquisition Regulation, both of which restrict purchasing from manufacturers in foreign countries (Shaban et al. 2018). A national survey of more than 1,000 providers conducted in 2010 identified no less than 1,000 errors and adverse patient outcomes due to drug shortages. These errors occurred mainly because less experienced prescribers were unfamiliar with alternative drugs and used the wrong dosage (Morrison and Molina 2011).

Drug shortages can force physicians to delay treatment for patients. This can be dangerous for patients who need immediate, life-saving treatments, such as patients with cancer and those undergoing surgery. A survey conducted in June 2011 found that 99.5% of the 820 responding hospitals had experienced one or more drug shortages in the previous 6 months. The survey also found that 78% of the hospitals nationwide were rationing drugs in short supply. In some instances, this led to patients waking up in the middle of a surgery because of insufficient anesthesia. Drug shortages also jeopardize the development of new treatments that could help patients. According to the U.S. Department of Health and Human Services, more than

300 clinical studies paid for by the National Cancer Institute involved a drug that was in short supply (Morrison and Molina 2011).

One cause of the drug shortages is an inadequate supply of generic medications. Many of the problems in the U.S. generic drug market can be attributed to a reduction in the number of suppliers, consolidation of production volumes, and a concentration of market pricing power (Business Wire 2018). To help patients by addressing the often unwarranted shortages and high costs of generic medications, Intermountain Healthcare is leading a collaboration with Ascension, SSM Health, and Trinity Health, in consultation with the VA, to form a new, not-for-profit generic drug company. The five organizations represent more than 450 hospitals around the United States. The new company intends to be an FDA-approved manufacturer and will either directly manufacture generic drugs or subcontract manufacturing to reputable contract manufacturing organizations, providing patients an affordable alternative to products from generic drug companies with inconsistent pricing practices that are damaging the generic drug market and hurting consumers. The company will also strive to steady the supply to hospitals of essential generic medications, many of which have fallen into prolonged shortage. The new initiative will result in lower costs and more predictable supplies of essential generic medicines, helping to ensure that patients and their needs come first in the generic drug marketplace (Business Wire 2018).

The FDA plays a crucial role in ensuring that patients have consistent access to their medicine. In 2018, the FDA commissioner announced the formation of a Drug Shortages Task Force that expanded on the work of the FDA Safety and Innovation Act of 2012. The task force included leaders from the FDA, VA, and CMS and focused on evaluating various aspects of the drug-shortage issue, such as reimbursement policies from CMS and other payers that are making it difficult to manufacture certain drugs profitably, along with incentives to encourage expansion of manufacturing capacity and enhanced quality (U.S. Food and Drug Administration 2018b). Patients expect and deserve high-quality drug products, and it is the manufacturer's responsibility to guarantee that its drug products are safe, effective, and of high quality. The FDA has established an emerging technology team to engage with companies to employ new production technologies that could prevent drug shortages caused by product quality and manufacturing problems. The FDA also implemented new initiatives regarding quality metrics, used in a variety of industries to monitor the quality-control systems and processes that ensure quality standards are met and to identify opportunities for manufacturing improvements. These scientific and regulatory advances can help address some conditions that can give rise to drug shortages (U.S. Food and Drug Administration 2018b).

I High quality Low cost	II High quality High cost
III Low quality Low cost	IV Low quality High cost

FIGURE 13–1. A four-quadrant model of evaluating treatments based on quality and cost.
Note. Quadrant I represents the best interventions, and Quadrant IV represents the worst.

Value in Prescribing Practices

To obtain good value from prescribing practices, it is important to understand what *value* means in psychiatric care. For our discussion, *value* is conceptualized as a balance between the quality of outcomes and the cost of treatment. A more thorough discussion regarding value can be found in Chapter 1 ("Defining and Measuring Value"). If a similar outcome can be achieved at a lower cost (e.g., by using a generic formulation rather than a brand-name medication), it would be considered a higher-value intervention. An intervention would also be considered higher value if the quality of the outcome increases but the cost remains the same. This approach can be represented in a simple four-quadrant model of evaluating treatments based on quality and cost, in which quality equals outcomes and alignment with patient expectations, and cost equals the sum of direct and indirect costs (Figure 13–1 and Table 13–1). Ideally, psychiatrists should aim for high-value care (Quadrant I), avoid low-value care (Quadrants III and IV), and pay special attention to more complex circumstances (Quadrant II).

High-value prescribing can be defined as using the simplest medication regimen that yields the best outcomes and simultaneously minimizes risk

TABLE 13–1. Variables in the four-quadrant model of determining value

Outcomes	Symptom reduction, minimal side-effect load, functional improvement
Patient experience	Shared goals, employment, housing, relationships
Direct cost	Health care resources used (inpatient, outpatient, medication)
Indirect cost	Decrease of work productivity or employment

(financial and medical). This can be achieved by implementing strategies in three general categories: decreasing the cost of the medication(s), minimizing the complexity of the regimen, and reducing the medical risk posed by the regimen (Moriates et al. 2015).

Vignette 2

The same psychiatry resident as in Vignette 1, now an attending physician, evaluates another patient for MDD. Based on the interview, she recommends an antidepressant medication. The patient has never used an antidepressant medication; however, he asks the physician for vilazodone (Viibryd) because "I've heard that it really works wonders" and mentions his concerns about sexual side effects. The attending queries him about his insurance benefits and learns that he has to pay the entire cost of most of his medications out of pocket. After they look up the price of Viibryd on GoodRx, the patient believes that even at the cheapest available cost, the medication is beyond his means. Together they review the safety, tolerability, efficacy, and cost of antidepressants and decide on a trial of extended-release bupropion.

Encouraging Communication

Shared decision making between physician and patient has become a more important subject in medicine. A well-established example is the Choosing Wisely campaign, an initiative of the American Board of Internal Medicine (2012). Its stated goal is "to promote conversations between clinicians and patients by helping patients choose care that is supported by evidence, not duplicative of other tests or procedures already received, free from harm, [and] truly necessary." The American Psychiatric Association (2013) contributed the following recommendations to this initiative:

- Don't prescribe antipsychotic medications to patients for any indication without appropriate initial evaluation and appropriate ongoing monitoring.
- Don't routinely prescribe two or more antipsychotic medications concurrently.

- Don't routinely use antipsychotics as first choice to treat behavioral and psychological symptoms of dementia.
- Don't routinely prescribe antipsychotic medications as a first-line intervention for insomnia in adults.
- Don't routinely prescribe an antipsychotic medication to treat behavioral and emotional symptoms of childhood mental disorders in the absence of approved or evidence-supported indications.

Discussing Cost With Patients

In addition to practicing the Choosing Wisely recommendations that discourage polypharmacy and prescribing for non-FDA-approved indications, prescribers can discuss cost with patients to inform decision making and thereby increase the value of a treatment. Eaddy and colleagues (2012) looked at the relationship between patient cost sharing and medication adherence, along with clinical, utilization, and economic outcomes. They found that increased cost to patients led to decreased adherence and worse health outcomes. Medication nonadherence can result in numerous unhealthy outcomes, such as poor symptom control and illness management, medical complications and comorbidities, and hospitalizations and emergency room visits for additional treatment.

Stern and colleagues (2017) created a training curriculum for psychiatry residents titled "Resource Management: Providing Psychiatric Care That Is 'Cost Effective.'" The curriculum was adopted as a model by the American Association of Directors of Psychiatric Residency Training (AADPRT) and is available to members on its Web site (https://www.aadprt.org/training-directors/curriculum). This curriculum is similar to the High-Value Care curriculum established by the American College of Physicians (2012) but focuses on psychiatry. Stern and colleagues suggest asking the following questions for cost-conscious prescribing to assess whether patients might become medication nonadherent because of cost: 1) What is your out-of-pocket expense for medications? 2) What might you have to give up to purchase the medication? 3) Have you ever stopped taking a medication because you could not afford it?

Ubel and colleagues (2013) argue that there are distinct advantages to discussing cost with patients. First, doing so presents the opportunity for patients to choose lower-cost alternatives when available. Second, the discussion helps patients to decide whether the potential medical benefit advantage is worth the financial distress they might incur. This choice empowers the patient to consider financial and medical alternatives, and ultimately reduces the overall cost incurred by patients and society overall. Barkil-Oteo and colleagues (2014) noted that although the cost of medication is the main reason for discontinued or inconsistent use of medication, only 15% of the patients who were surveyed recalled discussing medication cost with their physicians.

Educating Prescribers

Psychiatry residents have received little, if any, training in how to think about value concepts when treating patients. For example, in a survey of psychiatry residents by Arbuckle and colleagues (2014), only 38% of the residents identified being encouraged to consider value when thinking about patient care. This is important because psychiatrists should be well positioned to have discussions about cost. Barkil-Oteo and colleagues (2014) noted that although a discussion about cost may be uncomfortable, psychiatrists are skilled in allaying patient discomfort. The authors emphasized the importance of educating future psychiatrists about high-value care, especially in light of the survey findings noted above.

The AADPRT curriculum created by Stern and colleagues (2017) defines high-value care in psychiatry, emphasizes the role of psychiatrists in providing high-value care, and provides guidance on how to incorporate high-value care into practice. The curriculum notes the high variability of medication costs between retailers, and offers resources such as GoodRx (https://www.goodrx.com) as an example of how to work through problematic system issues. Physicians can inform their patients about such resources and also make information about them available at their offices.

As mentioned earlier, price transparency has traditionally been a barrier facing prescribers and patients when making informed decisions about treatment. We now review some common terms used in discussions about health care expenses. As defined by Arora and colleagues (2015), the *charge* (or price) is the amount asked by a provider for a health care good or service, which appears on a medical bill. The *reimbursement* (which may not be the same as the charge) is the payment made by a third party to a provider for services. The cost of health care can be thought of as the cost to providers, or "the expense incurred to deliver health care services"; the cost to payers, or "the amount paid to providers"; and the cost to patients, or "the out-of-pocket payment" (Arora et al. 2015, p. 1046). Most listed charges are inflated to give the hospital or health care delivery entity the opportunity to bargain with commercial insurers. For hospitals, these charges are listed on a charge description master (or "chargemaster") list. Medication prices are also included on such a list.

Famously, in 2013 Kathleen Sebelius, then secretary of the U.S. Department of Health and Human Services, released the chargemaster lists of hospitals for the 100 most common services. The documents revealed the great variability in the charging schema of different facilities and ignited the movement for greater transparency in health care delivery (Hixon 2013). There are now several online tools that can help patients compare costs of services, including those featured on insurer Web sites for their clients. Good Rx (www.goodrx.com) and Blink Health (www.blinkhealth.com) are two examples of online and mobile device application-based resources that help patients identify the lowest-cost medication, based on a person's location. Such tools are becoming essential in a climate of increasing cost and copays for patients. In addition to Web sites that help with price transparency, well-researched sites such as Mayo Clinic and Consumer Reports incorporate value into treatment decisions and provide reliable information on medication options.

Cost-Effectiveness Analysis

One challenge for physicians when prescribing medications is the large volume of information that needs to be incorporated into the decision. The task is more complicated when comparing therapeutically equivalent agents in the same medication class. Fischer and Avorn (2012) highlight three main challenges for physicians trying to incorporate existing data into their practice: dealing with the complexity of research data, assessing the credibility of sources, and translating the research into clinical practice. They present evidence for the use of academic detailing to address these challenges. Academic detailing provides in-person, unbiased reviews of a clinical topic and connects them to clinical recommendations based on the available data. Nurses, pharmacists, or physicians who are trained educators typically serve as academic detailers. Academic detailing has been shown to be well accepted by physicians, to improve clinical decision making, and to reduce health care costs. This component is used by governmental agencies (e.g., the VA), state governments, and private health care entities (e.g., Kaiser).

Even if a system has eliminated low-value decision making and incorporated high-value initiatives, there may still be questions regarding how to weigh the value of two different therapeutic options. Although such an occurrence is not common, physicians may not be well equipped to make such distinctions without assistance. Fortunately, there are resources available to address such situations. One example is the Cost-Effectiveness Analysis Registry, developed and maintained by the Center for the Evaluation of Value and Risk in Health. Founded in 2006 at Tufts University, the center analyzes the benefits, risks, and costs of strategies to improve health and health care. The center's registry is free to access online (https://cevr.tuftsmedicalcenter.org).

Deciding whether to pay for a new antipsychotic injectable medication for individuals with schizophrenia is an example of a challenging decision relating to cost of treatment. As discussed earlier (see section "Pharmaceutical Development, Marketing, and Pricing"), the CATIE trial found that older antipsychotic medications are as efficacious as newer antipsychotics. In certain circumstances, however, a hospital system might want to purchase a brand name, atypical, long-acting antipsychotic agent for $2,500 even when a comparable dose of a generic, typical, long-acting antipsychotic agent may cost 10–100 times less. One way to figure out when it might be appropriate to pay for more expensive medication is to compare all costs to outcomes. The cost considerations of treating someone with schizophrenia include not only the cost of medication, such as the $2,500 for Invega Sustenna, a monthly injectable version of paliperidone. If Invega Sustenna is shown to lower hospitalization, which is expensive, and the side-effect load, which is bothersome to the patient, then the $2,500 may be cost effective. High-value prescribing includes taking patient needs into account. Patients might feel quite strongly that side effects greatly affect their quality of life. They might want to eschew the difficulty of remembering to take medication daily, or they might want to reduce reminders of being "sick" and yet want the benefit of medication. If a system incorporates these issues into the decision-making process, a patient and physician might decide to spend money on Invega Sustenna. This example demonstrates the complexity of cost analysis decisions.

Evidence-Based Treatment

One example of evidence-based treatment is the STEPS approach instituted by the American Academy of Family Physicians in 2003. Incorporating the attributes of **S**afety, **T**olerability, **E**ffectiveness, **P**rice, and **S**implicity (STEPS), the initiative provides a framework when weighing the advantages of one drug over another. We consider, as an example, the antidepressant vilazodone, prescribed for the patient in Vignette 2 earlier in this chapter. In 2013, Gazewood and colleagues (2013) concluded from the STEPS approach that the available evidence did not support routine use of vilazodone in the treatment of MDD. They reported that the medication was significantly more expensive than generic alternatives and no more effective than selective serotonin reuptake inhibitors or tricyclic antidepressants for treating moderate to severe MDD. They also mentioned that, as of 2013, vilazodone had not been studied in the treatment of mild to moderate MDD, the kind most commonly seen by family physicians. They concluded that, although vilazodone appears to be safe for long-term use based on a small study of 1 year's duration, other antidepressants have much more research supporting their long-term safety.

Consideration of Ethical Implications

Maximizing value in patient care requires that physicians also address its ethical implications. DeCamp and Tilburt (2017) propose three ethical categories—obligatory, permissible, and suspect—to help physicians consider their obligations to patients and high-value care. In an ethically obligatory value-based recommendation, determination of value is based on strong and sound evidence, and the patient would receive equivalent or superior care at a lower cost. An example of this might be the doctor's allowing a generic medication by ensuring that the substitution box is marked "yes" on the prescription. In the case of an ethically permissible value-based recommendation, the care may be only slightly more beneficial, more expensive, or based on limited or inconsistent data, but it may still be beneficial for a given patient. An example of such an intervention might be the off-label use of a medication (with only perhaps a case series as evidence) to alleviate the symptoms of a refractory illness. The authors emphasize that the high-value care outcome in such a situation would not be determined only by whether the medication was prescribed, but also by the conversation that occurred as part of the shared decision-making process. Finally, in some circumstances, high-value care could be ethically suspect. These are cases in which the physician withholds a treatment by placing societal needs over the fiduciary responsibility to the patient. An example of such a practice would be a physician who does not offer a new brand-name medication with superior efficacy to a patient simply because of the cost.

Conservative Prescribing

An excellent way to avoid side effects, unnecessary costs, and adverse events due to medication prescribing is to be judicious in the use of medications. One byproduct of the idea that psychic pain is biological is the expectation that there is a medication that alleviates the pain. Physicians as well as patients have been taught that medication is the solution. Prescribing a medication can make physicians feel that they are able to "do something" for patients during a 15-minute visit. With depressive illnesses, however, there are certainly many times when, after careful evaluation, a "prescription" of psychosocial interventions such as increased social interactions, renewed interest in hobbies, or a resumption of physical activity can prove to be quite helpful. Those patients might not need medication and not need to take on the risk.

The reality is that things physicians can do in brief visits can be valuable to patients. This idea, called *conservative prescribing*, was formally introduced by Schiff and colleagues (2011). The approach encapsulates many high-value considerations, including consideration of nonpharmacological interventions, minimizing of agents, monitoring for side effects, collaborating with patients, and keeping the broader scope of the situation in mind. The following are some considerations for conservative prescribing:

- **Think beyond drugs:** Consider nondrug therapy, treatable underlying causes, and prevention.
- **Practice more strategic prescribing:** Defer nonurgent drug treatment, avoid unwarranted drug switching, be circumspect about unproven drug uses, and start treatment with only one new drug at a time.
- **Maintain heightened vigilance regarding adverse effects:** Suspect drug reactions, be aware of withdrawal syndromes, and educate patients to anticipate reactions.
- **Exercise caution and skepticism regarding new drugs:** Seek out unbiased information, wait until drugs have sufficient time on the market, avoid stretching indications, and beware of selective drug trial reporting.
- **Work with patients for a shared agenda:** Do not automatically accede to drug requests, consider nonadherence before adding drugs to regimen, avoid restarting previously unsuccessful drug treatment, discontinue treatment with unneeded medications, and respect patients' reservations about drugs.
- **Consider long-term, broader impacts:** Weigh long-term outcomes, and recognize that improved systems may outweigh marginal benefits of new drugs.

Decreasing Polypharmacy

An increasing number of people take more than one medication. Polypharmacy disproportionately affects older adults with multiple medical problems, especially in long-term settings, where the rate of polypharmacy is approximately 40% in the United States, 15.5% in Canada, and 24.3% in Europe (Kojima et al. 2012). The growing number of prescriptions has two effects on cost: an increase in the direct cost of medication expenditures and an increase in the cost of medication-related adverse events. In a report by the U.S. Department of Health and Human Services (2016), an estimated $457 billion was spent on retail and nonretail medications in 2015. This constituted approximately 17% of the entire sum spent on health care services.

Regarding indirect costs, in an analysis of adverse drug events in the outpatient setting over an 11-year period, Bourgeois and colleagues (2010) found that the number of outpatient visits for adverse drug events increased from 9/1,000 to 17/1,000 persons. The number of medications (more than five) was identified as a factor in the increase in these visits. Adverse drug events also resulted in 107,468 hospital admissions annually, with older adults at highest risk for admission.

Masnoon and colleagues (2017) conducted a systematic review of studies involving polypharmacy to gain an understanding of the definitions of *polypharmacy* in the literature. Among the 110 articles that met their inclusion criteria, 138 definitions of *polypharmacy* and associated terms were found. The most common definition of *polypharmacy* was five or more medications daily. What becomes apparent from the authors' review is that without careful attention to the nature of polypharmacy, comments about the appropriateness of the polypharmacy are difficult to make. Only a small minority of articles, 6.4%, distinguished between appropriate and inappropriate polypharmacy. Furthermore, only 3.6% of the studies used polypharmacy tools or criteria. Increasingly, the concept of rational polypharmacy is a valuable perspective for clinicians. Preskorn and Lacey (2007) provide an approach for rational copharmacy (using more than one medication for a single illness) whereby physicians can make safe, evidence-based decisions.

Clearly, polypharmacy significantly affects the cost and safety of delivery of health care. Unfortunately, there is no consensus on an evidence-based approach for systematically addressing polypharmacy to improve outcomes. In 2016, Johansson and colleagues performed a systematic review and meta-analysis on the impact of strategies to reduce polypharmacy. They evaluated the effect of the interventions on mortality, hospitalizations, and change in number of drugs. They concluded that no definitive evidence supports the hypothesis that the interventions reviewed were effective in reducing polypharmacy, mortality, or hospitalization. The authors did not review the impact of the interventions on cost.

Kojima and colleagues (2012) developed an intervention to address polypharmacy and specifically measured its impact on cost. In the Polypharmacy Outcomes Project, the authors used the Minimum Data Set to identify nursing home residents receiving nine or more medications. The medications were first reviewed using the 2003 Beers Criteria and then the Epocrates online drug-drug interaction program. Recommendations were then made to the attending physicians responsible for the care of the residents. The program resulted in a reduction of number of medications per resident (from 16.6 to 15.5), with a statistically significant cost savings of $22.43 per resident per month.

To assist physicians in incorporating cost-saving strategies into their clinical work, Moriates and colleagues (2015) formulated the mnemonic GOT MeDS. It stands for **G**enerics, **O**rder in bulk, **T**herapeutic alternatives, **Me**dication Review, **D**iscounted medication plans, and **S**plitting medications (use with caution and proper education).

Conclusion

The judicious prescribing of medication can make a major impact on value in psychiatric care. There are numerous contributors to the cost of a medication that begin with the research and development of the medication. Once the drug is available for sale, then marketing, systemic health care relationships and contracts, practice guidelines, and individual physician practices intersect to determine the ultimate cost borne by an individual patient and the system.

Physicians have an important role in high-value prescribing. Knowledge about the systemic approaches to medication cost containment allows physicians to advocate for more competitive contracts and pricing of medications in their health care setting. Awareness of current medical literature and practice guidelines, coupled with ongoing efforts to improve one's medical practice, can ensure rational pharmaceutical management. Discussion about medication costs with patients is a necessary part of developing a complete and collaborative treatment plan. Finally, balancing one's ethical responsibilities to the patient and to society at large is essential when weighing treatment recommendations.

A growing number of resources assist physicians and patients in managing cost. Increasingly, electronic medical records provide the cost for medications and guidance for high-value prescribing. At the same time, insurance companies, governmental agencies, and other private entities are hosting easily accessible Web sites that help patients make more high-value decisions. By becoming more adept at incorporating these resources in decisions about treatment, physicians and patients have the potential to increase the value of care delivered and move the health care industry to a higher-value approach.

References

Allan GM, Lexchin J, Wiebe N: Physician awareness of drug cost: a systematic review. PLoS Med 4(9):e283, 2007

American Board of Internal Medicine: Choosing Wisely campaign. 2012. Available at: www.choosingwisely.org/our-mission. Accessed March 5, 2020.

American College of Physicians: High Value Care Curriculum. 2012. Available at: www.acponline.org/clinical-information/high-value-care/medical-educators-resources/newly-revised-curriculum-for-educators-and-residents-version-40. Accessed June 19, 2020.

American Psychiatric Association: Five things physicians and patients should question. 2013. Available at: www.choosingwisely.org/societies/american-psychiatric-association. Accessed March 5, 2020.

American Society of Health System Pharmacists: ASHP guidelines on medication cost management strategies for hospitals and health systems. Am J Health Syst Pharm 65(14):1368–1384, 2008a

American Society of Health System Pharmacists: ASHP statement on the pharmacy and therapeutics committee and the formulary system. 2008b. Available at: www.ashp.org/-/media/assets/policy-guidelines/docs/statements/pharmacy-and-therapeutics-committee-and-formulary-system.ashx. Accessed March 7, 2020.

Arbuckle MR, Weinberg M, Barkil-Oteo A, et al: The neglected role of resource manager in residency training. Acad Psychiatry 38(4):481–484, 2014

Arora V, Moriates C, Shah N: The challenge of understanding health care costs and charges. AMA J Ethics 17(11):1046–1052, 2015

Askin E, Moore N: The Health Care Handbook: A Clear and Concise Guide to the United States Health Care System, 2nd Edition. St Louis, MO, Washington University, 2014, pp 106–134

Barkil-Oteo A, Stern DA, Arbuckle MR: Addressing the cost of health care from the front lines of psychiatry. JAMA Psychiatry 71(6):619–620, 2014

Beaton T: Public payer news: how pharmacy benefit managers lower prescription drug prices. September 19, 2017a. Available at: https://healthpayerintelligence.com/news/how-pharmacy-benefit-managers-lower-prescription-drug-prices. Accessed March 5, 2020.

Beaton T: Value-based care news: 3 value-based pharmaceutical contracting options for payers. November 1, 2017b. Available at: https://healthpayerintelligence.com/news/3-value-based-pharmaceutical-contracting-options-for-payers. Accessed March 5, 2020.

Bourgeois FT, Shannon MW, Valim C, et al: Adverse drug events in the outpatient setting: an 11-year national analysis. Pharmacoepidemiol Drug Saf 19(9):901–910, 2010

Bristol-Myers Squibb: U.S. Food and Drug Administration approves ABILIFY® (aripiprazole) as the first medication for add-on treatment of major depressive disorder (MDD). Press Release, November 20, 2007. Available at: https://news.bms.com/press-release/us-food-and-drug-administration-approves-abilify-aripiprazole-first-medication-add-tre. Accessed March 5, 2020.

Business Wire: Leading U.S health system announces plans to develop a not-for-profit generic drug company. January 18, 2018. Available at: www.businesswire.com/news/home/20180118005320/en/Leading-U.S.-Health-Systems-Announce-Plans-Develop. Accessed March 5, 2020.

Centers for Medicare and Medicaid Services: Newsroom fact sheet: indication-based formulary design beginning in contract year (CY) 2020. August 29, 2018. Available at: www.cms.gov/newsroom/fact-sheets/indication-based-formulary-design-beginning-contract-year-cy-2020. Accessed March 5, 2020.

Cleary EG, Beierlein JM, Khanuja NS, et al: Contribution of NIH funding to new drug approvals 2010–2016. Proc Natl Acad Sci U S A 115(10):2329–2334, 2018

Cutler DM, Rosen AB, Vijan S: The value of medical spending in the United States, 1960–2000. N Engl J Med 355(9):920–927, 2006
DeCamp M, Tilburt JC: Ethics and high-value care. J Med Ethics 43(5):307–309, 2017
Drug Topics: Chains and business. The evolution of group purchasing organizations. October 10, 2016. Available at: www.drugtopics.com/chains-business/evolution-group-purchasing-organizations. Accessed March 5, 2020.
Eaddy MT, Cook CL, O'Day K, et al: How patient cost-sharing trends affect adherence and outcomes: a literature review. P T 37(1):45–55, 2012
Fischer MA, Avorn J: Academic detailing can play a key role in assessing and implementing comparative effectiveness research findings. Health Aff (Millwood) 31(10):2206–2212, 2012
Flacco ME, Manzoli L, Boccia S, et al: Registered randomized trials comparing generic and brand-name drugs: a survey. Mayo Clin Proc 91(8):1021–1034, 2016
Gazewood JD, Slayton P, DeGeorge K: Vilazodone (Viibryd) for the treatment of depression. Am Fam Physician 88(4):263–264, 2013
Hixon T: What the government's big data dump tells us about the hospital market. Forbes, May 22, 2013. Available at: www.forbes.com/sites/toddhixon/2013/05/22/what-the-governments-big-data-dump-tells-us-about-the-hospital-market/#33838603b4a1. Accessed March 5, 2020.
IMS Institute of Healthcare Informatics: Medicine use and spending shifts: a review of the use of medicines in the U.S. in 2014. April 2015. Available at: www.iqvia.com/-/media/iqvia/pdfs/institute-reports/medicines-use-and-spending-shifts-in-the-us-in-2014.pdf. Accessed March 5, 2020.
Johansson T, Abuzahra ME, Keller S, et al: Impact of strategies to reduce polypharmacy on clinically relevant endpoints: a systematic review and meta-analysis. Br J Clin Pharmacol 82(2):532–548, 2016
Kesselheim AS, Avorn J, Sarpatwari A: The high cost of prescription drugs in the United States: origins and prospects for reform. JAMA 316(8):858–871, 2016
Kojima G, Bell C, Tamura B, et al: Reducing cost by reducing polypharmacy: the Polypharmacy Outcomes Project. J Am Med Dir Assoc 13(9):818.e11–818.e15, 2012
Larkin I, Ang D, Steinhart J, et al: Association between academic medical center pharmaceutical detailing policies and physician prescribing. JAMA 317(17):1785–1795, 2017
Lieberman JA, Stroup TS: The NIMH-CATIE schizophrenia study: what did we learn? Am J Psychiatry 168(8):770–775, 2011. Available at: https://ajp.psychiatryonline.org/doi/full/10.1176/appi.ajp.2011.11010039. Accessed March 28, 2020.
Lièvre M, Ménard J, Bruckert E, et al: Premature discontinuation of clinical trial for reasons not related to efficacy, safety, or feasibility. BMJ 322(7286):603–605, 2001
Masnoon N, Shakib S, Kalisch-Ellett L, et al: What is polypharmacy? A systematic review of definitions. Geriatrics 17(1):230, 2017
Moriates C, Arora V, Shah N (eds): Understanding Value-Based Healthcare. New York, McGraw-Hill, 2015, pp 253–278

Morrison R, Molina S: Health issue brief: the impact of drug shortages in health care. Florida Hospital Government and Public Affairs, October 2011. Available at: www.adventhealth.com/sites/default/files/assets/impact-of-drug-shortages-2011.pdf. Accessed March 5, 2020.

National Institute of Mental Health: Questions and answers about the NIMH Clinical Antipsychotic Trials of Intervention Effectiveness study (CATIE)—phase 1 results. September 2005. Available at: www.nimh.nih.gov/funding/clinical-research/practical/catie/phase1results.shtml. Accessed March 5, 2020.

Pew Charitable Trust: Persuading the prescribers: pharmaceutical industry marketing and its influence on physicians and patients. November 13, 2013. Available at: www.pewtrusts.org/en/research-and-analysis/fact-sheets/2013/11/11/persuading-the-prescribers-pharmaceutical-industry-marketing-and-its-influence-on-physicians-and-patients. Accessed March 5, 2020.

Physicians Payments Sunshine Act, Section 6002, Transparency Reports and Reporting of Physician Ownership or Investment Interest. The Patient Protection and Affordable Care Act, March 23, 2010. Addition to Part A of Title XI, Social Security Act (42 U.S.C. 1301 et seq)

Preskorn SH, Lacey RL: Polypharmacy: when is it rational? J Psychiatr Pract 13(2):97–105, 2007

Sarnak DO, Squires D, Bishop S: Paying for prescription drugs around the world: why is the U.S. an outlier? The Commonwealth Fund, October 2017. Available at: www.commonwealthfund.org/publications/issue-briefs/2017/oct/paying-prescription-drugs-around-world-why-us-outlier. Accessed March 5, 2020.

Schiff GD, Galanter WL, Duhig J, et al: Principles of conservative prescribing. Arch Intern Med 171(16):1433–1440, 2011

Shaban H, Maurer C, Willborn RJ: Impact of drug shortages on patient safety and pharmacy operation cost. Fed Pract 35(1):24–31, 2018

Shrank WH, Porter ME, Jain SH, et al: A blueprint for pharmacy benefit managers to increase value. Am J Manag Care 15(2):87–93, 2009

Steinbrook R: Future directions in industry funding of continuing medical education. Arch Intern Med 171(3):257–258, 2011

Stern DA, Barkil-Oteo A, Asghar-Ali AA, et al: Curriculum for SBP2: resource management. Model curriculum. American Association of Directors of Psychiatric Residency Training, 2017. Available at: www.aadprt.org. Accessed March 7, 2020.

Teagarden JR, Epstein RS: Pharmacy benefit managers and their obligations during serious prescription drug shortages. Clin Pharmacol Ther 93(2):143–145, 2013

Tigas M, Grochowski Jones R, Ornstein C, et al: Dollars for docs. ProPublica, 2018. Available at: https://projects.propublica.org/docdollars. Accessed March 5, 2020.

Ubel PA, Abernethy AP, Zafar SY: Full disclosure—out-of-pocket costs as side effects. N Engl J Med 369(16):1484–1486, 2013

U.S. Department of Health and Human Services: ASPE Issue Brief. Observations on trends in prescription drug spending. March 8, 2016. Available at: https://aspe.hhs.gov/system/files/pdf/187586/Drugspending.pdf. Accessed March 5, 2020.

U.S. Food and Drug Administration: Frequently asked questions about drug shortages. July 5, 2018a. Available at: www.fda.gov/Drugs/DrugSafety/DrugShortages/ucm050796.htm. Accessed March 5, 2020.

U.S. Food and Drug Administration: Statement by FDA Commissioner Scott Gottlieb, M.D., on formation of a new Drug Shortages Task Force and FDA's efforts to advance long-term solutions to prevent shortages. Press Release, July 12, 2018b. Available at: www.fda.gov/news-events/press-announcements/statement-fda-commissioner-scott-gottlieb-md-formation-new-drug-shortages-task-force-and-fdas. Accessed March 5, 2020.

Zaitchik A: How big pharma was captured by the one percent. New Republic, June 28, 2018. Available at: https://newrepublic.com/article/149438/big-pharma-captured-one-percent. Accessed March 5, 2020.

14

Diagnostic Reform

Wesley E. Sowers, M.D.
Elizabeth Janopaul-Naylor, M.D.
Joseph Battaglia, M.D.

A discussion of diagnostic reform should start with definitions. Dictionary definitions of *diagnosis* include 1) the art or act of identifying a disease from its signs and symptoms, 2) a scientifically determined description or classification of conditions, and 3) an answer or solution to a problematic situation. To *diagnose* is to 1) identify an illness by medical examination, 2) ascertain the cause or nature of a problem, and 3) classify or make a determination on the basis of a scientific investigation. In Part I, "Where We Have Been," we attempted to *diagnose* the problems with our current systems of health care and consider how they came about. We hoped that analyzing past and current systems would lead to the identification of appropriate solutions to existing value-related problems, and ultimately to enhanced value in the services provided. Ironically, one of the problems identified by that inquiry was the limited ability of the psychiatric diagnostic system to correctly identify psychiatric problems, thereby leading to inappropriate treatments.

The association between diagnosis and value is not immediately obvious. To solve any kind of problem, one needs to accurately identify or characterize what the problem is. In a general sense, diagnostic systems create a common language that facilitates communication between interested parties. In medicine, diagnoses are used to guide treatment. An erroneous diagnosis of a condition will lead to inappropriate, or even harmful, attempts to provide treatment. Even in the best-case scenario, proper treatment will be delayed, and the condition may worsen if the "wrong" diagnosis is made. Time, effort, and money will be wasted on an ineffective solution.

The integrity of the parameters used to define a diagnosis may be referred to as its *validity*. In some cases, the constructs defining a diagnosis may be valid, but if the diagnosis cannot be consistently applied or interpreted, the results will be unreliable and vary from rater to rater. This could result in inappropriate treatment when diagnosticians make an incorrect diagnosis. The degree of variance in arriving at a similar diagnosis is referred to as *reliability*. Diagnosis implies the discovery of the cause of a condition. When a cause is determined, a solution to the problem can more readily be identified. In the absence of a known cause, treatments are based on observations and serendipity rather than scientific discovery. The connection between a diagnosis and the cause of the condition is referred to as the *etiology*. A diagnostic system that delivers the greatest value ought to be valid, reliably applied, and based on the etiology of the identified conditions.

In this chapter, we consider the development of the two current most used psychiatric diagnostic systems, the *Diagnostic and Statistical Manual of Mental Disorders*, 5th Edition (DSM-5) (American Psychiatric Association 2013) and *International Classification of Diseases*, 10th Revision (ICD-10) (World Health Organization 1992). We describe various critiques of these systems and their implications for value. After exploring alternative diagnostic approaches, we reflect on systems that would be most appropriate for value-driven services. Finally, we discuss how these systems are appreciated by the various stakeholders.

Historical Context

The earliest historical record of treatment for mental illness dates back to the 1300s (Shorter 2008). Because of the lack of effective medicines and therapies, early interventions consisted of placing severely ill patients in asylums for much of their lives. By the late 1800s, physicians started detailing different case presentations, searching for commonalities among patients. In 1899, both Emil Kraepelin and Sigmund Freud published books describing their approaches to psychiatry and diagnoses (Freud 1899; Kraepelin 1899). These two approaches, taxonomic and analytic, greatly influenced the history of the American diagnostic system.

Debate in the beginning of the twentieth century continued over what approach diagnosticians should take in nosology. However, the majority of individuals with mental illness were never assessed, because therapy of any kind was inaccessible to them. The only standard treatment for those with severe mental illness was containment. Thus, the *Statistical Manual for the Use of Institutions for the Insane*, the first diagnostic manual released by the American Psychiatric Association (APA), in 1918, was intended solely for asylums and included only 22 psychiatric diagnoses (American Psychiatric Association 1918). Most of these initial diagnoses were various types of psychoses (e.g., traumatic psychoses, alcoholic psychoses, psychoses with cerebral syphilis).

After World War II, the World Health Organization included mental health disorders for the first time in ICD-6. In 1952, APA released DSM with 128 different diagnoses (American Psychiatric Association 1952). Two categories of disease emerged, reflecting the ongoing debate in the mental health community over Kraepelin's and Freud's ideas. These categories were organic brain dysfunction (Kraepelin) and environmental stress–related disorders called "functional" disorders (Freud). The latter category was then subdivided into psychotic and neurotic disorders.

By DSM-II, published in 1968, the number of diagnoses had increased to 193 (American Psychiatric Association 1968). Both the first and second editions of DSM were rooted in psychodynamic ideologies regarding etiology and diagnoses (Grob 1991). Both editions described disorders through a narrative paragraph of about 200 words, but ambiguity was evident. In 1973, Rosenhan conducted his now famous experiment of sending sane colleagues into psychiatric hospitals, all reporting the same symptom. They reported hearing a voice saying "thud" or "empty." All of the participants were admitted and diagnosed with schizophrenia. On the basis of his findings, Rosenhan argued that those using the diagnostic system adopted by the hospitals could not accurately differentiate individuals who were sane or insane.

In 1974, Robert Spitzer and Joseph Fleiss published a paper detailing the unreliability of DSM-II. Spitzer went on to lead the development of DSM-III, released in 1980 (American Psychiatric Association 1980). This edition was a drastic departure from its predecessors. DSM-III detailed specific criteria based on symptoms and observable behaviors. Most of the criteria came from the Research Diagnostic Criteria (Spitzer et al. 1978) and Feighner Criteria (Feighner et al. 1972). The number of diagnoses in DSM-III increased to 228. DSM-III was the first edition to introduce the multiaxial diagnosis system (Axis I, clinical disorders; Axis II, personality disorders/cognitive limitations; Axis III, medical diseases; Axis IV, social stressors; and Axis V, Global Assessment of Functioning). The multiaxial system was a way to describe a more holistic picture of a person and provided some indication of the interaction between these domains and their impact on health and functioning. Many, including the DSM-III lead author Spitzer, hoped to move psychiatry back into the realm of medicine by creating discrete "disorders" with clear interrater reliability and symptom thresholds (Kawa and Giordano 2012). A core feature of DSM-III was its focus on "dysfunction." Each disorder had to have an impact on the person's ability to function when the defining criteria were met. Critics of this edition decried the lack of a clear definition of what "dysfunction" entailed (Wakefield 1992). Even so, the clearer and more specific nosology created some opportunities for the pharmaceutical companies and insurance providers, because it enabled them to generate more specific quantitative data (Gambardella 1995; Mayes and Horwitz 2005). By doing so, drug companies could target the defined disorders for drug testing and create a research agenda to validate the efficacy of their products. Insurers could begin to set diagnostically based "medical necessity" criteria, indicating which treatments would and would not be reimbursed.

DSM-IV was released in 1994 under the direction of Allen Frances (American Psychiatric Association 1994). Other than undergoing an increase to 383 diagnoses, this version featured minimal revisions. It did attempt to add further clarification of the meaning of *distress* or *dysfunction*, stating that it must be "clinically significant." This concept remained vague, however, as this construct was not well defined either. DSM-IV continued to move toward a more medical model of illness, and one that was more focused on research as opposed to the original biopsychosocial model (Rogler 1997). The psychiatric field has repeatedly struggled with the tension between wanting to categorize mental health disorders as biologically based, concrete diseases and a more holistic and multifactorial concept of an individual and their dysfunction.

While numerous advances in neuroscience and public health have occurred since 1994, clinical demands have also evolved. Work on DSM-5, the current version of DSM, started in 2000 with hundreds of experts in a variety of fields, including psychiatry, neurology, psychology, primary care, pediatrics, statistics, and epidemiology, taking into consideration research findings from all over the world. David Kupfer was the chair of the DSM-5 Task Force. His vision for this iteration was to move DSM further toward a biological basis for the disorders. He had hoped to incorporate more understanding of etiologies, an issue that DSM-III and DSM-IV had never addressed. This revision also started with the stated goal of incorporating dimensional criteria into the diagnostic system (Wakefield 2015).

The DSM-5 Task Force comprised more than 160 clinicians and researchers. Several work groups were created for various diagnostic categories. The strength of the evidence for proposed changes was reviewed by an appointed scientific review committee. In an attempt to establish transparency, the work groups published drafts of the manual to elicit feedback from the mental health community in advance of publication. For many critics, these efforts were not enough, and the final product fell short of the vision for significant change that had been proposed. Many of the original goals for DSM-5 were rolled back, and instead of simplifying diagnosis, the edition expanded to 541 different diagnoses (Blashfield et al. 2014). The multiaxial assessment was eliminated from DSM-5. Although that assessment was imperfect, its deletion resulted in the loss of a multifactorial platform for the formulation of the defined conditions, as well as the loss of some index of the severity of impairment. This change effectively reinforced a biological reductionist perspective and deemphasized the interaction of mental and physical functioning.

In the next section we consider criticisms of DSM-5 further. Despite its faults, DSM-5 remains the way mental health providers, patients, public health officials, insurers, and researchers communicate about emotional health disturbances.

Critiques of DSM-5

Many psychiatrists, and stakeholders in general, have questioned and criticized current categorical diagnostic systems, each of which introduces many ways to diagnose any condition and presents significant difficulties in distinguishing one disorder from another. Consider DSM-5 criteria for major depressive disorder. There are 1,500 combinations of symptoms that meet the threshold for diagnosis of major depression, many of which overlap with the multitude of combinations that might meet criteria for anxiety. Many questions arise from this scenario. Are all criteria of equal importance? Do the system developers provide guidance for the selection of treatment options? What is the meaning of the extensive co-occurrence of defined disorders, and how do they interact?

Although modern psychiatry has advanced in many ways, and people who are distressed by emotional disturbances have many more options for treatment and community living than in the past, it is not clear that the diagnostic systems currently in use have contributed to these advances. Prevention of mental illnesses has been elusive, and the number of people with diagnosable conditions is growing (Timimi 2014). The critiques of DSM and ICD are very similar. The ICD is a product of the World Health Organization and has been used in general medicine since 1948. Mental health diagnoses were added to the classification in the sixth revision, after World War II. The diagnoses and their criteria are quite similar to those in DSM, and ICD codes are generally used for billing mental health issues in the United States because that classification is also used for other medical problems. Although this discussion is generally centered on DSM-5, most of the issues raised apply equally to ICD. The criticisms of these diagnostic systems can be considered in several categories.

Process

The process for the development of DSM-5 has come under fire from many critics for its secrecy and lack of documentation, despite the Task Force's assertions to the contrary (Schatzberg et al. 2009; Wakefield 2015). In most cases, the rationales for the changes adopted by the work groups have not been preserved or made available to the public. Wakefield (2015) points out that the confidentiality agreements that work group members were required to sign is an example of the secrecy surrounding their decisions. Most of the overarching goals set for the development of DSM-5, including distinguishing diagnosis from impairment and incorporating biomarkers into diagnostic criteria, were abandoned. The Task Force's primary goal of incorporating dimensional measures (Regier et al. 2009) ran into controversy related to the conflicting characteristics of dimensional descriptions of function or severity and defining discrete psychiatric disorders. The inclusion of dimensional ratings, suggested most strongly for the personality disorders, did not come to fruition, and the one dimension of function that was included in the two previous versions of DSM, the Global Assessment of Functioning (GAF), was eliminated (Wakefield 2015).

Validity

At the present time scientific research has not been able to identify any specific biological markers for psychiatric diagnoses, which is a perceived or seeming disadvantage with the rest of medical diagnosis (Timimi 2014). The common occurrence of comorbidity (the existence of two or more diagnoses concurrently) is an indication of the ambiguous boundaries between diagnoses and the inability of clinicians to clearly distinguish the source of observed symptoms (Anckarsater 2010; Middleton 2008). DSM-5 expanded criteria for many disorders in a way that pathologized many observed emotional reactions that were formerly considered to be normal reactions to various stressors (e.g., grief reactions vs. major depression). The failure to adequately distinguish the symptoms of many disorders results in false positives (making a diagnosis when it is not present). This issue has significant implications for psychiatric epidemiology research, which depends on the DSM classifications. As noted previously, the definitions of these conditions provide no explanation of their cause and give no indication of the severity of impairment associated with them (Wakefield 2015).

Reliability

Despite the fact that some degree of reliability (agreement among multiple users) has been established for the selection of many DSM-5 disorders, reliability has been established only under controlled conditions. Common diagnoses lose their meaning when psychiatrists are unable to agree on the significance of key symptoms. The symptom checklist approach of DSM was designed to reduce these potential disagreements, but it has not proven to be successful when applied in clinical settings (Freedman et al. 2013; Kirk and Kutchins 1994). Individuals in emotional distress often end up with as many diagnoses as they have had clinicians opining. The lack of reliability further undermines the validity of the diagnostic framework and results in many false positives and, by extension, inappropriate or excessive treatments (Wakefield 2015).

Etiology

The lack of any established biological or psychological markers for mental illnesses not only undermines the validity of their construction but also leaves psychiatrists with no way to verify their impressions. No reliable laboratory or imaging tests are available to pinpoint a diagnosis. Research groups have abandoned the use of DSM-5 because of the lack of validation for its designated disorders, in favor of classifications that attempt to identify the source of observed phenomena (National Institute of Mental Health 2018; Owen et al. 2011). The search for specific genetic underpinnings of any psychiatric disorder has not been fruitful (Timimi 2014).

Treatment

The ability of a diagnosis to identify specific and appropriate treatments for emotional health conditions would be very important to the consideration of value. Although a number of specific and effective treatment protocols have been developed for various conditions, evidence indicates that the therapeutic alliance is much more important than the details of the protocol (Duncan 2012) and that this relative importance accounts for the majority of variance in outcomes. Lack of specificity is also evident with the use of psychoactive medications. Several categories of medications are used for a wide variety of DSM-5 disorders; for example, selective serotonin reuptake inhibitors are used for the full range of mood disruptions, several types of anxiety, obsessions, eating disorders, and some conditions for which there is little evidence of their efficacy. Many medications may effectively alter the recipient's mental state, but they do not appear to correct "chemical imbalances" or act in a way that is specific to diagnosis (Moncrieff 2009; Timimi 2014). A large part of the variance in outcomes related to medication use, as with other types of clinical interventions, is attributable to placebo effects or a positive relationship with the prescriber (Sparks et al. 2008).

Prognosis

To date, the application of a psychiatric diagnosis gives little or no indication of what the course of the illness might be. A single diagnosis can be quite mild with only moderate impairment and a short course, or severe and disabling over the course of many years. Additionally, stigma associated with being labeled as someone with a mental health disorder might lead to reluctance to seek care even if there is a favorable prognosis (Angermeyer et al. 2011). These factors have implications for treatment options, patient expectations and life planning, and discrimination at work and social activities, all of which are related to quality of outcomes (Warner 2010). It is interesting to note that outcomes for persons with severe mental illness may be worse in more industrialized nations than in developing countries, where diagnoses are less frequently made, and treatments are less readily available when they are made (Jablensky 1992; Patel et al. 2006; Sartorius 2008).

Of these many criticisms, perhaps those most relevant to the discussion of value in psychiatric care are ones—such as false positives and overdiagnosis—that lead to overtreatment of various kinds. Even though treatments for emotional disturbances seem to be largely nonspecific with regard to outcomes, there are many instances in which interventions, particularly medications, can do more harm than good. The expansion of criteria and the number of individuals deemed to have a treatable diagnosis have grown, unnecessarily putting more people in harm's way and increasing the overall cost of care. In the following section, some alternatives for diagnostic thinking will be examined.

Alternative Diagnostic Systems

Since the inception of DSM, critics have called for alternative models. As detailed earlier in this chapter, DSM-III itself was an alternative diagnostic model that radically changed the course of psychiatry (Surís et al. 2016). The previous section discussed the many criticisms of the DSM series, and by extension ICD-10, over the last several decades. Despite long-standing criticism of these systems, few alternatives have gained traction. In 2011, the British Psychological Society published an open letter to the APA criticizing the proposed

DSM-5 (Kamens et al. 2017). The main concerns expressed in the letter included the lowering of diagnostic thresholds, leading to the pathologizing of normative behaviors, and the lack of scientific evidence for several new diagnostic categories. The criticisms spawned the Global Summit on Diagnostic Alternatives, which provides a forum for diagnostic reform discussions (Robbins et al. 2017). During the group's conference in 2014, a committee was created to establish recommendations for a future diagnostic model. A subsequent article outlined their major recommendations: "(1) valuing the whole person and recognizing the richness, complexity, and diversity of lived experience; (2) appreciating not only the biopsychosocial but also the sociopolitical context of emotional distress; and (3) valuing the plurality of theoretical perspectives and epistemic commitments of service users and other individuals with lived experience" (Kamens et al. 2018, p. 405–406).

When one is comparing alternative diagnostic models, it is helpful to consider the type of change from the current models of DSM-5 and ICD-10. *First-order change* is defined as a change within the system, while the system itself remains unchanged (Weakland et al. 1974). These types of changes are new formulations of problems within an existing framework developed through expert or professional consensus. This has been the approach used with the successive versions of DSM and ICD. *Second-order change* is transformational, with different principles guiding diagnoses. A description of some of the diagnostic systems proposed to improve or replace current systems follows. These alternative diagnostic models represent second-order changes.

Research Domain Criteria

For many diseases, medical advances were able to both identify etiology and yield effective treatments. In some cases, these discoveries proceeded in reverse order. For example, Edward Jenner's serendipitous discovery of cowpox's ability to provide vaccination against smallpox helped further the study of both virology and immunology. To date, although many pharmacological discoveries in psychiatry have provided treatment, few have offered insight into the elusive etiology of mental health disorders. Despite the many technological, genetic, and neurobiological advances that have occurred in recent years, little light has been shed on the pathophysiological causes of emotional disruptions. In 2008, the National Institute of Mental Health (NIMH) established a goal to "develop, for research purposes, new ways of classifying mental disorders based on dimensions of observable behavior and neurobiological measures" (Cuthbert and Insel 2013).

Bruce Cuthbert and Thomas Insel from NIMH launched the Research Domain Criteria (RDoC) in 2010. Their commentary to the *American Jour-*

nal of Psychiatry that year documents their reasoning (Insel et al. 2010). They state that clinical symptoms alone do not necessarily relate to distinct disease pathogenesis. They presented a new model to guide research, with the end goal of creating a more biologically based diagnostic system. Consequently, RDoC has drastically shifted the state of mental health research.

The RDoC Matrix (National Institute of Mental Health 2018) is an interactive framework. This matrix is broken into six "domains of functioning," listed below with some of their constructs (National Institute of Mental Health 2020):

- *Negative valence systems:* fear, anxiety, sustained threats, loss, frustrations
- *Positive valence systems:* reward responsiveness, reward learning, reward valuation
- *Cognitive systems:* perceptions, cognitive control, working memory
- *Systems for social processes:* social communication, perception of self and others
- *Arousal/regulatory systems:* arousal, circadian rhythms, sleep and wakefulness
- *Sensorimotor systems:* motor actions, agency and ownership, innate motor patterns, habit

According to RDoC, research projects that receive grant funding from NIMH must evaluate one or more of the above listed dimensions based on "Units of Analysis." These units include genes, molecules, cells that comprise circuits, physiological responses, behavior, self-report, and paradigms. The creators hoped that this matrix would allow researchers to take any element of the matrix and connect it to the neurophysiological circuits involved (Cuthbert 2014), the long-term goal being to characterize the biological underpinning of each domain of the matrix.

DSM has been criticized for overlap of symptoms across many supposedly distinct diagnoses (e.g., difficulty with sleep in depression and anxiety disorders). This overlap has made it difficult to correlate a particular diagnosis with distinct biological markers. Proponents of the RDoC system hope that its dimensional categorization, once fully elaborated, can provide more precision to diagnoses than can the phenomenological framework in DSM. If so, the RDoC system may open new doors to understanding disease etiology and pathophysiology. Unfortunately, the matrix is so broad and complex that it provides no practical framework to guide treatment.

A main criticism of the RDoC system is that it has funneled all funding for research into basic science studies and away from health services research. By NIMH's own estimation, many of the potential results from research using the RDoC system will likely be decades in the future. Critics and advocacy groups have decried the lack of funding for more pertinent and practical research, which is needed given the poor outcomes obtained from the current mental health care system (Frances 2014). Proponents feel that using the new RDoC system is the only way to move forward in understanding psychiatric illness.

In terms of value, RDoC to date has not impacted diagnosis or guided treatments. Should its aims be fulfilled, discovering the biological basis for mental illness has the potential to drastically change how we treat and understand mental health, but it does not appear to be a viable alternative system for clinical practice.

Hierarchical Taxonomy of Psychopathology

The Hierarchical Taxonomy of Psychopathology (HiTOP) was first introduced by Dr. Roman Kotov and colleagues (2017). The authors created HiTOP in response to the DSM-5 Task Force's failure to develop the dimensional approaches that had been promised for DSM-5. Their main argument was that DSM created an "artificial boundary" between wellness and mental illness; their second critique of DSM was the overwhelming prevalence of comorbidity when using the system. With these issues in mind, this group worked to create a simpler, evidence-based model using factor analysis. The researchers initially took the overarching concept of internalizing versus externalizing symptom clusters and then integrated Digman's (1990) five-factor model (five broad dimensions of personality characteristics: openness, conscientiousness, extraversion, agreeableness, and neuroticism). HiTOP is composed of five tiers: Spectra, Subfactors, Syndromes/Disorders, Components, and Symptoms. The HiTOP method starts with the top taxonomic rank, called "Spectra," which include internalizing (or negative affectivity), thought disorder (or psychoticism), disinhibited externalizing, antagonistic externalizing, detachment, and somatoform. The goal of HiTOP is to decrease the number of codes and current level of comorbidities involved in assigning diagnoses. For example, a patient with generalized anxiety disorder, major depressive disorder, and perhaps borderline personality disorder according to the DSM system, would be identified under the single HiTOP spectra of internalizing distress (Kotov et al. 2018).

Proponents of HiTOP say that using a hierarchical model helps clarify treatment because many of these now clustered diagnoses have similar treatments. The creators of this model believe this is valid because the disorders likely have shared biological and environmental etiologies (Lahey et al. 2017). They argue that RDoC has gone too far in breaking down mental health issues in its quest for understanding micro-level interactions between brain function and behavior. Instead, they believe that research should focus on zooming out to look at the larger-scale determinants of mental health disorders. Critics of this new model state that many people can have both internalizing and externalizing spectra, leading to the same failings noted for DSM-5, and therefore that HiTOP does not bring the field closer to understanding the etiology of symptom clusters or improving treatment planning for those conditions.

Unlike RDoC, the current iteration of HiTOP has the potential to reframe how we understand diagnosis. Simplifying the diagnostic system could improve ease of billing and insurance reimbursement. For patients, having one overarching diagnosis instead of four may be less confusing and more empowering. Indeed, researchers could focus more on how treatments work for overlapping symptoms instead of assuming they are all due to distinct causes.

Novel Approaches to Assessment and Classification of Emotional Disruptions

Classification and Statistical Manual of Mental Health Concerns

The *Classification and Statistical Manual of Mental Health Concerns* (CSM) was developed by Jeffrey Rubin and first presented at the American Psychological Association's annual convention in 2015. His reasoning for creating this alternative diagnostic model was in response to many criticisms of DSM, most notably the stigma associated with the DSM's definition of mental health disorders. The CSM is a patient-focused model that uses the word *concern* instead of *disorder* in describing emotional health issues. Concerns are broken down into concerns for self and concerns for others. Instead of receiving a specific diagnosis, each individual would be given a psychological formulation, based on the patient's reported concerns and expressed level of functioning in various aspects of life (Rubin 2018). To date, no recent presentations or work has been done to further develop this model, and thus no true evaluation has occurred. Critics point out that, whatever worth CSM might bring to clinical encounters, it does not actually provide a classification of emotional conditions that could be useful for communication and treatment guidance.

Power Threat Meaning Framework

In 2012, the British Psychological Society funded a project to create an alternative and nondiagnostic model to describe mental health. The current outline is called the Power Threat Meaning Framework (PTMF). The project's goal is to move away from a medical model toward a more conceptual understanding of patient experiences. To this end, many of those working on the framework are mental health users themselves. The creators argue that because of the multitude of human experiences, identifying specific etiologies of mental health issues is fruitless. In their words, "the factors that contribute to any aspect of human behavior, and their outcomes, are generally multiple, complex, highly interactive and overdetermined, and, crucially, always shaped by personal meaning and agency" (Johnstone and Boyle 2018). The model rejects the problem-centered approach used by other systems and moves toward a patient-focused understanding of experience and coping strategies. The term *power* is used to understand how individuals have faced adversities and social injustices. *Threat* refers to when persons experience loss or perceived threats to their core needs, including safety, security, and relationships. Finally, *meaning* refers to how individuals understand their lived experience. PTMF postulates that there are patterns of experiences that lead to regular behavioral responses, and that these patterns can be used to guide treatment. The framework also aims to be more inclusive of cultural aspects of emotional health that more biologically based models have struggled to incorporate. Most notably, PTMF is not a diagnostic model. Rather, PTMF is attempting to shift understanding of mental wellness toward a more subjective, individualistic framework of human experience. Elaboration of PTMF can be found on the society's Web site (British Psychological Society 2018).

PTMF is focused on increasing the value of diagnosis specifically for patients. In its current form, it is unlikely to be useful for insurers and providers in terms of their ability to communicate to one another. Although it would allow for a more comprehensive assessment of an individual, it would be difficult for research to clarify which groups of patients would benefit from particular treatments. Nonetheless, it may be of value in the context of patient-centered care.

A Multifactorial Model: "The Perspectives of Psychiatry"

The model that would become "The Perspectives of Psychiatry" was articulated by Paul McHugh and Phillip Slavney at Johns Hopkins University in 1998 (McHugh and Slavney 1998). Based on the concepts borrowed from Adolf Meyer and Karl Jaspers in the early twentieth century, the multifactorial model requires that a person's psychiatric condition be considered from four perspectives: disease, dimensional, behavior, and life story.

Disease refers to the biological components of the illness (i.e., pathology or etiology), as far as they are known. The *dimensional* perspective attempts to capture physical and psychological attributes that determine a person's interaction with their environment (e.g., strength, impulsivity, emotional stability). *Behavior* focuses on learned behaviors and conditioned responses, which determine what a person does and the choices they make. The *life story* is the personal narrative that people construct for themselves, and how the clinician understands the story and uses it to help clients "rescript" their life story in a way that is more functional (Peters et al. 2012).

This approach is considered to offer a more comprehensive understanding of a person's condition and to be a more useful construct to inform treatment planning. It is in many ways similar to the biopsychosocial approach proposed by George Engel at the University of Rochester in the 1970s (Engel 1977, 1980) or the discarded multiaxial system from previous editions of DSM. However, proponents of this model consider it to be better suited to combine these dimensions to formulate practical plans for individuals. Multifactorial approaches may be viewed as leading to comprehensive formulations of a person's condition, rather than to a diagnosis per se. Like PTMF, these approaches have limitations with regard to their usefulness for research, communication, and billing purposes.

The *p* Factor

Another model representing a radical departure from current constructs was put forth by Caspi and Moffitt (2018). It proposes using a single dimension to characterize all mental disorders. This dimension indicates an overall level of psychopathology, termed the *p* factor. The *p* factor unites all the diagnoses under categorical classifications of symptoms. In doing so, it eliminates much of the ambiguity and overlap of criteria for diagnoses in systems currently being used (Kotov et al. 2017) and focuses instead on the severity of psychopathology, from low (symptoms with limited impact on function) to high (psychotic-level symptoms interfering with activities of daily living). High *p* scores are correlated to family history of psychiatric illness, brain dysfunction, childhood developmental delays, and adult impairment. The primacy of this *p* factor may account for the extensive cooccurrence of disorders in categorical systems and the fact that many diagnoses share the same risk factors, biomarkers, and therapeutic response (Caspi and Moffitt 2018).

This single-dimensional model is a distillation of an earlier three-dimensional model, which designated three types of experiences: internalizing (anxious and depressive symptoms), externalizing (aggressive, impulsive, and hyperactive symptoms), and psychotic (dissociation, disorganization, and disturbances of perception and interpretation) (Krueger and Markon 2011). The *p* factor is derived from observations that many commonalities exist between these dimensions. The suggestion that a single factor—namely the quality of the therapeutic relationship—is most salient in the treatment of all emotional health disorders lends some credence to this construct. At present, the evidence supporting this model is not developed, and it remains a statistical abstraction of correlates. However, the hypothesis that *p* captures a disordered form and content of thought that permeates practically all diagnoses of psychopathology may have roots in genetics, epigenetics, and neurophysiology. Research would be needed to clarify the validity of this proposal. Whether or not this fascinating idea will one day be substantiated, the underlying concept provides one way to think about how psychiatric impairment may be quantified and used as an indicator of severity of impairment (Caspi and Moffitt 2018). Nonetheless, it does not appear that this one factor alone will meet all the interests of various stakeholders and the functions of diagnosis alluded to in earlier sections. The following section will examine the needs of the major stakeholders in emotional health services.

Stakeholders' Perspectives

The criticisms leveled at emotional health diagnostic systems have different implications for various stakeholders with respect to value. For those who pay for services, financial or market success is of primary concern to insurers and their investors. The first priority for private insurers is to make a profit. They incur a cost when an event (illness) occurs and treatment is rendered. They need to be able to predict, with some accuracy, the probability of an event occurring. Because they accept risk, in exchange for the inflow of income (either through premiums or contracts), they must be sure that expenses do not exceed income. If more events occur than predicted, they will be in danger of losing money rather than making a profit (Sowers 2012). They will only be secure if they reduce occurrences, reduce the amount they will pay per occurrence, or increase their revenues. Although premiums can be increased, that remedy will be limited by what purchasers would be willing or able to pay.

How is the insurance industry related to diagnosis? The use of a standard diagnostic system in the United States was mandated by the federal Health Insurance Portability and Accountability Act (HIPAA) of 1996 (U.S. Department of Health and Human Services 2015). The ICD coding system was adopted by the Department of Health and Human Services to specify psychiatric diagnoses. These ICD codes were matched to the corresponding DSM-IV diagnoses and subsequently to the DSM-5 classification. Theses codes are used for billing, so how they are applied will have a direct bearing on insurers by affecting their expenses. For example, an insurance company must be able to estimate the cost it would incur to treat depression. If it is determined that about 6.7% of the U.S. population ages 18 and older suffer from depression according to DSM criteria in a given year, and the average yearly cost of treatment for each person diagnosed is $4,500, an insurance company can calculate what their likely expenses will be. If this diagnosis is made more frequently than anticipated, expenses will be greater than predicted and the company will lose money. Insurance companies can try to reduce their expenses in various ways, such as through high deductibles, high copays, limiting the use of expensive interventions such as hospital-based care, and reducing access to certain medications and therapies. They can also attempt to reduce the incidence of depressive illnesses through health incentive programs, but they cannot control misdiagnosis. Overdiagnosis will have a significant impact on both quality and cost of care. Overall, given the primacy of financial concerns, insurance companies would value a diagnostic system that has fewer numbers of diagnoses, is clear on when interventions and treatments are required, and can be easily documented and reliably applied.

The priorities for health care providers will vary to some degree depending on whether they are for-profit or not-for-profit systems. The financial concerns considered above for private payers also apply to private providers. In the public sector, there will be greater emphasis on positive outcomes and patient satisfaction relative to costs. Diagnostic systems such as DSM-5 give little guidance with regard to treatment or severity of impairment in functioning. As a result, they are not very useful for predicting costs or treatment planning. Dimensional assessments of functioning in various domains would be more easily applied to these processes and better related to patient satisfaction. Complex diagnostic systems are also costly for providers because they require more extensive training and usually require more of the clinician's time for making a determination and documenting it. The possibility of inaccuracy of diagnosis also increases with complexity, which has implications for cost and quality (Wakefield 2015).

For people with emotional health disruptions, the stigma associated with diagnosis must be considered. Studies show that stigma and associated discrimination can result in reduced use of services and reduced engagement in recreational activities (Corrigan 2004). Stigma is also the greatest barrier to treating mental illness early and lowering treatment costs. Despite the possible effects of stigma, many people in emotional distress want to have some explanation for their suffering. Having a name for their condition may seem to legitimize their struggles and reduce their sense of self-blame (Boyle and Johnstone 2014; Timimi 2014). However, when they receive a different diagnosis each time they are assessed, the naming process becomes less compelling and undermines legitimacy, leaving them even more confused. Most people will not be familiar with the terminology and will have difficulty understanding what their various diagnoses mean unless they are highly motivated to read and comprehend the current DSM and ICD editions (DSM-5 and ICD-11, respectively). Receiving diagnoses that are not based on etiology and that provide little guidance for specific treatments will provide little satisfaction for most recipients.

Employers have a very different perspective with regard to value. Their priorities are efficiency, productivity, and outputs that will be attractive to their customers. Presently, about half of all Americans—some 156 million people—get their health insurance through employer-based plans (Henry J. Kaiser Family Foundation 2018), and this is a significant expense for employers. However, most employers have come to realize the importance of keeping their workers healthy. Workplace health is discussed in detail in Chapter 20 ("Health and the Workplace"), so it should suffice to say here that recent research shows that mental disorders, especially depression, have a greater impact on productivity in the United States than physical disorders and are the greatest cause of worker disability in the country (Brown et al. 2019). Employers incur costs due to employee absenteeism, presenteeism (being at work but not productive), and turnover. A survey of almost 35,000 employees from 10 companies revealed that depression ranked first and anxiety ranked fifth as causes for absenteeism or presenteeism. Employees with any mental disorder experienced more absenteeism days per year than individuals with no conditions, at a ratio of 31:1. Among all reasons for absenteeism, mental health conditions accounted for 62.2% of all days "out of role" (Cooper and Dewe 2008). Looking at direct (medical/pharmaceutical) and indirect (absenteeism/presenteeism) costs of each disorder, the highest total cost per worker per year is for mental disorders ($18,864 in 2002), which is $5,000 greater than the costs associated with the next most costly medical condition—breathing disorders (Starling Minds 2020). However, the current categorical diagnostic system says little about the degree of disability of a worker and provides no guidance to the employer with regard to reasonable accommodations or other actions that would enable affected workers to return to full productivity.

Conclusion

Although the priorities of various stakeholders may be disparate, there is a common thread with regard to the diagnosis of emotional health conditions. All stakeholders would seem to benefit from a system that could provide consistent, reliable results, as well as some indication of the severity of impairment and some estimate of prognosis. A simplified system in which the numbers and subdivisions of diagnoses are significantly reduced would improve the reliability of assessments and decrease time spent on training and deliberation over decisions. Such a system would also enhance one of the main functions of diagnosis—namely, communication between clinicians and people in services.

Returning to the opening of this chapter, where *diagnosis* was defined, it is unclear whether the DSM classification would objectively meet that definition. Although it is a process of identifying a "disease" from its signs and symptoms, in other parts of medicine the symptoms are derived from the disease. In psychiatry, the "disease" is derived from the signs and symptoms and has no other intrinsic elements. Additionally, although there have been investigations of the cause or nature of conditions, there are not yet any established conclusions. The scientific basis of the classification is dubious, and a diagnosis itself provides no specific answer or remedy for the identified condition. The preceding discussion indicated the limited utility of a system that generates more uncertainty that confidence, and its implications for value. Disorders defined by DSM-5 are not discrete, and severity of illness lies along a continuum that is not distinguished by the present structure. The incorporation of dimensional assessments would provide greater clarity and guidance for treatment planning. This includes the reintroduction of a more global approach to identifying factors that contribute to distress and dysfunction, such as environment, sociopolitical conditions, physical health, and other stressors.

To accomplish this system change, the field of psychiatry might do best to start from scratch, developing a system that is geared toward improving outcomes and guiding treatment while avoiding unnecessary labeling and inappropriate treatment. Elimination of possible conflicts of interest in that process would be imperative, and the inclusion of people who are, or who have been, affected by emotional health disruptions must be part of the process (Bracken 2012). While the efforts to develop a better understanding of the underlying causes of mental illness continue, psychiatry does not need to make itself appear more medical. Psychiatrists only need to do what they do best: develop a comprehensive understanding of the many forces that influence emotional health and communicate it in a simple and useful way to the people they serve.

References

American Psychiatric Association: Statistical Manual for the Use of Institutions for the Insane. New York, National Committee for Mental Hygiene, Bureau of Statistics, 1918

American Psychiatric Association: Diagnostic and Statistical Manual of Mental Disorders. Washington, DC, American Psychiatric Association, 1952

American Psychiatric Association: Diagnostic and Statistical Manual of Mental Disorders, 2nd Edition. Washington, DC, American Psychiatric Association, 1968

American Psychiatric Association: Diagnostic and Statistical Manual of Mental Disorders, 3rd Edition. Washington, DC, American Psychiatric Association, 1980

American Psychiatric Association: Diagnostic and Statistical Manual of Mental Disorders, 4th Edition. Washington, DC, American Psychiatric Association, 1994

American Psychiatric Association: Diagnostic and Statistical Manual of Mental Disorders, 5th Edition. Washington, DC, American Psychiatric Association, 2013

Anckarsater H: Beyond categorical diagnostics in psychiatry: scientific and medicolegal implications. Int J Law Psychiatry 33(2):59–65, 2010

Angermeyer M, Holzinger A, Carta M, et al: Biogenic explanations and public acceptance of mental illness: systematic review of populations studies. Br J Psychiatry 199(5):367–372, 2011

Blashfield RK, Keeley JW, Flanagan EH, et al: The cycle of classification: DSM-I through DSM-5. Annu Rev Clin Psychol 10:25–51, 2014

Boyle M, Johnstone L: Alternatives to psychiatric diagnosis. Lancet Psychiatry 1(6):409–411, 2014

Bracken P: Psychiatric power: a personal view. Ir J Psychol Med 29(1):55–58, 2012

British Psychological Society: Introducing the Power Threat Meaning Framework. February 1, 2018. Available at: www.bps.org.uk/news-and-policy/introducing-power-threat-meaning-framework. Accessed March 9, 2020.

Brown N, Gorsky A, Moynihan B: Mental health and the workplace: what employers must realize. FOXBusiness, March 12, 2019. Available at: www.foxbusiness.com/personal-finance/mental-health-and-the-workplace-what-employers-must-realize. Accessed March 9, 2020.

Caspi A, Moffitt T: All for one and one for all: mental disorders in one dimension. Am J Psychiatry 175(9):831–844, 2018

Cooper C, Dewe P: Well-being—absenteeism, presenteeism, costs and challenges. Occup Med (Lond) 58(8):522–524, 2008

Corrigan P: How stigma interferes with mental health care. Am Psychol 59(1):614–625, 2004

Cuthbert BN: The RDoC framework: facilitating transition from ICD/DSM to dimensional approaches that integrate neuroscience and psychopathology. World Psychiatry 13(1):28–35, 2014

Cuthbert BN, Insel TR: Toward the future of psychiatric diagnosis: the seven pillars of RDoC. BMC Med 11:126, 2013

Digman JM: Personality structure: emergence of the five-factor model. Annual Review of Psychology 41:417–440, 1990

Duncan B: The Partners for Change Outcome Management System (PCMS): the heart and soul of change project. Canadian Psychologist 53(4):93–104, 2012

Engel GL: The need for a new medical model: a challenge for biomedicine. Science 196(4286):129–136, 1977

Engel GL: The clinical application of the biopsychosocial model. Am J Psychiatry 137(5):535–544, 1980

Feighner JP, Robins E, Guze SB, et al: Diagnostic criteria for use in psychiatric research. Arch Gen Psychiatry 26(1):57–63, 1972

Frances A: RDoC is necessary, but very oversold. World Psychiatry 13(1):47–49, 2014

Freedman R, Lewis D, Michels R, et al: The initial field trials of DSM-5: new blooms and old thorns. Am J Psychiatry 170(1):1–5, 2013

Freud S: Die Traumdeutung. Leipzig, Germany, Franz Deuticke, 1899

Gambardella A: Science and Innovation: The U.S. Pharmaceutical Industry During the 1980s. Cambridge, MA, Cambridge University Press, 1995

Grob GN: Origins of DSM-I: a study in appearance and reality. Am J Psychiatry 148(4):421–431, 1991

Henry J Kaiser Family Foundation: Health insurance coverage of the total population. 2018. Available at: www.kff.org/other/state-indicator/total-population. Accessed June 20, 2020.

Insel T, Cuthbert BN, Garvey M, et al: Research Domain Criteria (RDoC): toward a new classification framework for research on mental disorders. Am J Psychiatry 167(7):748–751, 2010

Jablensky A: Schizophrenia: manifestations, incidence and course in different cultures. Psychol Med Monogr Suppl 20:1–95, 1992

Johnstone L, Boyle M: The Power Threat Meaning Framework: an alternative nondiagnostic conceptual system. Journal of Humanist Psychology August 5, 2018. Available at: https://journals.sagepub.com/doi/10.1177/0022167818793289. Accessed March 10, 2020.

Kamens SR, Elkins DN, Robbins BD: Open letter to the DSM-5. Journal of Humanist Psychology 57(6):675–687, 2017

Kamens SR, Cosgrove L, Peters SM, et al: Standards and guidelines for the development of diagnostic nomenclatures and alternatives in mental health research and practice. Journal of Humanist Psychology 59(3):401–427, 2018

Kawa S, Giordano J: A brief historicity of the Diagnostic and Statistical Manual of Mental Disorders: issues and implications for the future of psychiatric canon and practice. Philos Ethics Humanit Med 7:2, 2012

Kirk S, Kutchins H: The myth of reliability of DSM. Journal of Mind and Behavior 15(1&2):71–86, 1994

Kotov R, Krueger RF, Watson D, et al: The Hierarchical Taxonomy of Psychopathology (HiTOP): a dimensional alternative to traditional nosologies. J Abnorm Psychol 126(4):454–477, 2017

Kotov R, Krueger R, Watson D: A paradigm shift in psychiatric classification: the Hierarchical Taxonomy of Psychopathology (HiTOP). World Psychiatry 17(1):24–25, 2018

Kraepelin E: Psychiatrie, 6th Edition. Leipzig, Germany, Barth, 1899
Krueger R, Markon J: A dimension-spectrum model of psychopathology: progress and opportunities. Arch Gen Psychiatry 68(1):10–11, 2011
Lahey BB, Krueger RF, Rathouz PJ, et al: A hierarchical causal taxonomy of psychopathology across the life span. Psychol Bull 143(2):142–186, 2017
Mayes R, Horwitz A: DSM-III and the revolution in the classification of mental illness. J Hist Behav Sci 41(3):249–267, 2005
McHugh PR, Slavney PR: The Perspectives of Psychiatry. Baltimore, MD, Johns Hopkins University Press, 1998
Middleton H: Whither DSM and ICD, chapter V? Mental Health Review Journal 13(4):4–15, 2008
Moncrieff J: An alternative drug-centered model of action, in The Myth of Chemical Cure: A Critique of Psychiatric Drug Treatment. London, Palgrave McMillan, 2009, pp 14–15
National Institute of Mental Health: RDoC matrix. 2018. Available at: www.nimh.nih.gov/research/research-funded-by-nimh/rdoc/constructs/rdoc-matrix.shtml. Accessed March 9, 2020.
National Institute of Mental Health: RDoC matrix. 2020. Available at: https://www.nimh.nih.gov/research/research-funded-by-nimh/rdoc/definitions-of-the-rdoc-domains-and-constructs.shtml. Accessed July 29, 2020.
Owen M, O'Donovan M, Thapar A, et al: Neurodevelopmental hypothesis of schizophrenia. Br J Psychiatry 198(3):173–175, 2011
Patel V, Cohen A, Thara R, et al: Is the outcome of schizophrenia really better in developing countries? Braz J Psychiatry 28(2):149–152, 2006
Peters M, Taylor J, Lyketsos CG, et al: Beyond the DSM: the perspectives of psychiatry approach to patients. Prim Care Companion CNS Disord 14(1), 2012
Regier D, Narrow W, Kuhl E, et al: The conceptual development of DSM-5. Am J Psychiatry 166(6):645–650, 2009
Robbins BD, Kamens SR, Elkins DN: DSM-5 reform efforts by the Society for Humanistic Psychology. Journal of Humanist Psychology 57(6):602–624, 2017
Rogler L: Making sense of historical changes in the Diagnostic and Statistical Manual of Mental Disorders: five propositions. J Health Soc Behav 38(1):9–20, 1997
Rosenhan D: On being sane in insane places. Science 179(4070):250–258, 1973
Rubin J: The Classification and Statistical Manual of Mental Health Concerns: a proposed practical scientific alternative to the DSM and ICD. J Humanist Psychol 58(1):93–114, 2018
Sartorius N: Brief description of World Health Organization studies comparing mental health recovery in developed and developing nations. 2008. Available at: https://mindfreedom.org/kb/sartorius-on-who. Accessed March 9, 2020.
Schatzberg A, Scully J, Kupfer D, et al: Setting the record straight: a response to Frances commentary on DSM-V. Psychiatric Times, July 1, 2009. Available at: www.psychiatrictimes.com/dsm-5/setting-record-straight-response-frances-commentary-dsm-v. Accessed March 9, 2020.

Shorter E: Before Prozac: The Troubled History of Mood Disorders in Psychiatry. New York, Oxford University Press, 2008

Sowers WE: Affordable quality care: rational approaches to financing behavioral health. Journal of Psychiatric Administration and Management 1(2):81–88, 2012

Sparks J, Duncan B, Miller S: Common factors in psychotherapy: common means to uncommon outcomes, in 21st Century Psychotherapies, 2nd Edition. Edited by Lebow J. New York, Wiley, 2008, pp 453–498

Spitzer RL, Fleiss JL: A re-analysis of the reliability of psychiatric diagnosis. Br J Psychiatry 125(0):341–347, 1974

Spitzer R, Endicott J, Robins E: Research diagnostic criteria: rationale and reliability. Arch Gen Psychiatry 35(6):773–782, 1978

Starling Minds: The economic impact of mental illness: absenteeism and presenteeism. 2020. Available at: www.starlingminds.com/wp-content/uploads/2018/06/Starling-Minds-Research-Paper-The-Economic-Impact-of-Mental-Health.pdf. Accessed March 9, 2020.

Surís A, Holliday R, North CS: The evolution of the classification of psychiatric disorders. Behav Sci (Basel) 6(1), 2016

Timimi S: No more psychiatric labels: why formal psychiatric diagnostic systems should be abolished. Int J Clin Health Psychol 14(3):208–215, 2014

U.S. Department of Health and Human Services: The HIPAA privacy rule. April 16, 2015. Available at: www.hhs.gov/hipaa/for-professionals/privacy/index.html. Accessed March 9, 2020.

Wakefield JC: Disorder as harmful dysfunction: a conceptual critique of DSM-III-R's definition of mental disorder. Psychol Rev 99(2):232–247, 1992

Wakefield JC: DSM-5, psychiatric epidemiology and the false positives problem. Epidemiol Psychiatr Sci 24(3):188–196, 2015

Warner R: Does the scientific evidence support the recovery model? The Psychiatrist 34(1):3–5, 2010

Weakland JH, Fisch R, Watzlawick P, et al: Brief therapy: focused problem resolution. Family Process 13:141–168, 1974

World Health Organization: International Statistical Classification of Diseases and Related Health Problems, 10th Revision. Geneva, World Health Organization, 1992

15

Advocacy

Deepika Sastry, M.D., M.B.A., FAPA
Nubia Lluberes, M.D., CCHP-MH, FAPA
Colleen Bell, M.D., FACHE, FAPA

Advocacy Defined

The word *advocacy* comes from the Latin *advocatia*, which means to summon or to call to one's aid. It also refers to the act of speaking on behalf of or in support of another person, place, or entity. *Advocacy*, in layman's terms, is the provision of public support. In medicine, however, *advocacy* acquires a broader definition and a higher level of commitment, as it encompasses the provision of support to promote patients' health and their rights in relation to their health concerns. In many instances, advocacy aims to give patients a voice. Physicians have a duty to follow basic ethical principles, including beneficence (moral obligation to act in the benefit of the patient), nonmaleficence (moral obligation not to inflict harm), and justice (to equitably distribute benefits, risks, costs, and resources) (Jahn 2011). In doing so, they look after the well-being of their patients and thus are arguably well positioned to advocate on patients' behalf.

As society grew and matured, and as governments and political structures developed, the role of physicians gradually evolved to include a focus on not only the health of individual patients but also other health-related aspects of larger communities. Geraghty and Wynia (2000) opine that medicine's shift from political to religious goals in the eighteenth century heightened its prominence in social affairs, while simultaneously raising tension between physicians' obligations to individual patients and their obligations to the community. This expanded role has been especially apparent during public health crises, such as epidemics. Large-scale advocacy efforts with systemwide targets, including improvement of health care access and revamping of the health care system, are as important as individual-level efforts. Hubinette and colleagues (2017) proposed a conceptual model for medical advocacy based on two axes, with the horizontal axis representing who determines the need for advocacy, and the vertical axis representing the level at which advocacy occurs. They also propose training physicians to be responsive to the needs of patients, communities, and populations while paying attention to the dynamic role of physicians in the health care systems.

In psychiatry, the most obvious targets for advocacy are the needs of people suffering from mental illness (i.e., access to shelter, food, medication, and qualified treatment providers). Addressing these issues through any activity, large or small in scale, can have an impact on these individuals' well-being. Inequities in the availability or access to services ultimately affect the population as a whole, not only the individual who is denied care. Persons suffering from mental illness are stigmatized by society; they also face racial discrimination and other social disadvantages that limit access to services in many cases. Advocacy efforts aimed at reducing stigma can play an important role in mitigating some of these barriers to quality care to improve the quality of life of mentally ill patients and their families (Holubova et al. 2016).

The World Health Organization (WHO) points out that those lower in the social hierarchy are more likely to experience less favorable economic, social, and environmental conditions throughout life. In a 2014 publication, WHO released a multilevel framework for understanding social determinants of mental health and applying that understanding to promote strategies that can improve mental well-being, which include education, policy change, and advocacy (World Health Organization 2014).

Advocacy efforts have also evolved with changes in the values of the health care system. Once a paternalistic and doctor-centered discipline, medicine is now moving toward embracing a more egalitarian and patient-centered philosophy. This transformation has paved a path to a more unified advocacy platform in which a partnership among patients, their providers, and their families will produce the greatest impact.

A Brief History of Mental Health Advocacy

Looking at the timeline of mental health advocacy efforts in the United States, it is evident that the initial efforts were prompted by the deplorable conditions that patients had to endure in the asylum era. The first documented complaint was that of Elizabeth Stone, who in 1842 denounced the conditions of deprivation she suffered while hospitalized at McLean Asylum in Massachusetts. Since then, patients have advocated for their own causes; in some cases, their voices were so powerful that they led to new legislation protecting patients' interests.

One of the earliest advocacy efforts that had significant impact was led by Dorothea Dix. In a letter to the Massachusetts legislature in 1849, she wrote,

> I found, near Boston, in the Jails and Asylums for the poor, a numerous class brought into unsuitable connexion [sic] with criminals and the general mass of Paupers. I refer to Idiots and Insane persons, dwelling in circumstances not only adverse to their own physical and moral improvement, but productive of extreme disadvantages to all other persons brought into association with them.... I shall be obliged to speak with great plainness, and to reveal many things revolting to the taste, and from which my woman's nature shrinks with peculiar sensitiveness. ... If I inflict pain upon you, and move you to horror, it is to acquaint you with suffering which you have the power to alleviate, and make you hasten to the relief of the victims of legalized barbarity.... I proceed, Gentlemen, briefly to call your attention to the present state of Insane Persons confined within this Commonwealth, *in cages, closets, cellars, stalls, pens! Chained, naked, beaten with rods*, and *lashed* into obedience! (Dix 2006, p. 622)

Dorothea Dix drew attention to the painful reality of the asylum environment affecting the indigent mentally ill patients and championed this cause by addressing the legislators directly. Her letter is filled with detailed descriptions of the barbarities she observed and transmits a sense of urgency.

Important sociopolitical events such as the Civil Rights Movement helped pave the way for mental health advocacy (Figure 15–1). These social movements and landmark cases were frequently cited in the legislature changes related to the development of psychiatric advance directives that started in the 1990s. The Civil Rights Movement originated during a period of United States history in which there was increased awareness of issues related to social justice. Beginning in the 1950s and continuing through the 1960s, the African American community engaged in advocacy that resulted in a U.S. Supreme Court decision striking down forms of legalized racial discrimination and segregation known as the "Jim Crow" laws. The civil rights victories instilled hope for many groups that were discriminated against, facilitating a new appreciation of American civil liberties during this new era of activism.

Also during the 1960s, the Kansas case of *Natanson v. Kline* (1960) addressed patients' rights to informed consent. The court opined that patients

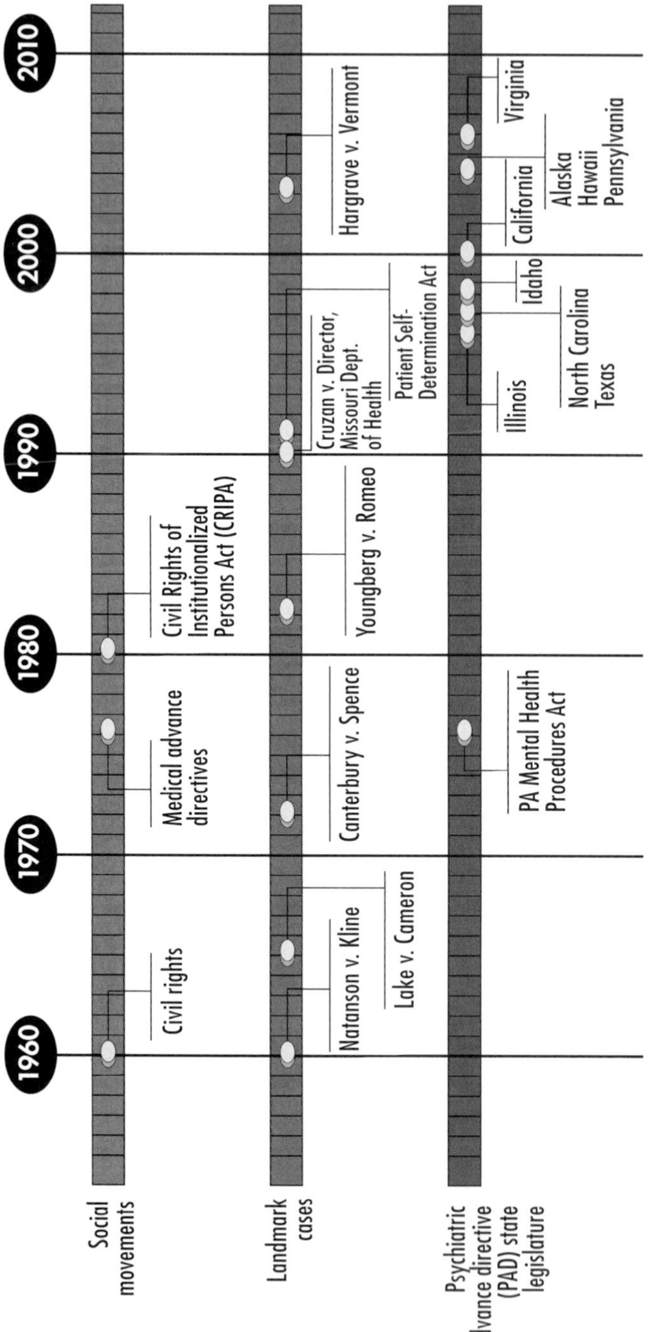

FIGURE 15–1. Parallel timeline of advocacy efforts.

Source. Graph by Gigi Polo.

should be apprised of information "a reasonable person" would want to know in making an informed decision about their health care. Moreover, the case of *Lake v. Cameron* (1966) addressed patients' rights during involuntary hospitalization due to mental illness. The advocacy for medical advance directives in the 1970s set the stage for the following 20 years of patient right advocacy.

In 1980, the Civil Rights of Institutionalized Persons Act (CRIPA) was passed as federal law for the protection of persons living in mental health facilities, nursing homes, and correctional institutions. It allowed the U.S. Attorney General to bring suit in the federal court on behalf of persons institutionalized by the states under unconstitutional conditions (Dean 1988). The case of *Youngberg v. Romeo* (1982) arose from CRIPA and addressed freedom from restraint and maintenance of safe conditions during confinement in those institutions. Under the authority of CRIPA, the Civil Rights Division of the U.S. Department of Justice has been able to bring the "right to treatment" closer to a reality for individuals in state psychiatric hospitals and in facilities for individuals with developmental disabilities by applying the standards of *Youngberg* (Geller 2017). For patients and families, this means that a person admitted to a psychiatric hospital has a right to receive—and should receive—the standard of care delivered in any accredited psychiatric setting (Sederer 2013). Later federal legislation, such as the Patient Self-Determination Act of 1990, addressed the rights of persons suffering from terminal illness. It was derived from the Supreme Court case *Cruzan v. Director, Missouri Dept of Health* (1990). (This act introduced the concepts of *advance directives* and *power of attorney*, which in turn led to the development of psychiatric advance directives.) More recently, in 2003, the case of *Hargrave v. Vermont* (2003) extended the validity of the durable power of attorney to individuals hospitalized for mental illness.

Types and Levels of Advocacy

Advocacy can take many forms and have varying degrees of intensity. Although various nomenclatures may be used, advocacy can be characterized in one of three ways: 1) *case advocacy*—lobbying for an individual, 2) *cause advocacy*—lobbying for services for groups of individuals, and 3) *guild advocacy*—lobbying on behalf of specific provider groups. Another approach is to divide advocacy into two arenas: *agency* ("working the system" to benefit the health of individual patients) and *activism* ("changing the system" to promote the health of populations) (Dobson et al. 2012). The latter serves as the bridge between clinical care and the social determinants of health. According to the Centers for Disease Control and Prevention (2018), *social determinants of mental health* refer to the conditions in which people live, work, learn, and play and the impact of these on overall health and well-being. For the sake of simplicity, we organize our discussion around the three primary advocacy realms, while acknowledging that some elements of agency and activism may overlap.

Case Advocacy

Advocacy at the individual patient level can be carried out by patients, physicians, and other interested parties. When patients advocate for themselves, they bring a unique and heartfelt understanding of the issue at hand. Their efforts, initially developed to address a problem or concern that affects them personally, sometimes translate into a larger activity with legal consequences and long-lasting repercussions. One such case was brought by Elizabeth Packard in the 1800s. Mrs. Packard was committed to an institution for the insane by her husband in 1860, on the grounds of an Illinois statute that specifically allowed husbands to commit their wives. Her experience led her to advocate for commitment law reform, paving the road to what we know today about involuntary commitment regulations (Pinals and Mossman 2012). More than 100 years later, in Wisconsin, the case *Lessard v. Schmidt* (1972), brought by Alberta Lessard, resulted in the court's reasoning that because involuntary hospitalization was a significant deprivation of liberty in civil commitment hearings, the state was required to prove mental illness and dangerousness beyond a reasonable doubt, and to ensure that less restrictive alternatives were not available in lieu of the commitment. The court also ruled that due process required that patients be given timely notice of their rights and that they have the right to legal counsel (Ford and Rotter 2014).

Nonprofessional advocates include family members and natural supports (e.g., clergy, coaches, mentors). To become effective advocates, individuals must gain and maintain the trust of the person for whom they are advocating and must become familiar with the person's desires and needs. Establishing communication with the treatment team is an important way to influence care and clarify the interests of the person being treated. These advocates may be able to supply information that an impaired individual cannot effectively relay to those providing care. Progressive organizations may include natural supports as part of the treatment team. This has been especially important in providing care for children and adolescents.

As Luft (2017) noted, it is incumbent on physicians to be very familiar with the concept of seeing patients' needs beyond a biomedical model and incorporating social factors of health into patient care, which forms the foundation of being an advocate. Psychiatrists are well positioned to be advocates when they are trained to treat their patients with a biopsychosocial perspective. In developing a treatment plan, they can take into account social, economic, environmental, and cultural factors that contribute to mental illness, as well as medical and psychological causes. In some cases, however, the psychiatrist may be constrained from engaging in advocacy for individuals. In forensic examinations, for example, the psychiatrist's primary role is to serve the justice system rather than the person being evaluated.

Psychiatrists who work in team-based settings can, with the collaboration of other mental health professionals, implement holistic treatment plans that address all factors contributing to a patient's mental illness. Other professionals enjoy roles with prominent advocacy elements that may be particularly helpful in this regard. These include nurses, peer professionals or navigators (a person who has experienced mental illness), care managers (a person who coordinates all health care needs of an individual), and rehabilitation specialists (Repper and Carter 2011).

Psychiatric advanced directives (PADs) were initially thought to be a byproduct of the antipsychiatry movement and not in the best interests of patients or society. A PAD allows patients to document their preferred treatment options in the event of a future crisis. The National Resource Center on Psychiatric Advance Directives provides state-specific information about PADs. Today, after many years of experience with PADs, most of the criticism associated with them has subsided. Many psychiatrists view this collaborative tool as a document to help facilitate communication. These documents are woefully underutilized. For example, in Texas, a state that has had PAD statutes in place since the early 2000s, the use of PADs is very rare (National Resource Center on Psychiatric Advance Directives 2018).

Case advocacy includes elements related to education, training, counseling, raising awareness, mediating, defending, and denouncing, with the goal of achieving positive incremental change (World Health Organization 2003). The broader use of PADs is an issue for cause advocacy, discussed next.

Cause Advocacy

In an attempt to change organizational operations and quality, agencies' use of resources, and governmental rules, laws, and policies, physicians have often engaged in advocacy reaching beyond the care of individual patients. Many choose to get involved in activities on a local, state, national, or even international level. Policy advocacy is a form of cause or system advocacy specifically related to the need for changes in laws, rules, and regulations.

It would be very challenging for individuals with other responsibilities to be effective lobbyists for legislative change to health policy. Psychiatrists and other physicians have organized to carry out lobbying activities collectively; indeed, this has become a preferred platform for taking action. Professional organizations such as the American Medical Association (AMA), American Psychiatric Association (APA), Group for the Advancement of Psychiatry, and many others have also made efforts to influence systemic changes through various types of advocacy. These organizations may advocate by promoting specific legislation, developing position papers, or developing informational materials to educate policy makers.

One example of this type of advocacy on a federal level is the 2017 position statement released by the APA opposing the American Health Care Act (AHCA) (American Medical Association 2017). The AHCA was a proposal released in 2017 by the Republican leadership to "repeal and replace" the Affordable Care Act (ACA). The bill passed in the House of Representatives in May 2017. Concerns arose about the effects the AHCA was expected to have by reversing the Medicaid eligibility expansion previously attained by the ACA, defunding Planned Parenthood, and abolishing the expansion of required benefits for mental health and addiction services under Medicaid (Civic Impulse LLC 2017). Dr. Maria Oquendo, then APA president, articulated the APA's position by explaining that removing insurance coverage would threaten millions of Americans (1.3 million Americans with serious mental illness and 2.8 million Americans with substance use disorders) and expressed the APA's willingness to work with members of both parties in Congress on finding a better solution (American Psychiatric Association 2017). Partly as a result of this effort, the AHCA did not pass the Senate. Some of the other key issues that the APA has tried to influence at a federal level include support of federal mental health and substance use disorders programs, criminal justice reform, and enhancing diversity and health equity.

The APA provides online resources regarding how to become successfully involved in advocacy at the state and federal levels. The APA's Advocacy Action Center, a resource that ensures the delivery of consistent messages to policy makers, the media, and the public and facilitates communication between psychiatrists and their elected officials. In another effort to influence policy, the APA organized a congressional briefing on Capitol Hill in 2018, partnering with the American Psychological Association. This briefing educated legislators on mental health services for people leaving prisons and the need for cutting-edge mental health practice, policy, and research related to reentering the community. This effort was intended to generate the support needed to provide more comprehensive services to a greater number of individuals (American Psychiatric Association 2019b). APA Government Relations advocates at both state and federal levels, advising Congress, the White House, and federal agencies on issues faced by psychiatrists, patients, and their families.

Another form of advocacy utilized by professional associations is the amicus brief. *Amicus curiae* (Latin for "friend of the court") briefs are legal documents filed in appellate court cases by nonlitigants who have a strong interest in the subject matter. The briefs advise the court of relevant and important information or arguments that the court should consider in its decision. A well-written amicus brief can have a significant impact on judicial decision making (Public Health Law Center 2019). One recent example is the amicus brief submitted to the Supreme Court in 2019 on the case *Kahler v. Kansas*. In it, the APA supports the recognition of an insanity defense broad enough to allow meaningful consideration of the impact of serious mental disorders on individual culpability (American Psychiatric Association 2019a).

Similar work has been done at state and local levels through the regional branches of the AMA and APA. One such initiative took place in 2003 when the Texas Medical Association (TMA) created an activity, First Tuesday at the Capitol, which allowed senators and representatives to listen to their hometown doctors who visited their offices in what is now known as "the white coat invasion." TMA's advocacy tools include a Grassroots Advocacy Guide that provides detailed examples on how to become an effective advocate and lobbyist (Texas Medical Association 2019). It also created the VoterVoice app that allows advocates to respond to action alerts in a timely manner.

Other organizations have had significant involvement in cause advocacy. One such organization is the National Alliance on Mental Illness (NAMI), which started in 1979 as a group of families advocating for the interests of their family members with mental illness. It has grown rapidly since that time, and now includes many professionals and people in recovery in its membership. NAMI has created a public policy platform providing direction and guidance on policy issues affecting people living with a mental illness. This platform addresses issues related to stigma and discrimination, early diagnosis, cultural awareness, special populations, and many more topics (National Alliance on Mental Illness 2016). NAMI has grown to become an association of more than 500 local affiliates, which operate semiautonomously and work in many communities across the nation, raising awareness and providing education and support (National Alliance on Mental Illness 2018).

Governmental advocacy and activism can present challenges related to the slow pace of policy change, scarcity of resources, and partisan politics. The decrease in the number of state hospital beds and the correlated over-representation of individuals with mental illness in emergency departments, jails, and prisons have resulted in several controversial issues for cause advocacy (Borja and Sharfstein 2010; Prins 2014; Steadman et al. 2009). These problems have prompted some organizations to study, monitor, and publish information that can be used to influence changes in the status quo. The Treatment Advocacy Center, founded in 1998, addresses opportunities it considers to be improvements in treatment systems and policy in the United States. It has produced manuals for specific system-related processes in clinical care that relate to public policy. One example is "A Guide for Implementing Assisted Outpatient Treatment" (Treatment Advocacy Center 2012). The Mental Illness Policy Organization is another entity with similar objectives. Founded in 2011, this organization provides information about the treatment that people with serious mental illness receive and makes the information available to policy makers and the media (Mental Illness Policy Org 2020). These organizations have been criticized for what many mental health advocates consider to be regressive and restrictive policies that threaten the civil rights of individuals with severe mental illness.

In many instances, an individual physician will be the engine for an organized group to start working on a systems issue by drawing attention to a problem that requires the revision of policies enacted by the government or by an agency. Many physicians begin their training with interest in social justice and activism. They might work in free clinics, volunteer in the community, or organize advocacy activities. Some physicians may pursue further training in public health or health policy. Despite the decline of these ideals and involvement over the course of training (Freeman 2014), there is still a subset of physicians who remain socially and politically active. These individuals can have significant impact on policy and procedures, whether individually or through professional organizations.

Many physicians have been vocal about the needs for oversight, change, and accountability related to immigration and border policy. Their voices have provided some insight regarding the precarious conditions in the immigration centers. In April 2019, one of these outspoken physicians, Pamela McPherson, M.D., received the 2019 Human Rights Hero Award and the 2019 Ridenhour Prize for Truth-Telling for exposing the conditions in immigrant detention centers (American Psychiatric Association 2019d).

In another example related to the LGBTQ+ population, advocacy efforts to raise awareness, decrease discrimination, and promote access to competent care has resulted in policy changes in many states. Since the 1970s, many groups have joined advocacy efforts for nondiscriminatory policies and protections for this population; however, their advances continue to be threatened. In May 2019, the U.S. Department of Health and

Human Services announced a plan to weaken the protections for LGBT individuals that were previously provided by the ACA. The APA joined a coalition of professional associations that advocated against these plans (American Psychiatric Association 2019c). Although these efforts do not appear to be directly connected to value, when successful, they can indirectly influence the overall quality of the population's health.

With regard to psychiatrists, physicians attempting advocacy for a particular cause within their work environment face a variety of challenges. Many physicians have opted to become employed by large systems of health care in part because the administrative burdens of medicine have become so great that it can be difficult for a solo provider to navigate the myriad rules of insurance and state and federal government requirements. These larger systems provide an infrastructure to facilitate this regulatory interface, and they present a plethora of issues that require attention to make them work more efficiently. In these organizations, physicians can advocate to improve processes, to transform the culture of the institution, or to improve the conditions of the work environment, among other issues. The overall culture of the agency, its mission and values, and the skills of its leaders can either facilitate or impede the success of efforts to improve the quality of care within the organization. One way to advocate for change within an organization is through quality improvement projects, which in many cases reduce the cost associated with inefficient or ineffective services.

Many large health care systems have administrative positions for physicians that provide protected time for advocacy work. The psychiatric administrator role has been controversial, because many detractors argue that the skill set of the psychiatrist is better suited for treating patients. Supporters, however, highlight the impact that administrators have on improving quality of care, health care policy, and advancing the profession (Kolodny 2007).

Guild Advocacy

Guild advocacy relates to issues in advancing professional interests. The biggest concern regarding this type of advocacy is whether the interests of the professionals align with value and with patients' interests. In most cases these interests are aligned, but this is not always the case. Many professional organizations provide protections to the interest of the group, including advocating for issues such as improved working conditions and income protection.

Some professional associations make their guild advancement efforts more explicit. For example, the AMA published a document explaining this role and its goals (American Medical Association 2017). The AMA advocates on a broad set of issues that directly affect physicians' private practice, including payment, reduced regulatory burdens, insurers' oversight, and medical liability reform. Some of these efforts, such as opposition to financing reform, have contributed to the high costs of medical care in the United States. Failure of these organizations to regulate their constituents' cost consciousness in the prescribing and use of expensive diagnostics and levels of care has been counterproductive, resulting in the imposition of externally enforced restrictions.

In 2017, Minkoff and Ecker wrote,

> When interests conflict, physicians must be cognizant of the forces at play, that is, self-interest or in-group interest on the one hand and obligations to the patients on the other. This entails recognition and negation of motivated reasoning. Often the most difficult calculus is evaluating proposed actions that would disadvantage physicians but advantage patients. In such cases, the health care provider must be aware not only of the temptation to oppose the action for financial reasons, but also the equally natural temptation to frame the proposal as a threat to patient well-being.

The risk of losing sight of this ethical conundrum has made involvement of physicians in politics a focus of criticism. According to Rothman (2000), physicians are more likely to engage their legislators on issues affecting their own well-being as opposed to issues related to professional responsibility or public health.

Many guild organizations limit their advocacy activities to those that are aligned with their interests in value. The 2011 announcement of massive budget cuts affecting the National Institutes of Health and other research agencies brought together many guild groups that did not traditionally get involved in external advocacy. By limiting the advancement of science and discovery, these cuts were unfavorable to the professional community and ultimately to the community at large (Feldman 2011). Organizations such as the American Association for Community Psychiatry and the Group for the Advancement of Psychiatry see their primary mission in terms of advancing knowledge, optimizing the quality of care, or improving practice processes, and recognize that these advances in quality will ultimately serve the interests of their members. They accomplish these goals through the production of policy position papers, practice guidelines, and clinical tools that promote value (American Association for Community Psychiatry 2019; Group for the Advancement of Psychiatry 2019). Both APA and AMA have a tradition of advocating for increasing the workforce. One example is AMA's Doctors Back to School program, which connects practicing physicians with schools in underserved areas in their communities. These volunteer physicians serve as role models to minority children, encouraging them to pursue a career in medicine (Hoven 2014).

Aligning the Interests of Health Care Stakeholders

Providing care that delivers high value is arguably a shared interest for all stakeholders. However, the specific views of what this means and how it should be measured is variable. The Institute for Healthcare Improvement categorized patient-centered care and satisfaction as one of the components of its highly regarded Triple Aim for quality health care (Institute for Healthcare Improvement 2019). Triple Aim encompasses eight principles, including respect for patient's values, coordination and integration of care, information and education, physical comfort, emotional support, involvement of family and friends, continuity and transitions, and access to care (Oneview 2015).

Patient-centeredness is one of the six dimensions of need or aims for improvement in health care related to individual care. The other five dimensions include safety, effectiveness, timeliness, efficiency, and equity. The concept of Triple Aim, developed by John Willington, M.D., and Tom Nolan, Ph.D., adds these individual components of care (individual care) to population components of care (population care) and lower per capita cost (Institute for Healthcare Improvement 2019). All aspects of the Triple Aim are subject to advocacy efforts, and these efforts can be performed by any of the stakeholders.

Although any of these "values" could be the focus of advocacy efforts, for psychiatrists, the goal of providing good patient care can often limit their capacity for advocacy activities. In mental health, high-value care means positive outcomes that are cost-effective and evidence based. Over the past few decades, physicians have been slowly buried under time constraints, documentation requirements, unwieldy electronic health records, regulations, and oversight by health systems, insurance companies, and licensing boards, leaving them with little time to spare for advocacy activities or even to offer the additional time that some patients need. Insurance companies and health care systems, preoccupied with cost considerations, often lose sight of this issue that directly affects quality of care. Therefore, advocating for protection against these constraints not only will reduce professional fatigue or burnout, but will ultimately improve the quality of care delivered.

Combating Burnout

There has been a marked increase in physician dissatisfaction, burnout, depression, and even suicide in the past decade. *Burnout* refers to a prolonged response to chronic emotional and interpersonal stressors on the job and is characterized by "overwhelming exhaustion, feelings of cynicism and detachment from the job, and a sense of ineffectiveness and lack of accomplishment" (Maslach 2016, p. 103). Burnout can detract from patient care, diminish health outcomes, and even increase costs by means of medical errors (Shanafelt 2010). Burnout places achievement of the Triple Aim in jeopardy. Given the pervasiveness of burnout in recent years, the Quadruple Aim was proposed as a response in 2014, with the fourth element being the improvement of the work life of physicians and other health care providers (Bodenheimer 2014). Rates of burnout are higher among physicians than professionals in other occupations, even when controlling for major demographic variables, with 54% of U.S. physicians endorsing at least one of the three primary symptoms of burnout: emotional exhaustion, depersonalization, or decreased personal efficacy (Shanafelt et al. 2015).

A 2017 Medscape survey found that 42% of physician respondents reported burnout, with 15% of all physicians reporting feeling down or clinically depressed. For comparison, 6.7% of all U.S. adults reported suffering from a major depressive episode that same year. Over half of the physician respondents (56%) cited too many bureaucratic tasks such as charting and paperwork as the cause of burnout, followed by long hours (39%), lack of respect from staff and colleagues (26%), and the electronic health record (24%) (Medscape 2018). Parks (2016) cited similar sources for burnout, which include excessive clerical work, depersonalization of the doctor-patient relationship, process inefficiencies, and clinician lack of control of daily and weekly schedules.

Konopasek and Bernstein (2016), among others, have advocated for a reduction of working hours to reduce burnout, especially for trainees. However, the reduction of job hours may not be the whole answer to solve this problem. In 2005, a burnout study conducted in a third-world country (Dominican Republic) found that among a sample of internal medicine and surgery residents from four different institutions, the residents with the highest levels of burnout were those who were being trained at institutions with poor funding and unclear job expectations (Lluberes 2007).

Recent advocacy efforts have focused on raising awareness of the potential danger of overwork during the years of residency training and the early years of practice and encouraging use of methods for protecting physicians' emotional health and managing obligations. The APA and other organizations have been active in this regard. Providing a safe environment for physicians to identify and discuss factors contributing to their stress is an essential element of strategies to reduce their susceptibility to being overwhelmed.

Reducing Stigma

The fight against the stigma surrounding psychiatric illness is an issue of concern that impacts the activities of all mental health professionals and their patients. The fact that stigma acts as a factor affecting treatment entry due to its negative effect on help-seeking behaviors is well established (Clement et al. 2015). When people sense or expect a negative labeling and judgmental reactions from providers, they are more likely to avoid treatment. Psychiatrists and other mental health professionals are acutely aware of and have spoken very openly about stigma and the need to counteract the stereotypes held by society overall. Educating about mental illness and its ramifications on human behavior, including demystifying old conceptions about mental illness and aggressive behavior, is an important way to begin this process. Confronting pejorative language when it is used in conversations about these disorders and about the people suffering from them is another important way to raise awareness and reduce stigma and marginalization.

Gronholm and colleagues (2017) have conceptualized various types of stigma. *Experiential stigma* consists of 1) perceived stigma (beliefs "most people" are thought to hold), 2) endorsed stigma (expressed agreement with stereotypes/prejudice/discrimination), 3) anticipated stigma (expected experiences of prejudice/discrimination), 4) received stigma (overt experiences of rejection or devaluation), and 5) enacted stigma (discriminatory behaviors). *Action-orientated stigma* consists of 1) public stigma (stereotypes, prejudice, and discrimination endorsed by the general population), 2) structural stigma (prejudice and discrimination through laws, policies, and constitutional practices), 3) courtesy stigma (stereotypes, prejudice, and discrimination acquired through an association with a stigmatized group/person), 4) provider-based stigma (prejudice and discrimination by occupational groups designated to provide assistance to stigmatized groups), and 5) internalized stigma (people who belong to a stigmatized group legitimize publicly held stereotypes and prejudice and internalize these by applying them to themselves).

Many psychiatrists have found opportunities through public engagement to fight stigma and to provide support and advocacy for patients' rights. The following are some examples:

1. Public speaking for the purpose of education.
2. Direct collaboration with media industry in the production of shows or movies having respectful portrayals of mental illness and the role of the professional. Some psychiatrists involved in these activities include Glen O. Gabbard (consultant in "The Sopranos"), Kenneth P. Rosenberg (producer of films for PBS and HBO), and Nubia Lluberes (consultant in the documentary "Madly Gifted").
3. Expressive art and creativity. A comic book depicting a superhero who also happens to have bipolar disorder (Fomich 2014) was created by

psychiatrist Vasilis Pozios who has pledged to destigmatize mental illness through the life of a superhero.

Technology and Advocacy

Although there has been some erosion of trust in medicine over the years, physicians still have a relatively strong social standing and engender high public trust. Psychiatrists and other physicians can leverage this favorable reputation to access legislators at the local, state, and national levels to effect policy change (Earnest et al. 2010). When combined with technology, advocacy efforts can become a powerful tool to challenge the status quo and ignite needed change. Among technological advancements, social media offers a wide platform for advocacy. Used wisely, social media can deliver great results by promoting engagement of larger groups and collective action. Some critics suggest that its effectiveness may be overblown, however, and that anecdotal evidence may actually be deceptive, masking the reality that social media does little to strengthen social movements and effect change (Obar et al. 2012).

Advocacy Strategies

Obviously, people and organizations advocate for what they value, and therefore advocacy is always to some degree self-serving. When evaluating advocacy efforts for any particular issue, one needs to look at who the various stakeholders are and examine their position. It is important to become familiar with both potential allies and adversaries. What is the basis for the positions taken? Is their position based on emotion, beliefs, money, influence, social justice, or prestige? Being aware of these motivations will be important for the formulation of effective strategies for advocacy efforts. Finding intersecting interests is often a critical element of change strategies. When parties are consumed by enmity, as has been the case in U.S. politics in the early twenty-first century, no compromise is possible and very little can be accomplished.

A variety of strategies may be employed in advocacy efforts. Education, demonstration, protest, promotion, and lobbying all have places in the advocacy playbook. The careful use of other individuals' stories and the use of self-disclosure can prove to be an effective way to engage targets of advocacy efforts. These stories and personal accounts can be even more effective when they are backed by data and written material that is concise and easy to understand. When interacting with legislators, for example, time is often of the essence, and supplying information that is easily digestible and appeals to their interests (i.e., getting reelected) can be most effective in winning them to the identified cause. Strategies must be tailored to the group being targeted. For instance, whereas cost savings may perk up a legislator's ears, patient outcomes will likely matter more to a clinical director.

It will also be important to consider the level of sophistication of the person or group being targeted. If one hopes for engagement, one should not assume that their knowledge of the issue being considered is materially deficient (resulting in a sense of condescension and insult) or that they are morally deficient (resulting in indignation and devaluation). Creating relationships is key for influencing those in a position to make changes. Gaining the trust of those individuals can go a long way in the process of evaluating various propositions. When they feel respected, they are more likely to seriously listen and consider what is being suggested. Taking the time to build relationships and interact with those one needs to win over is key. As with other change processes, motivational approaches are sometimes most effective, as they allow people to discover for themselves why taking the suggested position might benefit them. Developing coalitions and partnerships and defining shared interest are often key elements of successful advocacy efforts. Constancy, perseverance, and respect for others are core elements of the strategies that should remain in the forefront of any attempt to advocate.

Conclusion

In this chapter we have considered a number of ways that people and organizations can become involved in advocacy efforts to accomplish a variety of objectives. The advocacy of professionals, such as psychiatrists, is most often a voluntary activity, so there is virtually no expense involved for health care systems. Any contribution made through these voluntary activities to processes that impact the overall health and well-being of individuals and communities adds value by augmenting the numerator (quality) of the value equation without increasing the denominator (cost). Although psychiatrists can have a direct impact on the outcomes of the people they serve through advocacy within the organizations in which they work and local service agencies, they may be able to have an even greater impact by lending their weight to promoting grander issues that impact value. As practitioners of change processes, they are well suited to judge the motivations of the individuals to whom they are appealing and to discover the incentives that are most likely to persuade them. Although many of these activities do not have a direct impact on cost or quality, indirectly they can have a significant influence on a variety of issues related to the social, political, and environmental determinants of health. One cannot hope for a better value than that.

References

American Association for Community Psychiatry: Strategic Plan. 2019. Available at: www.communitypsychiatry.org/about/mission. Accessed June 15, 2020.

American Medical Association: Protecting physician practices. 2017. Available at: www.ama-assn.org/sites/ama-assn.org/files/corp/media-browser/specialty%20group/arc/protecting-physician-practices.pdf. Accessed March 11, 2020.

American Psychiatric Association: APA urges house to reject American Health Care Act (AHCA). March 2017. Available at: http://cqrcengage.com/psychorg/app/document/15697567. Accessed March 11, 2020.

American Psychiatric Association: Amicus briefs: Kahler v Kansas, U.S. Supreme Court, No. 18-6135. 2019a. Available at: www.psychiatry.org/File%20Library/Psychiatrists/Directories/Library-and-Archive/amicus-briefs/amicus-2019-Kahler-v-Kansas-No186135.pdf. Accessed March 11, 2020.

American Psychiatric Association: APA federal affairs. 2019b. Available at: www.psychiatry.org/psychiatrists/advocacy/federal-affairs/criminal-justice. Accessed March 11, 2020.

American Psychiatric Association: Diversity and health equity advocacy news. May 4, 2019c. Available at: www.psychiatry.org/psychiatrists/cultural-competency/advocacy-news. Accessed March 11, 2020.

American Psychiatric Association: Psychiatrist honored for blowing whistle on border policies. Psychiatric News, May 17, 2019d. Available at: https://psychnews.psychiatryonline.org/toc/pn/54/10. Accessed March 10, 2020.

Bodenheimer T: From the Triple to Quadruple Aim: care of the patient requires care of the provider. Ann Fam Med 12(6):573–576, 2014

Borja B, Sharfstein S: The role of emergency care, in the Disparities in Psychiatric Care. Edited by Ruiz P, Primm A. Baltimore, MD, Lippincott Williams & Wilkins, 2010, pp 248–256

Centers for Disease Control and Prevention: Social determinants of health. 2018. Available at: www.cdc.gov/socialdeterminants. Accessed March 11, 2020.

Civic Impulse LLC. H.R. 1628 (115th): American Health Care Act of 2017. July 28, 2017. Available at: www.govtrack.us/congress/bills/115/hr1628/summary. Accessed March 11, 2020.

Clement S, Schauman O, Graham T, et al: What is the impact of mental health-related stigma on help-seeking? A systematic review of quantitative and qualitative studies. Psychol Med 45(1):11–27, 2015

Cruzan v Director, Missouri Dept. of Mental Health, 497 U.S. 261, 110 S.Ct. 2841 (1990)

Dean S: The Civil Rights of Institutionalized Persons Act of 1980: a guide for clinicians. Developments in Mental Health Law, 1988. Available at: www.questia.com/magazine/1G1-233541891/the-civil-rights-of-institutionalized-persons-act. Accessed March 10, 2020.

Dix D: Voices from the past: "I tell what I have seen"—the reports of asylum reformer Dorothea Dix. Am J Public Health 96(4):622–625, 2006

Dobson S, Voyer S, Regehr G: Agency and activism: rethinking health advocacy in the medical profession. Acad Med 87(9):1161–1164, 2012

Earnest M, Wong S, Steven F: Perspective: physician advocacy: what is it and how do we do it? Acad Med 85(1):63–67, 2010

Feldman A: Advocacy: a new arena for the translational scientist. Clin Transl Sci 4(2):73–75, 2011

Fomich N: Mental illness, superheroes, and stereotypes—Vasilis Pozios on his new comic aura. 2014. Available at: www.bleedingcool.com/2014/09/16/mental-illness-superheroes-and-stereotypes-vasilis-pozios-on-his-new-comic-aura. Accessed March 11, 2020.

Ford E, Rotter M: Landmark Cases in Forensic Psychiatry. New York, Oxford University Press, 2014

Freeman J: Advocacy by physicians for patients and for social change. Virtual Mentor 16(9):722–725, 2014

Geller J: The right to treatment, in Principles and Practice of Forensic Psychiatry. Boca Raton, FL, CRC Press, 2017, pp 145–154

Geraghty K, Wynia M: Advocacy and community: the social roles of physicians in the last 1000 years, part II. MedGenM 2(4):1–4, 2000

Gronholm P, Thornicroft G, Laurens K, et al: Mental health–related stigma and pathways to care for people at risk of psychotic disorder or experiencing first-episode psychosis: a systematic review. Psychol Med 47(11):1867–1879, 2017

Group for the Advancement of Psychiatry: Mission. 2019. Available at: https://ourgap.org/Mission. Accessed June 15, 2020.

Hargrave v Vermont, 340 F3D 27 (2003)

Holubova M, Prasko J, Ociskova M, et al: Self-stigma and quality of life in patients with depressive disorder: a cross-sectional study. Neuropsychiatr Dis Treat 12:2677–2687, 2016

Hoven AD: Leadership viewpoints: how organized medicine is reducing health care disparities. May 2014. Available at: www.ama-assn.org/advocacy/leadership-viewpoints/how-organized-medicine-reducing-health-care-disparities. Accessed March 11, 2020.

Hubinette M, Dobson S, Scott I, et al: Health advocacy. Med Teach 39(2):128–135, 2017

Institute for Healthcare Improvement: The IHI Triple Aim Initiative. 2019. Available at: www.ihi.org/Engage/Initiatives/TripleAim/Pages/default.aspx. Accessed March 11, 2020.

Jahn W: The 4 basic ethical principles that apply to forensic activities are respect for autonomy, beneficence, nonmaleficence, and justice. J Chiropr Med 10(3):225–226, 2011

Kolodny A: Psychiatrists as administrators: the perspective of a mental health department psychiatrist. Psychiatr Q 78(3):193–198, 2007

Konopasek L, Bernstein C: Combating burn out, promoting physician well-being: building blocks for a healthy learning environment in GME. 2016. Available at: www.acgme.org/Portals/0/PDFs/Webinars/July_13_Powerpoint.pdf. Accessed March 11, 2020.

Lake v Cameron, 364 F.2d 657 (1966)

Lessard v Schmidt, 349 F.Suppl. 1078 (E.D. Wis. 1972)

Lluberes NG: Sindrome de burnout. Revista Electrónica de Medicina Neuropsicológica 2546–2601, 2007

Luft L: The essential role of physician as advocate: how and why we pass it on. CMEJ 8(3):e109–e116, 2017

Maslach C: Understanding the burnout experience: recent research and its implications for psychiatry. World Psychiatry 15(2):103–111, 2016

Medscape: Medscape national physician burnout and depression report 2018. January 2018. Available at: www.medscape.com/slideshow/2018-lifestyle-burnout-depression-6009235. Accessed March 11, 2020.

Mental Illness Policy Org: About Mental Illness Policy Org. 2020. Available at: https://mentalillnesspolicy.org/about.html. Accessed March 11, 2020.

Minkoff H, Ecker J: When guild interests and professional obligations collide. Obstet Gynecol 130(2):454–457, 2017

Natanson v Kline, 186 Kan. 393, 411, 350 P.2d 1093 (1960)

National Alliance on Mental Illness: Public policy platform. 2016. Available at: www.nami.org/getattachment/Learn-More/Mental-Health-Public-Policy/Public-Policy-Platform-December-2016-(1).pdf. Accessed March 11, 2020.

National Alliance on Mental Illness: About NAMI. 2018. Available at: www.nami.org/about-nami. Accessed March 11, 2020.

National Resource Center on Psychiatric Advance Directives: Texas. 2018. Available at: www.nrc-pad.org/states/texas/. Accessed March 11, 2020.

Obar JA, Zube P, Lampe C: Advocacy 2.0: an analysis of how advocacy groups in the United States perceive social media as tools for facilitating civic engagement and collective action. Journal of Information Policy 2(2012):1–25, 2012

Oneview: The eight principles of patient-centered care. May 2015. Available at: www.oneviewhealthcare.com/the-eight-principles-of-patient-centered-care. Accessed March 11, 2020.

Parks T: How the Mayo Clinic is battling physician burnout. March 2016. Available at: www.ama-assn.org/practice-management/physician-health/how-mayo-clinic-battling-physician-burnout. Accessed March 11, 2020.

Pinals D, Mossman D: Evaluation for Civil Commitment: Legal Context. New York, Oxford University Press, 2012

Prins SJ: The prevalence of mental illnesses in U.S. state prisons: a systematic review. Psychiatr Serv 65(7):862–872, 2014

Public Health Law Center: Amicus briefs. 2019. Available at: https://publichealthlawcenter.org/amicus-briefs. Accessed March 11, 2020.

Repper J, Carter T: A review of the literature on peer support in mental health services. J Ment Health 20(4):392–411, 2011
Rothman D: Medical professionalism—focusing on the real issues. N Engl J Med 342(17):1284–1286, 2000
Sederer L: Right to treatment and right to refuse treatment. August 2013. Available at: https://careforyourmind.org/the-right-to-treatment-and-the-right-to-refuse-treatment. Accessed March 11, 2020.
Shanafelt TD: Burnout and medical errors among American surgeons. Ann Surg 251(6):995–1000, 2010
Shanafelt TD, Hasan O, Dyrbye C, et al: Changes in burnout and satisfaction with work-life balance in physicians and the general U.S. working population between 2011 and 2014. Mayo Clin Proc 90(12):1600–1613, 2015
Steadman HJ, Osher FC, Robbins PC, et al: Prevalence of serious mental illness among jail inmates. Psychiatr Serv 60(6):761–765, 2009
Texas Medical Association: Texas Medical Association's Grassroots Advocacy Guide, 86th legislative session. 2019. Available at: www.texmed.org/uploadedFiles/Current/2016_Advocacy/Texas_Legislature/Get_Involved/First_Tuesdays/First_Tuesday_Handbook_Grassroots_Advocacy_Packet.pdf. Accessed March 11, 2020.
Treatment Advocacy Center: A Guide for Implementing Assisted Outpatient Treatment. 2012. Available at: www.treatmentadvocacycenter.org/storage/documents/aot-implementation-guide.pdf. Accessed March 11, 2020.
World Health Organization: Advocacy for mental health. 2003. Available at: www.who.int/mental_health/policy/services/1_advocacy_WEB_07.pdf. Accessed March 11, 2020.
World Health Organization: Social determinants of mental health. 2014. Available at: https://apps.who.int/iris/bitstream/handle/10665/112828/9789241506809_ eng.pdf;jsessionid=948C32D5F5F69EE40A5CF0B812B54DE7?sequence=1. Accessed March 11, 2020.
Youngberg v Romeo, 457 U.S. 307, 102 S.Ct. 2452 (1982)

16

Psychiatric Leadership

Wesley E. Sowers, M.D.

Since the 1960s, much has been discovered about the brain, pharmacology, and the biological processes contributing to behavioral health disorders. Those advances have been embraced by psychiatry and have created a great deal of excitement and hope for people striving to overcome the symptoms of mental illness. But during this same period, a variety of economic forces converged to constrict the scope of psychiatric practice around these biological aspects of illness, thereby reducing the role of psychiatry in consultation, prevention, and psychotherapeutic interventions. As psychiatric residency training programs began to focus a greater portion of their curricula on the biological aspects of illness, young psychiatrists were left less well prepared to contribute in other ways. One of the casualties of these changes was the exposure of psychiatrists to administrative activities and the development

---

Portions of this chapter were previously published in a 2016 article: Sowers W: "Psychiatric Leadership and the Implementation of Person-Centered, Recovery-Oriented Care. *Journal of Psychiatric Administration and Management* 5(2), 2016.

of leadership skills. Psychiatry is one of the most significant sources of revenue from billing for behavioral health organizations, but it is also a significant expense. In fee-for-service systems, organizations are reluctant to use psychiatric resources for nonbillable activities unless there are significant advantages and added value in doing so.

In Chapter 11, "An Expanded Role for Psychiatry," the advantages of a return to a broader scope of practice for psychiatrists were considered along with some of the circumstances that could facilitate those changes. In this chapter, we consider the advantages of reestablishing a more robust role for psychiatrists in leadership positions in this era of rapid evolution of health care systems, and the ways in which this would add to the value of the services offered. We first consider the incorporation of Recovery Oriented Care (ROC) into clinical practice. This is followed by a discussion of some of the recent opportunities that have been developed to provide psychiatrists with training that better prepares them for leadership roles. We then consider the skills that are useful in the exercise of leadership, whether formal or informal. These skills include systems assessment and strategic planning tailored to a system's culture, facilitation skills, and team building. The implementation of the ROC paradigm for the delivery of behavioral health services will then be considered as a specific example of applied leadership.

It has been some time since the release of the President's New Freedom Commission Report in 2003 (Hogan 2003). Its recommendation for a recovery oriented approach to treatment has been widely embraced by administrative entities, but application and implementation of ROC principles in everyday practice has proceeded slowly. The incorporation of this paradigm usually requires a shift in organizational culture and is a process in which well-trained psychiatrists can play significant leadership roles in facilitating this change. The principles highlighted in this chapter might be applied to any number of organizational or cultural change processes, but we chose the example of ROC because of its current prominence in mental health policy. This example is also particularly relevant because many ROC principles are also applicable to the exercise of leadership. The recovery paradigm adds quality to proffered services and can reduce the cost of care, both directly and indirectly (Sowers 2012). Transformational, managerial, and transactional aspects of leadership, which would be useful in the implementation of the essential elements of this paradigm, are described. Processes and instruments that could facilitate implementation of the American Association of Community Psychiatrists' (AACP's) Recovery Oriented Services are considered. Specifically, the Recovery to Practice Curriculum for Psychiatry (American Association of Community Psychiatrists and American Psychiatric Association 2011) can be used to develop a uniform understanding of recovery principles. Tools that can be employed to facilitate the implementation of ROC by leaders, even in the context of economic pressures and limited resources, include the AACP Guidelines for Recovery Oriented Services (American Association of Community Psychiatrists 2001a), Level of Care Utilization System (American Association of Community Psychiatrists 2016), Child and Adolescent Level of Care Utilization System (American Association of Community Psychiatrists 2019, Recovery Oriented Services Evaluation (American Association of Community Psychiatrists 2001b), and Psychiatric Recovery Oriented Practices Evaluation and Rating (American Association of Community Psychiatrists 2010). Each of these tools is discussed in some detail later in the chapter.

Taking on Leadership Roles

Sometimes medical leadership roles are thrust on psychiatrists who possess neither the skills nor the interest in being or learning to be leaders or managers. It is rarely advantageous to try to push these physicians into such positions. The focus in this section is on those who do have the talent, interest, and energy to accept these responsibilities when offered. Leadership roles vary widely. In some cases, psychiatrists have a nominal role that amounts to not much more than providing required signatures to treatment plans and other documents. In other cases, psychiatrists serve as medical directors who have a wide range of responsibilities, including supervision of the medical staff, recruitment and hiring, overall clinical oversight, clinical policy, and quality improvement, as well as other administrative roles (Ranz et al. 2000). Medical directors are often part of leadership teams and are usually the only individuals on a team who have an ongoing clinical role. Therefore, they provide a liaison between clinical activity and administration and can advocate for clinician- and client-friendly policies. Although there has been a trend of exclusion of psychiatrists from significant leadership roles in the past, many organizations are once again recognizing the value of having well-trained physicians in leadership roles.

A study by Ranz and colleagues (1997) demonstrated that having some kind of leadership role contributed to the job satisfaction of psychiatrists working in the public sector. Allowing psychiatrists to exercise a full range of clinical and administrative leadership activities, regardless of the level, will help prevent some of the burnout that has been a prominent concern for psychiatrists in recent years (see Chapter 11, "An Expanded Role for Psychiatry"). It is important to emphasize that in many cases psychiatrists may have limited defined authority but may still have a significant capacity to be influential or inspirational. One way they can do this is by demonstrating attentiveness to clinical systems and quality improvement. They can provide constructive criticism to identify both problems and solutions and can encourage engagement of others (Duncan and Warden 1999; Sowers et al. 2011). Leadership is seldom given blindly, and in most cases it must be earned, which is usually accomplished through work done beyond defined job descriptions and compensation arrangements. Often, the psychiatrists who demonstrate their knowledge and capacity on a voluntary basis are those who are recognized and considered for a wide range of opportunities that may arise subsequently.

Regardless of the route taken to leadership responsibilities, many psychiatrists who arrive in these roles will want to enhance their knowledge of effective leadership styles and strategies and the systemic issues to which they may be applied. The following section considers some of the options for doing so.

Leadership Training

As mentioned in the introduction to this chapter, leadership roles for psychiatrists diminished over the last few decades of the twentieth century, but interest in and opportunities for psychiatrists to enhance their leadership skills has been growing more recently. Opportunities are available to psychiatrists at various stages of their career development. Psychiatrists who have been placed in roles as medical directors or other leadership positions have often found that they are inadequately prepared to manage some of their expected responsibilities. For example, psychiatrists with experience working in organized systems of care were targeted for a training program developed by the National Council for Behavioral Health (NCBH) and the AACP, with support from the Substance Abuse and Mental Health Services Administration's (SAMHSA's) Center for Mental Health Services in 2008 (Sowers et al. 2011). During the first years of operation, it provided training to a significant number of these medical directors before morphing into what is now the NCBH's Executive Leadership Program (National Council for Behavioral Health 2020). This program trains leaders from all behavioral health professions, rather than focusing on psychiatrists in particular.

Some psychiatrists with interests in leadership choose to obtain a master's degree in business administration or public health management to augment their psychiatric training. Most leadership training programs designed specifically for physicians are not differentiated by specialty. Several physician leadership programs have been developed and are offered either as in-person trainings or online; in many cases, they are a combination of the two (Sobczak 2015). One example is the American College of Physicians' Certificate in Physician Leadership program, offered in conjunction with the American Association for Physician Leadership. It is an 18-month program that uses periodic in-person training and video conferencing with additional online content (American College of Physicians 2018). Several other options for leadership training are available through university programs. These courses are of variable length and intensity.

The preparation of psychiatrists to assume leadership roles has not been a prominent part of training programs in the past. In recent years there has been growing interest from early career psychiatrists in obtaining additional training in administrative skills. Although Columbia University's Public Psychiatry Fellowship has been in operation since 1981 (Ranz et al. 2008), it was not until the decade between 2008 and 2018 that more than 20 new fellowships in public and community psychiatry appeared, and the number has continued to grow. Although these training programs have been developed primarily for public and community psychiatrists, most aspects of the curricula address issues that would be relevant for any psychiatrist interested in taking on leadership roles in organized systems of care. These elements include person-centered care, health care administration, advocacy, leadership skills, program development and evaluation, quality improvement, advocacy, and teamwork. These are generally 1-year training programs that are available to psychiatrists in their first postgraduate year. Many of these programs also accept psychiatry residents in their final year of training (American Association of Community Psychiatrists 2008).

Because these fellowships are not accredited by the Accreditation Council for Graduate Medical Education, there is a great deal of flexibility in the structure and focus of the programs, allowing potential fellows to choose the training that best suits their needs. To provide some standards for existing and developing programs, Columbia University's Public Psychiatry Fellowship program developed a set of core elements that should be included in all of these programs (Ranz et al. 2008). The AACP's "Guidelines for Developing and Evaluating Public and Community Psychiatry Training Fellowships" elaborated these elements further and created a set of core competencies for their graduates (American Association of Community Psychiatrists 2008). Graduates of these programs have in most instances had significant leadership roles as part of their careers.

These fellowships have provided administrative and systems training to a growing number of psychiatrists. The graduates of these programs are well positioned to elaborate their own job descriptions and negotiate with potential employers regarding the activities they should include. To assist in that process, the AACP developed "AACP Guidelines for Psychiatric Leadership in Organized Delivery Systems for Treatment of Psychiatric and Substance Disorders" (American Association of Community Psychiatrists 2012). It provides a template for psychiatrists developing or evaluating job descriptions as they consider leadership roles. The AACP also developed its Board Certification in Community and Public Psychiatry, a certification examination for graduates of these fellowship programs and other experienced psychiatrists, in 2016. Certification does not necessarily bring additional financial benefits, but it does demonstrate interest in and knowledge of systems of care and methods used to improve them (Moran 2018).

Building a Base for Leadership

Organizational Assessment: The Context for Leadership

Leadership does not take place in a vacuum, so it is extremely important to understand the mechanics of the systems in which one is working. Although many leadership principles will apply across a variety of circumstances, specific strategies or leadership styles will be selected based on the structure and culture of an organization. Situations that require agility and urgency of decision making will be more successful if leadership is concentrated with a few people. Longer-term decisions will usually do better with more inclusive participation in developing a plan.

Organizations may be structured in various ways. Organizational theory dates back as far as Adam Smith in his landmark book *The Wealth of Nations* in 1776, in which Smith introduced the concept of a division of labor and the efficiencies derived from it. Classic organizational theory evolved in the industrial era, and the division of labor was conceptualized in four components: 1) hierarchy of authority, 2) span of control or supervisory range, 3) degree of centralization, and 4) degree of specialization (Docherty et al. 2001). Classically structured organizations employ a rigid hierarchy of authority, centralized decision making, a high degree of specialization, and a narrow span of control. In other words, power to make decisions is confined to a small group of people at the top of the pyramid, and there are narrowly defined roles for employees at the bottom, who are closely supervised and have little opportunity to participate in decision making of any kind (Taylor 1911). Although this arrangement allows decisions to be made quickly and with limited deliberation, the exclusion of the workforce often results in resentment and lack of investment in the work. This model has worked well in military organizations, however, in which there is a strong sense of mission and interdependence, and the need to make rapid decisions.

At the other end of the spectrum, more contemporary and horizontally structured organizations have a loose hierarchy of authority, decentralization of decision making, less specialization, and a broader span of control. In other words, there is broad participation in decision making, and much of it is delegated to those closest to the product. Employees have a high degree of diversity in their role and have a high degree of autonomy. There is an interactive leadership structure that includes participants from all aspects of the organization in decision-making processes; in medical facilities, this includes clients, family members, and nonclinical staff. This structure has the advantage of engaging all associates in a process that encourages their investment in the organization, and thereby gives them incentives to work hard to ensure its success (Senge 1990). These models generally perform very well for the development of a product. The disadvantages of these arrangements are that they are time consuming and reaching a consensus is often difficult. Because these models are time consuming, they can also be quite expensive.

The formal structure of an organization's administration and decision-making process provides an understanding of how issues are supposed to be addressed, but the reality of how the organization is governed may be something else entirely. Regardless of the leadership structure that is put on paper, power relationships within the organization and the ways in which they play out will impact decision making. Psychiatrists and anyone else wishing to make improvements within an organization, regardless of their position in it, will want to make an assessment of who has power, how much they have, and what factors provide motivation for them. Without this information, even the most earnest and well-reasoned initiatives will have limited chances for success. Having insight into an organization's politics and culture will allow potential leaders to develop strategies that are most likely to succeed. Most change processes within an organization require the collaboration of a number of individuals. Identifying those people who will be easiest to work with and who will invest in the objectives of a project will provide a good starting point for any initiative. Developing an awareness of those individuals who may be most resistant to the initiative will also be needed to develop sound strategies for implementation (Bell et al. 2012).

Team Building

As alluded to above, most work within a system requires the concerted effort of a number of individuals. Those who are attentive to group processes, and the methods for facilitating those processes, will be able to contribute to the smooth functioning of the team and the efficient pursuit of its objectives. Teams of which psychiatrists are most often members are those convened to deliver treatment. Psychiatrists may be involved in other types of teams as well. They may become part of a team or committee charged with developing a specific project or program. In many cases, psychiatrists may be asked to join a team to create specific policies or clinical protocols. As their experience and expertise increase, they will often be invited to become part of leadership teams for an organization. Regardless of the specific team setting, most of the principles for building a strong team process will apply. In the following discussion of these principles, the clinical treatment team is used as an example (Ranz and Stueve 1998).

Treatment teams are most highly developed in intensive treatment programs, such as inpatient or residential care. Partial hospital and Assertive Community Treatment teams (see Chapter 5, "Successful Approaches to Increasing Value") also require team approaches. It has been more difficult to establish teams for high-volume, low-intensity treatment programs. Most treatment teams today emphasize collaboration and employ an egalitarian structure. Although most teams designate a "team leader" to facilitate the group process, decisions are generally reached through a more or less consensual process. A psychiatrist may or may not have a designated leadership role, but when engaged and invested in the team, he or she will usually have significant influence. Psychiatrists will generally be most successful in exercising this influence when they maintain humility and display genuine interest in and respect for the input of other team members. Although the needs of the client should always be the top priority, consideration and accommodation of other team members' needs will ultimately advance the client's interests as well (Diamond 1996).

A treatment team that functions well will generally have well-defined roles for each member and will at the same time allow flexibility and interdependence in those roles. When arranged in this way, team members are best positioned to address urgent needs and other complex issues in a timely and effective manner. What conditions allow teams to function smoothly and effectively? The relationships that develop between team members are major determinants of team function (Covey 1989). Building and managing these relationships in a positive manner is a key to successful teamwork.

Lencioni (2002) identified five factors that create dysfunction in teamwork and that must be addressed in team building. First among them involves issues with trust. Team members must have confidence in their colleagues' good intentions toward one another, allowing them to be honest enough to address their shortcomings and ask for help. Leaders must create a nurturing environment in which all members' contributions are appreciated. Second, a fear of addressing conflict as it arises often leads to an erosion of trust and team function. Creating clear channels for communication that address differences of opinion allows growth and perspicacious decisions (Bell et al. 2012). Third, achievement of a goal or mission will be undermined if the entire team is not committed to it. An inclusive process in which all viewpoints are considered and respected will help create a shared vision in which teammates can invest. Fourth, issues regarding accountability must be addressed. Monitoring the results of the team's efforts will indicate whether progress is being made. When results are falling short of expectations, the team and the individuals involved in the operation of the project will be expected to find solutions. The fifth factor is a corollary to the fourth: the team must pay attention to the results of its evaluation processes. Keeping the team focused on outcomes and excellence, rather than individual interests is important to accomplish.

Many authors have described characteristics of leaders that facilitate the healthy function of treatment teams and organizations (Bell et al. 2012; Feldman 2012). It is not surprising that the qualities described are similar to those described for ROC. Both the described characteristics of successful leaders and those of clinicians practicing ROC emphasize empowerment, collaboration and delegation/autonomy, inspiration/hope, motivation, creative problem solving, and respect for each individual's strengths and abilities (Sowers 2012). Some of these characteristics may be seen as innate personality traits, but in most cases these skills are developed through interest, education, and experience. When conflicts, large or small, arise within the team, as they invariably will, they should be processed in a manner that allows everyone to gain something from the experience. An important role of leadership is to ensure that this happens.

Putting Recovery Oriented Care Into Practice

Implementation of Person-Centered, Recovery Oriented Care

In the context of productivity demands and liability fears, psychiatrists have had limited exposure to recovery concepts, and those who have been exposed are often reluctant to deviate from more directive and perceived low-risk approaches to care. Psychiatry training program milestones include exposure to recovery principles and humanistic aspects of care, but the quantity and quality of that exposure is variable, and their support in practice is limited by the availability of faculty who understand and incorporate this approach in their clinical activities. An emphasis on disease has not yet been balanced by a focus on wellness and maintaining health. The elements of ROC are multifaceted and deceptively complex and therefore require a solid conceptual foundation as well as ongoing support and supervision. Psychiatry has lacked a unifying conceptual framework to integrate the diverse circumstances and modalities in which its members work. The recovery philosophy provides a set of principles that psychiatrists can apply to biological and humanistic aspects of care, in mental health, physical health, and addictions, and all across the lifespan. Psychiatrists need to have a solid foundation in recovery oriented practice to provide care in the diverse settings of the evolving systems of care (Sowers et al. 2015). With this foundation, services become more coherent, efficient, and effective. Psychiatry plays an essential role in establishment and maintenance of such practice.

Developing strategies to achieve system transformations is essential. Psychiatrists who have administrative and supervisory roles must play a significant part in these strategies if a successful outcome is to be expected. Psychiatric leaders can facilitate the transformation process in a variety of ways, with or without defined responsibility or actual authority for doing so. The remainder of this chapter addresses some of the practices that psychiatric leaders may employ to influence colleagues and supervisees to incorporate the principles of ROC into their practices; examines some of the challenges to their implementation and various methods that may be used to help mitigate them; and describes several tools that can facilitate recovery oriented practices.

Transformational Leadership

Psychiatrists assuming leadership roles in systems that have maintained traditional service delivery methods will likely face many challenges to their attempts to change organizational culture. The establishment of recovery oriented services requires a major change in the way professionals have been trained to think about their roles. This reconceptualization will include an understanding that the role of clinicians should be facilitative rather than directive, hope inspiring rather than critical, autonomy enhancing rather than paternalistic, and collaborative rather than autocratic. Transformational leadership (Corrigan and Garman 1999) must be able to articulate the vision of recovery oriented services and inspire supervisees and colleagues to embrace it.

The process for accomplishing this task is, of course, very similar to that involved in helping individuals make changes for their personal recovery. An effective leader will often be able to assist individual clinicians to identify those personal values that support the principles of ROC. Motivational interviewing skills should serve leaders well in their efforts to effect collective changes in an organization's culture (Prochaska and DiClemente 1983). Motivational interviewing allows people to find logical responses to their circumstances based on their own preferences and values. These responses are often not easily realized by clinicians who have been acculturated in hierarchical, paternalistic systems. In leadership positions, they need to model the qualities that are envisioned for clinical interactions: communication, collaboration, information sharing, tolerance, and flexibility in efforts to help staff identify better ways to manage relationships with their clients. This approach will also result in greater investment of staff in the recovery paradigm.

Regardless of professional orientation, most clinicians take pride in their ability to form relationships, and this can often be a starting point for the examination of their current practices. Because they have at some point had extensive training in creating therapeutic relationships with patients and families, this can be framed as the basis for developing biopsychosocial assessments, making diagnoses, and planning a course of treatment. For most who have not become too jaded or burned out, these relationships are also among the primary sources of professional satisfaction. Even though some clinicians may be motivated only by altruistic impulses, or on the other extreme by prestige or monetary compensation, the recognition that most clinicians wish to improve their own quality of life will make an appeal to professional satisfaction a powerful approach. Through face-to-face collaborative care, in conjunction with promoting and facilitating treatment and recovery, clinicians encourage change through their growing relationships with their clients, their families, and their communities. This, along with an enhanced involvement with treatment teams and the health care system, will be a tremendous source of satisfaction for behavioral health professionals, in many cases markedly reducing the risk of burnout (Rosen and Callaly 2005).

An important part of recovery oriented care and the clinical relationship it promotes is inclusion and collaborative decision making. People pursuing recovery are encouraged to diversify resources they can use to support their efforts. Of great significance in this paradigm is the placement of the locus of responsibility with the person seeking recovery. An effective leader will eschew traditional hierarchical, authoritarian concepts of leadership, as discussed earlier (see section "Building a Base for Leadership"), and model an inclusive, collaborative approach to the transformation process. Psychiatrists and other clinicians should be encouraged to think creatively about problems related to service delivery and overcoming obstacles encountered in implementing their solutions. Delegation of responsibilities identified for the change process allows everyone to take pride in positive outcomes and motivate them to work diligently to achieve them (Aarons et al. 2017).

Developing, promoting, and modeling the vision of ROC requires the use of transformational leadership skills such as those described in this chapter. The idea of person centeredness, collaboration, and promotion of autonomy will not be foreign to many staff members, but the practical aspects of implementation can be daunting, and it will not take long for these obstacles to come to the surface. Some of the challenging systems issues that impact the implementation of recovery practices include brief scheduled visits, demands for productivity, lack of diversity in job activities, compassion fatigue, excessive paperwork, isolation, and working with people in punitive or restrictive environments. Likewise, there are several issues that cause psychiatrists to struggle in clinical applications. Challenges to the application of recovery oriented principles are especially likely when clinicians are working with people who have limited decision-making capacity; substance users who are ambivalent or uninterested in change; people who may be seeking and/or misusing medication, or are self-medicating with marijuana or alcohol; people who are easily agitated and who may become threatening or violent; and people who are deeply distrustful, frightened, or angry. After there has been significant success in moving staff toward a consensus on *what* the transformation should look like, the question then becomes "*How* do we do it?"

Managerial and Transactional Leadership

Leadership must do more than inspire staff to embrace a change in organizational perspective; it also requires developing the means for achieving that change (Rosen and Callaly 2005). Managing change includes the development of strategies and concrete tasks to be accomplished. This encompasses supervision with specific outcomes in mind and a process for evaluating progress toward those objectives. Providing constructive feedback for improving performance and creating incentives for continuing efforts is an important aspect of a transformation plan (Aarons et al. 2017; Rosen and Callaly 2005).

The following are some tools that could be employed in creating a plan for implementation of a recovery oriented, person-centered paradigm.

- **Setting the Benchmarks:** The basic principles of ROC can be grasped fairly easily, but not everyone will be able to visualize how they might look in practice within systems that adopt them. Creating the structures that are supportive of ROC can be a challenge, and referring to some descriptive materials can greatly expedite implementation and provide some standards against which progress can be gauged. The AACP Guidelines for Recovery Oriented Services is one tool that can be of value in this regard (American Association of Community Psychiatrists 2001a).

- **Workforce Training:** Staff psychiatrists need to be on the same page with regard to their understanding and practice of the principles of ROC. In many cases, psychiatrists may have a basic understanding of these concepts but may struggle with more complex or nuanced aspects of the model; this may result in a reluctance to confront perceived risks and to fully embrace these principles across service and population lines. The *Recovery to Practice Curriculum for Psychiatry* will provide a base for reaching a consensus among practitioners (American Association of Community Psychiatrists and American Psychiatric Association 2011).
- **Efficiency and Collaboration:** One of the great challenges to the recovery paradigm is a perception that time constraints make many of the principles impractical. Particularly in the fee-for-service structure of the current financial climate, psychiatrists and other clinicians often feel overwhelmed by productivity demands. The addition of more collaborative practices and the need to document them seems daunting if not impossible. It is clearly important to confront these challenges with solutions that will facilitate implementation of the clinical model. The Level of Care Utilization System (LOCUS) developed by the American Association of Community Psychiatrists (2016) is a comprehensive clinical assessment and organizational system.
- **Evaluation and Accountability:** Staff who have made a commitment to the implementation of ROC will want to be able to track the progression of change. The use of some simple tools created for this purpose will allow systems to monitor their progress toward a recovery environment and allow individuals to mark their own evolution in the clinical model. The AACP Recovery Oriented Services Evaluation (ROSE) is one instrument for measuring a system's adherence to the principles of ROC (American Association of Community Psychiatrists 2001b). The Psychiatric Recovery Oriented Practice Evaluation and Rating (PROPER; American Association of Community Psychiatrists 2010) was developed for the Recovery to Practice Curriculum for Psychiatry project (American Association of Community Psychiatrists and American Psychiatric Association 2011), with the contributions of many behavioral health stakeholders, to measure the psychiatrist's evolution in the implementation of practices that support recovery.

In the remainder of this chapter, the tools mentioned above are described in greater detail. These are not the only instruments available that may aid in the implementation process, but they are good examples of aids for beginning and sustaining the transformation process. Unlike many of the other available products, the tools described here are nonproprietary and easily accessible. Readers are encouraged to discover others that may suit their needs, and even to create their own tools to facilitate the implementation process.

Tools for Planning Implementation of a Recovery Oriented, Person-Centered Paradigm

AACP Guidelines for Recovery Oriented Services

The AACP Guidelines for Recovery Oriented Services were developed by the Quality Management Committee of the American Association of Community Psychiatrists (2001a). The committee was composed of psychiatrists working primarily in the public sector with extensive experience in a variety of clinical settings with multidisciplinary teams (Rosen and Callaly 2005). The guidelines were developed in partnership with an array of stakeholder and advocacy groups. The guidelines are divided into three domains of service systems: administration, treatment, and supports. Each domain is composed of several elements that are characteristic of recovery enhancing services. Each of these elements is described in detail, and indicators are included for each element. They are intended to provide a platform for systems wishing to develop standards for service delivery processes, and include some benchmarks to which their progress can be compared. They may be customized to meet specific circumstances unique to localities, but in most cases further refinement is not necessary. The domains and the elements of which they are composed are provided in Table 16–1.

Recovery to Practice Curriculum for Psychiatry

The Recovery to Practice project was initiated in 2008 to facilitate the system transformation envisioned by the President's New Freedom Commission Report in 2003 (Substance Abuse and Mental Health Services Administration 2003). Part of this initiative is the Recovery Oriented Care in Psychiatry Curriculum, a 5-year project of SAMHSA to increase aware-

TABLE 16–1. Recovery oriented services quality domains

Administration
Mission, Vision, and Strategic Planning
Organizational Resources—Peer Inclusion
Training and Continuing Education
Continuous Quality Improvement
Outcome Assessment
Treatment
Comprehensive Service Arrays
Advance Directives
Cultural Competence
Planning Processes
Integrated Care
Minimal Coercive Treatment
Supports
Advocacy and Mutual Support
Access Facilitating Processes
Family Services
Employment and Education
Housing

Source. American Association of Community Psychiatrists 2001a.

ness, acceptance, and adoption of recovery principles and practices among mental health providers (Sowers et al. 2015). The psychiatry section of the project was a collaborative effort of the AACP and the American Psychiatric Association, with assistance from an advisory group of psychiatrists, other mental health professionals, and people in recovery. After the first phase of the project, which was devoted to information gathering from a wide variety of sources and the development of a vision for the transformation of psychiatry derived from that process, the curriculum was designed.

The curriculum materials include a series of modules addressing specific aspects of recovery oriented practice that could be used in a series or independently. They were designed to be relevant to diverse psychiatric audiences (e.g., trainees, early career psychiatrists, senior community psychiatrists, supervising psychiatrists, teaching psychiatrists, hospital psychiatrists, addiction psychiatrists) without significant modification of the materials. The content of each of the nine modules (Table 16–2) is presented in a slide presentation with an audio narrative and video components.

TABLE 16–2. Recovery to Practice Curriculum for Psychiatry: modules

1.	Introduction to Recovery Oriented Care
2.	Engagement and Welcoming Environment
3.	Person-Centered Planning and Shared Decision-Making
4.	Peer Support in Recovery
5.	Role of Medication
6.	Health and Wellness Focused Care
7.	Developing Living Skills and Natural Supports
8.	Culturally Appropriate Care
9.	Trauma-Informed Care

Source. American Association of Community Psychiatrists and American Psychiatric Association 2011.

The modules can be viewed independently online (American Association of Community Psychiatrists and American Psychiatric Association 2011), but they are designed more specifically to provide a foundation for a live conversation among viewers. Facilitator teams (consisting of a psychiatrist and a person in recovery) have been trained to lead these discussions, the focus of which may be customized to meet the needs of the specific psychiatric subgroup participating. The modules include video clips of psychiatrists, other mental health professionals, and persons in recovery. Facilitators have additional materials available to them to stimulate discussion and challenge participants to think creatively. Each module takes 20–30 minutes to view, leaving 30–40 minutes for discussion in 1-hour sessions.

Continuing medical education credits may be arranged by sponsoring agencies for individuals who complete these sessions. Larger agencies might benefit from having facilitators trained within their organization to enhance the availability of training and provide ongoing coaching to the psychiatric staff as they attempt to incorporate these principles into their practice. PROPER, a self-assessment tool described later in this section, allows psychiatrists to mark their evolution. More information can be obtained at www.communitypsychiatry.org.

Level of Care Utilization System

Since the arrival of managed care programs and principles in the 1990s, the use of quantifiable measures to guide assessment, level of care placement decisions, and continued stay criteria, as well as to monitor clinical outcomes, has been increasingly important. Since 1996, LOCUS has provided a single instrument that can be used for these functions in diverse settings and systems. According to AACP records, as of 2019 it was used in 26 states and in several international locations. Because of its unique design and simplicity, LOCUS also provides a framework for facilitating clinical interactions and collaborative ROC. Since its inception, LOCUS has included content related to recovery status, stage of change, and choice. Its simple style and structure have invited use not only by a variety of clinicians with various levels of training, but also by service users themselves, allowing assessment to become a collaborative process. Engagement in this collaboration is central to person-centered treatment planning, and the language in the instrument accommodates that process (American Association of Community Psychiatrists 2016).

The document is divided into two main sections. The first section defines six evaluation parameters or dimensions: I) Risk of Harm; II) Functional Status; III) Medical, Addictive, and Psychiatric Co-Morbidity; IV) Recovery Environment, with two subscales—Level of Stress and Level of Support; V) Treatment and Recovery History; and VI) Engagement and Recovery Status. A 5-point scale is constructed for each dimension, and the criteria for assigning a given rating or score in that dimension are elaborated. The second section of the document defines six "levels of care" in the service continuum in terms of four variables: 1) Care Environment, 2) Clinical Services, 3) Support Services, and 4) Crisis Stabilization and Prevention Services. Each level describes a flexible or variable combination of specific service types and might more accurately be said to describe levels of resource intensity. Each level encompasses a multidimensional array of service elements, combining crisis, supportive, clinical, and environmental interventions, which may vary independently.

Following the level-of-care description, this section elaborates recommendations for the most appropriate level of care. These recommendations are based on the scores generated from each of the seven rating scales, using an algorithm. This decision can be reached using the paper version of the instrument or with the help of a computer-generated recommendation following the same algorithm but with somewhat greater speed. LOCUS 20, the most recent revision of the tool, provides a comprehensive clinical system that extends throughout the continuum of care. When implemented to its full potential, LOCUS 20 can be used from the initial assessment through treatment planning, progress monitoring, and finally transition management. It provides an easy platform for tracking needs over time, a clear rationale for recommendations when interacting with managed care organizations, and a time-saving individualized documentation system, allowing more time for clinical interaction. A worksheet provided in LOCUS 20 is useful for tabulating scores during the initial assessment (Figure 16–1).

Please check the applicable ratings within each dimension and record the score in the lower right hand corner. Total your score and determine the recommended level of care using the Placement Grid or the Decision Tree.

I. Risk of harm — Criteria

- ☐ 1. Minimal risk of harm ______
- ☐ 2. Low risk of harm ______
- ☐ 3. Moderate risk of harm ______
- ☐ 4. Serious risk of harm ______
- ☐ 5. Extreme risk of harm ______

Score ______

II. Functional status — Criteria

- ☐ 1. Minimal impairment ______
- ☐ 2. Mild impairment ______
- ☐ 3. Moderate impairment ______
- ☐ 4. Serious impairment ______
- ☐ 5. Severe impairment ______

Score ______

III. Comorbidity — Criteria

- ☐ 1. No comorbidity ______
- ☐ 2. Minor comorbidity ______
- ☐ 3. Significant comorbidity ______
- ☐ 4. Major comorbidity ______
- ☐ 5. Severe comorbidity ______

Score ______

IV-A. Recovery environment—level of stress — Criteria

- ☐ 1. Low stress environment ______
- ☐ 2. Mildly stressful environment ______
- ☐ 3. Moderately stressful environment ______
- ☐ 4. Highly stressful environment ______
- ☐ 5. Extremely stressful environment ______

Score ______

IV-B. Recovery environment—level of support — Criteria

- ☐ 1. Highly supportive environment ______
- ☐ 2. Supportive environment ______
- ☐ 3. Limited support in environment ______
- ☐ 4. Minimal support in environment ______
- ☐ 5. No support in environment ______

Score ______

V. Treatment and recovery history — Criteria

- ☐ 1. Fully responsive ______
- ☐ 2. Significant response ______
- ☐ 3. Moderate or equivocal response ______
- ☐ 4. Poor response ______
- ☐ 5. Negligible response ______

Score ______

VI. Engagement and recovery — Criteria

- ☐ 1. Optimal engagement and recovery ______
- ☐ 2. Positive engagement and recovery ______
- ☐ 3. Limited engagement and recovery ______
- ☐ 4. Minimal engagement and recovery ______
- ☐ 5. Unengaged and stuck ______

Score ______

Composite score ☐

Level of care recommendation ☐

Rater name ______________________

FIGURE 16–1. LOCUS Worksheet, Version 20.

Source. American Association of Community Psychiatrists. https://www.communitypsychiatry.org/resources/locus.

The Child and Adolescent Level of Care Utilization System (CALOCUS) was developed in collaboration with the American Academy of Child and Adolescent Psychiatry a few years after the initial release of the adult version. As with the adult version, the most recent revision, CALOCUS 20 (American Association of Community Psychiatrists 2019; see also Stroul and Friedman 1986) reflects 20 years of use in the field. CALOCUS 20 follows the same format as LOCUS 20 and uses the same scoring algorithm to make level of care recommendations . The instrument was developed from a systems-of-care perspective, incorporating Child and Adolescent Service System Program principles in both evaluation criteria and level of care descriptions. One departure from the adult format is the addition of a Dimension VI subscale for the assessment of family acceptance and engagement for use with children who are not yet independent. As in the adult version, CALOCUS 20 integrates mental health, physical health, and addiction variables, and also factors in developmental disabilities. When used as designed, it allows clinicians more time to focus on their clinical work.

It should be noted that there are other approaches that will also facilitate a person-centered, recovery oriented model of care. Surveys completed before visits, with or without the assistance of a peer advisor, can be helpful to expedite clinical transactions, leaving more time for the psychiatrist to develop a relationship with the client and to address more existential concerns. These previsit questionnaires can be completed with paper and pencil, but there are also computerized versions that can be incorporated into the electronic medical record. Perhaps the best known of these programs is "Common Ground," developed by Patricia Deegan (2010). Personal recovery plans are commonly used to enhance a person's sense of agency by identifying actions and people that can be stabilizing when stressors become overpowering. These are most commonly completed with the assistance of a peer or counselor, but psychiatrists can encourage their use and utilize them as one way to create a connection with clients. The best known of these personal recovery plans is the Wellness Recovery Action Plan developed by Mary Ellen Copeland (1997).

Psychiatric Recovery Oriented Practice Evaluation and Rating

Once psychiatric staff have been effectively engaged and invested in a recovery oriented approach to care, and they have participated in relevant training, it will be important to provide ongoing reinforcement and support for technical improvement. Opportunities for peers and supervisors to observe staff and provide feedback can be a very valuable part of a transformation process. To record and monitor progress, use of measurable, quantifiable indices will be very useful.

Psychiatric Recovery Oriented Practice Evaluation and Rating (PROPER) was developed as a tool as part of the Recovery to Practice project, discussed earlier in this section (American Association of Community Psychiatrists 2010; Sowers et al. 2015). PROPER includes three scales, each containing 27 questions, to be completed by different individuals: 1) psychiatrist (self-rating), 2) colleagues and supervisors, and 3) service recipients. Each item in the scales is rated from 1–5, from *strongly agree* to *strongly disagree*, and the total yields a composite score for each scale. Four domains of recovery oriented practice in psychiatry are defined and used to frame the items in the evaluation: I) Relationship Builder, II) Facilitator of Collaborative Interactions, III) Planner and Problem Solver, and IV) Promoter of Population Health, derived from the work of the Mental Health Services Committee of the Group for the Advancement of Psychiatry (Ranz et al. 2012). Use of this tool within a practice allows psychiatrists to see how their own perceptions of their practice compare with those of their peers and people who receive mental health services. The tool was vetted by both behavioral health professional and advocacy groups and went through several iterations to incorporate valuable feedback.

PROPER is intended to be administered to participants prior to taking part in ROC training, and again later to gauge the effectiveness of training and to monitor an individual psychiatrist's growth over time. Although there may be structural administrative issues that interfere with implementation and that are beyond an individual psychiatrist's ability to change, periodic administration of PROPER will increase awareness of system issues that must be addressed for a successful system transformation. Figure 16–2 shows the first 8 items from Domain I to provide a basic representation of how the instrument is structured. PROPER with all three versions can be viewed at www.communitypsychiatry.org/resources/proper.

Conclusion

Strong leadership is critical in order for change processes to be successful. Creating health care systems that deliver better value is one of the greatest challenges currently facing our society and perhaps the most fundamental for its well-being. This chapter has considered various aspects of leadership in general, and psychiatric leadership in particular. When psychiatrists are well trained to take on leadership roles, they are uniquely positioned to provide a broad vision of how diverse elements of behavioral health systems can interact effectively to provide the optimal outcomes with the resources

Please rate yourself on each of the following statements from 1–5 based on the following key:
5 = Agree strongly, or I do this all the time
4 = Agree, or I am able to do this most of the time
3 = Sometimes, or when I can
2 = Disagree, or I rarely do this
1 = Strongly disagree, or I never do this

Item number	Item	Score
I. Relationship builder		
1	My clients believe that I value my relationship with them.	
2	My clients feel that I understand them.	
3	I emphasize the value of having adequate information to make good choices.	
4	I am dependable with regard to my availability and commitments.	
5	I do all I can to help get clients what they need.	
6	I consider how culture, spirituality, and experience affect my client's behavior and perceptions.	
7	I assist clients in the identification of their strengths and assets.	
8	I am aware of my personal challenges in developing positive relationships with clients.	

FIGURE 16–2. PROPER psychiatrist version: relationship builder
Source. American Association of Community Psychiatrists (https://www.communitypsychiatry.org/resources/proper).

available. Changing aspects of an organization's culture is a difficult task regardless of the rationale for change. Successful transition to new organizational paradigms will benefit from the strong leadership and interpersonal skills psychiatrists can provide. Although one aspect of that leadership is selling a vision and inspiring staff to invest in it (Ranz et al. 2000), provision of the methods and structure for realizing that vision is probably equally important.

The recovery paradigm becomes more compelling as our health care systems evolve to deliver greater value. The transition to ROC provided an example of systems change, and how psychiatric leadership could contribute to it in several ways. Using existing tools and products, and possibly creating others, psychiatrists can greatly facilitate these processes. When psychiatrists take a step beyond inspirational leadership, more efficient practices and measurements can be employed to help assure the success of initiatives and establish the value of psychiatric inclusion in leadership roles (Peebles et al. 2009).

References

Aarons G, Ehrhart M, Torres MS, et al: The humble leader: association of discrepancies on leader and follower ratings of implementation leadership with organizational climate in mental health. Psychiatr Serv 68(2):115–122, 2017

American Association of Community Psychiatrists: AACP Guidelines for Recovery Oriented Services. 2001a. Available at: www.communitypsychiatry.org/resources/recovery-to-practice. Accessed June 21, 2020.

American Association of Community Psychiatrists: AACP ROSE—Recovery Oriented Services Evaluation. 2001b. Available at: https://drive.google.com/file/d/0B89glzXJnn4cZDRxVDBoMExtb2s/view. Accessed March 12, 2020.

American Association of Community Psychiatrists: Guidelines for developing and evaluating public and community psychiatry training fellowships. May 2008. Available at: https://drive.google.com/file/d/0B89glzXJnn4cVjZ3bX-dPS21VUlE/view. Accessed March 12, 2020.

American Association of Community Psychiatrists: PROPER: Psychiatric Recovery Oriented Practice Evaluation and Rating. 2010. Available at: www.communitypsychiatry.org. Accessed April 8, 2020.

American Association of Community Psychiatrists: AACP guidelines for psychiatric leadership in organized delivery systems for treatment of psychiatric and substance disorders. 2012. Available at: https://drive.google.com/file/d/0B89glzXJnn4cVG1JNzJRY0JReGM/view. Accessed March 12, 2020.

American Association of Community Psychiatrists: LOCUS: Level of Care Utilization System for Psychiatric and Addiction Services, Adult Version 20. 2016. Available at: www.communitypsychiatry.org/resources/locus. Accessed April 8, 2020.

American Association of Community Psychiatrists: CALOCUS: Child and Adolescent Level of Care Utilization System—Child and Adolescent Version 20. July 2019. Available at: www.communitypsychiatry.org/resources/locus. Accessed March 12, 2020.

American Association of Community Psychiatrists, American Psychiatric Association: Recovery to Practice Curriculum for Psychiatry. 2011. Available at: https://www.communitypsychiatry.org/resources/recovery-to-practice. Accessed June 21, 2020.

American College of Physcians: Certificate in Physician Leadership Program. 2018. Available at: www.acponline.org/meetings-courses/acp-courses-recordings/acp-leadership-academy/certificate-in-physician-leadership-program. Accessed June 2020.

Bell C, McBride D, Redd J, et al: Team-based treatment, in Handbook of Community Psychiatry. Edited by McQuistion H, Sowers W, Ranz J, et al. New York, Springer Science+Business Media, 2012, pp 211–221

Copeland M: Wellness Recovery Action Plan. Dummerston, VT, Peach Press, 1997

Corrigan P, Garman A: Transformational and transactional leadership skills for mental health teams. Community Mental Health J 35(4):301–312, 1999

Covey SR: The seven habits of highly effective people. New York, Simon & Schuster, 1989, pp 13–33

Deegan PE: A Web application to support recovery and shared decision making in psychiatric medication clinics. Psychiatr Rehabil J 34(1):23–28, 2010

Diamond RJ: Multidisciplinary teamwork, in Practicing Psychiatry in the Community: A Manual. Edited by Clark G, Vacarro J. Washington, DC, American Psychiatric Press, 1996, pp 51–69

Docherty JP, Surles RC, Donovan CM: Organizational theory, in Textbook of Administrative Psychiatry: New Concepts for a Changing Behavioral Health System, 2nd Edition. Edited by Talbott JA, Hales RE. Washington DC, American Psychiatric Publishing, 2001, pp 33–42

Duncan EA, Warden GL: Influential leadership and change environment: the role leaders play in the growth and development of the people they lead. J Healthc Manag 44(4):225–226, 1999

Feldman JM: Exercising effective leadership, in Handbook of Community Psychiatry. Edited by McQuistion H, Sowers W, Ranz J, et al. New York, Springer Science+Business Media, 2012, pp 523–531

Hogan MF: New Freedom Commission Report: the President's New Freedom Commission: recommendations to transform mental health care in America. Psychiatr Serv 54(11):1467–1474, 2003

Lencioni P: The Five Dysfunctions of a Team. San Francisco, CA, Jossey-Bass, 2002, pp 23–52

Moran M: AACP offers certification exam in community psychiatry. Psychiatric News, November 8, 2018. Available at: https://psychnews.psychiatryonline.org/doi/10.1176/appi.pn.2018.11b2. Accessed March 12, 2020.

National Council for Behavioral Health: Executive leadership program. 2020. Available at: www.thenationalcouncil.org/training-courses/executive-leadership-program. Accessed March 12, 2020.

Peebles S, Mabe P, Fenley G, et al: Immersing practitioners in the recovery model: an educational program evaluation. Community Mental Health J 45(4):239–245, 2009

Prochaska JO, DiClemente CC: Stages and processes of self-change of smoking: toward an integrative model of change. J Consult Clin Psychol 51(3):390–395, 1983

Ranz J, Stueve A: The role of the psychiatrist as program medical director. Psychiatr Serv 49(9):1203–1207, 1998

Ranz J, Eilenberg J, Rosenheck S: The psychiatrist's role as medical director: task distributions and job satisfaction. Psychiatr Serv 48(7):915–920, 1997

Ranz J, McQuistion H, Stueve A: The role of the community psychiatrist as medical director: a delineation of job types. Psychiatr Serv 51(7):930–932, 2000

Ranz J, Deakins S, LeMelle S, et al: Core elements of a public psychiatry fellowship. Psychiatr Serv 59(7):718–720, 2008

Ranz J, Wienberg M, Arbuckel M, et al: A four factor model of system-based practices in psychiatry. Acad Psychiatry 36(6):473–478, 2012

Rosen A, Callaly T: Interdisciplinary teamwork and leadership: issues for psychiatrists. Australas Psychiatry 13(3):234–240, 2005

Senge PM: Fifth Discipline: The Art and Practice of the Learning Organization. New York, Doubleday, 1990, pp 3–55

Sobczak A: 10 key leadership programs for physicians. Beckers ASC Review, December 30, 2015. Available at: www.beckersasc.com/asc-turnarounds-ideas-to-improve-performance/10-key-leadership-programs-for-physicians.html. Accessed March 12, 2020.

Sowers W: Recovery and person-centered care: empowerment, collaboration, and integration, in Handbook of Community Psychiatry. Edited by McQuistion H, Sowers W, Ranz J, et al. New York, Springer Science+Business Media, 2012, pp 79–89

Sowers W, Pollack D, Everett A, et al: Progress in workforce development 2000–2010: advanced training opportunities in public and community psychiatry. Psychiatr Serv 62(7):782–788, 2011

Sowers W, Primm A, Cohen D, et al: Transforming psychiatry: a curriculum on recovery-oriented care. Acad Psychiatry 40(3):461–467, 2015

Stroul BA, Friedman RM: A system of care for severely emotionally disturbed children & youth. July 1986. Available at: https://www.ncjrs.gov/pdffiles1/Digitization/125081NCJRS.pdf, Accessed June, 2020

Substance Abuse and Mental Health Services Administration: President's New Freedom Commission Report. 2003. Available at: https://store.samhsa.gov/shin/content/SMA03-3831/SMA03-3831.pdf. Accessed March 12, 2020.

Taylor FW: Scientific Management. New York, Harper & Row, 1911, pp 23–39

Part IV

Special Value Opportunities

17

Addiction Treatment and Harm Reduction

Maria A. Sullivan, M.D., Ph.D.
Gabrielle Marzani, M.D.
Collins Lewis, M.D.
Arthur Robin Williams, M.D., M.B.E.
Frances R. Levin, M.D.
Zev Labins, M.D.
Ashwin A. Patkar, M.D.
Elie G. Aoun, M.D.

There is widespread recognition that substance use disorders (SUDs) have a neurobiological basis and represent chronic brain diseases leading to behaviors with adverse consequences (Volkow et al. 2016a). Despite this acknowledgment, the adoption of evidence-based treatment has not been widely realized. Access to care for SUDs is somewhat limited and such care is often sequestered from general health care treatment settings, compounding the stigma associated with these disorders.

SUDs contribute substantially to both the U.S. public health burden (Degenhardt et al. 2013; Whiteford et al. 2013) and the economic costs of health care (Gryczynski et al. 2016; Rehm et al. 2009). In 2018, an estimated 164.8 million people age 12 or older in the United States (60.2%) were past-month substance users (i.e., tobacco, alcohol, or illicit drugs). Approximately 20.3 million people had a past-year SUD, including 14.8 million people who had an alcohol use disorder (AUD) and 8.1 million people who had an illicit drug use disorder (Substance Abuse and Mental Health Services Administration 2018a). Alcohol, tobacco, and illicit drugs are major risk factors for disability and premature loss of life (Lim et al. 2012). More than 25% of Americans, an estimated 66.9 million people, currently use tobacco products; despite significant declines in cigarette smoking, it is still the leading cause of preventable death in the United States, accounting for more than 480,000 deaths every year (U.S. Department of Health and Human Services 2014). Also, the current opioid crisis is associated with a range of public health issues, including opioid use disorder (OUD), opioid overdoses, neonatal abstinence syndrome, and increased spread of infectious diseases such as HIV and hepatitis C (National Institute on Drug Abuse 2016).

The health burden of SUDs is accompanied by significant economic costs, including health care and law enforcement costs, lost productivity, and other direct and indirect costs, such as harm to others (Rehm et al. 2009). Using the 2009–2013 National Surveys on Drug Use and Health, Gryczynski and colleagues (2016) examined all-cause hospitalizations and estimated costs across substance use profiles for alcohol, marijuana, and other illicit drugs. The authors found that people with SUDs involving illicit drugs other than marijuana had substantially elevated rates of hospitalization. Among working-age adults (20- to 64 years-old), 1 in 10 deaths can be attributed to excessive alcohol use (Stahre et al. 2014), and fatal drug overdoses have risen sharply during the past decade (Dart et al. 2015). From 1999 to 2016 in the United States, drug overdoses resulted in 632,331 deaths, of which 351,630 were due to opioid overdoses (Seth et al. 2018). In the United States, the annual economic impact of substance abuse on crime, productivity losses, and health care costs totals in the hundreds of billions of dollars (National Drug Intelligence Center 2011).

In this chapter, we consider prevention, treatment, and harm reduction strategies aimed at reducing the adverse impacts of SUDs. Because SUDs are a major source of impairment and disability, all efforts to reduce substance use or to mitigate its direct and indirect effects on health will have a positive impact on population health and the overall value created for the system. All of these interventions will reduce harms associated with SUDs, but the greatest impact on value may be derived from strategies focused on reducing the harm of ongoing substance use, and that is the major focus of our discussion. We review evidence indicating that an abstinence-only approach poses a barrier to many patients seeking treatment to mitigate addiction-related harms. We highlight the value of a harm reduction approach as facilitating entry into treatment and allowing patients to choose a pathway to recovery, including one of abstinence, when they are prepared to make this commitment.

Prevention

An important approach to reducing the disease burden and health care costs associated with SUDs is the use of prevention strategies. These interventions carry great value with respect to protecting the health of individuals at risk for SUDs and the population's health in general. Preventive strategies include education, universal screening, and brief intervention, which can lead to timely access to evidence-based treatments. Screening and early detection of psychiatric disorders can prevent or mitigate the risk of developing an SUD, since these conditions often occur concurrently (Volkow et al. 2019). When co-occurring psychiatric illnesses are identified and treated early, outcomes for the treatment of SUDs improve. Other prevention strategies target the initial stages of alcohol or substance use. Screening and brief interventions can be implemented in both primary care (Palacio-Vieira et al. 2018) and emergency department settings (Barata et al. 2017). Screening and brief interventions in primary care settings are valuable ways of identifying individuals engaging in risky patterns of alcohol or substance use (Hargraves et al. 2017).

In light of the frequent co-occurrence of mental health and substance use disorders, accurate diagnosis requires a comprehensive assessment. Empirically validated screening and diagnostic instruments may be helpful in this regard. Of the screening and diagnostic tests available, Larun et al. (2007) recommend 1) the CAGE questionnaire to identify AUD, both current and lifetime and 2) the Alcohol Use Disorders Identification Test (AUDIT). Although these tools provide an initial indication of the presence of an SUD, they cannot replace the role of the more sophisticated assessment skills provided by a well-trained psychiatrist. Early identification and treatment of psychiatric conditions, which pose a risk for alcohol or substance misuse, may prevent the later development of comorbid SUDs.

Student- and parent-based programs in the school setting have also shown promise for preventing and reducing alcohol and drug use (Newton et al. 2017). Universal (addressing an entire population) school-based interventions that emphasize protective factors have been shown to be effective in reducing illicit substance use in adolescents. This finding is more robust than those for similar interventions related to tobacco or alcohol use, which may require different approaches. Selective or indicated interventions for students at elevated risk for misuse of these substances or for those who have already initiated use may be more beneficial. These interventions have a more targeted emphasis on known risk factors (Hodder et al. 2017).

Prescriber-targeted interventions have included recently published guidelines on safer opioid prescribing (Centers for Disease Control and Prevention 2018). Other prevention strategies include increasing taxes on tobacco and alcohol products to reduce use, particularly among young people, and restricting advertising and marketing of addictive substances to youth. One example of this is the 2020 U.S. Food and Drug Administration (FDA) decision to restrict the marketing of all flavored (other than tobacco and menthol) electronic nicotine delivery systems (ENDS) targeting minors, or any other ENDS product for which the manufacturer has failed to take adequate measures to prevent minors' access. This is an attempt to reduce the potential harm associated with the legalization of a substance for which the medical and neurobiological effects of its use are not well understood.

The history of alcohol and drug legislation in the United States suggests that the complete prohibition of a widely used substance (e.g., alcohol) does not succeed. More recently, another example of unsuccessful prohibition has been visible. In the current opioid overdose epidemic, deaths from natural (e.g., morphine, codeine) and semisynthetic opioids (heroin) are stabilizing, while deaths from synthetic opioids (e.g., fentanyl, oxycodone) are rising at an alarming rate (Rudd et al. 2016). Novel synthetic opioids present extraordinary challenges for regulators and law enforcement, as small amounts routinely escape detection when they enter the country through the U.S. Postal Service. Thus far, prohibition strategies have proved ineffective at stemming the tide of novel synthetic opioids, as demonstrated by the rapid rise in mortality rates from overdoses. Public health would be better served by other strategies, including education, increased availability of naloxone for overdose reversal, and other medications (e.g., buprenorphine or methadone) that reduce or effectively eliminate dangerous opioid and alcohol use. Partial disincentives for use, through taxes and regulation of distribution, might be successful as long-term strategies.

Medication-Assisted Treatment

Medication-assisted treatment incorporates both medication and behavioral therapies and has an evidence base for its use in treating AUD and opioid dependence. There is a relative paucity of approved pharmacological treatments for SUDs, compared to other illnesses. Although a small number of medications have FDA approval for AUD (disulfiram, oral naltrexone, acamprosate, extended-release injectable naltrexone/XR-NTX) or OUD (methadone, buprenorphine, XR-NTX), there are currently no approved medications for stimulant or cannabis use disorders. This paucity of available medications contrasts with over 115 agents for hypertension and diabetes. Meanwhile, there has been considerable progress in the development of behavioral therapies for SUDs. Among the empirically validated therapies are motivational interviewing, cognitive-behavioral therapy, relapse prevention therapy, contingency management (e.g., voucher incentives), and couples and family therapy. Combining efficacious pharmacological treatment and effective psychosocial therapy has produced better outcomes than using either type of treatment alone (Carroll 2005).

Currently, the most pressing issue that medication-assisted treatment must address is the opioid crisis. The opioid abuse and overdose epidemic is considered to be one of the largest public health crises facing the United States today. The strategy for mitigation of harm associated with opiate addiction is to employ prevention efforts and to provide timely access to effective treatment for all affected individuals. The current evidence-based treatment strategy recommended by the Substance Abuse and Mental Health Services Administration (SAMHSA) includes FDA-approved medications in combination with behavioral therapies and counseling to provide a biopsychosocial approach (Substance Abuse and Mental Health Services Administration 2020). Approved medications for OUD include sublingual buprenorphine-naloxone and long-acting injectable buprenorphine, methadone, and oral and long-acting injectable naltrexone formulations. Evidence-based behavioral approaches include motivational enhancement therapy, drug counseling, cognitive-behavioral therapy, and relapse prevention strategies.

Medications for OUD have been shown to 1) reduce opioid overdose deaths, 2) decrease rates of infectious disease transmission, 3) improve retention in treatment, 4) improve social functioning, 5) decrease criminality, 6) increase patients' ability to gain and maintain employment, and 7) improve birth outcomes among women who have SUDs and are pregnant. A recent meta-analysis of 17 different cohorts with over 120,000 people showed that retention in methadone or buprenorphine treatment is associated with substantial reductions in the risk for all causes of overdose mortality in people with opioid dependence (Sordo et al. 2017).

Unfortunately, medications for OUD have been greatly underused. Of 13,084 facilities providing substance abuse services in the United States, less than 50% offer an FDA-approved medication for OUD, and less than 10% offer all three forms of approved opiate pharmacotherapy (amfAR 2020). The slow adoption of these evidence-based treatment options for opioid dependence is partly due to misconceptions about substituting one drug for another. Discrimination against patients receiving medication for OUD is also a factor, despite state and federal laws prohibiting employers from discriminating against OUD patients in treatment. (For example, the Americans with Disabilities Act makes it illegal for employers to discriminate against recovering individuals with alcohol or substance use disorders who have already sought treatment for their addiction.) Other factors include physicians' lack of training about, and health care professionals' negative attitudes toward, medications for OUD. These negative attitudes are particularly prominent in some segments of the addiction treatment community.

Treatment as an Alternative to Punishment

The relationship between untreated SUD and illegal behavior is well established and is further cemented by a set of socioeconomic circumstances including unhealthy living conditions, poverty, and immersion in a criminal culture. Models of diversion to treatment as an alternative to incarceration for persons with SUD have been implemented at every level of the justice continuum. Such interventions are offered by law enforcement agents at the prebooking level or at the judicial level. Prebooking diversion is typically encouraged through provision of Crisis Intervention Training for police officers. Crisis Intervention involves collaboration between police officers and behavioral health service providers to serve the needs of individuals in crisis. Officers may also be provided support from behavioral health professionals in mobile crisis teams to ensure that individuals are evaluated for treatment rather than being arrested and jailed (Steadman and Naples 2005). Judicial-level diversion is subclassified as preadjudication diversion and postadjudication intervention. In the former, prosecution may be deferred pending the offender's successful completion of an SUD treatment program. In the latter, offenders are diverted from incarceration via probation (Mitchell et al. 2012; Shafer et al. 2004). Overall, outcomes from these interventions suggest that diversion interventions engage persons with SUDs in treatment, and some studies demonstrate significant reductions in criminal recidivism (Mitchell et al. 2012).

A limited number of programs involve alternative sentencing or a judicial mandate as part of their referral to services. The successful San Diego Serial Inebriate Program (SIP) encourages individuals transported by emergency medical services (EMS) more than five times in a 30-day period for "public intoxication" to enter treatment rather than face escalating jail terms (City of San Diego 2008). SIP has partnered with the San Diego Fire-Rescue Department and Rural/Metro Ambulance to form a paramedic-coordinated project for "superusers" of EMS services. There was a 50% decline in EMS, emergency department, and inpatient services among SIP participants, which resulted in an estimated mean decrease in monthly charges of $5,662 (EMS), $12,006 (emergency department), and $55,684 (inpatient). For individuals who refused SIP treatment, there was no change in the use of these EMS, emergency department, and inpatient services (Dunford et al. 2006).

Harm Reduction

Harm reduction is a strategy with an overarching goal of minimizing harms caused by substance use, including psychosocial consequences, without requiring abstinence. This approach is based on the premise that substance use is a complex societal problem that, in addition to biological and/or psychiatric vulnerabilities, often interacts with poverty, social isolation, and discrimination (see Chapter 4, "Social Determinants of Health"). Intrinsic to this strategy is respect for the autonomy of the individual. Harm reduction emphasizes the possibility of change for an individual by reducing the psychiatric, psychosocial, and medical problems caused by the substance. To increase participation and access, harm reduction employs a "low-threshold" approach to treatment entry. It is fundamentally a collaborative practice in which the mental health practitioner or substance abuse counselor partners with addicted individuals and accepts them "where they are" (Logan and Marlatt 2010). Harm reduction also addresses the medical and social consequences of substance use. It encompasses goals related to a reduction in the risk level associated with continued use. One example of a harm reduction strategy is the use of extended-release injectable naltrexone (XR-NTX) to reduce an individual's desire to drink. It has been found to decrease the number of heavy drinking days in individuals who have not yet achieved abstinence (Garbutt et al. 2005). Still understudied in the field of addiction treatment, harm reduction holds significant potential for improving treatment engagement, health, and quality of life outcomes.

The core principles of harm reduction, as set forth by Marlatt and Tapert (1993), are as follows:

1. Drug use is a complex problem influenced by other quality of life issues such as poverty, class, racism, social isolation, and discrimination.

2. Moral neutrality is essential; a person's choices in consumption should not be condemned.
3. Respect for both the dignity and autonomy of the individual is required. This approach accepts the reality that individuals will always make their own choices regarding drug use.
4. Working with the individual collaboratively forms the basis of all harm reduction practice.
5. Participation should be a goal of treatment; thus, a low-threshold approach to entry is part of the engagement strategy.

Successful programs, which embody these core principles, enable individuals to access services despite continued alcohol consumption or drug use. This low-threshold approach uses alternative service elements such as drop-in centers, impromptu intake mechanisms, information groups, active recruitment in the field, and continual encouragement of clients who have relapsed and/or are actively using substances. Harm reduction interventions are characterized by a multidisciplinary approach and continuity of engagement (Graham et al. 1995), and are mindful of the social and medical consequences of substance use (Bergeron and Kopp 2002). These interventions occur on a continuum, ranging from safer use to managed use to complete abstinence from use (Peterson et al. 2006).

Substance Use Management is a harm reduction approach that focuses on a range of options for improvement. It may also include the following alternatives:

1. Abstaining from one or more drugs for a limited or open period of time
2. Switching routes of administration
3. Decreasing frequency of use and, by extension, finding joy or pleasure in other activities (e.g., hobbies, sports, social relationships)
4. Switching drugs consumed both in formal drug substitution therapies (e.g., methadone maintenance) and through informal, unprescribed substitutions (e.g., cannabis for cocaine or heroin)
5. Considering risks and benefits of combining drugs
6. Learning drug purification and drug purity testing measures

The harm reduction model also respects the ambivalence inherent in the stages of change model. This model is also known as the transtheoretical model of behavior change. Although first developed for smokers, this model has been embraced more broadly as an explanatory framework for addiction and the struggle to change. It proposes that individuals move through predictable psychological stages related to making changes in behavior that contribute to poor health and other negative consequences (Prochaska et al. 1992). These stages are precontemplation, contemplation, preparation, action, and maintenance. Relapse is often a part of this process. Readiness to change is a key aspect of this model as well. Strategies such as motivational interviewing complement this model by helping individuals to move from one stage in the change process to the next.

Motivational interviewing is a therapeutic technique that can be effectively employed in most harm reduction efforts, including Substance Use Management. Motivational interviewing is a client-centered, nonadversarial psychological approach used to help individuals increase awareness of the impact that their illness has on their lives and the lives of others (Miller and Rollnick 1991). Taking a nonjudgmental stance, the therapist uses a cognitive-behavioral approach to highlight ambivalence ("rolling with resistance"; i.e., avoiding direct confrontation and instead eliciting the patient's intrinsic motivation) and to harness patients' strengths in reaching their goals in recovery. Motivational interviewing is future oriented and encourages envisioning the positive consequences of behavioral change. This technique minimizes client resistance. Strategies include reflective listening, focusing on processes of change, and goal planning. The therapist must accept patients' perceptions of the effects of their addiction, but also uses methods of questioning, provision of information, and logic to help clarify the validity of their choices. A brief intervention based on motivational interviewing was found to be more effective than a brief educational intervention at reducing some high-risk injecting behaviors (Bertrand et al. 2015).

The remainder of this chapter focuses on various approaches to harm reduction and its impact on population health and enhancement of value in our health care systems.

Harm Reduction in Opioid Use Disorders

While U.S. governmental policies were espousing "Just say no" in the 1980s, Europe began to embrace a pragmatic, harm reduction focus on preventing or reducing the consequences of infectious disease and overdose deaths. This approach can be traced to the response in the Netherlands and Britain in the late 1980s to hepatitis outbreaks and the AIDS epidemic; in these contexts, harm minimization became the overriding goal in the interests of public health (Price 1996; Van Wormer 1999). The European Monitoring Centre for Drugs and Drug Addiction (2020) currently lists harm reduction standards and guidelines for many European countries. The vast majority of Western European countries have an explicit supportive reference to harm reduction in their national policies on HIV and/or drugs (Harm Reduction International 2020). Harm reduction measures include needle and syringe exchanges, opioid substitution therapy, and safe drug consumption rooms.

Although harm reduction is now an integral part of drug policy in the European Union, it is implemented differently in various countries. In the Netherlands, harm reduction has been part of an official policy for decades and has received state support for encouraging and maintaining drug users' contact with services. "Injection rooms," which allow people to use heroin safely, were first developed in England and subsequently adopted by Switzerland. Also, trials of heroin prescribing started in Switzerland and have now been adopted in other countries such as the Netherlands, Germany, and Denmark. Several European countries have syringe exchange programs, which have resulted in the reduction of needle and syringe sharing over the past decade. The National Institute on Drug Abuse (NIDA) recommends this strategy as well, although the adoption has been less formal and more variable throughout the United States (National Institute on Drug Abuse 2018). The more global adoption of these public health interventions and their expansion to most European Union countries in the 1990s had a significant impact on the prevalence of needle-related illnesses (Kinnunen and Nilson 1999). In Spain, the lack of success of abstinence methods in the 1990s and the ensuing rapid expansion of AIDS among intravenous drug users triggered the adoption of more pragmatic harm reduction policies. These intervention strategies brought about a significant reduction in new reported cases of AIDS, from a peak of 7,116 cases in 1994 to 4,867 cases in 1997 (Kinnunen and Nilson 1999). Controversy persists regarding the relative safety provided by injection facilities and needle exchange programs. The United States has been slower to accept harm reduction models.

Opioid medication therapies can be used to support abstinence from illicit or misused opioids, but also may be used as a harm reduction strategy to decrease health-related harms associated with opioid misuse. Buprenorphine-naloxone is used to avoid opioid withdrawal as well as for maintenance treatment (Furst 2013). Opioid substitution therapy with methadone or buprenorphine is considered a low-threshold treatment. It aims to engage in treatment those patients who are not prepared to undergo detoxification and to become abstinent from opioids (Kourounis et al. 2016). Patients who choose agonist maintenance are seeking to avoid the risk of opioid withdrawal, or the financial pressures associated with continuing use of illicit drugs. In many cases, they continue to use other substances, such as benzodiazepines or cocaine. They may wish to avoid other risks associated with relapse, such as exposure to infectious diseases, health complications, and overdose. Office-based buprenorphine treatment has become a more convenient option for patients with OUD and can also be seen as a harm reduction approach (Korthuis et al. 2010). The introduction of efficacious medications for OUDs, and more broadly the disease model of SUDs, has moved clinical and societal perceptions further away from an outdated moral model.

Harm Reduction in Alcohol Use Disorders

The acceptability of harm reduction models differs according to the class of drug and is influenced by national policies and politics. In the United States and in Europe, public opinion has vacillated and is often tied to the particular substance under discussion. For example, in the United States, even when there is a less punitive attitude toward illicit substances and a movement away from punishment and toward treatment, AUD tends to remain an issue in which there is less acceptance of harm reduction, and complete abstinence is usually the goal of treatment. The prevailing U.S. attitude of abstinence only harkens back to Alcoholics Anonymous as an anchor for this paradigm (Magura 2007). Americans' relationship to alcohol remains ambivalent: social drinking is widely engaged in and accepted, but complete abstinence is expected of so-called alcoholics. It is still widely believed that any alcohol use leads individuals with AUD (i.e., alcoholics) to uncontrolled use, and that there is no safe level of consumption for those who are dependent. Traditional 12-step programs frown upon nonabstinent approaches even when associated with reduced harms, and this perceived censure can be distressing for individuals who would like to take advantage of the social support provided by these fellowship programs.

Substance use professionals often oppose nonabstinence-based interventions as well. In a recent large (N=913) survey of addiction professionals, one-third of respondents viewed nonabstinence as an acceptable final outcome goal. This view was more prevalent among those working in independent or outpatient practice settings (Davis et al. 2016). In a subsequent survey (N=432) by the same researchers, a larger proportion of respondents rated nonabstinence as an acceptable final treatment goal for clients diagnosed with alcohol abuse (30%) or cannabis abuse (24%) than for clients diagnosed as abusing other drugs (11%–13%) (Rosenberg and Davis 2014).

An analysis of the National Epidemiologic Survey on Alcohol and Related Conditions found that for current drinkers in this U.S. survey, reductions in the four-level World Health Organization (WHO) drinking risk categories are meaningful indicators of how individuals feel and function, and could serve as nonabstinence targets in clinical trials (Knox et al. 2018). The WHO risk levels of drinking specify associated ranges of daily alcohol consumption: low risk (males 1–40 g; females 1–20 g), medium risk (males 41–60 g; females 21–40 g), high risk (males 61–100 g, females 41–60 g), and very high risk (males 101+ g, females 61+ g). The authors noted that when abstinence is identified as the only treatment aim for AUDs, this may deter those individuals who prefer drinking reduction goals from entering treatment. They further observed that using abstinence alone as a significant outcome in clinical trials may prevent potentially useful new pharmacotherapies from receiving FDA approval (Knox et al. 2018). Effective treatments for AUD and SUD should encompass flexible goals that encourage treatment engagement and improve the health and functioning of affected individuals.

In contrast to the prevailing treatment paradigm in the United States, harm reduction principles in Europe have frequently been applied to individuals with AUD. Revised primary outcomes are being considered in alcohol studies. One example is the "percentage of subjects with no heavy drinking days." Studies using this percentage as an outcome include abstinent individuals as well as individuals who engage in "low-risk drinking behavior" (nonabstinence and no days of five or more drinks during the prior 30 days) (Falk et al. 2010). The European Medicines Agency accepts intermediate harm reduction goals as clinically sustained reduction in alcohol consumption. These goals describe changes from baseline measurements of total consumption of alcohol per month as well as reduction in number of heavy drinking days, defined as five or more drinks per day for men and four or more drinks per day for women. These intermediate goals are used as optional endpoints in clinical trials for new pharmacotherapies (Mann et al. 2017). These alternative endpoints reflect the recognition that heavy drinking days are associated with acute cardiovascular outcomes, accidents, and other adverse health events.

Medications that decrease craving and drinking urges allow some individuals to decrease binge use and successfully moderate consumption. In 1951, disulfiram (Antabuse) was approved by the FDA; its use was intended to enforce abstinence by causing an aversive effect if alcohol was taken. This strategy of developing medications for abstinence prevailed in the United States for the next 50 years. The FDA historically reflected this intent by requiring that clinical trials supporting new medications identify abstinence, or an absence of heavy drinking days, as endpoints. In recent years, however, several federal agencies (e.g., NIDA, SAMHSA, FDA) have promoted new guidelines, reflecting a paradigm shift by incorporating the principles of harm reduction. These guidelines acknowledge that certain levels of nonabstinence may sometimes represent a positive treatment outcome. Meaningful clinical endpoints now include outcomes related to a patient's quality of life, such as work productivity and other social, occupational, and legal metrics. These guidelines recommend strategies ranging from safer use to substitution treatments, all with a patient-centered approach. Medications such as topiramate, acamprosate, and naltrexone may also be used and have been shown to decrease number of drinks per drinking day (Johnson 2020).

XR-NTX is an injectable medication available for the treatment of AUD in nonabstinent individuals seeking to reduce their drinking. XR-NTX has been shown to reduce the number of heavy drinking days in people with AUD (Garbutt et al. 2005). An opioid antagonist, XR-NTX has been shown to reduce the reinforcing effects of alcohol and the incentive to drink (O'Malley 1996). In a study of XR-NTX for the treatment of alcohol dependence in primary care, among patients (n=40) receiving three injections, median drinks per day decreased from 4.1 (95% confidence interval=2.9–6) at baseline to 0.5 (0–1.7) during the third month (O'Malley et al. 2007). In patients able to abstain from alcohol before treatment initiation, XR-NTX (compared with placebo) has been found to increase the rate of abstinence several-fold, as well as to substantially reduce the median number of any drinking days per month and increase the time to any heavy drinking day.

A combination of XR-NTX and other harm reduction strategies (i.e., case management and supportive housing) has been demonstrated to significantly decrease alcohol craving, frequency and quantity of consumption, and alcohol-related problems in chronically homeless individuals with alcohol dependence, over a 12-week course of treatment (Collins et al. 2015b).

Harm Reduction for Severe Alcohol Dependence: Housing Models

Although harm reduction is only now gaining an evidence base as a valid treatment goal for AUD, this model has already been applied to one group of individuals with AUD. A subpopulation of chronically homeless individuals with severe AUD and a high burden of comorbid mental and physical disorders is well known to treatment and social service providers (see Table 17–1 for studies attempting to define this population of homeless individuals with chronic public inebriation). This complex population with severe AUD, often middle-aged males ages 30–50, represents a fraction of chronically homeless people; 60% have a lifetime history of severe AUD and 40% have past-year occurrence (Koegel et al. 1999; North et al. 2010). Largely alienated from society and unconnected to longitudinal care, this population consumes great amounts of high-acuity services: emergency response teams, ambulance transports, emergency room visits, detoxification

TABLE 17–1. Descriptions of the population of homeless individuals with chronic public inebriation

Study	Setting/population	Assessment methods	Observations
High service utilizers			
Doupe et al. 2012	Manitoba ED patients (province wide, 17% of population resides in urban Winnipeg district, otherwise in rural areas)	Health care use records of 105,000 patients with 200,000 ED visits in Winnipeg; analyzed from most recent visit of 2004 and the preceding 365 days; triangulation of ICD-9 codes from prior physician/clinic/inpatient visits	Substance abuse distinguished *highly* frequent ED users (18+ visits/year) from frequent ED users (7–17 visits); 67.3% versus 35.9% of patients in the ED user groups were substance users. Highly frequent users disproportionately used ED as main care delivery option compared to frequent users. 90% of highly frequent users with dementia had SUDs.
LaCalle and Rabin 2010	Systematic review of literature	Review of 25 articles, most based on analyses of hospital databases of ED patients	4.5%–8% of patients utilize 21%–28% of visits. Patients are often white, with public insurance (60%), ages distributed bimodally 25–44 or >65. Few remain high utilizers long term. An outlier 4% of patients visit 5+ ED locations and tend to have a recurring singular complaint (often injury-related).
Homeless high service utilizers			
Chambers et al. 2013	Urban homeless in Toronto with universal health insurance, randomly sampled over 12 months in shelters (90%) and meal programs (10%)	4-year prospective study with 892 homeless participants; province-wide ED visits reviewed via administrative databases over study period	77% of homeless adults used ED once/year, average was twice/year (adjusted), and the top 10% used 12.1 times/year. Risk factors for high use were greater monthly income, lower health status, perceived unmet mental health needs, and perceived external health locus of control, as well as isolation.

TABLE 17–1. Descriptions of the population of homeless individuals with chronic public inebriation *(continued)*

Study	Setting/population	Assessment methods	Observations
Homeless high service utilizers *(continued)*			
Hall et al. 2015	San Francisco "superusers" of EMS transport (15+ rides/year)	Retrospective cross-sectional study based on 1 year of data from an urban EMS system	"Superusers" comprised 0.3% of the study population but over 6% of annual EMS charges. Superusers mostly comprised younger males with AUDs.
Chronically intoxicated in public			
City of San Diego 2008	San Diego Serial Inebriate Program (SIP): arrestees, chronically homeless, with severe AUD and "revolving door syndrome" (local EDs, jail)	In-custody screening interviews with potential clients (*N*=184) conducted by SIP Case Manager of Mental Health Systems Inc., the County of San Diego substance abuse treatment provider for SIP	87% male, 50% ages 40–49; 100% unemployed. 70% of "chronic public inebriates" have additional SUDs, 90% have co-occurring mental illness (38% psychosis rate).
McCormack et al. 2013	New York City psychiatric emergency room patients at a large public hospital	Chart review of hospital electronic medical record and coordinated data sharing with department of homeless services	51 patients identified with 10+ visits in two consecutive years (annual mean of 37 visits) with average of $75,723 in hospital costs. They had an average of 6 medical comorbidities, and 92% had psychiatric comorbidity.

Note. AUD=alcohol use disorder; ED=emergency department; EMS=emergency medical services; SUD=substance use disorder.

admissions, and frequent cycles through the criminal justice system (Collins et al. 2012). Despite incurring substantial costs, this population has poor outcomes and elevated annual mortality rates, approximately 10% higher than the general population. This increase is due to physical injury and self-neglect (McCormack et al. 2013). Therefore, targeting effective treatments for this population is important.

A report by the National Institute on Alcohol Abuse and Alcoholism (NIAAA), regarding alcohol and drug treatment programs, showed that treatment engagement with chronically homeless populations decreases as program demand characteristics—particularly abstinence from substances—increase (Orwin et al. 1999). This finding has been corroborated by research showing greater retention and decreased substance use among participants (often with many prior treatment failures) in Housing First programs than among those in abstinence-based housing programs (Larimer et al. 2009; Padgett et al. 2011). Housing First programs have a low threshold for program entry and no requirement for abstinence. This approach quickly and successfully connects individuals who are homeless, and who have significant behavioral difficulties, to permanent housing without preconditions such as sobriety or service participation requirements. It is based on the construct that housing is a necessary component to the decrease or cessation of alcohol consumption. This model originated with the establishment of Pathways to Housing, which was founded in New York City in 1992 (Tsemberis and Eisenberg 2000). Pathways to Housing established a new paradigm for supportive housing that upended the linear or continuum-of-care model that required clients to move through stages of mental health treatment adherence and sobriety before being eligible for long-term housing placements. A housing-first model has been adopted in many locations across the country and is thought to have been responsible for a 10% reduction in chronic homelessness nationwide from 2007 to 2011. By 2009, over 350 municipalities had changed to Housing First models for chronically homeless populations with mental illness and SUDs. Studies have found that chronically homeless individuals often do not find abstinence-based goals and treatments acceptable or desirable in initial phases of intervention (Collins et al. 2012; Padgett et al. 2008). Engagement in these housing programs allows homeless individuals with AUDs to stabilize and increases the likelihood of their moving from the precontemplative stage of change ("Problem? What problem?") to more active stages of the change process (Griffith 2008).

Beyond housing, innovative interventions have blended case management and harm reduction strategies to improve treatment retention, reduce acute service utilization, decrease heavy drinking days, and improve health outcomes. These models have had mixed results due to nonstandardized assessment procedures and the difficulty in assessing the fidelity of self-described "housing first" or "harm reduction" programs (Table 17–2). However, intensive case management, consistent with the newer Health Home models under the Affordable Care Act, have shown promise for reducing cost and improving outcomes among homeless or marginally housed patient populations with significant substance (e.g., alcohol, opioid, cocaine) use disorders and serious medical comorbidities (Raven et al. 2011). A computer-assisted social media motivational interviewing intervention has shown promise for homeless adults transitioning into a Housing First program. Participants reported that visualization of their social network was helpful in initiating thoughts about changing their alcohol, drug use, and HIV risk behaviors (Osilla et al. 2016).

Harm Reduction for Marijuana Use

Public opinion about cannabis legalization has become considerably more progressive since the 1990s in the United States. An empirically based study using data from population surveys and media word searches identified causes for this change in public attitudes. They include a decline in support for punitive approaches, a decrease in religious affiliation, and a shift in media framing (Felson et al. 2019). In the past decade, certain states have begun to legalize the possession of small amounts of marijuana for personal use, beginning with Colorado in 2012. Several other states have subsequently enacted similar laws.

Historically, cannabis has been used in various cultures and populations as indigenous therapy for a range of medical conditions (e.g., fever, headache, insomnia, cachexia, constipation, rheumatic pain) and diseases (venereal diseases, malaria) (Svrakic et al. 2012). Cannabis is currently the most widely used illegal drug in European countries. Prevalence of use is *not* lower in those countries with repressive cannabis policies than in those with tolerant laws (Ogrodnik et al. 2015). Legalization of marijuana significantly reduces the expenses for repressive cannabis policies and law enforcement, allowing more resources to be allocated to prevention and treatment. A legal market will also create employment and generate tax revenues to support prevention efforts (Ogrodnik et al. 2015). Also, for individuals engaged in the use of cannabis, legalization removes the range of harms associated with legal sanctions. In addition, there are potential public health benefits associated with marijuana legalization—specifically, the potential for marijuana to be used as a substitute to opioids and other hazardous substances (Lake and Kerr 2016).

It is important to note that the harms reduced by the legalization and normalization of cannabis are counterbalanced by evidence of the physical

TABLE 17–2. Community-based interventions for chronic public intoxication

Study	Setting/population	Intervention	Outcomes	Significance
Housing				
Collins et al. 2012	U.S. Pacific Northwest/currently/formerly chronically homeless with alcohol problems (*N*=31) from two community-based agencies	Naturalistic observation of verbal exchanges between staff and residents in a project-based HF program, in the context of a larger program evaluation.	Important to take into account residents' motivations for alcohol use: both perceived positives and negative consequences. HR was reported to facilitate housing attainment and maintenance, but residents remained affected by an internalizing moral model of AUD. Some reported less need to be highly intoxicated as in the past in order to gain access to sobering centers to have an indoor bed.	Despite HR-based care in HF sites, patients continued to feel stigmatized under a moral model of addiction.
Greenwood et al. 2013; see also Padgett et al. 2008	New York City/(often chronically) homeless individuals with mental illness and/or SUDs	Pathways Housing First (PHF): Review of creation/evolution and spread of PHF with ACT weekly model or ICM (twice/month with CM visits). Assess compliance with PHF Fidelity Scale as model is widely spreading throughout world.	PHF reduced homelessness faster and at higher rates than more traditional programs, and was associated with longer tenure in stable housing arrangements and reduced time spent in institutions such as psychiatric hospitals; consumers experienced greater choice in service delivery, and PHF cost less to administer.	Led to 250 cities with HF components after a federal campaign funded 11 sites; PHF is now the model for VA Health System since 2012.

TABLE 17–2. Community-based interventions for chronic public intoxication *(continued)*

Study	Setting/population	Intervention	Outcomes	Significance
Housing *(continued)*				
Larimer et al. 2009	Seattle, Washington/ super high utilizers, chronically homeless individuals with SUDs	Project-based HF model: Residents are provided with individual units (e.g., private studio apartments or semiprivate cubicles) within a single housing project that does not require abstinence. In this approach, residents can elect to receive on-site case management and other supportive services.	Cut costs for intervention/HF residents by 53% ($2,449/month); increased housing stability; reduced utilization of publicly funded services; and reductions in alcohol use and alcohol-related problems.	Nonabstinence housing models can be associated with less drinking and lower care costs.
Podymow et al. 2006	Ottawa, Ontario/ chronic homeless individuals with severe AUD, failed abstinence attempts, and referred by social worker (*N*=17, average participant is white male, age 50)	Managed Alcohol Program: Alcohol distributed to residents in 15-bed special section of shelter in amounts and at intervals agreed upon in residents' alcohol management plans (typically up to 2 drinks/hour from 7 A.M. to 10 P.M. 7 days/week) and withheld if resident deemed too impaired.	Mean daily consumption fell from 46 to 8 drinks/day. Residents had more frequent contact with staff, which provided more points for micro-interventions, including check-ins with residents about their current alcohol use, medication compliance, mental status, and interpersonal situations. Police encounters were cut 50% and ED visits by 36%.	Providing alcohol on a managed schedule can greatly reduce consumption over time and significantly reduce acute care utilization and police encounters.

TABLE 17–2. Community-based interventions for chronic public intoxication *(continued)*

Study	Setting/population	Intervention	Outcomes	Significance
Housing *(continued)*				
Tsemberis and Eisenberg 2000	New York City 1990–2000; homeless individuals with psychiatric disabilities	Pathways to Housing scatter-site Hf model; residents offered choice of individual housing units throughout larger community; supportive ACT services accessible.	Improved retention in housing and lowered costs. Resident perceptions of greater choice compared to linear models/continuum of care programs (which require abstinence before transition allowed to independent housing from temporary shelter).	Key features for HF: 1) direct housing with little or no requirements; 2) choice of supportive services; 3) ACT; 4) HR for SUDs; 5) supportive services continued even if resident is hospitalized or jailed.
Harm reduction case management and counseling				
Raven et al. 2011	New York City/19 patients (17 homeless, 15 specifically AUD, 18 other SUDs); validated projected risk of readmission at a large public hospital; all had Medicaid exclusively	ICM (11 hours/month), nonsober housing, prepaid cell phones, weekly conference calls with all providers, entitlement/benefit assistance.	Patients had a total of 64 inpatient admissions in the year before the intervention, versus 40 in the following year, a 37.5% reduction. Most patients (73.3%) had fewer inpatient admissions in the year after than the year prior. ED visits decreased, while outpatient clinic visits increased. Yearly Medicaid reimbursements fell an average of $16,383/patient.	ICM with nonsober housing can greatly reduce service utilization and costs.

TABLE 17–2. Community-based interventions for chronic public intoxication *(continued)*

Study	Setting/population	Intervention	Outcomes	Significance
Harm reduction case management and counseling *(continued)*				
Watson et al. 2013	Large Midwestern city/ chronically homeless individuals with dual diagnosis, in single- or multiple-site HF programs	Integrated study design combining elements of case study and grounded theory. Comparative assessments of core elements within four community-based HF programs via interviews and focus groups conducted with 60 informants (staff and consumers).	Qualitative analysis demonstrated six program ingredients to be essential: 1) a low-threshold admissions policy, 2) HR, 3) eviction prevention, 4) reduced service requirements, 5) separation of housing and services, and 6) consumer education.	Low-threshold admissions policies and harm reduction approach of providing a more flexible service structure than a Treatment First model is associated with improved outcomes.
Alternative treatment				
Dunford et al. 2006	San Diego Serial Inebriate Program (SIP), 2000–2003/ *N*=529, 92% male, 75% white, mostly ages 35–50	Judge offers arrestees (repeat offenders of public intoxication arrests with 5+ Inebriate Reception Center visits in 30 days) 6-month outpatient treatment in lieu of escalating jail time. Arrestees are more likely to accept once sentence is over 150 days. Of note, nonambulatory "chronic public inebriates" are not taken to Inebriate Reception Center, go to ED instead.	Offered to 268, and 156 (58%) accepted treatment. Use of EMS, ED, and inpatient services declined by 50%, resulting in an estimated decrease in total monthly average charges of $5,662 (EMS), $12,006 (ED), and $55,684 (inpatient). There was no change in use of services for individuals who refused treatment.	This community-supported 6-month SIP treatment strategy reduced the use of emergency medical services, ED visits, and inpatient resources by individuals repeatedly intoxicated in public.

TABLE 17–2. Community-based interventions for chronic public intoxication *(continued)*

Study	Setting/population	Intervention	Outcomes	Significance
Alternative treatment *(continued)*				
Tadros et al. 2012	San Diego, California/ urban chronically homeless individuals with AUDs	Resource Access Program is an EMS-based surveillance case management system. This paramedic-coordinated project is for those who repeatedly access 911.	During the first 2 years of using this case management method, program demonstrated significant improvements for 51 clients, reducing the number of ambulance transports (736 to 459), task time (263 hours), miles (1,939), and charges ($314,306).	An EMS-based case management and referral program was effective at decreasing EMS transports by frequent users, but had only a limited impact on use of hospital services.
Pharmacotherapy				
Collins et al. 2015a	U.S. Pacific Northwest city/currently/ formerly chronically homeless, alcohol-dependent individuals (N=31) from two community-based agencies	Randomized controlled trial had four treatment arms: a) XR-NTX+HR, b) placebo+HR, c) HR only, and d) community-based, supportive-services treatment as usual.	Participants evinced decreases in alcohol craving (33%), typical (25%) and peak (34%) use, frequency (17%), problems (60%), and ethyl glucuronide from baseline to the 12-week follow-up (P<0.05).	Extended-release naltrexone and harm reduction counseling may support reductions in alcohol use and alcohol-related harm among chronically homeless, alcohol-dependent individuals.

Note. ACT=assertive community treatment; AUD=alcohol use disorder; CM=case management; ED=emergency department; EMS=emergency medical services; HF=Housing First; HR=harm reduction; ICM=intensive case management; XR-NTX=extended-release naltrexone; SUD=substance use disorder.

and especially psychological harms associated with cannabis smoking. Earlier age of initiation and an increase in consumption are among the unplanned consequences of legalization (Ogrodnik et al. 2015). Research on the effects of the legalization of marijuana has noted significant increases in poison center calls and marijuana-related hospital discharges (Davis et al. 2016). Other public health effects of the legalization of marijuana include increased accidental pediatric exposures (Wang et al. 2017). Particular risks for adolescents include altered brain development, leading to psychiatric sequelae that may include persisting psychosis; behavioral effects such as impaired driving; and a greater risk of developing cannabis use disorder (D'Amico et al. 2017). There is strong physiological and epidemiological evidence supporting a mechanistic link between cannabis use and schizophrenia (Volkow et al. 2016b); frequent use of cannabis with high tetrahydrocannabinol (THC) potency increases the risk of schizophrenia sixfold. A recent study of population-level effects of recreational cannabis legalization in Colorado also found an increase in hospitalizations for motor vehicle accidents, alcohol abuse, and overdose injury, along with reductions in chronic pain admissions (Delling et al. 2019).

These emerging data may help to guide future decisions regarding cannabis policy, with the goal of protecting society from, on the one hand, the costs associated with repressive policies and, on the other, the harms and costs associated with cannabis use disorder and an increased risk of chronic persisting psychosis.

The Role for the Psychiatrist

Psychiatrists and other mental health providers are in a unique position to identify SUDs and to assess patients' motivation for entering treatment. Compared to other medical providers, a therapist or psychiatrist typically spends substantially more time with a patient and engages in more frequent treatment sessions. This extended therapeutic contact often leads to a trusted relationship, which may permit a patient to make an honest disclosure of an at-risk pattern of alcohol or substance use. In the context of therapy, the patient and psychiatrist have the opportunity to define whether the initial goal of treatment is abstinence or harm reduction.

Psychiatrists are aware of the effects of substance use, including substances' mechanisms of dependence and associated comorbid psychiatric conditions, as well as strategies for prevention and management. They thus have an important role to play in communicating to their patients the risks associated with psychoactive substance use. Psychiatrists also have access to evidence-based treatments guided by research in the field. Both independently and through their professional associations, psychiatrists can contribute to the education, training, and support of the public and other health care professionals, particularly those in primary care, to increase their ability to identify and manage SUDs. Through these interventions, psychiatrists have the potential to reduce the health burden associated with SUDs (Poznyak 2005).

Interests of Patients, Providers, and Payers in Treatment Outcomes

Although abstinence has historically been the treatment goal in the United States, recent research suggests that an exclusive focus on this aim may be counterproductive. Those individuals whose preferred goal is nonabstinence may be more likely to avoid entering treatment (Knox et al. 2018). Data from the National Survey on Drug Use and Health from 2002 to 2016 show that among adults age 18 and older who reported that they needed substance use treatment, the most common reason for not receiving treatment at a specialty facility was that they were not ready to stop using (38.1%) (Park-Lee et al. 2017). Abstinence-only treatment programs may not help a large number of individuals who recognize a need for some treatment but who are not initially seeking abstinence. In particular, patients with no prior treatment history, higher levels of functioning, higher family income, and lower levels of negative consequences are more likely to have the goal of controlled use (De Martini et al. 2014). However, it is important to recognize that patients' treatment goals may change over time, and it is not unusual for individuals who enter treatment with the aim of moderating drinking to later recognize that they should in fact seek a goal of complete abstinence. Once these individuals are engaged in a treatment relationship, motivational techniques may facilitate this transition.

From the standpoint of providers (physicians, nurses, counselors, therapists, social workers) in a variety of treatment settings (inpatient, outpatient, supervised housing facilities), the goal of harm reduction increases the acceptability of treatment and encourages individuals to engage more collaboratively in addiction treatment. Trying to convince individuals that they are not able to control their behavior is not likely to be successful, as changes in addictive behavior are usually self-initiated and self-driven (Peele 2016). Controlled studies have shown sustained improvements in drinking reductions for many patients following behavioral treatments (e.g., cognitive-behavioral therapy) and pharmacotherapy (e.g., oral or long-acting injectable naltrexone, topiramate) (Mann et al. 2017).

In a follow-up study of adults with AUDs in outpatient treatment, individuals with lower-risk drinking did not have significantly different medical costs compared with those who were abstinent over 5 years (Kline-Simon et al. 2014). These results suggest that a harm reduction approach to AUD affords comparable health care utilization cost reduction compared to abstinence-based treatment.

Recommendations for Policy and Practices

Harm reduction models, in conjunction with motivational interviewing, can inform policy and practice guidelines. This combination provides an opportunity for an individual with ambivalence to contemplate and accept treatment. Understanding of the psychological basis of illness and the patient's perspective is more likely to lead to realistic treatment goals and retention in care. Harm reduction can offer guidance for policy makers in terms of where to place resources. This strategy is practical and acceptable to the affected population and has shown financial benefits for health care utilization costs. Harm reduction acknowledges the importance of abstinence but does not make it a primary goal. It draws on an understanding of the neurobiology of addiction and the critical role that pharmacotherapy plays in the treatment of SUDs.

A collaborative strategy improves treatment retention and health-related outcomes. The patient-doctor relationship plays a key role in this approach. The effectiveness of collaboration has been demonstrated by evidence-based approaches that include pharmacotherapy, motivational interviewing, and other therapies, as well as housing models and other support services. FDA-approved medications can serve an important role in reducing craving, decreasing alcohol or substance use, or supporting abstinence. Substance Use Management focuses on a range of options for improvement. These may include changing routes of administration; decreasing frequency of use; switching drugs via formal substitution therapies (e.g., methadone maintenance) or informal, private substitutions (e.g., cannabis for alcohol); and reducing infectious risk (e.g., through use of clean needles).

Alternatives to incarceration, such as legally mandated drug courts, have been shown to be more effective, because incarceration rarely has recovery-centered resources or incentives on which the individual can focus during confinement. Decriminalization of certain drug offenses represents an effort to reduce the negative legal consequences of SUDs and encourages individuals to seek recovery without fear of reprisal.

Conclusion

We have reviewed the many unique challenges that confront individuals seeking treatment for AUDs or SUDs. Among these are the paucity of FDA-approved pharmacotherapies, the stigma and discrimination experienced by those who develop an addictive disorder, and difficulty accessing evidence-based treatments. Individuals seeking treatment must overcome both internal barriers (e.g., ambivalence, alienation) and external barriers (e.g., lack of trained providers, legal punishment). Given the enormous toll that AUDs and SUDs impose on affected individuals, including the unprecedented mortality associated with the current opioid epidemic, it is imperative that treatment access be expanded. We have reviewed evidence demonstrating the value of an inclusive, low-threshold approach to those with SUDs who may not be able to fully commit to abstinence at present.

Client satisfaction with treatment is an important outcome indicator for the quality of service. A treatment plan that is aimed at attaining the patient's own goals is one pathway to achieving this, facilitated by empathic listening and motivational techniques that clarify those goals. In the context of the current emphasis on a more patient-centered approach to medicine, harm reduction strategies offer a cost-effective way of creating a pathway to substance use treatment. Approaches such as low-threshold treatment entry can increase patient access to FDA-approved pharmacotherapies with demonstrated efficacy (Han et al. 2017; Luquiens and Aubin 2014).

Although sustained abstinence may represent the safest outcome for individuals with an AUD or SUD, the goal of complete abstinence is often not desired or considered attainable by more severely affected populations. These high service utilizers—such as those with chronic AUD—warrant a comprehensive approach to improve their health care and contain its costs. When considering interventions for affected individuals, therefore, policy makers, social service providers, and clinicians should draw on successful precedents from the alcohol and illicit drug harm reduction literature. Promising examples for severe AUD include provision of low-threshold stable housing with community support and judicious management of access to alcohol for residents. Recent guidance from SAMHSA and NIDA indicate that the benefits of harm reduction, with respect to broader outcomes for health and social functioning, are being recognized as valid treatment goals for AUDs and SUDs, beyond that of sustained abstinence. Harm reduction represents an understudied and underemployed treatment strategy in the field of addiction treatment, and one that has the potential to significantly improve rates of treatment engagement, health outcomes, and quality of life for those suffering from AUDs and SUDs. It will ultimately reduce both the direct and indirect costs associated with substance use.

References

amfAR: Opioid and health indicators database. 2020. Available at: https://opioid.amfar.org/. Accessed March 16, 2020.

Barata IA, Shandro JR, Montgomery M, et al: Effectiveness of SBIRT for alcohol use disorders in the emergency department: a systematic review. West J Emerg Med 18(6):1143–1152, 2017

Bergeron H, Kopp P: Policy paradigms, ideas, and interests: the case of the French public health policy toward drug abuse. Annals of the American Academy of Political and Social Science 582(1):37–48, 2002

Bertrand K, Roy É, Vaillancourt É, et al: Randomized controlled trial of motivational interviewing for reducing injection risk behaviours among people who inject drugs. Addiction 110(5):832–841, 2015

Carroll KM: Recent advances in the psychotherapy of addictive disorders. Curr Psychiatry Rep 7(5):329–336, 2005

Carroll KM, Onken LS: Behavioral therapies for drug abuse. Am J Psychiatry 162(8):1452–1460, 2005

Centers for Disease Control and Prevention: Quality improvement and care coordination: implementing the CDC guideline for prescribing opioids for chronic pain. 2018. Available at: www.cdc.gov/drugoverdose/pdf/prescribing/CDC-DUIP-QualityImprovementAndCareCoordination-508.pdf. Accessed March 17, 2020.

Chambers C, Chiu S, Katic M, et al: High utilizers of emergency health services in a population-based cohort of homeless adults. Am J Public Health 103 (suppl 2):S102–S310, 2013

City of San Diego: Serial Inebriate Program fiscal year 2007/2008. 2008. Available at: www.sandiego.gov/sites/default/files/legacy/sip/pdf/SDPD%2007-08%20SIP%20Report.pdf. Accessed March 17, 2020.

Collins SE, Clifasefi SL, Dana EA, et al: Where harm reduction meets Housing First: exploring alcohol's role in a project-based Housing First setting. Int J Drug Pol 23(2):111–119, 2012

Collins SE, Duncan MH, Smart BF, et al: Extended-release naltrexone and harm reduction for chronically homeless people with alcohol dependence. Subst Abus 36(1):21–33, 2015a

Collins SE, Grazioli VS, Torres NI, et al: Qualitatively and quantitatively evaluating harm-reduction goal setting among chronically homeless individuals with alcohol dependence. Addict Behav 45:184–190, 2015b

D'Amico EJ, Tucker JS, Pedersen ER, et al: Understanding rates of marijuana use and consequences among adolescents in a changing legal landscape. Curr Addict Rep 4(4):343–349, 2017

Dart RC, Surratt HL, Cicero TJ, et al: Trends in opioid analgesic abuse and mortality in the United States. N Engl J Med 372(3):241–248, 2015

Davis JM, Mendelson B, Berkes JJ, et al: Public health effects of medical marijuana legalization in Colorado. Am J Prev Med 50(3):373–379, 2016

Degenhardt L, Whiteford HA, Ferrari AJ, et al: Global burden of disease attributable to illicit drug use and dependence: findings from the Global Burden of Disease Study 2010. Lancet 382(9904):1564–1574, 2013

Delling FN, Vittinghoff E, Dewland TA, et al: Does cannabis legalisation change healthcare utilisation? A population-based study using the healthcare cost and utilisation project in Colorado, USA. BMJ Open 9(5):e027432, 2019

De Martini KS, Devine EG, DiClemente CC, et al: Predictors of pretreatment commitment to abstinence: results from the COMBINE study. J Stud Alcohol Drugs 75(3):438–446, 2014

Doupe MB, Palatnick W, Day S, et al: Frequent users of emergency departments: developing standards and defining prominent risk factors. Ann Emerg Med 60(1):24–32, 2012

Dunford JV, Castillo EM, Chan TC: Impact of the San Diego Serial Inebriate Program on use of emergency medical resources. Ann Emerg Med 47(4):328–336, 2006

European Monitoring Centre for Drugs and Drug Addiction: Standards and guidelines for practices. 2020. Available at: www.emcdda.europa.eu/best-practice/standards/harm-reduction. Accessed March 18, 2020.

Falk D, Wang XQ, Liu L, et al: Percentage of subjects with no heavy drinking days: evaluation of an efficacy endpoint for alcohol clinical trials. Alcohol Clin Exp Res 34(12):2022–2034, 2010

Felson J, Adamczyk A, Thomas C: How and why have attitudes about cannabis legalization changed so much? Soc Sci Res 78:12–27, 2019

Furst RT: Suboxone misuse along the opiate maintenance treatment pathway. J Addict Dis 32(1):53–67, 2013

Garbutt JC, Kranzler HR, O'Malley SS, et al: Efficacy and tolerability of long-acting injectable naltrexone for alcohol dependence: a randomized controlled trial. JAMA 293(13):1617–1625, 2005

Graham K, Timney C, Bois C, et al: Continuity of care in addictions treatment: the role of advocacy and coordination in case management. Am J Drug Alcohol Abuse 21(4):433–451, 1995

Greenwood RM, Stefancic A, Tsemberis S: Pathways Housing First for homeless persons with psychiatric disabilities: program innovation, research, and advocacy. Journal of Social Issues 69(4):645–663, 2013

Griffith LJ: The psychiatrist's guide to motivational interviewing. Psychiatry (Edgmont) 5(4):42–47, 2008

Gryczynski J, Schwartz RP, O'Grady KE, et al: Understanding patterns of high-cost health care use across different substance user groups. Health Aff (Millwood) 35(1):12–19, 2016

Hall MK, Raven MC, Yeh C: EMS-STARS: emergency medical services "Superuser" transport associations: an adult retrospective study. Prehosp Emerg Care 19(1):61–67, 2015

Han JK, Hill LG, Koenig ME, et al: Naloxone counseling for harm reduction and patient engagement. Fam Med 49(9):730–733, 2017

Hargraves D, White C, Frederick R, et al: Implementing SBIRT (Screening, Brief Intervention and Referral to Treatment) in primary care: lessons learned from a multi-practice evaluation portfolio. Public Health Rev 38:31, 2017

Harm Reduction International: Western Europe—harm reduction programmes. 2020. Available at: www.hri.global/western-europe-harm-reduction-programmes. Accessed March 18, 2020.

Hodder RK, Freund M, Wolfenden L, et al: Systematic review of universal school-based "resilience" interventions targeting adolescent tobacco, alcohol or illicit substance use: a meta-analysis. Prev Med 100:248–268, 2017

Johnson BA: Medication treatment of different types of alcoholism. Am J Psychiatry 167(6):630–639, 2010

Kinnunen A, Nilson M: Recent trends in drug treatment in Europe. Eur Addict Res 5(3):145–152, 1999

Kline-Simon AH, Weisner CM, Parthasarathy S, et al: Five-year healthcare utilization and costs among lower-risk drinkers following alcohol treatment. Alcohol Clin Exp Res 38(2):579–586, 2014

Knox J, Wall M, Witkiewitz K, et al: Reduction in nonabstinent WHO drinking risk levels and change in risk for liver disease and positive AUDIT-C scores: prospective 3-year follow-up results in the U.S. general population. Alcohol Clin Exp Res 42(11):2256–2265, 2018

Koegel P, Sullivan G, Burnam A, et al: Utilization of mental health and substance abuse services among homeless adults in Los Angeles. Med Care 37(3):306–317, 1999

Korthuis PT, Gregg J, Rogers WE, et al: Patients' reasons for choosing office-based buprenorphine: preference for patient-centered care. J Addict Med 44(4):204–210, 2010

Kourounis G, Richards BD, Kyprianou E, et al: Opioid substitution therapy: lowering the treatment thresholds. Drug Alcohol Depend 161:1–8, 2016

LaCalle E, Rabin E: Frequent users of emergency departments: the myths, the data, and the policy implications. Ann Emerg Med 56(1):42–48, 2010

Lake S, Kerr T: The challenges of projecting the public health impacts of marijuana legalization in Canada; comment on "Legalizing and regulating marijuana in Canada: review of potential economic, social, and health impacts." Int J Health Policy Manag 6(5):285–287, 2016

Larimer ME, Malone DK, Garner MD, et al: Health care and public service use and costs before and after provision of housing for chronically homeless persons with severe alcohol problems. JAMA 301(13):1349–1357, 2009

Larun L, Helseth V, Bramness JG, et al: Dual Diagnoses—Substance Use Disorder and Severe Mental Illness: Part I—Accuracy of Screening and Diagnostic Instruments. Report from Norwegian Knowledge Centre for the Health Services (NOKC) No 21-2007. Oslo, Norway, Knowledge Centre for the Health Services at the Norwegian Institute of Public Health, 2007

Lim SS, Vos T, Flaxman AD, et al: A comparative risk assessment of burden of disease and injury attributable to 67 risk factors and risk factor clusters in 21 regions, 1990–2010: a systematic analysis for the Global Burden of Disease Study 2010. Lancet 380(9859):2224–2260, 2012

Logan DE, Marlatt GA: Harm reduction therapy: a practice-friendly review of research. J Clin Psychol 66(2):201–214, 2010
Luquiens A, Aubin H-J: Patient preferences and perspectives regarding reducing alcohol consumption: role of nalmefene. Patient Prefer Adherence 8:1347–1352, 2014
Magura S: Drug prohibition and the treatment system: perfect together. Subst Use Misuse 42(2–3):495–501, 2007
Mann K, Aubin H-J, Witkiewitz K: Reduced drinking in alcohol dependence treatment: what is the evidence? Eur Addict Res 23(5):219–230, 2017
Marlatt GA, Tapert SF: Harm Reduction: Reducing the Risks of Addictive Behaviors. Thousand Oaks, CA, Sage, 1993
McCormack R, Williams AR, Ross S, et al: Committing to assessment and treatment: comprehensive care for patients gravely disabled by alcohol use disorders. Lancet 382(9896):995–997, 2013
Miller WR, Rollnick S: Motivational Interviewing: Preparing People to Change Addictive Behavior. New York, Guilford, 1991
Mitchell O, Wilson DB, Eggers A, et al: Assessing the effectiveness of drug courts on recidivism: a meta-analytic review of traditional and non-traditional drug courts. Journal of Criminal Justice 40(1):60–71, 2012
National Drug Intelligence Center: The economic impact of illicit drug use on American society. April 2011. www.justice.gov/archive/ndic/pubs44/44731/44731p.pdf. Accessed March 17, 2020.
National Institute on Drug Abuse: 2016–2020 NIDA strategic plan. Goal 4: increase the public health impact of NIDA research and programs. 2016. Available at: www.drugabuse.gov/about-nida/strategic-plan/goal-4-increase-public-health-impact-nida-research. Accessed March 16, 2020.
National Institute on Drug Abuse: Request for information (RFI): the HEALing Communities Study: developing and testing an integrated approach to address the opioid crisis. Notice number: NOT-DA-18-023. June 29, 2018. Available at: https://grants.nih.gov/grants/guide/notice-files/NOT-DA-18-023.html. Accessed March 16, 2020.
Newton NC, Champion KE, Slade T, et al: A systematic review of combined student- and parent-based programs to prevent alcohol and other drug use among adolescents. Drug Alcohol Rev 36(3):337–351, 2017
North CS, Eyrich-Garg KM, Pollio DE, et al: A prospective study of substance use and housing stability in a homeless population. Soc Psychiatry Psychiatr Epidemiol 45(11):1055–1162, 2010
Ogrodnik M, Kopp P, Bongaerts X, et al: An economic analysis of different cannabis decriminalization scenarios. Psychiatr Danub 27(Suppl 1):S309–S314, 2015
O'Malley SS: Opioid antagonists in the treatment of alcohol dependence: clinical efficacy and prevention of relapse. Alcohol Alcohol Suppl 31(1):77–81, 1996
O'Malley SS, Garbutt JC, Gastfriend DR, et al: Efficacy of extended-release naltrexone in alcohol-dependent patients who are abstinent before treatment. J Clin Psychopharmacol 27(5):507–512, 2007

Orwin RG, Garrison-Mogren R, Jacobs ML, Sonnefeld LJ: Retention of homeless clients in substance abuse treatment. Findings from the National Institute on Alcohol Abuse and Alcoholism Cooperative Agreement Program. J Subst Abuse Treat 17(1–2):45–66, 1999

Osilla KC, Kennedy DP, Hunter SB, et al: Feasibility of a computer-assisted social network motivational interviewing intervention for substance use and HIV risk behaviors for Housing First residents. Addict Sci Clin Pract 11(1):14, 2016

Padgett D, Henwood B, Abrams C, et al: Engagement and retention in services among formerly homeless adults with co-occurring mental illness and substance abuse: voices from the margins. Psych Rehab J 31(3):226–233, 2008

Padgett D, Stanhope V, Henwood BF, et al: Substance use outcomes among homeless clients with serious mental illness: comparing Housing First with Treatment First programs. Community Ment Health J 47(2):227–232, 2011

Palacio-Vieira J, Segura L, Anderson P, et al: Improving screening and brief intervention activities in primary health care: secondary analysis of professional accuracy based on the AUDIT-C. J Eval Clin Pract 24(2):369–374, 2018

Park-Lee E, Lipari RN, Hedden SL, et al: Receipt of Services for Substance Use and Mental Health Issues Among Adults: Results From the 2016 National Survey on Drug Use and Health. CBHSQ Data Review. Rockville, MD, Substance Abuse and Mental Health Services Administration, September 2017. Available from: www.ncbi.nlm.nih.gov/books/NBK481724. Accessed March 17, 2020.

Patkar AA, Weisler RH: Opioid abuse and overdose. J Clin Psychiatry 16(8):1–7, 2017

Peele S: People control their addictions. Addict Behav Rep 4:97–101, 2016

Peterson J, Mitchell SG, Hong Y, et al: Getting clean and harm reduction: adversarial or complementary issues for injection drug users. Cad Saude Publica 22(4):733–740, 2006

Podymow T, Turnbull J, Coyle D, et al: Shelter-based managed alcohol administration to chronically homeless people addicted to alcohol. CMAJ 174(1):45–49, 2006

Poznyak VB: The role of psychiatrists in prevention of psychoactive substance use and dependence: beyond clinical practice. World Psychiatry 4(1):31–32, 2005

Price C: Putting the harm in harm reduction: toward a new social policy. Harm Reduction Communications 2(5), 1996

Prochaska DO, DiClemente CC, Norcross JC: In search of how people change: applications to addictive behaviors. Am Psychol 47(9):1102–1114, 1992

Raven MC, Doran KM, Kostrowski S, et al: An intervention to improve care and reduce costs for high-risk patients with frequent hospital admissions: a pilot study. BMC Health Serv Res 11:270, 2011

Rehm J, Mathers C, Popova S, et al: Global burden of disease and injury and economic cost attributable to alcohol use and alcohol-use disorders. Lancet 373(9682):2223–2233, 2009

Rosenberg H, Davis AK: Differences in the acceptability of non-abstinence goals by type of drug among American substance abuse clinicians. J Subst Abuse Treat 46(2):214–218, 2014

Rudd RA, Seth P, David F, Scholl L: Increases in drug and opioid-involved overdose deaths—United States, 2010–2015. MMWR Morb Mortal Wkly Rep 65(50–51):1445–1452, 2016

Seth P, Scholl L, Rudd RA, et al: Overdose deaths involving opioids, cocaine, and psychostimulants—United States, 2015–2016. MMWR Morb Mortal Wkly Rep 67(12):349–358, 2018

Shafer MS, Arthur B, Franczak MJ: An analysis of post-booking jail diversion programming for persons with co-occurring disorders. Behav Sci Law 22(6): 771–785, 2004

Sordo L, Barrio G, Bravo MJ, et al: Mortality risk during and after opioid substitution treatment: systematic review and meta-analysis of cohort studies. BMJ 357:j1550, 2017

Stahre M, Roeber J, Kanny D, et al: Contribution of excessive alcohol consumption to deaths and years of potential life lost in the United States. Prev Chronic Dis 11:130293, 2014

Steadman HJ, Naples M: Assessing the effectiveness of jail diversion programs for persons with serious mental illness and co-occurring substance use disorders. Behav Sci Law 23(2):163–170, 2005

Substance Abuse and Mental Health Services Administration: Key Substance Use and Mental Health Indicators in the United States: Results From the 2018 National Survey on Drug Use and Health. August 2019. Available at: www.samhsa.gov/data/sites/default/files/cbhsq-reports/NSDUHNationalFindingsReport2018/NSDUHNationalFindingsReport2018.pdf. Accessed July 10, 2020.

Substance Abuse and Mental Health Services Administration: Medication assisted treatment. 2020. Available at: www.samhsa.gov/medication-assisted-treatment. Accessed June 28, 2020.

Svrakic DM, Lustman PJ, Mallya A, et al: Legalization, decriminalization and medicinal use of cannabis: a scientific and public health perspective. Mo Med 109(2):90–98, 2012

Tadros AS, Castillo EM, Chan TC, et al: Effects of an emergency medical services-based resource access program (RAP) on frequent users of health services. Prehosp Emerg Care 16(4):541–547, 2012

Tsemberis S, Eisenberg RF: Pathways to Housing: supported housing for street-dwelling homeless individuals with psychiatric disabilities. Psychiatr Serv 51(4):487–493, 2000

U.S. Department of Health and Human Services: The Health Consequences of Smoking—50 Years of Progress: A Report of the Surgeon General. Atlanta, GA, U.S. Department of Health and Human Services, Centers for Disease Control and Prevention, National Center for Chronic Disease Prevention and Health Promotion, Office on Smoking and Health, 2014. Available at: www.ncbi.nlm.nih.gov/books/NBK179276. Accessed June 28, 2020.

U.S. Food and Drug Administration, Center for Tobacco Products: Enforcement Priorities for Electronic Nicotine Delivery Systems (ENDS) and Other Deemed Products on the Market Without Premarket Authorization (Revised): Guidance for Industry. Washington, DC, U.S. Department of Health and Human Services, April 2020. Available at: www.fda.gov/media/133880/download. Accessed June 28, 2020.

Van Wormer K: Harm induction vs harm reduction: comparing American and British approaches to drug use. Journal of Offender Rehabilitation 29(1/2):35–48, 1999

Volkow ND, Koob GF, McLellan AT: Neurobiologic advances from the brain disease model of addiction. N Engl J Med 374(4):363–371, 2016a

Volkow ND, Swanson JM, Evins AE, et al: Effects of cannabis use on human behavior, including cognition, motivation, and psychosis: a review. JAMA Psychiatry 73(3):292–297, 2016b

Volkow ND, Jones EB, Einstein EB, et al: Prevention and treatment of opioid misuse and addiction: a review. JAMA Psychiatry 76(2):208–216, 2019

Wang GS, Heard K, Roosevelt G: The unintended consequences of marijuana legalization. J Pediatr 190:12–13, 2017

Watson DP, Wagner DE, Rivers M: Understanding the critical ingredients for facilitating consumer change in Housing First programming: a case study approach. J Behav Health Serv Res 40(2):169–179, 2013

Whiteford HA, Degenhardt L, Rehm J, et al: Global burden of disease attributable to mental and substance use disorders: findings from the Global Burden of Disease Study 2010. Lancet 382(9904):1575–1586, 2013

18

Impact of Climate Change

Elizabeth Haase, M.D.

Climate change will be the greatest public health and mental health challenge of the twenty-first century (Costello et al. 2009). The main environmental drivers of its health impacts are higher global temperatures, poorer air quality, and warmer oceans. These three factors have already led to habitat losses from natural disasters, sea level rise, and depletion of soil, water, fish, and animal life (Ebi et al. 2018). Psychic distress will increase with each rise in temperature (Obradovich et al. 2018). Lesser quality and quantity of food, shifts in infectious disease patterns, poorer health, and psychosocial unrest will worsen with passing years. There will be increasing refugee crises, civic conflicts (Smith et al. 2018), and changes in the experience of self and community (Asugeni et al. 2015). These factors will have direct effects on health, but the main cause of climate change health impacts will be human behavior, which has proved to be refractory to decades of warnings about the coming devastation from use of fossil fuels. This chapter lays out the public health implications of climate change and considers how value-driven mental health care can mitigate the impact of climate change on population mental health.

Physical and Mental Health Impacts of Climate Change

Heat Impacts

Currently, there are relatively more deaths and injuries from cold exposure than from heat. Later in this century, heat-related morbidity and deaths will increase, with total impact dependent on geographic region (Gosling et al. 2009a; Vardoulakis et al. 2014). The elderly, who will make up 32% of the world's population by the end of this century (Lutz et al. 2008), will be particularly vulnerable to heat impacts. For example, the elderly accounted for 80% of heat-related deaths in the European heat wave of 2003 (Fouillet et al. 2006).

Climate models use four representative concentration pathways, or RCPs, that assume four levels of radiant heat forcing that will result depending on how greenhouse gas emissions are controlled and use these to predict the consequences for global warming. These climate models predict an average global rise in temperature of 1–4°C (1.8–7.2°F) by 2100 (Collins et al. 2013). (1°C equals 1.8°F.) This increase in global temperature will be unevenly distributed, with increases predicted of 10°C (18°F) at the poles (Vose et al. 2017) and greater warming in cities and places with more air pollution or fewer natural "carbon sinks" such as tree cover. Heat waves have been increasing steadily in frequency, with a projected number of events of at least one per year predicted for the United States by 2050, compared with less than one per year in 20 years in 2017 (Wuebbles et al. 2014).

Direct health effects of hotter temperatures will come primarily from the impacts of extreme heat on the human body and changes in other ecosystems from the shift in ratio of cold to warm days. The ability of the body to cope with hotter temperatures by releasing heat is dependent on the gradient between core body temperature and a measure that combines environmental temperature and humidity; this is called the "wet bulb index" to reflect the inclusion of humidity in the thermometer "bulb" reading. It is a measurement of the capacity of the body to reduce its temperature through evaporation of sweat. Human survival is threatened when body temperatures rise over 40.6°C (105°F). The cardiovascular system fails, cells lose the ability to function, and enzymatic lysis begins. Cognition and other physical functions become impaired when core temperature surpasses 38°C (100.4°F). It is important to note that physical acclimatization, or adaptation of the body to a changed heat environment, can significantly improve human heat tolerance by 25%–65% (Hanna and Tait 2015).

Individuals with mental illness are more than three times more vulnerable to direct heat-related morbidity and mortality than others (Bouchama et al. 2007). Cognitive deficits, amotivation, low energy, and other symptoms that impair judgment and effort may decrease attention to the warning signs of overheating. Those with mental illness are more likely to use substances that impair hydration (e.g., alcohol) and decrease heat tolerance (e.g., stimulants). They have more psychosocial difficulties that predispose to overheating, such as homelessness, and poor access to transportation to help them escape urban heat islands where they often live. Financial hardship may limit access to cooling measures such as air conditioning.

Because they are more likely to be taking psychiatric medications that impair heat tolerance, individuals with mental illness are also at higher risk for the medical comorbidities that increase with heat. Heat causes dilation of peripheral blood vessels and constriction of cerebral and other blood vessels. Renal vessels constrict with heat via a serotonergic mechanism, and platelets are activated by heat (Thulius 2006). Psychiatric medications that raise and lower dopaminergic and adrenergic vessel tone impair the flexibility of this response, increasing cardiovascular heat impacts such as heat stroke and myocardial infarction. In a meta-analysis of short-term consequences of increased temperature, Schwartz and colleagues (2015) found an increase in ischemic stroke of 1.2% per 1°C. Li and colleagues (2018) made near-term projections by 2050 of an increased risk of 5%–20% for myocardial infarction and of 20%–40% for ischemic stroke for the median-risk (RCP 4.5) and high-risk (RCP 8.5) scenarios of climate warming. Parasites and microbes, which adapt more flexibly to heat than do multicellular organisms, will sometimes have advantages over humans as temperatures rise, increasing the likelihood of opportunistic diseases, such as Lyme disease, that impact brain function (El-Sayed and Kamel 2020). Renal vessel constriction and dehydration will create increased risks of toxicity and renal failure for individuals taking lithium (Knowlton et al. 2016).

In a study that might be suggestive of the magnitude of these impacts, Martin-Latry and colleagues (2007) compared individuals who came to the emergency room with heat-related illness with those who came to the emergency room for other reasons during a heat wave. Patients taking psychotropic medications were at much higher risk for heat-related emergency room visits. Anticholinergics, antipsychotics, or benzodiazepines were among the medications most commonly associated with this risk, raising the likelihood of an emergency room visit for patients taking one of these medications two- to sixfold higher than for patients not taking one of these medications.

Mental health disorders also increase with hotter temperatures. Completed suicides increase when there is an increase in temperature, both on a seasonal level and with progressive increases in temperature above annual means for a given geographic zone. Rates of suicide increase in different studies have been variable but averaged 1% per 1°C in one recent meta-analysis, separate from other meteorological variables that have been linked to suicide risk (Gao et al. 2019). In another study, climate accounted for up to 37.6% of the variance among suicides, which was greater than economic distress (Fountoulakis et al. 2016). Burke and colleagues (2018) estimated that by 2050, if climate change continues on its current course, an additional 14,020 temperature-based suicides would occur in the United States alone, a number that would nullify the gains of all current suicide prevention programs.

Studies have suggested an association of suicides not only with temperature directly but also with emotional distress about climate changes. For example, for every 1°C that the temperature was higher than 20°C (68°F) during the growing season, over a time frame of approximately 50 years, Tamma Carleton (2017) documented an average of 68 extra suicides per year above the usual annual means in Indian farmers. These suicides occurred only during the growing season and showed an inverse relationship to crop yield and were not present when temperatures rose without associated crop damage. This study is significant because it helps tease apart how suicides increase because of factors that impact psychological distress when it is hot. If a person is a farmer, distress associated with crop yield exacerbates the direct effects of heat itself on the biology of suicidal behavior. This study and others (Barreau et al. 2017; Bhise and Behere 2016) illustrate the connection between social determinants of health and psychiatric symptoms in the context of the complex systemic impacts that characterize climate change and are critical for value-based assessments of what psychiatric responses may be helpful.

Another psychiatric consequence of heat is its impact, directly and indirectly, on aggressive behavior (Carleton et al. 2016). With every 1°C increase in temperature, there is a 4% increase in interpersonal and intergroup violence. This can be seen in behavior in a wide range of circumstances, from aggression on the baseball field (Larrick et al. 2011) to homicide and violence rates in domestic settings (Hsiang et al. 2013). Projections indicate nine excess violent crimes per 100,000 people per 2°F temperature rise (Anderson 1989). Projections also suggest that by 2099, the United States will have seen 22,000 murders, 180,000 rapes, 1.2 million aggravated assaults, 2.3 million simple assaults, 260,000 robberies, 1.3 million burglaries, 2.2 million cases of larceny, and 580,000 cases of vehicle theft in excess of what would be expected at current temperatures (Ransom 2014). Studies suggest that this increase in conflict and aggression might be higher in agricultural areas where production is more affected by unfavorable climate conditions, such as excess rainfall or drought, leading to greater economic stress and unemployment (Crost et al. 2017; Jun 2017).

In summary, direct effects of heat on the overall population are considerable. People are likely to have significantly higher rates of suicide, violent behavior, and risk of victimization from violent conflict with others as temperatures rise. Those who have a mental illness are at even greater risk of adverse consequences. They will suffer more heat stroke, heat exhaustion, and heat-related death due to medications or psychosocial circumstances. They will also suffer medical complications from heat, including stroke, myocardial infarction, renal failure, and others.

Air Pollution Impacts

Global warming is caused by burning too much fossil fuel, creating carbon particles that trap solar radiation (Hayhoe et al. 2018). Air pollution is a mix of these carbon particulates and other fuel derivatives, such as ozone, heavy metals, nitrous oxide, and sulfur dioxide, as well as carbon fuel byproducts released by the increasing numbers of fires that result from hotter and drier forests. Ground ozone is also increased by heat. The effects of air pollution are therefore inseparable from those of climate change.

The most obvious and immediate health impacts of air pollution are on the respiratory system. Fuel-based irritants increase rates of asthma and other respiratory illness and also inhibit lung development in children. The resulting smaller total lung volumes are associated with poorer overall health and brain health (Perera 2017).

The smaller carbon particles in air pollution, those 2.5 microns or less in diameter, are also capable of entering the brain via uptake into the vasculature and transport across the blood-brain barrier. They can also be taken up by olfactory neuronal transport into the brain, in a manner similar to retrograde transport of herpes simplex virus along neuronal pathways. These carbon particles can also be taken up via pulmonary and vagal neurons. The pathophysiological impacts on brain tissue include increased inflammatory and oxidative changes and cellular apoptosis. Such damage has been shown to occur from smaller particles of various sizes and across a wide variety of settings. These include proximity to coal plants, freeways, and areas of high ambient air pollution of multiple types. They can be measured over time frames ranging from several days to decades (Calderón-Garcidueñas et al. 2016). By virtue of downward socioeconomic drift, those with mental illness are more likely to live in these unhealthy air environments. They are also more likely to smoke cigarettes and be vulnerable to the cumulative impacts of the two types of toxic inhalants.

The magnitude of cerebral damage associated with this carbon-based air pollution cannot be overstated. Starting in utero and progressing through childhood and the adult lifespan, this neuronal damage has been associated with greater rates of intrauterine growth retardation, smaller brain volume, and increased rates of autism and behavioral disorders such as attention-deficit/hyperactivity disorder. As a result, there are decreases in childhood and adult IQ scores, increases in adult depression, and earlier onset of dementia. One study showed that compared to children raised in clean air environments, those raised in the highly polluted environment of Mexico City have relatively smaller brain volumes beginning in utero and reaching a volume deficit of 25% by teen years (Calderón-Garcidueñas et al. 2016; Perera 2017). In several large population studies (Chen et al. 2015; Weuve et al. 2012), rates of dementia are two to four times greater in persons living in polluted environments compared with those from cleaner air environments. This effect is particularly marked if genetic risk for early dementia is present. For example, in a study by Cacciottolo et al. (2017), a woman who carried two copies of the APOE*E4 allele (alleles producing the ε4 type of apolipoprotein E, associated with risk for Alzheimer's disease) and who was exposed to highly polluted air, was four times more likely to progress to dementia over the 8-year study than a woman with no air pollution exposure and no APOE*E4 alleles. This level of risk is greater than most of the major risk factors for dementia, including lower educational attainment, hypertension, diabetes, obesity, smoking, deafness, and inactivity (Livingston et al. 2017).

Acute psychiatric impacts of air pollution have also been demonstrated. These included elevated risk of the onset of depression (Gu et al. 2019) and bipolar disorder (Khan et al. 2019), as well as increased risk of completed suicide (Bakian et al. 2015; Kim et al. 2018).

Although the economic and mortality burdens of brain impacts from air pollution have not been studied, the total mortality burden of particle and ozone pollution overall has been estimated at about 4 million premature deaths per year (Global Burden of Disease Collaborative Network 2017). Air pollution continues to add $130 billion per year in damages to the U.S. economy, most of which are health costs (Jaramillo and Muller 2016). The psychosocial impacts of respiratory illness, particularly for children and families, contribute significantly to the damage from air pollution, leading to hundreds of dollars per year in medical costs, lost work and school days, and impaired capacity to participate in exercise and social activities, all of which are vital for mental well-being and development. In contrast, air pollution control policies save $30 for every $1 invested, and have returned $1.5 trillion to the U.S. economy since the passage of the Clean Air Act in the 1970s (Landrigan et al. 2018). The inclusion of brain impacts in these numbers will add both to the impressive social costs of unrestrained fossil fuel use and the innumerable benefits of protecting air quality in value-based mental health care.

Extreme Weather Impacts

The third major health impact of carbon-based fuel derives from changes in global weather resulting from higher average oceanic and atmospheric temperatures. These changes result in more volatile precipitation patterns, causing both drought and flooding. Hurricanes have become more frequent and intense, steadily increasing over the last 15 years, and causing damage totaling $326 billion in the United States in 2017 (Hayhoe et al. 2018). Loss of life, injury, exposure to environmental toxicity, and property loss are the acute stressors associated with these changes.

The major mental health impacts, however, come from the longer-term traumatic stress that a natural disaster places on psychosocial functioning (Johannesson et al. 2015;Thoresen et al. 2019). For example, after flooding in England, residents whose homes flooded had 2–5 times greater mental health symptoms than those whose homes were unaffected, particularly if the former had financial hardship (Paranjothy et al. 2011).

In the immediate wake of a disaster, most of those affected develop mental symptoms including insomnia, hyperarousal, dissociation, difficulties with concentration and memory, and somatic complaints such as headache and diarrhea. Although affected individuals may not meet full criteria for a DSM-5 diagnosis (American Psychiatric Association 2013), their symptoms are important for value-based care because they cause up to 70% of acute disaster-related distress in an affected population. In the subsequent months after the disaster, however, many are able to cope reasonably well, buoyed by a "honeymoon phase" of public support as well as the belief that life will soon return to "normal." Later, when social support wanes and difficulties with loss of property, insurance complications, and lack of housing, electricity, food, and water continue, the individuals experience demoralization and depression. Substance use disorders, domestic violence, child abuse, anxiety disorders, and posttraumatic stress disorder (PTSD) increase. Rates vary from 9% to 90% for PTSD to 40% for depression and alcohol use disorders. Rates of violence against women and children also increase (Norris and Elrod 2006; North and Pfefferbaum 2013).

In developing countries, natural disasters and rising water levels from melting oceanic ice also lead to mass migrations and refugee crises. Such refugee populations have high rates of trauma, anxiety, and depressive disorders, as both a direct result of climatic events and the associated exposure to politically motivated violence and social unrest (Li et al. 2016; Porter and Haslam 2005). The issues of these displaced populations will increasingly impact the United States, as will the plight of similar migrants within U.S. borders, as the impacts of climate on coastal regions force relocation of the country's citizenry.

Finally, extreme weather damages soil and habitats, changing the food supply, animal life, and other patterns of disease. Not only are there food shortages from destruction of crops and diarrheal illness from contaminated water supplies, but plants themselves are changed. When grain fields are flooded with salinated water or displaced toxic waste, existing strains of these crops may not flourish, demanding the development of new strains of grain. Even the more rapid growth of plants at higher temperatures can be problematic. Plants that grow more rapidly have higher carbohydrate count and less time to absorb soil minerals such as iron and zinc. Because such micronutrients are important for psychiatric illness (e.g., low zinc is associated with depression, and depletion of B vitamins is associated with schizophrenia and depression), these dietary changes may raise base rates of mental illness (Firth et al. 2018; Wang et al. 2018).

The total costs of extreme weather are high, totaling $306 billion in 2017 and $91 billion in 2018 (NOAA National Centers for Environmental Information 2020). Rosenheim and colleagues (2019) demonstrated that the medical destabilization associated with disasters is also significant and costly. Among Medicare users, even extreme disaster victims received only $68.32 per capita in all forms of governmental support yet had an average increase in health care costs ranging from $323 to $2,140 in the first year. Although this study did not differentiate mental and physical health visits, clearly there is value to be added in disaster-prevention and postdisaster health intervention.

Psychological Impacts

The slower environmental changes that occur with climate disruption are also leading to high rates of psychic distress and suicide—so called "ecoterratic syndromes" (Albrecht et al. 2007). As habitats change, loss of familiar landscapes and life forms shift personal identity and are associated with a sense of mourning. This syndrome has been called *solastalgia*, to reflect nostalgia for past environmental conditions and the associated way of life. Solastalgia is particularly evident in communities where contact with the natural world is an integral part of daily experience and livelihood (Ostapchuk et al. 2015). Examples of such cultures include the Inuits (Cunsolo-Willox et al. 2012) and Australian aborigines (Ellis and Albrecht 2017). Both ethnographic and demographic studies show higher rates of depressive symptoms, alcohol use, and suicide in these groups, which are linked, sometimes linearly, to losses and changes in the environment.

Two important psychological drivers of climate distress include helplessness and guilt. U.S. surveys of attitudes toward climate change show that the majority of the population worry that climate change is causing harm and believe that more government action and policy change are needed to reverse it (Marlon et al. 2018). The denial of politicians and awareness of personal complicity in climate destruction can lead to frustration, hopelessness, and despair, as well as other maladaptive psychological responses such as disavowal and denial. Case reports suggest clinical manifestations of climate distress, including obsessive-compulsive symptoms related to particular climate actions (Jones et al. 2012), self-destructive behaviors such as unsafe sex practices to express the nihilistic beliefs about the future (Janet Lewis, personal communication, September 16, 2018), and extremes of self-denial or social activism followed by burnout or suicide (Robbins and Ransom 2018).

To assess the overall magnitude of mental health distress related to rising temperature, Obradovich and colleagues (2018) compared self-reported data on personal mental health for 2 million U.S. residents, reported by the Centers for Disease Control and Prevention, with meteorological data from 2002 to 2012. The authors showed that with temperatures over 30°C, a 1° temperature rise was associated with 0.5% increase in self-perceived mental distress. Notably, 30°C is 86°F, a moderate temperature, showing that climate distress mounts even without extreme weather events. These data are in line with the findings of Noelke and colleagues (2016), who reported that ambient temperatures over 70°F decrease positive emotions, increase negative emotions, and increase fatigue, and are also in line with the general trend of other work (Baylis et al. 2018; Denissen et al. 2008).

Assessing the Magnitude of Climate Change Impacts on Mental Health

Climate change causes declining conditions that lead to morbidity and mortality as well as distress and specific mental disorders. The field of psychiatry needs to know the overall magnitude of psychiatric illness and services that will be necessary to address this unprecedented mental health challenge. Little research has been done toward this goal, with the articles already discussed by Burke and colleagues (2018), estimating the increased number of suicides, and by Obradovich and colleagues (2018), estimating the increase in total mental distress, as notable exceptions and excellent examples of the type of work that is urgently needed. Engagement with a robust research agenda to model and predict the psychiatric impacts of climate change and the location-specific services that will be needed is a critical piece of U.S. psychiatry's role in providing valuable mental health services in this era. This section addresses how psychiatry should participate in projective climate research.

Climate change research is coordinated globally through a research consortium. The Intergovernmental Panel on Climate Change (IPCC) is a body that was established by the United Nations in 1988 that meets every 5–7 years to assess climate change science and to estimate global climate impacts, adaptation, and vulnerabilities. The IPCC also predicts global climate risk, defined as "the potential for consequences when something of human value, including humans themselves, is at stake and where the outcome is uncertain" (Intergovernmental Panel on Climate Change 2014, p. 6). Risks are stratified by degrees of confidence in the statement made depending on the consistency and certainty of the data and predictions. IPCC assessments are conducted by hundreds of scientists reviewing the scientific literature and are published as reports that are used for climate needs assessment and response. Their predictions have been impressively accurate but have also commonly underestimated the rapidity of change (Scherer 2012).

Data for global climate change research are stored by the Earth System Grid Federation (ESGF; https://esgf.llnl.gov), an international, decentralized, and collaborative database that consists of software protocols and interfaces. The ESGF is supported by the Program for Climate Model Diagnosis and Intercomparison (https://pcmdi.llnl.gov/about.html), an organization that works to provide and improve tools to model and compare simulations of climate impacts. These data sets and modeling tools are publicly available for projective research. They can be applied to unique climate data from particular geographic cells under different local parameters of climate change for a given health condition. In other words, they provide estimates of how a specific mental health measure might change in places with various climate conditions. These geographically enriched outcomes can then be averaged to reach a conclusion about national trends.

Because of the complexity and uncertainty of climate outcomes, an iterative risk assessment strategy is used, in which the projected cost of a climate event and key climate variables that can be monitored are identified, then extrapolated through a series of "what if" scenarios. These potential climate scenarios are used to identify points at which a system is unable to adapt. At these points, new strategies can be considered to enhance adaptation to these new climate conditions. Researchers can next change decision variables one at a time to assess how each would affect the overall climate impact (Ranger and Surminski 2013). This iterative process allows for the inclusion of new knowledge and provides a range of probabilities for expected outcomes. It is a way of making predictions in complex evolving scenarios and also helps validate the multiple strategies tested according to the internal consistency of results.

As an example, to calculate future risk of suicide in the current "business as usual" global warming scenario, Burke and colleagues (2018) used projections from 30 climate models and local climate data predictions for each U.S. county. From this, the researchers were able to get a summary average of climate effects on local temperature for the country. They then used historical data on how suicide rates since 1968 by county have varied with temperature, and they calculated projected suicide rates based on the likely increase in temperature and the predicted future population by county. All in all, the group ran approximately 30,000 possible projections. They additionally controlled for and studied the impact of air conditioning, gun ownership, and other variables. Their initial strategy, using direct climate data and calculation of mental health impacts is known as "top-down, impacts-first, science-first, or standard" research (Jones et al. 2014, p. 208). This kind of research can examine, for example, how a 50% increase in exposure to hurricanes will change the prevalence of PTSD, or help estimate how many more emergency mental health visits will be generated by the 16% predicted increase in interpersonal violence when the temperature has increased 4 degrees.

The next level of complexity in climate modeling includes determinations about how changing social conditions, particularly economics and climate mitigation strategies, might change projected climate impacts (Dittrich et al. 2015). Burke and colleagues (2018) did not model how changes in local or national social norms, suicide rates, or climate interventions would modify their data, but the flexibility of this iterative, multimodel approach would allow them to do so. In one study aiming to discover how social attitudes can be included in climate modeling, Carleton and colleagues (2018) wanted to know the economic value that people would place on a ton of carbon if they knew that reducing carbon would extend their lives. They asked how much people would pay for practical adaptations, such as an air conditioner, to prevent loss of lives due to hotter temperatures. They asked this question across specific regions and by age category across 41 countries. They also adjusted their cost analysis for future costs relative to predicted changes in income. Carleton et al. then evaluated how this amount of adaptation spending would impact predicted heat mortality. This value can then be used to make economic and marketing arguments for global policy decisions. For example, one can make the statement, "Citizens place a value of $39 per ton of carbon." This estimate could then be used to support spending on climate initiatives, such as the use of alternative fuel resources, to improve health.

A similar approach can be used to provide value-based psychiatric service delivery for climate change. For example, the acceptable value per ton of carbon, as discussed above, could be used to figure out how much spending would be needed to implement climate initiatives that would reduce heat-related suicides and violence compared to the costs of doing nothing. One could compare the financial costs of lost life years for a suicide victim and the impacts of distress over that suicide on health morbidity and work productivity for family and friends, and the costs to a community and its law enforcement related to violent acts, and then one could compare these costs to the costs of carbon-saving measures that would keep temperatures lower through clean energy initiatives. This could truly be a value-based population mental health intervention, with the extensive cobenefits of a healthier planet.

Climate change psychiatric research will also require the use of scenario-based research to study how changes in group *psychological* variables that impact mental health indirectly, such as values, context, or emotion, might change rates of mental disorders as climate is further disrupted. This scenario-based approach is variably known as "context-first, decision scaling, bottom up, vulnerability, tipping point, or policy-first" research (Jones et al. 2014, p. 208). To give several examples, climate psychiatric research can ask how the preexisting emotional state of solastalgia changes the impact of flooding on mental health, and how a shorter interval from an extreme weather event impacts mental health costs of a subsequent extreme weather event both at psychiatric service and intrapsychic levels. Other questions include how participation in social climate mitigation efforts changes population-wide mental health outcomes, or how mandated conflict-resolution education changes interpersonal aggression on hot days.

Establishing the Stakeholders and Values to Guide the Climate Mental Health Response

Climate *health* outcome research has the advantage of *relative* agreement about the value of health and the systemic tools used to monitor it. Climate *mental health* outcome research, in contrast, will be difficult to carry out because good mental outcomes are defined differently by different social groups and individuals. An environmental change may have no impact on one person but a dramatic impact on another. A loss of a national park to mining may increase depressive symptoms in a mother who is an environmentalist but have a positive impact on a father who now has a job. They may both have increased depressive symptoms from the lost opportunity for exercise. There are a wider variety of root inputs to mental health and a greater number of ways to mitigate them than for physical health. For example, if the parents' children in the park scenario above show an increase in mental symptoms, it may be difficult to discern the relative impacts of parental conflict from differing values, increased parental neglect due to time at work, loss of contact with nature increasing inattention and aggression, or other possibilities.

Complex problems such as these are called "wicked problems," defined in decision science as problems that cannot be easily or completely solved because of changing or contradictory requirements. Climate change prediction itself is a wicked problem. Wicked problems also arise when solving one problem creates others, as when clean energy initiatives threaten coal plant jobs or the actions of one nation impacts the survival of others. Understanding sociocultural and cognitive-behavioral contexts helps reduce the complexity of wicked problem solving. Wicked problems also become simpler when there is a shared set of social values among members of a group for what constitutes a good society. If they can be identified, commonly accepted values and outcomes, which can be monitored in a relatively straightforward way, help reduce conflict among members of a group deciding how to proceed (Jones et al. 2014, p. 202).

Establishing shared social views of how to view and respond to climate change has therefore become a focus of significant climate mitigation investment. Until recently, however, the impacts of climate change have not been concrete enough for many to grasp, a problem that has been theorized to have four core dimensions: temporal, geographic, social, and climate uncertainty (Spence et al. 2012). These impacts will manifest in a distant future. Intervening weather fluctuations will make it difficult to see the impacts as part of a larger pattern. The paradox that climate impacts evolve slowly but are acutely determined by people's actions now is difficult to grasp. Individual greed and political attitudes also work against establishing a shared moral understanding for how humanity should respond.

Centers such as the Yale Program on Climate Change Communication and George Mason University Center for Climate Change Communication have attempted to determine what characterizes the climate understanding, risk assessment, and behavioral responses of different groups of Americans. Perceived risks of climate change vary significantly (Ballew et al. 2019). There continue to be deficits in understanding, capacity for complex and abstract thought, and cognitive and defensive mechanisms that make it hard to take in climate change impacts fully.

In this behavior-driven planetary climate crisis, psychiatrists and patients, along with all of humanity, are equal stakeholders in the outcomes. Psychiatrists have a critical role in lowering the mental health impacts of climate change, particularly for those who are most vulnerable. This effort should include attention to people of countries that are disproportionately impacted by climate disruption. As a professional group, psychiatrists have not had adequate decision support—defined by the National Research Council as "processes intended to create the conditions for the production of decision-relevant information and for its appropriate use" (Jones et al. 2014, p. 202)—to begin to define what values and professional activity should be part of our climate response. The American Psychiatric Association, National Institute for Mental Health, and other organizations must study and explain how psychiatric epidemiology may change in coming decades. Ethically, they must establish a clear set of principles and goals for our involvement with climate change.

These principles and goals should guide assessment processes, communication, and interdisciplinary collaboration. They will enable climate research to be relevant and practical for psychiatry and other mental health professions (Jones et al. 2014, pp. 202–203). The IPCC suggests that a climate response developed by any professional body is helped by institutional flexibility, integration into existing policy and programs, and coordination with multiple stakeholders (Jones et al. 2014, p. 206).

In developing a value-based culture for these decisions, several guidelines can be considered:

1. Psychiatry should devote resources to climate impacts in proportion to the impact of climate on mental symptoms.
2. Psychiatry should base its organizational response to climate mental health impacts on biomedical science.
3. Psychiatry should practice in such a way as to promote safety and viable living conditions for patients consistent with planetary science.
4. Psychiatry should protect from harm those who are most vulnerable.

The physician's role includes an obligation to do no harm oneself and to dissuade people and institutions from doing harm. Science has clearly established that air pollution causes brain pathology in children and that fossil fuel particulates are the major source of the air pollution and heat that double rates of dementia and PTSD, and contribute to approximately 10% more suicides (Burke et al. 2018) and 20% more violence (Ransom 2014). These facts suggest that psychiatrists have an obligation to advocate for sound climate policies and to reduce our professional and personal carbon footprints.

A new system of psychiatric values requires significant personal change on the part of all psychiatrists to decrease the unsustainable habits of living in the industrial age. Personal values that have been shown to influence the interpretation and response to climate change risk include 1) the presence or absence of an implicit association between self and nature, 2) seasonal fluctuations in perceived climate significance, 3) explicit environmental values, 4) level of public activism, 5) "protected" values such as political or religious beliefs that people will not compromise or change, and 6) cultural values based on nature (Jones et al. 2014, p. 203). Holistic and analytical thinking modes will also influence whether an individual is oriented to take action for the benefit of all or only for themselves. Place attachment, political affiliation, perceived costs and benefits, higher perceived personal risk, and attitude toward time play a role in climate values, as does perceived personal risk. Psychiatrists are cut from the same cloth as the rest of humanity, so it is to be expected that adjustment of personal values will play a large role in our professional response to climate disruption.

To find these shared psychiatric values for our response to climate change, we as psychiatrists must make a paradigm shift from a biopsychosocial model to a biopsychosocial-*environmental* model of promoting mental health. We must redefine what it means for psychiatrists to be stakeholders in our own and our patients' health, just as we shifted in the last century from psychoanalytical to biological models of mental illness. This paradigm shift requires us to understand that to have a stake in population health, we must also have a significant, and in fact equal, stake in the health of the earth. The scope of concern for practitioners must expand from a focus on sustaining human life to sustaining all life and habitats. Making this shift will immediately orient mental health leaders toward mental health policy and advocacy work that reduces global warming and improves the health of the environment. Protection of the natural world and its inhabitants becomes an urgent aspect of service delivery to our clients, supporting the profession's ethical mandate to protect our patient population from preventable health effects.

This shift in focus and value also means that we must shift our clients' belief system toward greater valuation of nonhuman life. It begins to frame the health of the self, a core concept for psychiatry, more interdependently. The assessment "Does this person sustain the planetary community in their behavior?" becomes as important an assessment of a patient's psychic health as "Does this person function well independently and in relationships?" The definition of the *self* in this paradigm is much closer to that of Asian and indigenous cultures than to those of the West.

The health of this biopsychosocial-*environmental* self is fundamentally dependent on an attachment model for human psychic development that places as much importance on secure attachment to planetary life as on secure relationships with individuals. Just as any loving attachment facilitates appropriate care and concern, an understanding of our interdependency on and symbiotic relationship to nature can facilitate a mutually sustaining relationship to our environment. Embracing this health paradigm as clinicians means that a strong attachment to the natural world must become an important clinical goal for our patients. It asserts that having a healthy planet to live *on* is as essential to clients' survival and health as having a healthy body to live *in*. Addressing excess time indoors, animal and germ phobias, and nonsustainable behavior become important *clinical* goals. Bringing many more animals and plants into care settings might be part of a shift to emphasize relationships other than that between client and provider. Agoraphobia might come to be seen as a nature-attachment disorder, and the care of an animal or garden part of the therapeutic process of cure. Excessive consumptive behavior, such as flying multiple times per year, may come to be seen as pathological, reflecting denial or masochistic self-destructive behavior, as well as a lack of concern for others.

Another value-based mode of climate response is organized around the goal of maximizing human survival by preventing harm particularly to those most vulnerable to climate impacts. According to this view, psychiatrists should focus attention on areas of greatest unpredictability and vulnerability, such as places where catastrophes are more likely to occur if people are not prepared. Issues needing urgent attention to the system's capacity to respond include the following: 1) the increasing incidence of cumulative or recurrent meteorological hazards (e.g., recurrent flooding); 2) single extreme events that overwhelm a health system (e.g., the European heat wave); 3) changes in ecosystems critical to health (e.g., fish populations); and 4) abrupt environmental shifts (e.g., emergence of a disease a thousand miles north of where it has been previously identified) (Hess et al. 2012). In this view, psychiatrists should be focused on areas where social determinants create vulnerable populations with poor health, which will be further threatened when they intersect with areas of high climate disruption. Although it is certainly true that vulnerable populations will be more impacted by climate disruption, this mode of climate response hinges on a pathological grandiosity asserting than one can escape one's dependency on planetary health if one is not a minority. It also tends to promote paradoxical increases in injustice to minority populations. For example, resources might be spent on rocket development (so that the elite can avoid climate impacts by escaping to other planets) rather than on development of airplane engines that do not use nonrenewable fuel sources.

As these two value-based modes of climate response demonstrate, in crafting any research and response agenda, psychiatry will face the epistemological and practical tensions that arise over use of resources in response to this particular public health challenge. Hess and colleagues (2012) lay out two core ideologies of climate response. The first expects that climate change will amplify *known* public stressors, with particular impacts on vulnerable populations. This conceptualization is easier to understand, because we already have experience with these stressors and impacts. In setting priorities, it suggests that we should expand existing public health strategies. This orientation is likely to be favored by those looking to fund existing public health research and programs that address immediate mental health priorities, whether from climate or other short-term public mental health concerns (Hess et al. 2012).

The second ideology holds that climate disruption will be so multifactorial, novel, and complex in its impacts that it will destabilize public infrastructure of all kinds. Current social and institutional structures that contribute to mental health will also be destabilized, and potentially irrelevant. In this conceptualization, climate changes, as well as the types of "treatments" that will be needed to address them, are much more difficult to predict using current data. This perspective—that climate impacts are unpredictable, novel, and chaotic—requires innovative response strategies and innovative preparations of infrastructure. However, this second ideology may feel somewhat overwhelming, and cause policy makers to retreat to a focus on the short-term threats. As an example, the current emphasis on disaster preparedness in organized psychiatry leaves less room for innovative work on climate preparedness. For some, future climate changes are an abstract distraction from urgently needed disaster training. For others, disaster training distracts from addressing the actual problem of climate change. This is the kind of "wickedness" that makes climate response difficult.

A variety of guidelines and tools have been suggested by the IPCC to help psychiatric and other leaders make good climate policy decisions under these types of complex circumstances. They recommend that good climate policy be based on information that is credible, legitimate, actionable, and salient for users. Good climate policies should strive to promote institutional stability and learning in the systems set up to address the issue, so that stakeholders have a stable structure within which to engage their own problems over time. Robustness is another criterion of good climate policy decisions. Robust decisions can be recognized by their tendency to produce decent outcomes under a wide variety of scenarios, including those that are unanticipated or uncertain, or those for which a decision needs to be reversed (Jones et al. 2014, pp. 203, 209, 210). The IPCC has also supported the use of multicriteria decision analysis (MCDA), a mathematical analytical method for complex decision making, for climate decisions (Jones et al. 2014). These guidelines provide criteria to evaluate the psychiatric climate response.

Adapting Psychiatric Practice to Respond to Climate Change

Both the strategy of expanding existing programs and that of preparing for chaotic change recognize that the entire population faces climate impacts. General preventive measures for climate health impacts should therefore be underway as a standard part of health care delivery.

Adaptive capacity has been defined as the ability to adjust, to take advantage of opportunities, or to cope with consequences (Adger et al. 2008; Masson-Delmotte et al. 2018, p. 214). Interventions that combine adaptation and mitigation, and that lead to sustainable development going forward, are considered the most adaptive climate responses. Adaptation leads to resilience, the capacity to overcome adversity while also preserving identity—that is, to "bounce back." Adaptation measures would include provision of clean water and sanitation, basic health care and child health services, increased disaster preparedness and capacity for response, and alleviation of poverty. Public health efforts toward these ends have been shown to be the most effective overall ways to reduce general climate health vulnerability (Jones et al. 2014, p. 214).

Mitigation either prevents climate impacts or lessens the severity of those that occur (e.g., control of population growth through access to family planning services). Examples of mitigations that lower carbon and also promote sustainable growth include reducing emissions of climate-altering air pollutants through shifts to clean energy sources, decreasing methane production by decreasing food waste in landfills and shifting food consumption away from ruminant animals such as cattle, and designing transportation systems that reduce use of vehicles dependent on fossil fuels (Masson-Delmotte et al. 2018, p. 714).

Including attention to climate disruption in routine psychiatric care will involve educating all patients about the impact of climate change on their health and mental health, through public health campaigns and in the office. Psychiatric residencies should include training in the mental health impacts of climate change. Patients should have specific information about relationships between heat and mental symptoms and between heat and psychiatric medication. General medical counseling should inform patients about the neurological damage of air pollution, just as patients are educated about other dementia risk factors. As a profession, psychiatry should standardize clinical interventions that will help patients avoid climate-related morbidity, such as by recommending cooling devices or air filters.

Research supports the use of carbon-neutral nonmedication interventions, such as gardening and exercise, for mental health treatment. Nature-based interventions have the co-benefits of improving physical health. Climate-informed, value-based health insurance coverage would compare the costs of medication to the costs of nonpharmacological depression treatment, including nature exposure, biking, or other carbon-neutral measures. These calculations would not merely include comparing the cost of a medication against, for example, the cost of a bicycle program. Sophisticated calculations would also include the health cost improvement to the insurance plan of the reductions in the carbon footprint. Insurance plans would calculate whether it would be cost effective to cover biking programs based not only on how much medication cost would be avoided, but also by factoring in the decreased health costs of the insured population when the air quality has benefited from the lower fossil fuel emissions associated with bicycle use, for example.

Because climate disruptions cause acute and chronic fear responses that are fundamentally different from the anxiety disorders that are a psychiatrist's bread and butter, psychotherapy techniques will also need to be reconsidered. Patients will face two extremes that cause anxiety: responding rapidly to dangerous and continually evolving conditions, and tolerating the complexity of climate change and slow pace of natural cycles. Existing tools for anxiety management and resilience, such as psychological first aid, mindfulness, meditation, and many others, will add value to the public health response to climate for both rapid and gradual adaptation. Dialectical behavior therapy skills for interpersonal effectiveness can be adapted to help with assessment and management of intrapsychic and interpersonal complexities when usual systems are down or emotions are heightened because of rapid change.

Distinct from what psychiatrists do when focusing on reducing anxiety when treating panic attacks or other anxiety disorders, management of the stress response to real and urgent threats requires people to translate fear into effective *action*, whether they are reacting to an imminent threat, such as a tornado, or a more existential, but equally reality-based fear, such as the possibility of mass extinction. Under imminent threats, such as the very high-distress, high-threat conditions of a tornado, the cortex goes "offline," and only trained adaptive automatic responses can be relied upon to react (Ripley 2009). Effective actions under such circumstances include drilled responses, such as rapidly moving to an underground shelter, that create procedural memory. Less imminent threats, such as political actions that actively threaten one's planetary future, also require an active response. Developing personal empowerment in the face of environmental degradation and societal inaction may help prevent climate burnout syndromes and promote hope (Macy 2012). Examples of effective actions include confronting distortions of facts in the media, starting local initiatives for cleaner energy mandates, participation in lawsuits seeking environmental justice, and civil disobedience.

Psychiatrists can help patients identify when a threat is real versus exaggerated, avoid pathological denial of a real urgent threat, and implement effective safety measures, whether for an imminent or slowly evolving disaster. They can help develop behavior-based public training that will propel people to employ automatic actions when faced with extreme threat. Under more chronic fear conditions, they can help people identify maladaptive chronic defenses such as disavowal, and a long list of cognitive biases that may prevent patients from assessing real climate threats in an adaptive way. For example, a person operating under the cognitive bias of the gambler's fallacy might believe they could buy coastal property after a hurricane because "the last one was here, so the next one won't be." Psychiatrists can contribute by pointing out this kind of distorted thinking, which can lead to negative personal and social outcomes.

Psychiatry as a field must also be prepared for severe chaotic climate impacts. The possibilities of population-wide annihilation anxiety and sudden catastrophic events that render existing psychiatric systems inactive are real. Psychiatrists should be able to identify what they and their institutions will do during a catastrophic climate event. Facilities will face choices about how to use space and whom to help. For example, a space might be used as a shelter, or as a group meeting spot for first responders or other groups needing a headquarters for their outreach. Psychiatrists will need to plan for what registration paperwork will be most essential under duress. As a group, patients with mental illness will be extremely vulnerable and may lose access to their medications, so teaching patients to keep a backup supply of medication and working with pharmacies on strategies for emergency prescription overrides are important. Minorities, women, children, and older adults will be at increased risk of poor outcomes. Systemic measures, such as identifying sources of backup medication in advance and implementing call programs that use staff or automated systems to contact patients and their advocates to warn them of imminent climate health risks, can reduce the amount of injury from such catastrophes.

Confronted by the possibility of global existential distress, psychiatrists must also ask how people are *feeling* as their planet declines and life forms are extinguished. Younger generations are increasingly angry and despairing about the future, feeling abandoned and neglected by older generations. Older generations are struggling with feelings of failure and guilt for leaving their offspring with decline and suffering. Psychiatrists must contribute by designing coping strategies for people mourning planetary decline. A number of nonacademic models have been suggested, such as the Good Grief 10-step program (www.goodgriefnetwork.org) for mourning habitat loss. The SPIKES palliative care intervention (Balle et al. 2000), a program that has been demonstrated to help those facing early cancer death, has also been used as a model to mourn losses in the natural world due to climate change.

Anyone distressed by the actualities of global warming must first come to terms with deeply disturbing and complicated realities. Reflection on the real possibility of environmental and social collapse can initiate this process of acceptance, so-called "deep adaptation" (Bendell 2018). Psychiatrists must help patients process this traumatic reality and come to new sustainable ways of thinking and acting. General psychology programs such as transformational resilience and positive trauma therapy, a program for posttraumatic growth, have been developed to promote the new modes of living that can come from such deep processing.

Climate change adaptation also requires acting now for distant results, effectiveness in the face of helplessness, decision making when socio-environmental assumptions no longer hold, and other complicated dialectics. Psychiatrists can facilitate the process of deep reflection on these complexities by providing a holding environment that contains the patient's contradictory anxieties. and keeps the extreme ends of such dialectics in contact with each other. For example, a patient may simultaneously grieve a daughter's decision not to put children into the declining world and the suffering that children born now will face. Allowing the patient to hold both in mind can be a first step toward building the capacity to think about the problems ahead without traumatic affective responses or disavowal. This dialectical strategy can also increase the capacity for containment of uncertain and complex realities (Lewis et al. 2020). The psychiatrist can provide value by helping the patient cultivate a sense of self that can be a safe haven regardless of the level of external threat. This can often be facilitated by cognitive-behavioral techniques that review exactly how one might think or feel even under the worst-case scenario. Spiritual growth that distances survival of the epistemological self from physical survival or physical change can reduce anxiety in this way. Values from older cultures such as the Native Americans or religions such as Buddhism that define the individual as part of a larger and cyclical natural community, including plants, animals, and the cosmos, can also reduce the anxiety about threats to the self and promote peaceful adaptation amidst difficulty (Nadel 2018).

Through acceptance of and reflection upon the traumatic losses of climate change, patients can be helped to see what is happening and their own role in it as part of a cohesive narrative about our modern situation, without disavowal, denial, or catastrophic anxiety. This can then become a starting point for further behavioral change and growth, whether toward eco-friendly preindustrial ways of living, or toward the creative use of technological and biotechnological innovations that will contribute to the paradigm shift away from continual exploitation of nature's resources.

Value in Mitigating Carbon Impacts of Psychiatric Service Delivery

In designing these new systems, psychiatrists must reconsider the carbon footprint of all aspects of care delivery and must be prepared to significantly shift the financial and professional benefits obtained from how mental health care is practiced. A variety of radical changes must be proposed.

The maintenance of inpatient units, travel to and from psychiatric sessions, and the number of pharmaceuticals prescribed are factors that significantly impact the carbon footprint of mental health care (Yarlagadda et al. 2014). Pharmaceuticals are the most important source of emissions, followed by business services, equipment, electricity, and gas (Maughan 2015). Psychiatrists can cut the carbon impacts of pharmaceuticals in practice by giving smaller initial prescriptions, minimizing polypharmacy, and avoiding use of medications with low therapeutic yield (Morden et al. 2014).

Mobile mental health teams, family members, or peer psychosocial support can keep patients safe outside the hospital (Pfeiffer et al. 2011). Decreasing length of stay and referral to outpatient programs, if locally available, can also lower the number of inpatient days, and thus psychiatric beds necessary. Efforts can be taken to reduce the carbon costs of maintaining heat and electricity and staff, all of whom must travel to work, for 24 hours per day. Units can also be "greened" to reduce their carbon footprint by lowering food waste, decreasing the use of disposable items, and improving energy efficiency.

Patient travel to a medical clinic has also been estimated to use approximately four times the carbon as treatment conducted remotely (Holmner et al. 2014). Telephone-based treatment has been shown to be as effective as office visits and is carbon-neutral (Hilty et al. 2013), but it needs to be reimbursed by its length and content to the same degree as in-person treatment. Geographically distributed care, collaborative care, and telemedicine can further dramatically decrease the carbon costs of patients getting to doctors' visits, but with the slight sacrifice of one-to-one experience, which has value outside of treatment outcome (see Chapter 10, "Applications of Technology"). Taking the psychiatrist to the patients or using flexible office models, in which provider schedules are staggered or offices are shared, can maximize the use of available physical space and minimize energy usage.

One psychiatrist driving to a rural office to see 15 patients uses only 6% of the fossil fuel that is used if those patients drive to see the psychiatrist. The psychiatrist must be supported to achieve the same comfortable holding environment and sense of stability that are known to be therapeutic in adapting to these new practices, perhaps through telephone contact, placing familiar items in the office on visit days, or continuity of local staff.

Professional organizations currently receive significant benefits from carbon-intensive practices. Conferences generate a good deal of income for professional societies, and the number of people who fly to attend them and associated food waste are substantial. These events are encouraged by more favorable rates from airlines and conference centers, but they generate high levels of carbon waste. Reducing the number of conferences per year, investing in high-quality online programming, with monitoring and rewards for completion equivalent to the social rewards of professional travel and networking, and increased support for local professional organizations, are all ways of decreasing the carbon costs of professional education.

Conclusion

The mental health impacts of climate change require us as psychiatrists to develop specific medical expertise in heat-related illness, air pollution impacts, and treatment of environmental conditions and traumas. More importantly, they require a paradigm change in how we conceptualize health that includes care-giving attachment to the natural world and a greater emphasis on prevention of damage to environmental determinants of human health. Organized psychiatry must identify professional values associated with climate preservation and develop a research and response agenda for climate-related impacts on mental health. Using established international databases and models, we must both prepare for increasing service demand, particularly of vulnerable populations, and innovate changes to service delivery in chaotic or rapidly evolving conditions. To do no harm, we must reduce our professional carbon footprint to serve our patients sustainably, and work to promote a national psychology that improves human health through a secure attachment to nature and pro-environmental psychological traits. We must use our knowledge of denial, disavowal, cognitive biases, and anxiety to help patients align climate-relevant behaviors with their own health interests, and to tolerate difficult climate realities without annihilation of the psychological self and with the preservation of active hope. Embedded within these goals is the value of using our scientific expertise and our understanding of how the human mind can work against itself to prevent suffering and deliver care where it will waste least and work best, by shifting our understanding of what is truly valuable from a consumption-oriented individualistic model to one that encompasses a broader view of life and time.

References

Adger WN, Goulden M, Lorenzoni I, et al: Are there social limits to adaptation to climate change? Climatic Change 93(3):335–354, 2008

Albrecht G, Sartore G-M, Connor L, et al: Solastalgia: the distress caused by environmental change, Australas Psychiatry 15(1):S95–98, 2007

American Psychiatric Association: Diagnostic and Statistical Manual of Mental Disorders, 5th Edition. Washington, DC, American Psychiatric Association, 2013

Anderson CA: Temperature and aggression: ubiquitous effects of heat on occurrence of human violence. Psychol Bull 106(1):74–96, 1989

Asugeni J, MacLaren D, Massey P: Mental health issues from rising sea levels in a remote coast region of the Solomon Islands: current and future. Australas Psychiatry 23(6):22–25, 2015

Bakian AV, Huber RS, Coon H, et al: Acute air pollution and risk of suicide completion. Am J Epidemiol 181(5):295–303, 2015

Balle WF, Buckman R, Lenzi R, et al: SPIKES—a six step protocol for delivering bad news: application to the patient with cancer. Oncologist 5(9):302–311, 2000

Ballew MT, Leiserowitz A, Roser-Renouf C, et al: Climate change in the American mind: data, tools, and trends, Environment: Science and Policy for Sustainable Development 61(3):4–18, 2019

Barreau T, Conway D, Haught K, et al: Physical, mental and financial impacts from drought in two California counties. Am J Public Health 107(5):783–790, 2017

Baylis P, Obradovich N, Kryvasheyeu Y, et al: Weather impacts expressed sentiment. PLoS One 13(4):e0195750, 2018

Bendell J: Deep adaptation: a map for navigating climate tragedy. IFLAS Occasional Paper 2. July 27, 2018. Available at: www.lifeworth.com/deepadaptation.pdf. Accessed March 23, 2020.

Bhise MC, Behere PB: Risk factors for farmers' suicides in central rural India: matched case-control psychological autopsy study. Indian J Psychol Med 38(6):560–566, 2016

Bouchama A, Dehbi M, Mohamed G, et al: Prognostic factors in heat wave–related deaths: a meta-analysis. Arch Intern Med 167(20):2170–2176, 2007

Burke M, Gonzalez F, Baylis P, et al: Higher temperatures increase suicide rates in the United States and Mexico. Nature Climate Change 8:723–729, 2018

Cacciottolo M, Wang X, Driscoll I, et al: Particulate air pollutants, APOE alleles and their contributions to cognitive impairment in older women and to amyloidogenesis in experimental models. Transl Psychiatry 7(2):e1022, 2017

Calderón-Garcidueñas L, Leray E, Heydarpour P, et al: Air pollution, a rising environmental risk factor for cognition, neuroinflammation and neurodegeneration: the clinical impact on children and beyond. Rev Neurol (Paris) 172(2):69–80, 2016

Carleton TA: Crop-damaging temperatures increase suicide rates in India. Proc Natl Acad Sci 114(33):8746–8751, 2017

Carleton TA, Hsiang SM, Burke M: Conflict in a changing climate. European Physical Journal Special Topics 225(3):489–511, 2016

Carleton TA, Delgado M, Greenstone M, et al: Valuing the global mortality consequences of climate change accounting for adaptation costs and benefits. Climate Impact Lab Consortium, Becker Friedman Institute for Economics. Working Paper No 2018-51, 2018. Available at: https://epic.uchicago.edu/wp-content/uploads/2019/07/Working-Paper-2.pdf. Accessed March 23, 2020.

Chen JC, Wang X, Wellenius GA, et al: Ambient air pollution and neurotoxicity on brain structure: evidence from Women's Health Initiative Memory Study. Ann Neurol 78(3):466–476, 2015

Collins M, Knutti R, Arblaster J, et al: Long-term climate change: projections, commitments and irreversibility, in Climate Change 2013: The Physical Science Basis. Contribution of Working Group I to the Fifth Assessment Report of the Intergovernmental Panel on Climate Change. Edited by Stocker TF, Qin D, Plattner G-K, et al. Cambridge, UK, Cambridge University Press, 2013

Costello A, Abbas M, Allen A, et al: Manage the health effects of climate change: Lancet and University College London Institute for Global Health Commission. Lancet 373(1):1693–1733, 2009

Crost B, Duequennois C, Felter JH, et al: Climate change, agricultural production and civil conflict: evidence from the Philippines. Journal of Environmental Economics and Management 88(C):379–395, 2017

Cunsolo-Willox A, Harper S, Ford JD, et al: From this place and of this place: climate change, sense of place, and health in Nunatsiavut, Canada. Soc Sci Med 75(7):538–547, 2012

Denissen JJA, Penke L, Penke L, et al: The effects of weather on daily mood: a multilevel approach. Emotion 8(5):662–667, 2008

Dittrich R, Wreford A, Moran D: A survey of decision making approaches for climate change adaptation: are robust measures the way forward? Ecological Economics 122:79–89, 2015

Ebi KL, Bole JM, Crimmins A, et al: Human health, in Impacts, Risks, and Adaptation in the United States: Fourth National Climate Assessment, Volume II. Edited by Reidmiller DR, Avery CW, Easterling DR, et al. Washington, DC, U.S. Global Change Research Program, 2018, pp 572–603

Ellis NR, Albrecht GA: Climate change threats to family farmers' sense of place and mental wellbeing: a case study from the Western Australian Wheatbelt. Soc Sci Med 175:161–168, 2017

El-Sayed A, Kamel M: Climate changes and their role in the emergence and re-emergence of disease, Environmental Science and Pollution Research 27:22336–22352, 2020

Firth J, Rosenbaum S, Ward PB, et al: Adjunctive nutrients in first episode psychosis: a systemic review of the efficacy tolerability and neurobiological mechanisms. Early Interv Psychiatry 12(5):774–783, 2018

Fouillet A, Rey G, Laurent F, et al: Excess mortality related to the August 2003 heat wave in France. Int Arch Occup Environ Health 80(2):16–24, 2006

Fountoulakis KN, Chatzikosta I, Pastiadis K, et al: Relationship of suicide rates with climate and economic variables in Europe during 2000–2012. Ann Gen Psychiatry 15:19, 2016

Gao JJ, Cheng Q, Duan J, et al: Ambient temperature, sunlight duration, and suicide: a comprehensive review and meta-analysis. Sci Total Environ 646:1021–1029, 2019

Global Burden of Disease Collaborative Network: Global Burden of Disease Study 2017: Burden by Risk 1990–2018. Seattle, WA, Institute for Health Metrics and Evaluation, 2017

Goldman E, Galea S: Mental health consequences of disasters. Annu Rev Public Health 35:169–183, 2014

Gosling SN, Lowe J, McGregor GR, et al: Associations between elevated atmospheric temperature and human mortality: a critical review of the literature. Climatic Change 92(3–4):299–341, 2009a

Gosling SN, McGregor GR, Lowe JA: Climate change and heat-related mortality in six cities. Part 2: climate model evaluation and projected impacts from changes in the mean and variability of temperature with climate change. Int J Biometeorol 53(1):31–51, 2009b

Gu X, Liu Q, Deng F, et al: Association between particulate matter air pollution and risk of depression and suicide: systematic review and meta-analysis. Br J Psychiatry 205(3):256–267, 2019

Hanna EG, Tait PW: Limitations to thermoregulation and acclimatization challenge human adaptation to global warming. Int J Environ Res Public Health 12(7):8034–8074, 2015

Hayhoe K, Kossin JP, Sweet WV, et al: Our changing climate, in Impacts, Risks, and Adaptation in the United States: Fourth National Climate Assessment, Volume II. Edited by Reidmiller DR, Avery CW, Easterling DR, et al. Washington, DC, U.S. Global Change Research Program, 2018, pp 72–144

Hess JJ, McDowell JZ, Luber G: Integrating climate change adaptation into public health practice: using adaptive management to increase adaptive capacity and build resilience. Environ Health Perspect 120(2):171–179, 2012

Hilty DM, Ferrer DC, Parish MB, et al: The effectiveness of telemental health: a 2013 review. Telem J E Health 19(6):444–454, 2013

Holmner A, Ebi KL, Lazuardi L, et al: Carbon footprint of telemedicine solutions: unexplored opportunity for reducing carbon use in the health sector. PLoS One 9(9):e105040, 2014

Hsiang SM, Burke M, Miguel E: Quantifying the influence of climate on human conflict. Science 341(6151):1235367, 2013

Intergovernmental Panel on Climate Change: Summary for policymakers, in Climate Change 2014: Impacts, Adaptation, and Vulnerability: Part A: Global and Sectoral Aspects. Contribution of Working Group II to the Fifth Assessment Report of the Intergovernmental Panel on Climate Change. Edited by Field CB, Barros VR, Dokken DJ, et al. Cambridge, UK, Cambridge University Press, 2014, pp 1–32.

Jaramillo P, Muller NZ: Air pollution emissions and damages from energy production in the U.S.: 2002–2011. Energy Policy 90:202–211, 2016

Johannesson KB, Arinell H, Arnberg FK: Six years after the wave: trajectories of posttraumatic stress following a natural disaster. J Anxiety Disord 36:15–24, 2015

Jones MK, Wootton BM, Vaccaro LD, et al: The impact of climate change on obsessive compulsive checking concerns. Aust NZ J Psychiatry 46(3):265–270, 2012

Jones RN, Patwardhan A, Cohen SJ, et al: Foundations for decision making, in Climate Change 2014: Impacts, Adaptation and Vulnerability, Part A: Global and Sectoral Aspects. Contribution of Working Group II to the Fifth Assessment Report of the Intergovernmental Panel on Climate Change. Edited by Field CB, Barros VR, Dokken DJ, et al. New York, Cambridge University Press, 2014, pp 195–228

Jun TK: Temperature, maize yield, and civil conflicts in sub-Saharan Africa. Climatic Change 142(1):183–197, 2017

Khan A, Plana-Ripoll O, Antonsen S, et al: Environmental pollution is associated with increased risk of psychiatric disorders in the U.S. and Denmark. PLOS Biology 17(8):e3000353, 2019

Kim YH, Chris Fook Sheng Ng, Antonsen S, et al: Air pollution and suicide in ten cities in Southeast Asia, a time-stratified case-crossover analysis. Environ Health Perspect 126(3):37002–37019, 2018

Knowlton K, Rotkin-Ellman M, Galatea K, et al: The 2006 California heat wave: impacts on hospitalizations and emergency room visits. Environ Health Perspect 117(1):61–67, 2016

Landrigan P, Fuller R, Acosta NJR, et al: The Lancet Commission on Pollution and Health. Lancet 390(10119):462–512, 2018

Larrick RP, Timmerman TA, Carton AM, et al: Temper, temperature, and temptation: heat-related retaliation in baseball. Psychol Sci 22(4):423–438, 2011

Lewis J, Haase E, Trope A: Climate dialectics in psychotherapy: holding open the space between abyss and advance, Psychodyn Psychiatry 48(3), 2020

Li SS, Liddel BJ, Nickerson A: The relationship between post-migration stress and psychological disorders in refugees and asylum seekers. Curr Psychiatry Rep 18(9):82, 2016

Li T, Horton RM, Bader DA, et al: Long term projections of temperature related mortality risks for ischemic stroke, hemorrhagic stroke, and acute ischemic heart disease under change climate in Beijing, China. Environment International 112:1–9, 2018

Lian H, Ruan Y, Liang R, et al: Short-term effect of ambient temperature and the risk of stroke: a systematic review and meta-analysis. Int J Environ Res Public Health 12(8):9068–9088, 2015

Livingston G, Sommerlad A, Orgeta V, et al: Dementia prevention, intervention, and care. Lancet 390(10113):2673–2734, 2017

Lutz W, Sanderson W, Scherbov S: The coming acceleration of global population ageing. Nature 451(7179):716–719, 2008

Macy J: Active Hope: How to Face the Mess We're in Without Going Crazy. Novato, CA, New World Library, 2012, pp 2–3, 35

Marlon J, Howe P, Mildenberger M, et al: Yale climate opinion maps 2018. Yale Program on Climate Communications, 2018. Available at: https://climatecommunication.yale.edu/visualizations-data/ycom-us-2018/?est=happening&type=value&geo=county. Accessed March 23, 2020.

Martin-Latry K, Goumy MP, Philippe L, et al: Psychotropic drug use and risk of heat-related hospitalization. Eur Psychiatry 22(6):335–338, 2007

Masson-Delmotte V, Zhai P, Portner HO, et al (eds): Global Warming of 1.5°C: an IPCC special report on the impacts of global warming of 1.5°C above pre-industrial levels and related global greenhouse gas emission pathways, in the context of strengthening the global response to the threat of climate change, sustainable development, and efforts to eradicate poverty. Intergovernmental Panel of Climate Change, 2018. Available at: www.ipcc.ch/site/assets/uploads/sites/2/2019/06/SR15_Full_Report_Low_Res.pdf. Accessed March 20, 2020.

Maughan D: Sustainability in psychiatry. Occasional paper #97. Center for Sustainable Healthcare, March 2015. Available at: https://networks.sustainablehealthcare.org.uk/file/9617/download?token=TDD6IeZf. Accessed March 23, 2020.

Morden NE, Colla CH, Sequist TD, et al: Choosing wisely—the politics and economics of labeling low-value service. N Engl J Med 370(7):589–592, 2014

Nadel L: The Five Gifts: Discovering Hope, Healing, and Strength When Disaster Strikes. Deerfield Beach, FL, Health Communications, 2018, pp 171–240

NOAA National Centers for Environmental Information: U.S. billion-dollar weather and climate disasters. 2020. Available at: www.ncdc.noaa.gov/billions. Accessed July 2019.

Noelke C, McGovern M, Corsi DJ, et al: Increasing ambient temperature reduced emotional well-being. Environ Res 151:124–129, 2016

Norris F, Elrod C: Psychosocial consequences of disaster: a review of past research, in Methods for Disaster Mental Health Research. Edited by Norris F, Galea S, Friedman M, et al. New York, Guilford, 2006, pp 20–42

North CS, Pfefferbaum B: Mental health response to community disasters: a systematic review. JAMA 310(5):507–518, 2013

Obradovich N, Migliorini R, Paulus MP, et al: Empirical evidence of mental health risks posed by climate change. Proc Natl Acad Sci USA 115(43):10953–10958, 2018

Ostapchuk J, Harper S, Rigolet Inuit Community Government: Exploring elders' and seniors' perceptions of how climate change is impacting health and well-being in Rigolet, Nunatsiavut. International Journal of Indigenous Health 9(2):6–24, 2015

Paranjothy S, Gallacher J, Amlôt R, et al: Psychosocial impact of the summer 2007 floods in England. BMC Public Health 11(145):1–8, 2011

Perera FP: Multiple threats to child health from fossil fuel combustion: impacts of air pollution and climate change. Environ Health Perspect 125(3):141–148, 2017

Pfeiffer PN, Heisler M, Piette JD, et al: Efficacy of peer support interventions for depression: a meta-analysis. Gen Hosp Psychiatry 33(2):29–36, 2011

Porter M, Haslam N: Pre-displacement and post-displacement factors associated with mental health of refugees and internally displaced persons. JAMA 294(5):602–612, 2005

Ranger N, Surminski S: A preliminary assessment of the impact of climate change on non-life insurance demand in the BRICS economies. International Journal of Disaster Risk Reduction 3(1):14–30, 2013

Ransom M: Crime, weather, and climate change. Journal of Environmental Economics and Management 67:274–302, 2014

Ripley A: The Unthinkable: Who Survives When Disaster Strikes. New York, Three Rivers Press, 2009, pp 57–75

Robbins L, Ransom J: He called out sick then apologized for leaving this world. New York Times, April 16, 2018. Available at: https://main-viral-news.blogspot.com/2018/04/the-new-york-times-he-called-out-sick.html. Accessed March 20, 2020.

Rosenheim N, Grabick S, Horney JA: Disaster impacts on costs and utilization of Medicare. BMC Health Serv Res 18(89):3–9, 2019

Scherer G: IPCC predictions: then versus now. The Daily Climate, December 11, 2012. Available at: www.climatecentral.org/news/ipcc-predictions-then-versus-now-15340. Accessed April 13, 2020.

Schwartz JD, Mihye L, Kinney PL, et al: Projections of temperature-attributable premature deaths in 209 U.S. cities using a cluster-based Poisson approach. Environ Health 14:85, 2015

Smith JB, Alpert A, Buizer JL, et al: Climate effects on U.S. international interests, in Impacts, Risks, and Adaptation in the United States: Fourth National Climate Assessment, Volume II. Edited by Reidmiller DR, Avery CW, Easterling DR, et al. Washington, DC, U.S. Global Change Research Program, 2018, pp 604–637

Spence A, Poortinga W, Pidgeon N: The psychological distance of climate change. Risk Anal 32(6):957–972, 2012

Thoresen S, Birkeland MS, Arnberg FK, et al: Long-term mental health and social support in victims of disaster: comparison with a general population sample. BJPsych Open 5(2):e22, 2019

Thulius O: Thermal reactions of blood vessels in vascular stroke and heatstroke. Med Princ Pract 15(4):316–321, 2006

U.S. Global Change Research Program: Climate Science Special Report: Fourth National Climate Assessment, Volume I (Wuebbles DJ, Fahey DW, Hibbard KA, et al, editors). Washington, DC, U.S. Global Change Research Program, 2017

Van Vuuren DP, Edmonds J, Kainuma M, et al: The representative concentration pathways: an overview. Climatic Change 109:5–31, 2011

Vardoulakis S, Kear K, Hajat S: Comparative assessment of the effects of climate change on heat and cold-related mortality in the United Kingdom and Australia. Env Health Perspect 122(22):1285–1292, 2014

Vose RS, Easterling DR, Kunkel KE, Wehner MF: Temperature changes in the United States, in Climate Science Special Report: A Sustained Assessment Activity of the U.S. Global Change Research Program. Edited by Wuebbles DJ, Fahey DW, Hibbard KA, et al. Washington, DC, U.S. Global Change Research Program, 2017, pp 267–300

Wang J, Um P, Dickerman BA, Liu J: Zinc, magnesium, selenium and depression: a review of the evidence, potential mechanisms, and implications, Nutrients 10(5):584, 2018

Weuve J, Puett RC, Schwartz J, et al: Exposure to particulate air pollution and cognitive decline in older women. Arch Intern Med 172(3):219–227, 2012

Wuebbles DJ, Meehl G, Hayhoe K, et al: Climate model analysis: climate extremes in the United States. Bulletin of the American Meteorological Society 95:571–658, 2014

Yarlagadda S, Maughan D, Lingwood S, et al: Sustainable psychiatry in the U.K. Psychiatric Bull 38(6):285–290, 2014

19

Incarceration Reform

Michelle Joy, M.D.

The United States has an enormous and complex correctional system. Rates of incarceration in the United States are almost five times the global average and are higher than those of any other country (Adler et al. 2016; Dvoskin et al. 2017). The number of incarcerated people in America quadrupled between 1982 and 2007 (Swanson et al. 2013). Swelling of the justice-involved population has disproportionately affected racial/ethnic minorities, particularly young Black men, with as many as 1 in 3 men in their 30s incarcerated at any given time (Mauer 2011). In 2010, approximately 2.3 million individuals were incarcerated and many more were under community supervision (Barboriak 2017).

Presently, the criminal justice system is the largest provider of behavioral health treatment in the United States. Conservative estimates suggest that approximately 10%–15% of persons behind bars have a primary mental health problem that would benefit from treatment and that 7%–9% of persons on probation or parole have serious mental illness (Pinals 2017). Schizophrenia and major mood disorders are two to three times more prevalent in jails than in the general population (Dvoskin et al. 2017). In addition, over two-thirds of people in jail and half of people in prison have substance use disorders (Peters et al. 2015).

Since 1970 and the widespread closure of psychiatric facilities, individuals with mental illness have increasingly been housed in jails and prisons rather than in hospitals (Munetz et al. 2001; Rich et al. 2011; Torrey et al. 2014). This trend was exacerbated by the failure to establish a community mental health system adequately equipped to meet the needs of people with mental illness. In 2012, there were 10 times more people with severe mental illness in jails and prisons than in state hospitals (Torrey et al. 2014). The correctional system implicitly functions in ways that adversely affect mental health due to both undertreatment and exacerbation of illness. Compared with other individuals with mental health problems, those with forensic involvement have more disrupted care, poorer outcomes, and a higher risk of mortality (Pinals 2014). For these reasons, justice-involved mental health care is an important topic to discuss, with a focus on the delivery, costs, and outcomes in which psychiatrists can play a significant role.

Theories of Punishment

The criminal justice system theoretically serves a multiplicity of purposes. Deterrence, isolation, retribution, restitution, and rehabilitation are all goals of the courts, and through them, goals of society. Although psychiatrists are most likely to focus on potential rehabilitative opportunities of criminal justice, it is important to understand the system's many purposes. For one, the possibility of punishment is thought to deter individuals from enacting future crimes as well as to deter other individuals in society from ever committing a crime. Second, incarcerated individuals are removed from society and therefore unable to enact harm to society at large. One goal of the courts is to enact justice or to provide fair punishment for wrongs, through incarceration, probation, fines, and other penalties. Last, and most important for psychiatrists, the criminal justice system may provide treatment to reduce psychological suffering and/or the probability of future crimes.

Although criminal justice systems put forth various goals for incarceration, there are reasons to be critical of its outcomes. Indeed, at times the term *criminal justice* appears to be an oxymoron for those affected by arrest, incarceration, and probation. There are various negative outcomes that can accompany arrest. To commit a crime is to transgress the boundaries of social morality, but it is questionable whether justice is truly served by punitive approaches. Is the legal system effective at deterrence and rehabilitation, or are the only effectively achieved aims of the system those of isolation, retribution, and restitution? There are reasons to believe that the system prioritizes punishment over the more constructive goals, although this opinion is clearly opposed by some people.

Negative Outcomes of Punitive Approaches

To properly consider these questions, one must weigh the evidence for positive change against the various costs of punitive approaches. Potential harms include social disruption, reinforcement of antisocial behaviors, traumatization, exacerbation of mental illness, worsened physical health outcomes, recidivism, and social unrest, as explored in this chapter. Similarly, it is important to examine whether the goals of punishment, including deterrence of future crime, are achieved.

Although it is true that incarcerated individuals are taken away from communities in which they might cause harm, they are also removed from their community social systems. For example, parents who are incarcerated can no longer provide income or child-rearing for their families. Incarceration adversely affects the mental and behavioral health of individuals' family members in the community (Massoglia and Pridemore 2015). These effects are particularly profound in minority communities, given the astounding rates of arrest and incarceration of people who live in them (Massoglia and Pridemore 2015). Compared with white children, African American and Hispanic children, respectively, are 7.5 and 2.5 times more likely to have an incarcerated parent (Adler et al. 2016). Disruption of productive activity further pushes communities toward poverty and neglect, which are often driving factors in future criminal behavior.

Time spent incarcerated may also further the learning and expression of antisocial behaviors. When a person enters jail or prison, the individual's community or culture instantly becomes one of other inmates. A portion of antisocial behavior is learned socially, and during incarceration, one's peers consist entirely of those who have been accused of crimes. This observation is particularly important for juveniles, adolescents, and young adults who are most susceptible to the social learning of criminal behavior. Peer groups serve as very strong motivators of behavior in younger individuals, and their patterns of behavior (and even neurological functioning) are not yet formalized or set. The societal structures that exist within incarcerated settings are often strongly linked to criminal behavior (or criminal posturing). As a result, expression of criminality is often learned, supported, and valued during incarceration.

Incarceration can also have traumatizing effects. Some of these outcomes occur because of the value on and exposure to criminal behavior in such settings, as discussed above. Violence occurring in correctional settings includes victimization from staff and other inmates, as well as the witnessing of such violence. Inmate assaults on staff also occur. Confinement in an overcrowded and isolative environment can be traumatic even in the absence of specific incidents of trauma such as assault. Given that incarcerated individuals already have higher than average exposure to previous traumas, they are also sensitive to the effects of repeat or compounded traumatization.

The trauma of incarceration can affect anyone who enters the walls of a jail or prison. The very process of arrest and subsequent loss of rights, autonomy, and privacy can be distressing. However, the effects of incarceration on those with mental illness are particularly profound. The effects, including loss of community, antisocial learning, and traumatization, have exacerbating effects on those struggling with mental health problems (Kirk and Wakefield 2018; Rich et al. 2011; Sugie and Turney 2017). As state hospitals closed across the country and community mental health services struggled toward optimal implementation of community supports and services, the criminal justice system became a primary location for housing, supervision, and treatment of those with mental health problems. This process has commonly been described as *transinstitutionalization* (Primeau et al. 2013) and has been associated with significant cost expenditures. In Pennsylvania alone, transinstitutionalization was estimated to cost $82.3 million annually over 32 years (Primeau et al. 2013).

Although treatment of mental illness is available and improving in jails and prisons, efficacy is limited by low rates of identification and limited treatment modalities. There is a particularly glaring lack of available treatment for individuals who have substance use disorders (Belenko et al. 2013), although this has been improving in response to the opioid epidemic through the implementation of medication-assisted treatment (MAT). Rates of suicide and self-harm are also high among incarcerated individuals. In addition, solitary confinement often has a profound impact on mental illness (Kupers 2017).

There is a trend toward change, however. Correctional health and behavioral health organizations have denounced the use of solitary confinement, particularly for those with mental health problems, and have developed position papers and guidelines to limit its use (Garcia et al. 2016). Nonetheless, the lack of treatment persists and is complicated by the fact that researchers conduct very few studies on treatment of incarcerated individuals due to ethical protections for persons behind bars. Thus, psychosocial and biological therapies often lack a firm evidence base with respect to helping this specific population, which may have unique characteristics and needs that would be best served by specific treatments.

In addition to having effects on mental health, incarceration can have a negative impact on physical health. Being behind bars is associated with worsened mortality rates, chronic health problems, obesity, and increased transmission of infectious diseases such as HIV, tuberculosis, and hepatitis (Adler et al. 2016; Massoglia and Pridemore 2015). Health needs for inmates are often affected by treatment delays, restrictive prescription formularies, and lack of access to emergency and specialty services. Apart from the direct effects of incarceration on mental health, difficulties with physical aspects of health indirectly impact emotional well-being, adding to the overall mental health burden. Undertreatment of both mental and physical health problems is more pronounced for minorities and juveniles, especially African American and Hispanic youth (Davis and Shlafer 2017).

The question of whether incarceration increases or decreases recidivism of criminal behaviors is particularly important. Deterrence of future crime is one of the highest goals of the criminal justice system; however, the impact of incarceration on recidivism is not well understood. On the one hand, it may create a fear of going back to jail. On the other hand, it may result in normalization and acculturation to incarceration, learning of antisocial behavior, increased poverty and stigma, and social disruption—factors that have the potential to increase crime and recidivism. Overall, research on incarceration's effects on recidivism is mixed, with some studies supporting increases, others decreases, and some no change at all (Mears et al. 2015). The severity and length of penalties can variably affect outcomes (Mears and Cochran 2018), as can the type of crime that is punished—for example, incarceration does not decrease recidivism for drug offenses (Mitchell et al. 2017).

However, viewing recidivism through the lens of how incarceration impacts an individual's tendency to commit future crime is short-sighted in its singular focus. Such analyses typically concentrate on the individual, when in fact incarceration must also be viewed in terms of its effects on larger communities. Thus, an important additional question is whether the societal practice of incarceration works to prevent crime within the larger contexts of neighborhoods, cities, states, and even countries, and whether any benefits outweigh negative impacts on such social sectors as education, employment, housing, families, communities, and society. Weighing the costs and benefits of incarceration stands at the heart of this chapter and its proposed models, which are discussed in subsequent sections.

Prevention

The array of possible outcomes associated with incarceration makes it a particularly fruitful—though complex—ground for examination. As stated in the introduction to this chapter, rates of incarceration in the United States are the highest in the world. Given this high rate (partly due to high rates of recidivism), it appears that goals such as deterrence and rehabilitation are not—or at best only somewhat—attained. If that is the case, then the associated social disruption, reinforcement of antisocial behaviors, traumatization, exacerbation of mental illness, and social unrest make it a very costly and ineffective intervention that is hard to justify.

Of course, the various goals of the criminal justice system are valued to different extents by distinct sections of society. For example, political candidates often make statements strongly valuing deterrence, isolation, restitution, and retribution. Victims and victims' rights advocates might support similar goals. Different communities and neighborhoods may vary in the amount that they value deterrence versus rehabilitation depending on the social makeup of their constituents. Psychiatrists have a clear role in evaluating the effect of incarceration on potential rehabilitation, as well as some of the system's negative social and behavioral repercussions. Removing individuals from their community and placing them in a stressful, isolated, and antisocial context is not inherently restorative. Incarceration is intended to be unpleasant in order to deter and punish. Without these characteristics, those goals would not be perceived as achieved by many Americans. Thus, jail or prison is not often an ideal setting for a process of recovery from psychiatric difficulties. Some incarcerated persons with behavioral problems may be positively impacted by various elements of structure, hierarchy, and contingency, but it is safe to say that incarceration, in and of itself, is not fundamentally rehabilitative. Therefore, it is important to assess complements and changes to current criminal justice practices that might enhance rehabilitative aims.

One way to do this is by looking at model programs that function at different points throughout the criminal justice system and benefit from the engagement of psychiatrists. This chapter proposes roles for psychiatrists using the model of primary, secondary, and tertiary prevention. Primary prevention aims to prevent disease or injury before it occurs, secondary prevention reduces the impact of disease or injury, and tertiary prevention reduces the impact of such impairments. (See Chapter 8, "Prevention and Health Promotion," for additional information on this general topic.) In this chapter, the three levels of this prevention model typically used for disease or injury are adapted and used instead for primary, secondary, and tertiary prevention of *incarceration* (and related crimes). The chapter employs the framework of 1) preventing crime before it occurs, 2) identifying those committing early or low-level crimes before committing other crimes, and 3) controlling potential harms of involvement in the criminal justice system. Each program addressing health and crime must be viewed not only for its impact on rehabilitation outcomes (and possibly the other goals of criminal justice) but also for its impacts on financial systems, mental health providers, and of course, service users themselves.

Primary Prevention of Crime

Prevention of crime should be an attractive solution for everyone and may occur through various means. Prevention is a proactive, public health approach that exists outside the predominantly punitive methods of the criminal justice system. Given the high and rising costs of this system, effective prevention programs are usually cost-effective, especially when compared with imprisonment (Welsh and Farrington 2018; Welsh et al. 2015).

The most helpful population to intervene with prevention efforts is youth. Even in 1967, the U.S. President's Commission on Law Enforcement and Administration of Justice put forth that "America's best hope for reducing crime is to reduce juvenile delinquency and youth crime" (p. 55). In the United States, juvenile actions account for approximately 11% of all crime, 18% of property crimes, and 12% of violent crimes (Sawyer et al. 2015). Working with youth, at a time when behavior and life trajectory are still quite adaptable, can allow for intervention before criminal behavior occurs.

Antisocial Behavior

Antisocial personality traits are a clear target for crime prevention, given their association with participation in unlawful behaviors. Antisocial behaviors begin in childhood and develop over time. Their numerous neuropsychological and environmental risk factors include genetics, peer influence, male gender, low socioeconomic status, poor parent-child relationships, and early abuse (Douglas and Bell 2011; Moffitt 2017; Raine 2002). Antisocial behavior is described as the costliest of juvenile mental health problems, making prevention a promising, cost-effective approach to mental health services, juvenile justice, and education (Sawyer et al. 2015). Although antisocial personality disorder is viewed as relatively fixed once established, the trajectories of children's behavior problems toward persistent pathology are malleable if addressed early (Reidy et al. 2015). Numerous psychosocial interventions, although rarely implemented, have shown efficacy for longer-term modification of antisocial behavior (Dodge et al. 2014; Kingston et al. 2016; Sawyer et al. 2015). Public health approaches are aimed toward individuals embedded in social networks and aim to enhance positive community relationships, increase self-esteem, minimize trauma, and enhance social and emotional skills (Douglas and Bell 2011). Intervention is most successful in programs that are multimodal, involve caregivers, and occur across social contexts and developmental stages. Family-based interventions, including parenting and child-rearing classes, are particularly helpful for female and minority populations. There is some risk in utilizing group formats because antisocial behavior can be supported by peers or transmitted through these interventions. Young children, such as those in preschool, however, do benefit from group formats for preventing antisocial behavior as compared with other age groups (Sawyer et al. 2015).

Research has shown that community-based developmental programs, whether implemented with individuals, families, or schools, are effective at preventing antisocial behavior (Farrington et al. 2017; Sandler et al. 2014). These interventions are useful in reducing future aggression, violence, delinquency, and criminal offenses. The content and format of programs may vary but often include teaching children social, behavioral, and cognitive skills, as well as approaches to interpersonal problem solving. Other programs may work with families, including parenting and child-rearing classes. In school, programs may address elements of the educational culture, including the behaviors of teachers and peers. Table 19–1 lists a variety of interventions that have been effective as antisocial behavior interventions.

In an analysis of 50 systematic reviews of developmental programs, every type of prevention intervention was found to be effective in reducing antisocial behavior (Farrington et al. 2017). A focus on prevention would better enable the criminal justice system's goal of deterrence to be achieved, without the negative outcomes associated with incarceration.

Gun Violence

Another avenue for preventing crime is aimed specifically at reducing violence—particularly gun violence. The United States has much higher rates of homicide than comparable nations, and homicide is a leading cause of death for young males (Miller et al. 2002; Webster et al. 2014). Homicide is a major cause of racial disparities in life expectancies for African American men. Despite the way such events are portrayed by media, most shootings are nonrandom, and up to 85% occur within existing social networks. Homicides are most often committed by relatives, friends, enemies, and acquaintances rather than by unknown, solitary psychopaths (Metzl and MacLeish 2015).

Most homicides are committed with firearms, particularly handguns. Rates of homicide by firearm are 25 times higher in the United States than in similarly economically advantaged countries. There are extensively documented relationships between homicides and gun possession, in both region- and state-level analyses (Metzl and MacLeish 2015). States with more guns have more homicides, homes with guns have more homicides, people with guns are more likely to commit homicide, and purchasing a gun from a licensed dealer is associated with becoming a homicide victim (Webster et al. 2014).

TABLE 19–1. Community-based antisocial behavior interventions

Mentorship
Enrichment programming
Substance use prevention
Family-based counseling
Mental health promotion events
Occupational therapy
Parent and teacher trainings
Outreach to homeless youth
Behavior contracts
Officer education
Reading and music groups
Cognitive-behavioral therapy
Dialectical behavior therapy

Although there is a small epidemiological link between mental illness and violence, it is often grossly overestimated by the public (Rozel and Mulvey 2017). The overwhelming majority of persons with mental health diagnoses are not violent. Only about 4% of criminal violence can be attributed to those with mental illness, and having a diagnosis is 3 times more strongly linked with being a victim than being a perpetrator of crime. The number of people who are simultaneously mentally ill, armed, and potentially violent is actually quite small, although the number varies depending on the nature of the diagnosis. For example, substance abuse, personality disorders, attention-deficit/hyperactivity disorder (ADHD), and possibly initial episodes of psychosis have more significant associations with violence than do serious mental illnesses such as schizophrenia or major depression (Rozel and Mulvey 2017; White 2016).

The high rates of gun violence and homicide in the United States are more closely tied to the presence and availability of guns than to mental illness. Given the public health crisis surrounding firearm violence, psychiatrists have a role in advocating for policy and research interventions for these problems. A 2018 viral social media tag #thisisourlane has brought increasing attention to the role that physicians play in understanding gun violence, suicide by gunshot wound, and firearm injury prevention (Ranney et al. 2018; Taichman et al. 2018). The Black Lives Matter movement—#BlackLivesMatter or #BLM—has advocated for critical inquiry into the increased rates of police violence against Black and other marginalized people since 2013.

Despite these high rates, there have been significant federal limitations of funding for research on guns and public health, due in large part to lobbying efforts by the gun industry and the National Rifle Association. Psychiatrists need to understand the evidence that does exist and to educate others about what is understood among the links (or lack thereof) between violence, firearms, racism, and mental illness. Interventions that focus on the links between mental illness and violence are unlikely to have significant impact (Rozel and Mulvey 2017).

Conservative estimates indicate more than 300 million civilian guns in this country—similar to, or above, the number of people (Rozel and Mulvey 2017). Access to guns can be linked to violence against any person in an individual's social network, including the self. Although self-harm is not the focus of this chapter, such an approach also works to reduce suicide rates. Educating patients about the links between gun ownership and violence is important, as are conversations about safe storage (e.g., locks, safes, smart gun technology). Discussions should be open and fact based without seeming off-putting or threatening to gun owners, many of whom incorporate gun ownership as important parts of their identities and cultures. Psychiatrists should operate under the assumption that patients possess gun(s) even when ownership is not known or denied. Multiple studies have shown that counseling patients about guns, while providing safety devices (e.g., locks or safes), effectively changes people's practices (Rowhani-Rahbar et al. 2016).

Substance Abuse

Substance use has been independently linked to enacting violence, the presence of firearm violence, being a victim of violence, and accidental injury by firearms (Rozel and Mulvey 2017). A strong correlation also exists between substance abuse and criminal offending (White 2016). Substance abuse is also associated with higher rates of income-generating crime and other nonviolent offenses, such as theft, robbery, intoxication, and driving under the influence, as well as drug possession and distribution. The link between mental illness and arrest, especially for drug-related and nonviolent offenses, is largely mediated by co-occurring substance abuse (Swartz and Lurigio 2007). Furthermore, substance use disorders are associated with significant economic and social costs outside of the criminal justice arena, making prevention of substance use very cost-effective for the government and society in general (Committee on Prevention Diagnosis Treatment and Management of Substance Use Disorders in the U.S. Armed Forces et al. 2013).

For prevention of the development of substance use disorders in youth, after-school programming, mentoring, social-emotional learning instruction, and peer support have been found to have small but significant—and sustainable—effects (Sandler et al. 2014). The results are more impactful when the format is interactive rather than didactic. Communities That Care is one program that has been found to be particularly effective in sustainably preventing substance use and violence (Hawkins et al. 2007; Oesterle et al. 2018). Grounded in prevention science, the model works to engage and organize communities for successful implementation of programs that provide prosocial activities, skills training, promotion of bonding, clear standards for behavior, and personal validation.

Overall, the evidence base for prevention of substance use disorders supports programs that address risk and protective factors, and consider developmental stages. These programs effectively use the settings in which they are implemented and have effective management and oversight (Committee on Prevention Diagnosis Treatment and Management of Substance Use Disorders in the U.S. Armed Forces et al. 2013). Teaching skills (e.g., resisting peer pressure, avoiding risky situations, bonding with prosocial peers, regulating emotions and impulses) is more effective than education about facts or attempting to change individual attitudes. Effective interventions for substance use disorders are listed in Table 19–2.

Attention-Deficit/Hyperactivity Disorder

ADHD is associated with a twofold increase in arrests, convictions, and incarcerations, as well as increased risk for earlier and multiple offenses (Mohr-Jensen and Steinhausen 2016). Conceptually, the impulsivity, reward deficiency, and attentional deficits of this disorder correlate with acting out and potentially being incarcerated. Also, individuals with ADHD are at higher risk for developing other comorbid disorders associated with crime, including substance abuse and antisocial personality disorder (Asherson et al. 2016). The prevalence of ADHD in children is approximately 8%, making it the most common mental health diagnosis in this population (Wolraich et al. 2011). Given the high occurrence of this disorder, it is an appropriate target for intervention.

Positive short-term effects of the treatment of ADHD on conduct problems are well known (Lichtenstein et al. 2012). Epidemiological studies show that pharmacological treatment for ADHD is associated with fewer criminal convictions and reduced rates of substance abuse when an individual is maintained on the medication, but this association is not necessarily seen after medication management has ended (Asherson et al. 2016). Because ADHD typically manifests itself in younger individuals, they are an important target for prevention interventions. In this population, another relevant outcome of treating ADHD involves peer influence. Both stimulants and behavior modification treatments reduce rates of reinforcement for deviant peer behavior in children (Helseth et al. 2015). Although

TABLE 19–2. Effective interventions for substance use disorders

Contingency management
Motivational interviewing
Cognitive-behavioral therapy
Relapse prevention training
Family-based counseling
Supported housing
Drug counseling (individual and group)
12-step facilitation
Medication-assisted treatment
Screening, brief intervention, and referral to therapy
Psychodynamic psychotherapy

children with ADHD support the expression of deviant behavior in their peers at higher rates, this can be mediated by pharmacological or therapeutic intervention.

Community Mental Health System

People with mental illness are more likely to be incarcerated for a variety of reasons related to their symptoms or other psychosocial factors leading to their arrest. This reality calls for an accessible, comprehensive, and well-developed mental health system that delivers evidence-based care throughout the United States. It should include a continuum of crisis services, such as warmlines, hotlines, mobile crisis outreach, respite services, recovery centers, crisis stabilization beds, detoxification services, crisis residences, and psychiatric hospitals. Unfortunately, very few people with serious mental illness have had treatment in the year prior to an incarceration (Swartz and Tabahi 2017). Inadequate access to mental health care has been described as a primary contributor to incarceration of persons with mental illness (Committee on Psychiatry and the Community of the Group for the Advancement of Psychiatry 2016), although some analyses create doubt that undertreatment through conventional methodologies causes much crime (Wolff 2018).

The mental health system also needs to be aware of and respond to social determinants of mental health that are also associated with the potential for criminal justice involvement. Socioeconomic status—especially long-term unemployment and limited education—is strongly associated with criminal offending (Aaltonen et al. 2011). Studies have shown that increased spending on social services and public health is correlated with lower crime, including homicide, in the United States (Sipsma et al. 2017).

Similar socioeconomic variables, such as poverty, education, and housing, among others, influence both quality of health and levels of crime (Caruso 2017). Involvement in the criminal justice system is also an independent social determinant of health. Therefore, "upstream" social service interventions aimed at reducing crime can affect health outcomes through a number of routes. Realization of such a system is only likely to be achieved through close examination and reevaluation of financial models for health care funding.

Secondary Prevention of Crime: Jail Diversion

Despite interventions to prevent criminal activity, crime will occur. The goal of secondary prevention of crime is to reduce incarceration of those involved in low-level criminal activities. The way to approach this is to divert individuals who commit crimes into treatment rather than jails. Given the potential negative outcomes associated with incarceration, this approach aims to deter further crime without the costs of more punitive approaches.

Efforts to divert individuals with mental health or substance abuse problems from incarceration may take a variety of forms, although the shared goal is to redirect persons into treatment rather than jail. Persons with mental illness often decompensate from the stress of incarceration and are more sensitive to negative outcomes of incarceration (Dvoskin et al. 2017; Haney 2017). Because of the limited availability of mental health services behind bars, all treatment needs are unlikely to be met (Dvoskin et al. 2017). Untreated mental health needs contribute to longer periods of incarceration (and overcrowding of jails and prisons), disturbance of other inmates and correctional staff, and potential for violence against others. There is also a greater likelihood of victimization, placement in solitary confinement, and recidivism (Torrey et al. 2014). Treatment delivered in correctional settings is also more expensive than treatment delivered in the community (Skeem et al. 2018). Unfortunately, people with serious mental illness are often incarcerated for low-level misdemeanors, such as trespassing, panhandling, or petty theft (Fisher et al. 2006; Iglehart 2016). Approximately 2 million people with serious mental illness are arrested in the United States each year (Iglehart 2016). Finding ways to keep people who have mental illness out of jail and prison when they commit petty crimes will improve outcomes and reduce costs.

An organized framework for understanding efforts to keep those with mental health and substance use needs out of jail is the Sequential Intercept Model described by Munetz and Griffin (2006). This approach suggests five points at which to intercept people with mental health needs to community treatment instead of incarceration. The locations for intercepts are 1) law enforcement and emergency services, 2) booking and initial court appearance, 3) jails and courts, 4) jail and prison reentry, and 5) community corrections, probation, and parole. First intercept strategies may consist of specialized police responses, coordinated police-clinician outreach efforts, or transport to emergency mental health services. These have potential for significant savings related to costs of jail and policing (Pinals 2017).

The point of contact with the most potential efficacy is during individual interactions with police. Overall, approximately 7%–10% of persons who encounter police have a mental illness (Munetz and Griffin 2006). Those with untreated serious mental illness are at 16 times greater risk of being killed by law enforcement (Fuller et al. 2015), while Black men are at double the risk of men in general (Edwards et al. 2019). Officers are often called as first responders to individuals experiencing mental health emergencies. Police officers serve as gatekeepers and have significant discretion regarding decisions for arrest or diversion to treatment. Such choices require officers to have awareness of psychiatric symptomatology, although in many areas, little training is available in this regard. Without such training, police have a reduced capacity to appropriately handle persons with mental illness (Lamb et al. 2002). Some of the considerations that arise when officers make contact with persons who have mental illness include 1) severity of exhibited symptoms, 2) officers' attitudes about mental illness, 3) neighborhood characteristics, and 4) availability of disposition alternatives (Lamb et al. 2002; Pinals 2017). When they are unfamiliar with the context of the symptoms exhibited, officers often regard people with mental illness as dangerous (Lord and Bjerregaard 2014). Cross-system collaboration may involve education and training of police officers about mental health and substance abuse diagnoses and treatment needs. Advocating for improved mental health and social resources is crucial, and the United States has recently seen calls for transfer of funding from police budgets to other services in the midst of widespread protests in 2020 following the death of George Floyd.

Within the current system, the most well-known program for specialized police interventions is the Crisis Intervention Team (CIT), which was developed in Memphis and has been initiated in hundreds or even thousands of communities. The 2015 President's Task Force on 21st Century Policing called for mandatory CIT training of officers (Ramsey and Robinson 2015). The core of the standard format is 40 hours of training for certain police officers who become part of a dedicated team that responds to situations involving persons with potential mental health needs (Pinals 2017). The model also involves improving ease of police linkage to treatment in psychiatric emergencies and other cross-system collaborations. In fact, the program's founder, Sam Cochran, has said, "CIT is more than just training, it is a community program" (Steadman and Morrissette 2016).

CIT officer training has been found to increase officers' knowledge about psychiatric symptoms, improve confidence when responding to situations involving mental illness, enhance comfort when utilizing verbal deescalation skills, and decrease stigma about mental health problems and their treatments (Compton et al. 2014; Davidson 2016). Implementation has also been associated with fewer police and civilian injuries, more referrals to treatment, and reduced use of deadly force (Parent 2011; Pinals 2017). However, solid evidence for CIT's effectiveness is still lacking, so further research to illuminate longer-term outcomes is needed (Peterson and Densley 2018).

For diversion to be effective, there must be easily accessible treatment options to which individuals can be diverted before or following police contact. Mental health professionals go into the field for more effective deescalation and coordination of resources for treatment and other follow-up needs. These might include ensuring timely availability of community-based alternatives to jail as well as respite options for people with mental health needs (Steadman and Morrissette 2016). However, there are obstacles to redirecting individuals to mental health treatment. The time and energy required to connect someone with services may make some officers reluctant or resentful of taking a role in triaging individuals according to their mental health needs (Lamb et al. 2002). Efforts to make their jobs easier may enhance buy-in. More knowledge, training, and resources for working with people with mental health problems may help mitigate those attitudes (Reuland et al. 2009). National attention to police violence toward persons with mental illness and use of CIT may drive changes in police practices, reducing the likelihood that people with mental illness will be harmed or killed during interactions with police (Saleh et al. 2018).

Another early intercept strategy for diversion from jail involves police-based, specialized mental health services. These crisis services have been widely implemented (Pinals 2017). In this format, co-responder teams of mental health clinicians and police respond to calls involving persons with mental illness. Mental health professionals go into the field to assist police with deescalation and to coordinate resources for treatment and other follow-up needs. Sometimes they provide triage via phone lines or colocated mental health services in police stations (Heyman and McGeough 2018). Mental health professionals on co-responder teams provide treatment at the scene and attempt to resolve mental health issues and avoid use of emergency room or inpatient treatment (Meehan et al. 2019). Preliminary evidence suggests that such crisis programs reduce arrests as well as injuries and are experienced as less distressing to civilians (Abreu et al. 2017; Puntis et al. 2018).

A continuum of emergency mental health services can also be used to keep people with mental illness out of jail. Mobile crisis teams (MCTs) respond to emergencies with the goal of deescalation and linkage to service in the least restrictive way possible. These teams may include registered nurses and psychiatrists. Compared with patients in hospital emergency rooms, individuals served by mobile crisis units are more likely to have histories of violence, to have more complex mental health needs, and to be homeless. They often refuse formal treatment (Lord and Bjerregaard 2014). Calls for MCTs often involve suicidality, psychosis, and substance use and can be initiated by the person with mental health needs or other community members (Lord and Bjerregaard 2014). MCTs and law enforcement often arrive at the scene simultaneously, but MCTs are not directly embedded in the police department, as are co-responder teams. Mobile crisis interventions are associated with fewer psychiatric admissions and lower costs compared to routine police responses (Lord and Bjerregaard 2014). However, one study found mobile crisis units to be less effective at reducing arrest than crisis intervention teams (Steadman et al. 2000). Nevertheless, patients and their supports, as well as law enforcement officers, view mobile crisis units as being helpful (Lord and Bjerregaard 2014).

Tertiary Prevention of Crime

Various interventions, discussed below, are aimed at reducing length of involvement in, recidivism to, and negative impact of the correctional system. They take place in courts, behind bars, and through community reintegration.

Court-Based Interventions

In addition to the Sequential Intercept Model's secondary prevention and prebooking interventions designed to reduce incarceration (discussed in the previous section), its court-based, tertiary interventions can reduce criminal justice involvement for individuals with mental health needs. Participation in court-monitored mental health or substance use treatment can reduce or eliminate jail time, but at times can inadvertently lengthen jail stays by imposing additional demands that individuals can be reincarcerated for violating (Skeem et al. 2018). Miami-Dade County, Florida, established the first drug court in 1989 (Pinals 2017), and Broward County, Florida, created the first mental health court in 1997 (Wolff 2018). Participation in specialty courts is voluntary; nonadversarial criminal justice and behavioral health teams work to connect participants with mental health and social resources. The courts monitor defendants and utilize systems of sanctions and rewards to encourage adherence to court-ordered treatment plans. A document titled *Improving Responses to People With Mental Illnesses: The Es-*

sential Elements of a Mental Health Court was created by the Council of State Governments Justice Center for the U.S. Department of Justice (Thompson et al. 2008). It was adapted from a 1997 publication by the Department of Justice: *Defining Drug Courts: The Key Components* (National Association of Drug Court Professionals, Drug Court Standards Committee 1997).

The 2008 guideline describes 10 important features to be incorporated into mental health courts:

1. There must be collaboration between criminal justice, mental health, substance abuse treatment, and other stakeholders involved in planning and administration.
2. Eligibility for participation should consider public safety, community treatment capacity, and any relationship between mental illness and alleged offenses.
3. Screening, referral, and linkage to treatment should occur rapidly.
4. Successful engagement in treatment (following clearly communicated expectations) should be linked to positive legal outcomes.
5. Defendants demonstrate informed consent about their decisions to participate, are competent to do so, and have the assistance of specialized legal counsel for assistance.
6. Community treatment plans are comprehensive, individualized, and evidence-based.
7. Participants' confidentiality and constitutional rights should be protected.
8. Specialized, ongoing training is provided to team members.
9. Participants' compliance is monitored while incentives and sanctions are used to encourage adherence.
10. Courts collect data to analyze their impact and make appropriate modifications.

Research related to outcomes of mental health courts has varied depending on their fidelity to foundation principles of the model, as well as the specific populations and communities studied. On balance, the research has demonstrated that these courts increase treatment engagement and decrease individual recidivism when compared to referral to treatment as usual (Han and Redlich 2015; Kubiak et al. 2015). Decreased recidivism was demonstrated in courts that used intensive monitoring, personalized treatments, and teams with both correctional and mental health professionals (Bullard and Thrasher 2016). Studies have also found that mental health courts are associated with significant cost savings, extending beyond program completion, including savings from avoiding subsequent court and criminal justice costs (Kubiak et al. 2015). More studies of this type are necessary to firmly establish the value of the mental health courts.

Given that drug courts have a longer history, there is more evidence supporting their cost-effectiveness (Belenko et al. 2013; Carey and Finigan 2003; Marchand et al. 2006). Despite the strong evidence base for the safety and efficacy of using methadone, buprenorphine, or naltrexone for opioid addiction (MAT), a 2013 study found that only about half of drug courts offered at least one of these treatment options (Matusow et al. 2013). Although the incorporation of MAT might extend the success of this intervention, courts are often unfamiliar and/or uncomfortable with these valuable options.

In 2000, a judge in Florida's Miami-Dade County began a broader court-based decriminalization model—the Criminal Mental Health Project—with both secondary and tertiary measures of intervention (Iglehart 2016). Judge Steve Leifman developed and oversees this model, which utilizes multiple modalities of diverting persons with serious mental illness away from incarceration. The county utilizes extensive police CIT training, which has reduced the number of persons injured or killed by police (Iglehart 2016). At and after police contact, attempts are made to refer people with behavioral health needs to treatment and housing resources in lieu of being booked. Once taken into the county jail, persons are again screened for behavioral health needs, and judges are able to transfer them to a mental health crisis unit. Successful participation in crisis and future treatment is tied to dropping or lowering of legal consequences. Research on this system has shown decreases in recidivism by individuals arrested for both misdemeanors and nonviolent felonies (Iglehart 2016).

Correctional Psychiatry

Despite efforts taken to prevent crime and incarceration of people with mental illness, some people with mental health problems will still be incarcerated. Efforts must be undertaken to improve correctional psychiatric treatment and decrease recidivism for people with mental health difficulties. Correctional quality improvement plans should be established and regularly updated to review and improve quality, involving all levels of health care staff and including correctionals. Inmates do not usually have choices regarding providers or other elements of treatment while behind bars, and correctional mental health care should be held to the same quality standards as community-based services (American Psychiatric Association 2015). These programs are particularly needed with regard to reduction in the use of force for inmates with mental health issues.

Clinical psychiatry is practiced in lockups, jails, juvenile detention centers, prisons, and community-based programs that follow incarceration. These sites all provide opportunities for improvement in treatment, starting with appropriate screening and assessment. Best practice for correctional screening involves early assessment following intake, with rapid and appropriate follow-up for any identified problems. Trained staff, emphasizing a low threshold for referral, should be involved in the screening process (Dvoskin et al. 2017). Although treatment needs can be illuminated by communication between community and correctional providers, such communication rarely occurs (Munetz and Griffin 2006).

Inmates do not usually have choices regarding providers or other elements of treatment while behind bars, but correctional mental health care should be held to the same quality standards as community-based services (American Psychiatric Association 2015). Both the American Psychiatric Association and the National Commission on Correctional Health Care recommend that mental health treatment be overseen by a central correctional authority (Dvoskin et al. 2017). They also support collaboration between mental health and correctional authorities and clinical autonomy for practitioners' decisions. Adequate treatment requires sufficient staffing for the prescription of medications and various psychological and social interventions. More research regarding effective staffing and treatment is needed to establish adequate standards of care (Way and Candilis 2017). There is a need for development, evaluation, and dissemination of programs to reduce antisocial behavior once an individual is incarcerated. One such program is START NOW, a skills-based group therapy program in corrections that has been associated with fewer incidents of disciplinary infractions and days of postrelease psychiatric hospitalization (Cislo and Trestman 2015; Kersten et al. 2015).

The appropriate treatment of substance use disorders in correctional settings is also extremely important. The ability to engage inmates may vary significantly because of high turnover in jails. Screening, Brief Intervention and Referral to Treatment (SBIRT) interventions are often most appropriate for these settings. Prisons are more likely to incorporate services of higher intensity, such as residential therapeutic communities and daily group treatments (Belenko et al. 2013). Expansion of MAT beyond pregnancy or short-term detoxification in correctional settings would improve outcomes, but it is vastly underused (Friedmann et al. 2012). Negative attitudes about this treatment modality, including those of politicians and correctional staff, are the major barriers to its use.

Community Transition

Other than those individuals who die while incarcerated, inmates will de facto return to the community. Any effort to rehabilitate individuals during incarceration would be practically meaningless if not continued when the individual is no longer behind bars. Individuals with serious mental illness are at high risk for reincarceration (Munetz et al. 2001). However, continuity of care between corrections and the community rarely exists. One best practice model developed for individuals with co-occurring mental health and substance use problems is the APIC model: Assess, Plan, Identify, and Coordinate (Osher et al. 2003). The first step is to assess biopsychosocial needs and strengths to prepare the incarcerated individual for transition to the community. Planning should pay attention to short- and long-term needs, including benefits, clothing, housing, transportation, and an adequate supply of medication(s). Identification of appropriate community referrals (to whom discharge summaries should be forwarded) is important for continuity of care. Coordination of case management, family members, and other supports can help to facilitate the transition.

Other approaches to transition management include Risk-Need-Responsivity (RNR), Shared Responsibility and Interdependent (SRI), Critical Time Intervention (CTI), Sensitizing Providers to the Effects of Correctional Incarceration on Treatment and Risk Management (SPECTRM), Adult Cross-Training Curriculum (AXT), and Re-entry After Prison/Jail (RAP) (Osher and King 2015). RNR is particularly effective for individuals with substance use disorders (Belenko et al. 2013); this model places emphasis on matching individuals with the appropriate level of service, addressing criminogenic factors, and considering cognitive abilities. More research is needed, however, on the effectiveness of reentry programs in general.

Community-based mental health treatment for individuals with a history of incarceration is another piece of a comprehensive approach. When probation or parole is revoked, individuals are reincarcerated. Given the very high number of individuals on probation and parole, specialized community supervision services are prime targets for tertiary prevention of crime. Officers working in this system can benefit from education about mental health needs. Mental health probation programs add rehabilitation and reduced recidivism to supervision goals, and studies indicate that they are effective (Skeem et al. 2018). One example is high-intensity, multidisciplinary Forensic Assertive Community Treatment (FACT) programs, which require significant financing but are effective for individuals with serious mental illness (Pinals 2017). Despite significant cost savings when compared with traditional probation, specialty mental health programs are not widely used (Skeem et al. 2018). Returns on investment from these programs come in the form of reduced costs due to lower rates of incarceration and of emergency, residential, and inpatient treatments. Probation and parole officers often appreciate these programs and perceive them as helpful. Therefore, the success of mental health probation programs should be supported by psychiatrists to increase their availability and potential for benefit. It is important to note that in community corrections, as in many other settings, MAT for substance use disorders is vastly underused, a situation that needs to change (Friedmann et al. 2012).

Role of Psychiatrists

The correctional system is extensive and expensive and a ripe area for the involvement of psychiatrists. Psychiatrists can help to prevent and reduce crime as well as to lessen the potential negative impacts of incarceration on individuals and society. Professionals must first educate themselves on criminal justice issues in order to advocate for change. Psychiatrists have a unique role in implementing programs, educating and overseeing other professionals, and promoting and conducting research on these issues. Resources must be allocated for prevention science and cost studies. Attention must be paid to the comprehensive architecture of services before, during, and following incarceration that allows for integrative, cross-disciplinary work, including collaboration with allied health professionals. Because of the complexity of the correctional system, change requires substantial political will. Psychiatrists can also be effective advocates at the intersectional issues of mass incarceration and socioeconomic burdens, especially of minority populations.

Conclusion

The extensive numbers of people with mental illness behind bars lead to significant resources spent on incarceration in the United States. Although punishment can be a societal goal of imprisonment, it can also be associated with various negative outcomes for individuals, communities, and the country at large. A public health approach looks at reducing rates of incarceration for those with behavioral health problems and treating those health issues. Crime can be prevented through addressing antisocial behavior, substance abuse, ADHD, and gun violence. After the commission of low-level crime, individuals with mental illness can be diverted into treatment rather than into jail. Furthermore, if a person with mental illness is incarcerated, specialty courts, evidence-based correctional psychiatry, and reintegration services can all work toward reducing negative outcomes. This approach is predicated on an accessible and comprehensive mental health system that can be used to prevent crime, decrease the negative impact of incarceration, and improve quality of life for those with mental health problems and other marginalized populations.

References

Aaltonen M, Kivivuori J, Martikainen P: Social determinants of crime in a welfare state: do they still matter? Acta Sociologica 54(2):161–181, 2011

Abreu D, Parker TW, Noether CD, et al: Revising the paradigm for jail diversion for people with mental and substance use disorders: Intercept 0. Behav Sci Law 35(5–6):380–395, 2017

Adler NE, Cutler DM, Jonathan J, et al: Addressing Social Determinants of Health and Health Disparities: A Vital Direction for Health and Health Care. National Academy of Medicine Perspectives Discussion Paper. Washington, DC, National Academy of Medicine, 2016

American Psychiatric Association: Psychiatric Services in Correctional Facilities. Washington, DC, American Psychiatric Publishing, 2015

Asherson P, Buitelaar J, Faraone SV, et al: Adult attention-deficit hyperactivity disorder: key conceptual issues. Lancet Psychiatry 3(6):568–578, 2016

Barboriak PN: The history of correctional psychiatry in the United States, in Principles and Practice of Forensic Psychiatry, 3rd Edition. Edited by Rosner R, Scott CL. New York, CRC Press, 2017, pp 511–520

Belenko S, Hiller M, Hamilton L: Treating substance use disorders in the criminal justice system. Curr Psychiatry Rep 15(11):414, 2013

Bullard CE, Thrasher R: Evaluating mental health court by impact on jurisdictional crime rates. Criminal Justice Policy Review 27(3):227–246, 2016

Carey SM, Finigan MW: A detailed cost analysis in a mature drug court setting: a cost-benefit evaluation of the Multnomah County Drug Court. Journal of Contemporary Criminal Justice 20(3):315–338, 2003

Caruso GD: Public Health and Safety: The Social Determinants of Health and Criminal Behavior. Burnley, Lancashire, UK, ResearchersLinks, 2017, pp 1–38

Cislo AM, Trestman RL: Psychiatric hospitalization after participation in START NOW. Psychiatr Serv 67(1):143, 2015

Committee on Prevention Diagnosis Treatment and Management of Substance Use Disorders in the U.S. Armed Forces; Board on the Health of Select Populations, Institute of Medicine: Best practices in prevention, screening, diagnosis, and treatment of substance use disorders, in Substance Use Disorders in the U.S. Armed Forces. Edited by O'Brien CP, Oster M, Morden E. Washington, DC, National Academies Press, 2013, pp 97–136

Committee on Psychiatry and the Community of the Group for the Advancement of Psychiatry: People With Mental Illness in the Criminal Justice System: Answering a Cry for Help. Washington, DC, American Psychiatric Association Publishing, 2016

Compton MT, Bakeman R, Broussard B, et al: The police-based crisis intervention team (CIT) model: I. Effects on officers' knowledge, attitudes, and skills. Psychiatr Serv 65(4):517–522, 2014

Davidson ML: A criminal justice system-wide response to mental illness: evaluating the effectiveness of the Memphis Crisis Intervention Team training curriculum among law enforcement and correctional officers. Criminal Justice Policy Review 27(1):46–75, 2016

Davis L, Shlafer RJ: Mental health of adolescents with currently and formerly incarcerated parents. J Adolesc 54:120–134, 2017

Dempsey C: Beating mental illness: crisis intervention team training and law enforcement response trends. Southern California Interdisciplinary Law Journal 26(2):323–339, 2016

Dodge KA, Bierman KL, Coie JD, et al: Impact of early intervention on psychopathology, crime, and well-being at age 25. Am J Psychiatry 172(1):59–70, 2014

Douglas K, Bell CC: Youth homicide prevention. Psychiatr Clin North Am 34(1):205–216, 2011

Dvoskin JA, Brown MC, Metzner JL, et al: The structure of correctional mental health services, in Principles and Practice of Forensic Psychiatry, 3rd Edition. Edited by Rosner R, Scott CL. New York, CRC Press, 2017, pp 529–549

Edwards F, Lee H, Hedwig L, Esposito M: Risk of being killed by police use of force in the United States by age, race-ethnicity, and sex. Proc Natl Acad Sci USA 116(34):16793–16798, 2019

Farrington DP, Gaffney H, Lösel F, et al: Systematic reviews of the effectiveness of developmental prevention programs in reducing delinquency, aggression, and bullying. Aggression and Violent Behavior 33:91–106, 2017

Fisher WH, Roy-Bujnowski KM, Grudzinskas J Jr, et al: Patterns and prevalence of arrest in a statewide cohort of mental health care consumers. Psychiatr Serv 57(11):1623–1628, 2006

Friedmann PD, Hoskinson R Jr, Gordon M, et al: Medication-assisted treatment in criminal justice agencies affiliated with the Criminal Justice-Drug Abuse Treatment Studies (CJ-DATS): availability, barriers, and intentions. Subst Abus 33(1):9–18, 2012

Fuller DA, Lamb HR, Biasotti M, Snook J: Overlooked in the Undercounted: The Role of Mental Illness in Fatal Law Enforcement Encounters. Office of Research & Public Affairs, Treatment Advocacy Center, December 2015. Available at: www.treatmentadvocacycenter.org/storage/documents/overlooked-in-the-undercounted.pdf. Accessed August 7, 2020.

Garcia M, Cain CM, Cohen F, et al: Restrictive housing in the U.S.: issues, challenges, and future directions. November 2016. Available at: www.ncjrs.gov/pdffiles1/nij/250315.pdf. Accessed March 24, 2020.

Han W, Redlich AD: The impact of community treatment on recidivism among mental health court participants. Psychiatr Serv 67(4):384–390, 2015

Haney C: "Madness" and penal confinement: some observations on mental illness and prison pain. Punishment and Society 19(3):310–326, 2017

Hawkins JD, Smith BH, Hill KG, et al: Promoting social development and preventing health and behavior problems during the elementary grades: results from the Seattle Social Development Project. Victims and Offenders 2:161–181, 2007

Helseth SA, Waschbusch DA, Gnagy EM, et al: Effects of behavioral and pharmacological therapies on peer reinforcement of deviancy in children with ADHD-only, ADHD and conduct problems, and controls. J Consult Clin Psychol 83(4):280–292, 2015

Heyman I, McGeough E: Cross-disciplinary partnerships between police and health services for mental health care. J Psychiatr Ment Health Nurs 25(5–6):283–284, 2018

Iglehart JK: Decriminalizing mental illness—the Miami model. N Engl J Med 374(18):1701–1703, 2016

Kersten L, Cislo AM, Lynch M, et al: Evaluating START NOW: a skills-based psychotherapy for inmates of correctional systems. Psychiatr Serv 67(1):37–42, 2015

Kingston BE, Mihalic SF, Sigel EJ: Building an evidence-based multitiered system of supports for high-risk youth and communities. Am J Orthopsychiatry 86(4):132–143, 2016

Kirk DS, Wakefield S: Collateral consequences of punishment: a critical review and path forward. Annual Review of Criminology 1:171–194, 2018

Kubiak S, Roddy J, Comartin E, et al: Cost analysis of long-term outcomes of an urban mental health court. Eval Program Plann 52:96–106, 2015

Kupers TA: Solitary: The Inside Story of Supermax Isolation and How We Can Abolish It. Berkeley, CA, University of California Press, 2017

Lamb HR, Weinberger LE, DeCuir WJ Jr: The police and mental health. Psychiatr Serv 53(10):1266–1271, 2002

Lichtenstein P, Halldner L, Zetterqvist J, et al: Medication for attention deficit-hyperactivity disorder and criminality. N Engl J Med 367(21):2006–2014, 2012

Lord VB, Bjerregaard B: Helping persons with mental illness: partnerships between police and mobile crisis units. Victims and Offenders 9(4):455–474, 2014

Marchand G, Waller M, Carey SM: Kalamazoo County Adult Drug Treatment Court: Outcome and Cost Evaluation. Portland, OR, NPC Research, 2006

Massoglia M, Pridemore WA: Incarceration and health. Annu Rev Sociol 41:291–310, 2015

Matusow H, Dickman SL, Rich JD, et al: Medication assisted treatment in U.S. drug courts: results from a nationwide survey of availability, barriers and attitudes. J Subst Abuse Treat 44(5):473–480, 2013

Mauer M: Addressing racial disparities in incarceration. The Prison Journal 91 (3, suppl):87S–101S, 2011

Mears DP, Cochran JC: Progressively tougher sanctioning and recidivism: assessing the effects of different types of sanctions. J Res Crime Delinq 55(2):194–241, 2018

Mears DP, Cochran JC, Cullen FT: Incarceration heterogeneity and its implications for assessing the effectiveness of imprisonment on recidivism. Criminal Justice Policy Review 26(7):691–712, 2015

Meehan T, Brack J, Mansfield Y, et al: Do police-mental health co-responder programmes reduce emergency department presentations or simply delay the inevitable? Australas Psychiatry 27(1):18–20, 2019

Metzl JM, MacLeish KT: Mental illness, mass shootings, and the politics of American firearms. Am J Public Health 105(2):240–249, 2015
Miller M, Azrael D, Hemenway D: Rates of household firearm ownership and homicide across U.S. regions and states, 1988–1997. Am J Public Health 92(12):1988–1993, 2002
Mitchell O, Cochran JC, Mears DP, et al: The effectiveness of prison for reducing drug offender recidivism: a regression discontinuity analysis. Journal of Experimental Criminology 13:1–27, 2017
Moffitt TE: Adolescence-limited and life-course-persistent antisocial behavior: a developmental taxonomy, in Biosocial Theories of Crime. Edited by Beaver KM, Walsh A. New York, Routledge, 2017, pp 69–96
Mohr-Jensen C, Steinhausen H-C: A meta-analysis and systematic review of the risks associated with childhood attention-deficit hyperactivity disorder on long-term outcome of arrests, convictions, and incarcerations. Clin Psychol Rev 48:32–42, 2016
Munetz MR, Griffin PA: Use of the Sequential Intercept Model as an approach to decriminalization of people with serious mental illness. Psychiatr Serv 57(4):544–549, 2006
Munetz MR, Grande TP, Chambers MR: The incarceration of individuals with severe mental disorders. Community Mental Health Journal 37(4):361–372, 2001
National Association of Drug Court Professionals, Drug Court Standards Committee: Defining drug courts: the key components. U.S. Department of Justice, January 1997. Available at: www.ncjrs.gov/pdffiles1/bja/205621.pdf. Accessed March 25, 2020.
Oesterle S, Kuklinski MR, Hawkins JD, et al: Long-term effects of the Communities That Care trial on substance use, antisocial behavior, and violence through age 21 years. Am J Public Health 108(5):659–665, 2018
Osher F, King C: Intercept 4: reentry from jails and prisons, in The Sequential Intercept Model and Criminal Justice: Promoting Community Alternatives for Individuals With Serious Mental Illness. Edited by Griffin PA, Heilbrun K, Mulvey EP, et al. New York, Oxford University Press, 2015, pp 95–117
Osher F, Steadman HJ, Barr H: A best practice approach to community reentry from jails for inmates with co-occurring disorders: the APIC model. Crime and Delinquency 49(1):79–96, 2003
Parent R: The police use of deadly force in British Columbia: mental illness and crisis intervention. Journal of Police Crisis Negotiations 11(1):57–71, 2011
Peters RH, Wexler HK, Lurigio AJ: Co-occurring substance use and mental disorders in the criminal justice system: a new frontier of clinical practice and research. Psychiatr Rehabil J 38(1):1–6, 2015
Peterson J, Densley J: Is crisis intervention team (CIT) training evidence-based practice? A systematic review. Journal of Crime and Justice 41(5):521–534, 2018
Pinals DA: Forensic services, public mental health policy, and financing: charting the course ahead. J Am Acad Psychiatry Law 42(1):7–19, 2014

Pinals DA: Jail diversion, specialty court, and reentry services: partnerships between behavioral health and justice systems, in Principles and Practice of Forensic Psychiatry, 3rd Edition. Edited by Rosner R, Scott CL. New York, CRC Press, 2017, pp 237–246

President's Commission on Law Enforcement and Administration of Justice: The Challenge of Crime in a Free Society. Washington, DC, U.S. Government Printing Office, 1967

Primeau A, Bowers TG, Harrison MA, et al: Deinstitutionalization of the mentally ill: evidence for transinstitutionalization from psychiatric hospitals to penal institutions. Comprehensive Psychology 2:1–10, 2013

Puntis S, Perfect D, Kirubarajan A, et al: A systematic review of co-responder models of police mental health 'street' triage. BMC Psychiatry 18(1):256, 2018

Raine A: Biosocial studies of antisocial and violent behavior in children and adults: a review. J Abnorm Child Psychol 30(4):311–326, 2002

Ramsey C, Robinson L: Interim Report of the President's Task Force on 21st Century Policing. Washington, DC, Office of Community Oriented Policing Services, 2015

Ranney ML, Betz ME, Dark C: ThisIsOurLane—firearm safety as health care's highway. N Engl J Med 380(5):405–407, 2018

Reidy DE, Kearns MC, DeGue S, et al: Why psychopathy matters: implications for public health and violence prevention. Aggress Violent Behav 24:214–225, 2015

Reuland M, Schwarzfeld M, Draper L: Law Enforcement Responses to People With Mental Illnesses: A Guide to Research-Informed Policy and Practice. New York, Council of State Governments Justice Center, 2009

Rich JD, Wakeman SE, Dickman SL: Medicine and the epidemic of incarceration in the United States. N Engl J Med 364(22):2081–2083, 2011

Rowhani-Rahbar A, Simonetti JA, Rivara FP: Effectiveness of interventions to promote safe firearm storage. Epidemiol Rev 38(1):111–124, 2016

Rozel JS, Mulvey EP: The link between mental illness and firearm violence: implications for social policy and clinical practice. Annu Rev Clin Psychol 13:445–469, 2017

Saleh AZ, Appelbaum PS, Liu X, et al: Deaths of people with mental illness during interactions with law enforcement. Int J Law Psychiatry 58:110–116, 2018

Sandler I, Wolchik SA, Cruden G, et al: Overview of meta-analyses of the prevention of mental health, substance use, and conduct problems. Annu Rev Clin Psychol 10:243–273, 2014

Sawyer AM, Borduin CM, Dopp AR: Long-term effects of prevention and treatment on youth antisocial behavior: a meta-analysis. Clin Psychol Rev 42:130–144, 2015

Sipsma HL, Canavan ME, Rogan E, et al: Spending on social and public health services and its association with homicide in the USA: an ecological study. BMJ Open 7(10):e016379, 2017

Skeem JL, Montoya L, Manchak SM: Comparing costs of traditional and specialty probation for people with serious mental illness. Psychiatr Serv 69(8):896–902, 2018

Steadman HJ, Morrissette D: Police responses to persons with mental illness: going beyond CIT training. Psychiatr Serv 67(10):1054–1056, 2016

Steadman HJ, Deane MW, Borum R, et al: Comparing outcomes of major models of police responses to mental health emergencies. Psychiatr Serv 51(5):645–649, 2000

Sugie NF, Turney K: Beyond incarceration: criminal justice contact and mental health. American Sociological Review 82(4):719–743, 2017

Swanson JW, Frisman LK, Robertson AG, et al: Costs of criminal justice involvement among persons with serious mental illness in Connecticut. Psychiatr Serv 64(7):630–637, 2013

Swartz JA, Lurigio AJ: Serious mental illness and arrest: the generalized mediating effect of substance use. Crime and Delinquency 53(4):581–604, 2007

Swartz JA, Tabahi S: Community-based mental health treatment preceding jail detention among adults with serious mental illness. International Journal of Forensic Mental Health 16(2):104–116, 2017

Taichman D, Bornstein SS, Laine C: Firearm injury prevention: AFFIRMing that doctors are in our lane. Ann Intern Med 169(12):885–886, 2018

Thompson M, Osher FC, Tomasini-Joshi D: Improving Responses to People With Mental Illnesses: The Essential Elements of a Mental Health Court. New York, Council of State Governments Justice Center, 2008

Torrey EF, Zdanowicz MT, Kennard AD, et al: The Treatment of Persons With Mental Illness in Prisons and Jails: A State Survey. Arlington, VA, Treatment Advocacy Center, 2014

Way BB, Candilis PJ: Correctional psychiatry research, in Principles and Practice of Forensic Psychiatry, 3rd Edition. Edited by Rosner R, Scott CL. New York, CRC Press, 2017, pp 563–572

Webster D, Crifasi CK, Vernick JS: Effects of the repeal of Missouri's handgun purchaser licensing law on homicides. J Urban Health 91(2):293–302, 2014

Welsh BC, Farrington DP: Assessing the economic costs and benefits of crime prevention, in Costs and Benefits of Preventing Crime. Edited by Welsh B, Farrington DP, Sherman L. New York, Routledge, 2018, pp 3–19

Welsh BC, Farrington DP, Gowar BR: Benefit-cost analysis of crime prevention programs. Crime and Justice 44(1):447–516, 2015

White HR: Substance use and crime, in The Oxford Handbook of Substance Use and Substance Use Disorders, Volume 2. New York, Oxford University Press, 2016, pp 347–378

Wolff N: Are mental health courts target efficient? Int J Law Psychiatry 57:67–76, 2018

Wolraich M, Brown L, Brown RT, et al: ADHD: clinical practice guideline for the diagnosis, evaluation, and treatment of attention-deficit/hyperactivity disorder in children and adolescents. Pediatrics 128(5):1007–1022, 2011

20

Health and the Workplace

Ben W. Hunter, M.D.
Kenneth G. Hunter

In terms of financial and emotional capital, there is no greater battleground than the workplace. An individual's occupation is a source of meaning and social connection, of livelihood and value. We spend years, and often decades, in the educational system preparing to enter the workforce. Work is a major way that people define themselves and relate to one another. With 40 or more hours per week dedicated to work and a high level of emotional and social value assigned to professional life, it is no surprise that the workplace can also represent one of our primary stressors, often resulting in anxiety, depression, and drug and alcohol abuse. It may also contribute to physical health issues, such as hypertension, heart disease, and diabetes, and in rarer cases, interpersonal conflict and violence. To ensure that work remains a wellspring of purpose, engagement, and value, it is necessary to minimize the sources of stress in the workplace.

Mental Health in the Workplace

The dichotomous role of work in our lives—as a stressor and a source of meaning—combined with growing awareness of mental health issues worldwide presents a unique challenge for the employer. A 2015 report by the American Psychological Association's American Institute of Stress listed "job pressure" as the leading driver of stress among thousands of demographically representative Americans polled during 2014. The inherently linked factor of "money" followed close behind. A full 76% of respondents cited job or lack of money as their primary stressor, 77% reported physical symptoms associated with stress, 73% identified regular psychological symptoms associated with stress, and 30% said they "always" or "often" felt under stress at work. Seven of the top nine preventable health issues affecting job performance are related directly to mental health. As of 2010, employers' annual burden due to major depression alone was estimated at $210.5 billion, an increase of 21.5% from just 5 years prior (Greenberg et al. 2015). These figures are only shocking to the minority of the workforce who have not experienced the detrimental effects of workplace stress. However, the fact that these data are available and have started discussions of the importance of mental health maintenance in the workplace, is a monumental step toward improving the situation.

Beyond an increase in awareness, a subtle but appreciable shift in ethos has begun to take hold. Amid the many domains of work culture and the multitude of factors determining the health of employees, work-life balance and the time burden of work are a demonstrative place to begin the discussion of workplace mental health. In the current world of work, a walk around a typical office at 7:00 P.M. will not likely reveal many employees banging out e-mails over takeout dinners, as might have been the case in the past. Fewer workers are overheard glorifying long work hours, sleep deprivation, and dinners at the office. Although dedication and perseverance remain critical to success in most industries, lack of work-life boundaries and neglect of self-care have been repeatedly demonstrated to lead to dissatisfaction, decreased productivity, and lower-quality work. Some would argue that industry or employer expectations of "hard work" or "high achievement" should override attempts to maintain balance, and that these values justify lost time and health. However, employees are often disappointed to learn that their boss may not even notice their exceptional efforts, let alone direct silent or audible praise toward them. A study conducted in the global strategy consulting industry, considered to be a bastion of "old school" martyrdom, demonstrated that managers could not tell the difference between associates who worked 80-hour weeks and those who simply pretended to do so (Reid 2015). Moreover, with a generational emphasis on efficiency spreading through major industries, these indefatigable office warriors are increasingly likely to be seen as inefficient and, by extension, less competent.

Example: Doctors on the Brink

Perhaps the best-studied example of systematic overwork and the consequences thereof lies in medical residency training. Following undergraduate education and 4 years of medical school, resident physicians undergo the most labor-intensive years of their life, carrying the bulk of the patient care responsibilities at hospitals large and small. In an age not so long past, it was common for residents to work upward of 80 hours per week for the bulk of the 3–9 years that made up their training. Some participated voluntarily, considering the ridiculous work hours as a "badge of honor" or "trial by fire" that would lead to superior skill and, perhaps equally important, admission to the ranks of the elite. Doctors not so strongly compelled by ego were, in any case, forced to acquiesce to the same demanding schedule under threat of poor evaluations and the career implications they would carry. The issue was pervasive, a culturally condoned rite of passage that was allowed to persist for generations.

After much debate, residency programs finally addressed overwork of physicians-in-training by instituting major changes for its 2003 Common Program Requirements, released by the Accreditation Council for Graduate Medical Education (ACGME) and recapitulated in its 2020 guidelines (Accreditation Council for Graduate Medical Education 2020). The highly controversial "restrictions" included an 80-hour weekly limit, 1 day off in 7, and in-house call duties no more often than every 3 days, averaged over 4 weeks. The fact that these 80-hour work weeks represented a significant reduction, and that doctors were "forced" to leave the hospital once a week, should have been disconcerting, with the health of patients hanging in the balance. However, some senior physicians who cut their teeth under the old rules were appalled at the changes and the perceived lack of dedication of this generation's health care trainees. These stalwarts largely missed the point. Although improving quality of life for residents was a welcome byproduct, the ACGME created these rules with the primary intention of responding to concerns about patient safety and outcomes. Study after study proved that the traditionally inhuman residency work hours were hurting doctors, who in turn were hurting patients (Brown et al. 2015; Ouyang et al. 2016). Physicians became tired, nonempathic, forgetful, and inaccurate. This phenomenon of "burnout" directly affects patient care, and serves as an independent predictor of both medical errors (Shanafelt et al. 2010) and involvement in malpractice lawsuits (Balch et al. 2011).

Industry leaders hypothesized that rest, recovery, and balance would lead to better patient outcomes, not to mention higher profitability and less litigation for hospitals. The ACGME had no choice but to respond, and the results have been positive—for both physicians and patients alike. Mortality for patients treated by residents has decreased (Jena et al. 2014; Volpp et al. 2007, 2009; Shetty and Bhattacharya 2007), and residents are happier and healthier (Brunworth and Sindwani 2006; Reed et al. 2010). Moreover, fear of inferior training and poorer outcomes posttraining appears largely unfounded (Jena et al. 2014).

Origins of Workplace Wellness

A big surprise is that evidence-based, performance- and profit-enhancing changes in the culture of professional fields such as medicine were delayed until the early twentieth century. The connection between work conditions (as a proxy for worker satisfaction) and productivity began almost two centuries ago. In the early days of the industrial revolution, two major factors—safety and work hours—dictated workplace culture for the manual laborer. Beginning in the early nineteenth century, U.S. and U.K. unions fought for 8-hour work days. As laborers cried out for 8-hour days, employers grudgingly agreed after long and bitter disputes. What was seen as a socialist experiment had surprising economic merit, and to the surprise of the industry, profit and productivity rose. Seminal industrial psychology work of the early twentieth century included that of Frederick W. Taylor, the originator of "scientific management," which prescribed reduced work times and attained remarkable increases in per-worker output (Taylor 1911). At some level, employers began to understand that happier and healthier workers led to a stronger bottom line.

Stress, Mental Health, and the Modern Workplace

The rise of technology during the early to mid-twentieth century brought a new class of employee and a greater understanding of the relationship between health, happiness, and profitability. The writer Upton Sinclair is widely credited with coining the term "white collar" in the 1930s to describe professional, managerial, or administrative workers (BBC 2014). Sinclair's nomenclature indicated a significant change in the way business was conducted. Corporate function became dependent on multiple employees with diverse personalities, backgrounds, and skills. As a result, a much greater percentage of the average worker's day began to rely heavily on interpersonal communication, demanding competence in negotiating relationships and tasks alike. These interactions began to occur in many forms, from one-on-one conversations to group meetings to company-wide communications, functionally redefining the workplace. The product of these interactions, the manner in which they were interpreted and handled by management, and the explicit pronouncements of corporate leadership created a shared set of values, beliefs, and attitudes. These elements defined the concept of corporate culture, and the study of its impact on employees and organizations began.

Whereas measuring physical stress in manual laborers is a relatively simple task, measuring cognitive stress and the resulting performance impairment is a more complicated process. Some level of stress is inherent to any job and may be seen as the reaction of an individual in response to a demand. Work, at its core, is nothing more than a set of demands placed on an individual—and agreed on by the individual—in exchange for compensation. Indeed, healthy stress in response to reasonably challenging demands is a key driver of performance and engagement. What differentiates "healthy" or "positive" stress from "negative" or "unhealthy" stress? In healthy stress, or *eustress*, the associated stressor has been cognitively appraised as positive or challenging. Marriage, caring for a new baby, athletic competition, the financial burden of purchasing a new home, an increase in responsibilities associated with a promotion, and the challenge of transition into retirement are typical examples of eustress.

Distress, on the other hand, is the stress reaction to those stressors appraised as being negative or threatening. When conceptualizing distress, most people think about those times when they are under unpleasant pressure to perform, when catastrophe looms, or when they are dealing with the everyday stressors that seem unchanging or out of their control (Colligan and Higgins 2006). Positive work cultures, or corporate environments that promote mental health and happiness among employees, are those in which eustressors dominate over distressors. Improvements in culture result from thoughtful addition of eustress, reduction of distress, or ideally a combination of the two.

Volumes of research have led to a clear and meaningful set of conclusions about mental health in the workplace. Happy and confident employees show increased creativity, productivity, and overall performance (Amabile et al. 2005; Compte and Postlewaite 2004; Oswald et al. 2015). Mentally healthy workers produce more, cost less, and perpetuate a positive corporate culture that begets continued progress. With this in mind, this chapter will demonstrate that the burden of negative workplace culture, occupational stress, and unhealthy workers, is profound. From this starting point, the common strategies for successful interventions, from the global level of cultural change down to the point of access for specific mental health services, will be identified.

If there is one takeaway point, it is this: creating a positive corporate culture and improving workforce psychology will lead to happier, healthier employees, higher morale and productivity, and a staggering array of economic benefits. In other words, investing in the mental health of employees is not a tradeoff or a necessary expense—it is one of the most profitable investments a company can make.

The Cost of Disengagement

Employee disengagement can be either the cause or the result of mental health issues in the workplace. Disengagement is now recognized as a worldwide epidemic. Gallup's (2017) "State of the Global Workplace" report suggested that only 15% of employees worldwide were engaged—that is, involved in and enthusiastic about their work. Disengaged workers had 37% higher absenteeism, 47% more accidents, and 60% more errors and defects in their work. Organizations with low engagement scores showed 18% lower productivity, 16% lower profitability, 37% lower job growth, and 65% lower share price over time. On the other hand, businesses with highly engaged employees garnered twice as many applications from prospective employees (Seppala and Cameron 2015).

Although *engagement* is not synonymous with *health*, it might as well be. Another report by Gallup (Crabtree 2005) found that 62% of engaged employees felt that their work positively affects their physical health. However, for employees who were not engaged, this number drops to 39%, and for those who self-reported as actively disengaged, a mere 22%. Among those not engaged and actively disengaged, 54% said their work life has a negative effect on their health, whereas 51% reported a negative effect on their well-being. The combined math is concerning, as Gallup's polls suggest that over 40% of all employees worldwide see work as a detriment to their health and well-being.

The results were equally concerning when it came to employees' psychological health. Gallup found that 78% of engaged workers, but a mere 48% of disengaged employees and 15% of actively disengaged employees, felt that their work lives benefit them psychologically. Unsurprisingly, 51% of actively disengaged employees believed their work lives had a negative effect on their psychological well-being, compared with 20% of disengaged workers and only 6% of engaged workers (Crabtree 2005).

Disengaged employees are clearly unhappy, unhealthy, and unproductive. Unfortunately, most employees are disengaged. The news is not all bad, however, because an increasing number of companies are beginning to understand the link between corporate culture, employee engagement, mental health, and profitability. Engagement represents exceptionally low-hanging fruit for any firm looking to bolster their bottom line. The following subsections cover a variety of issues that affect costs related to mental health in the workplace.

Occupational Stress and Mental Health

When it comes to assessing the impact of work culture on individual psychology, traditional medical diagnostics prove cumbersome. At what exact point does a "bad week" end and a "major depressive episode" begin? How do we quantify the role of a raging boss in the variegated psychosocial picture of an individual with generalized anxiety disorder? And how can we expect employees to differentiate these points, which often elude even skilled providers? Fortunately, when it comes to the impact of mental health issues in the workplace, these fine distinctions appear to be less than critical. For demonstration purposes, enter the world of V codes.

In medical billing, V codes are used to highlight factors unrelated to an individual's primary diagnosis that nonetheless affect mental or physical health. For example, a patient with a primary psychiatric diagnosis of major depressive disorder may also qualify for V code 61.1, partner relational problem, if the psychiatrist feels that marital issues are contributing significantly to depression. V coding covers a wide range of factors, including nonadherence with treatment, religious problems, neglect, and occupational problems. As it turns out, these oft-neglected "secondary" factors in a patient's medical workup warrant greater attention, particularly in the work environment. In a 2008 study on employee assistance programs, individuals with V code diagnoses experienced losses in productivity similar to those with primary mental diagnoses. These individuals proved equally lucrative targets for intervention, because the "V code only" employees experienced benefits on par with their primary diagnosis counterparts when engaged in employee assistance (Hargrave et al. 2008). The significance of diagnosis is considered in greater detail in Chapter 14 ("Diagnostic Reform"), but this brief discussion should provide an adequate background for this discussion.

Although workplace stress is not tantamount to a mental health diagnosis, the effects of unmitigated stress can be similarly damaging for the average employee and potentially catastrophic for those already suffering from psychiatric concerns. With this reasoning in mind, we will use the terminology and concepts of *distress* and *mental health issues* interchangeably.

Absenteeism and Presenteeism

In terms of disengagement, *absenteeism* and *presenteeism* are the most direct measures at our disposal. Put simply, *absenteeism* considers the cost of missed work days, whereas *presenteeism* examines the cost of working while sick. For the organization, high rates of absenteeism result in lower levels of productivity and performance as well as globally diminished engagement. For example, employees who are not themselves absent feel the effects of missing coworkers. Erosion of camaraderie, loss of sense of personal investment, and ultimately souring of corporate culture are natural downstream effects. Estimates project the number of missed work days in the United States at $550 million per year, representing a massive financial burden for the national economy (American Psychological Association 2015). Unfortunately, this is just the tip of a large and destructive iceberg.

Consider this hyperbolic-sounding figure: $212 billion. That is the inflation-adjusted cost of absenteeism calculated in the 2001 American Productivity Audit (Stewart et al. 2003). Even more concerning is that for every dollar lost to absenteeism, many more are squandered on presenteeism. In a classic study at Bank One, the difference was 10-fold (Burton et al. 1999). A 2015 study calculated the employer burden of absenteeism due to major depressive disorder alone at $22 billion, which pales in comparison to the $74 billion tab associated with presenteeism (Greenberg et al. 2015). The insidious effects of presenteeism are partially to blame for this astronomical cost. A company can tell when an employee stays home due to illness, but it cannot easily measure the burden of workers showing up in impaired health. Showing up and "pushing through" might seem like the admirable option to some, but the data are clear: showing up to work when ill actually costs the employer more than having an employee stay home to attend to his or her health (Hemp 2004). Not only are employees who push self-care and medical attention down the road less efficient and productive, but their health care costs are compounded because they are not managed in the early stages at which interventions are most effective.

Disability

The majority of absenteeism due to mental health issues comes in the form of sporadic missed days, a combination of paid time off and earned time off. In rarer cases, however, the severity of the functional impairment may necessitate short- or long-term disability claims. Short-term disability claims due to mental health–related conditions are growing steadily—up to 10% annually—and can account for more than 30% of the total disability burden for the typical employer (Marlowe 2002). Add in the estimated 60%–80% of workplace accidents attributable to stress-induced factors, such as distractibility, and you will find that almost all causes of disability that occur at work may be traced, directly or indirectly, to workplace culture (Seppala and Cameron 2015).

The unfortunate consequence of limits to short-term disability and mental health benefits is that many workers who are suffering psychologically are forced to return to work before they are adequately treated, a situation that contributes to the aforementioned burden of presenteeism and, in some cases, long-term disability claims down the road. All in all, psychiatric and substance use disorders are the fifth leading cause of short-term disability and the third leading cause of long-term disability costs for employers in the United States (Leopold 2003). Moreover, 53% of employers found that return to work is more difficult for employees following an absence for psychiatric disability as opposed to general medical disability (Watson Wyatt Worldwide 1998). Whereas physical injuries and the resulting necessary accommodations are fairly easy to identify, it is much more difficult to quantify, isolate, and remedy the psychological burden that contributes to workers' psychiatric disability claims. More often, workers perceive an increased burden in returning to work due to a combination of stigma and the extra effort required to catch up with coworkers and projects.

In addition to direct payouts for disability, there are innumerable secondary consequences. Temporary absences lead to the offloading of assignments onto coworkers, generating resentment and stress. Hiring replacement labor is an even more unattractive option. To hire new employees and bring them up to expected performance standards, employers should prepare to write off 8 weeks for clerical jobs, 20 weeks for professional roles, and 26 weeks or more for executive positions (Williams 2003). More frequent hiring will invariably arise in companies with toxic culture or excessive job stress, classically associated with higher rates of turnover. Compounded by the negative impact of churning employees on company morale, accelerating levels of stress, disability, and attrition occur.

Attrition

The endgame of excessive workplace stress, and a nightmare for human resources directors worldwide, is attrition. The time, effort, and expense involved in replacing an employee are extensive. An average firm spends between 1% and 2.5% of total revenue on bringing new hires up to speed (Williams 2003), and that fails to include the cost of separation for the outgoing employees. Stated differently, the Society for Human Resource Management estimates cost of turnover at 6–9 months' salary for the average employee, or a range of 20% of annual salary for midrange employees to 213% for highly educated executives, who also typically command the highest salaries (Glynn and Boushey 2012). Keep in mind, if stress and mental health issues are the reason for separation, a company may have already paid out directly for health care costs and disability accommodations, compounding the economic burden.

In a company with toxic culture and overstressed employees, it is expected that in the worst-case scenario there will be continuous cycles of short-term disability to long-term disability to attrition, accelerating over time. Fortunately, key factors affecting employee turnover are highly modifiable, and they include organizational commitment and job satisfaction, quality of the relationship between employees and immediate supervisors, role clarity, job design and sense of mobility, and workgroup cohesion (Allen 2008). Executives and human resource directors will recognize these factors as the cornerstone of all corporate wellness and culture improvement initiatives. There is a reason why employee retention is tracked almost universally: it is a lagging indicator of firm culture and a leading indicator for profitability. Attrition affects the company globally. Damage to the firm's "brand" further dilutes its ability to attract top talent. Workplaces with rapid turnover rates foster a downward spiral of decreased collegiality, isolation, disengagement, and turnover.

Accidents and Workers' Compensation

The inception of industrial psychology in the nineteenth century was driven largely by recognition of the link between safety and profitability. Even before the modern concept of occupational safety and the ethical imperatives that govern business in the twenty-first century, factory owners and manufacturers began to understand that overstressed and injured workers—or in the worst case, employee fatalities—were bad for business. Efficiency slowed, mistakes were made, time and expensive raw materials were wasted, and the company's cost structures were severely threatened. Since the initiation of the 40-hour work week, it has gradually become clear that rested employees were happier, were more productive, and made fewer preventable mistakes.

After Otto von Bismarck's Workers' Accident Insurance system was instituted in 1881 and began to serve as the model for workers' compensation in the United States and Europe, the stakes grew significantly (Boggs 2015). In 2013, nonfatal injuries alone resulted in $62 billion in direct workers' compensation costs. This figure is staggering but pales in comparison to the indirect costs—increasing insurance premiums, replacement labor, lost time and institutional knowledge, and numerous other factors—which are estimated at four times direct costs. The Centers for Disease Control and Prevention estimates that a fatal injury carries an average cost of $991,027 in hospital expenses alone (Liberty Mutual 2016), and a National Safety Council model places the average occupational fatality's cost to society at $1.42 million (Morrison 2018). In 2017, workers killed on the job totaled 5,147 (3.5 per 100,000 full-time equivalent workers). This equates to more than 99 deaths per week or 14 per day (Bureau of Labor Statistics 2019). The cost of unmitigated workplace risk is unsustainable.

There is a temptation to place the responsibility for costly mistakes on employee negligence: "He should have been paying more attention" or "She was just clumsy." However, because excessive stress has been clearly demonstrated to impair such cognitive domains as motivation, arousal, attention, vigilance, and memory (Bourne and Yaroush 2003), psychologists and the Occupational Safety and Health Administration (OSHA) are united in refuting these formulations. In OSHA's recommendations for employers with regard to workplace safety, not a single reference is made to disciplining inattentive employees or hiring more resilient workers. Every item on the list suggests that employers and the workplace culture are the primary drivers of occupational safety and therefore they should bear the burden of responsibility for injuries and mistakes (Occupational Safety and Health Administration 2020). The health care industry specifically was shocked to learn that those residents who were tested after a long and stressful night call shift performed worse on tests of vigilance and cognition than a cohort who had consumed alcohol (Arnedt et al. 2005). Patients' lives were essentially in the hands of physicians who were functionally drunk. Few would blame these doctors for the demands placed on them by an apparently toxic system, and the same should be true for employees in other industries facing a different set of occupational hazards. Creating a culture of safety and a foundation of trust is the imperative of the organization.

Litigation

In situations where workers' compensation does not apply, litigation is a potential hazard for employers. Discrimination, harassment, and retaliation are only a few of the many points of exposure a company faces when workplace toxicity begets outright damages. Particularly in settings where negative management culture reigns, there is a twofold risk of exposure: employees are more likely to incur damages as harmful behavior is habitually tolerated, and greater disengagement leads to increased likelihood of the employee seeking legal recompense. According to the U.S. Equal Employment

Opportunity Commission (EEOC), mental health disabilities ranked behind only orthopedic injuries in terms of sheer volume of legal action under the Americans With Disabilities Act. Mood disorders accounted for 7.3% of all cases and anxiety disorders for 6.4%. In total, mental health issues represented more than 1 in 7 charges filed with the EEOC in 2017 (U.S. Equal Employment Opportunity Commission 2020).

Significant costs are associated with legal action resulting from negative workplace culture. A representative study of 1,214 closed claims reported by small- to medium-sized enterprises with fewer than 500 employees showed that 24% of employment charges resulted in defense and settlement costs averaging $160,000. On average, those matters took 318 days to resolve (Hiscox 2017). Add this to the cost of replacing disenfranchised employees, temporarily and permanently, and the cost to employers grows exponentially.

Health Care and Insurance Costs

Direct costs of employee health care and insurance have been intentionally left for last in this discussion of costs, because they represent only a fraction of employer costs. However, that is not meant to diminish the economic impact of mental health issues, which we have shown to be directly mediated by workplace stress in many cases. For example, in regard to depression, the National Institute of Mental Health (2019) posited that in the year 2016, about 16.2 million American adults experienced at least one major depressive episode—not merely a "few bad days," but 2 or more weeks with demonstrable deficits in functioning due to symptoms. With a full 6.7% of adults affected, clinical depression was a relevant factor in virtually every U.S. workplace. Research indicates that the average employed person with major depression accrued average annual health care costs of $10,836, as of 2016. A similar employed person without major depression experienced a cost of only $4,584. Thus, the incremental difference added by major depression is $6,252 per depressed employee per year, with $2,469 (39%) of that cost dedicated to treatment. Note that this conservative estimate only includes direct treatment of depression and other medical issues directly linked to depression, such as musculoskeletal pain (Greenberg et al. 2015).

Employers are rarely aware of the direct economic burden of treating mental health disorders such as depression, anxiety, and other issues created or exacerbated by workplace stress, but they bear the burden of increased insurance premiums. To avoid costly coverage for employees, companies have often tried to skimp on mental health services when selecting their plans. It has been over a decade since the Mental Health Parity and Addiction Equity Act of 2008 was passed, with its promise to make mental health and substance abuse treatment equally accessible to the insured as general physical health care. However, progress is slow. A 2017 study indicated that in fiscal year 2015, behavioral care was 4–6 times more likely than medical or surgical care to be classified as out of network. Insurers paid primary care providers 20% more for the same types of care than they paid addiction and mental health care specialists, including psychiatrists (Melek et al. 2017). A 2014 study in *JAMA Psychiatry* suggested that only 55.3% of psychiatrists accepted insurance versus 88.7% of providers in other specialties (Bishop et al. 2014). Thus, even for workers with decent mental health benefits, provider options are highly limited.

The results of systemic issues with insurance coverage and lack of functional mental health parity are absenteeism, presenteeism, higher rates of disability and attrition, and costly mistakes and injuries. Merely "checking the box" and providing nominal mental health coverage for employees will do little to defray the costs of unmitigated stress and negative workplace culture. Companies must commit themselves to actively pursuing improvements in the workplace—transforming corporate culture, reducing stress and stigma, and becoming accountable for ensuring that employees can access adequate mental health services.

Approaches to Enhance Value

Well-designed employee wellness programs should benefit all stakeholders. In this section, we are primarily discussing costs and benefits to employers and employees. However, as demonstrated, the effects of occupational stress on the workforce, health care system, and global economy are profound. Thus, the potential benefit of widespread implementation of such programs is equally enticing. Although every executive should ideally strive to build a company full of happy, productive employees, the cost-benefit analysis of an employee wellness program is where the rubber meets the road. As we have discussed, the cost of ignoring corporate culture and employee wellness is simply too much to bear. Additionally, employee wellness programs are both inexpensive—$12–$40 per employee year—and profitable for employers, with an estimated return on investment of $3–$10 for every $1 spent (Attridge et al. 2009).

Creating Healthy Workplaces—Acceptance, Empowerment, and Resources

To reduce the burden of stress and mental illness in the workplace, a company must begin by evaluating and addressing its culture. Cultural change is driven from the top down. Executives must embrace and exemplify the message, communicating the prime importance of employee wellness in the company's identity and day-to-day operations. They must be visibly dedicated to creating a workplace that will promote, support, and improve the mental health of employees and their families. Moreover, leadership must be visibly and genuinely engaged at multiple levels within the organization. Culture is driven not only by C-suite executives carving the company values statement into stone, but also by the day-to-day attitudes and management styles of leaders at all levels. If each successive tier of managers supports the wellness of those who report directly to them, the resulting cascade reaches every corner of the organization. Additionally, supervisors are in a prime position to recognize the signs of stress and other mental health issues in their direct reports and assist them in the process of engaging company wellness resources.

As a firm assesses the state of the organization in terms of employee wellness, it may recognize inconsistencies in the following critical domains:

- **Identity:** Who are we, as a company? Why were we founded? What characteristics unite our employees and our product? Does the image we portray, in both our outward branding and internal processes, align with the concept of employee wellness?
- **Mission Statement:** Why do we exist? What are our goals, and how will we get there? Do we measure ourselves by results alone, or are we invested in a sustainable process that promotes wellness of the company as reflected by its workforce and business practices?
- **Values:** At the end of the day, what matters most? What principles do we hold in highest regard? What ideals are we unwilling to sacrifice, even for profit? Is employee well-being on this list? If so, are there other "competing" values on the list that may compromise dedication to wellness?

Using the items above as a "temperature check" for corporate culture is a great way to identify the broader nature of the problem. This type of critical self-appraisal will often demonstrate the need for, and overarching goals of, an employee wellness effort.

The next step is identifying the scope of the problem.

- **Breadth:** How widespread is the problem, or how much change needs to occur to meet our wellness goals? How many departments are affected, or is the issue global? Are there any obvious gaps in corporate ideology or methodology that might compromise the long-term viability of change?

- **Depth:** Will the program meet the needs of employees at all levels of the organization? Is the company vertically integrated in a way that will allow spread of cultural change, monitoring of progress, identification of problems, and mobilization of resources at any level? If not, how will this issue be addressed?
- **Impact:** To what degree are health issues impacting productivity? How much are employees engaging their health care benefits? Does pharmacy spending data reflect adequate treatment of health care issues and adherence with recommended treatment? How is the company affected in terms of short- and long-term disability?

With the nature of the problem identified and the scope assessed, a company can begin to consider options for intervention. This will typically involve outside consultation and/or implementation of a predesigned and industry-proven wellness program. The following considerations will help guide the process of designing a program:

- **Fit:** How much time, money, and other resources can be dedicated to improving corporate wellness? Do the proposed interventions line up with the identified problems? Does the plan reflect corporate values and identity? Will the employees of this company understand, appreciate, and engage the effort and its associated interventions? Does the scope of the program reflect projected growth, or contraction, of the company?
- **Quality:** Have the proposed strategies been successful at other businesses, or at the current business in the past? If a consulting firm or established program is being utilized, does its track record suggest results on par with identified company goals? Have past results led to accelerating positive change and thus been deeply transformative and long-lived?
- **Integration:** Does the plan allow for cultivation of relationships with resources such as health care providers, insurance/benefits providers, fitness centers, nutritionists, and local foundations? Will employees be able to access the outside resources necessary to maintain wellness? Is the healthy lifestyle promoted by the program attainable and in line with broader cultural values?

If there is one factor known to consistently sabotage implementation and access for corporate wellness initiatives, it is stigmatization. Despite extraordinary efforts by the mental health community and a resulting increase in awareness, the stigma associated with mental health diagnosis and treatment remains a key barrier to engagement in wellness programs. Even for employees with subclinical issues—for example, an employee who uses an assistance program to deal with workplace stress that does not require medical intervention—the concept of "admitting weakness" or "needing help," along with fear of being perceived as "weak" or "soft" by coworkers, is often enough to deter the employees from accessing the very programs that would address these anxieties. The following principles are recommended to promote success and reduce stigma:

- **A Focus on Wellness:** Designing a program that promotes wellness and prevents illness implicitly includes every employee. An intervention designed to help sick or stressed workers risks alienating all those who are paying in but not seeing benefits. Not everyone suffers from mental or physical health issues, but everyone wants to feel secure, valued, and free. Wellness programs are not limited to health care access—they should promote ideal work conditions for all employees through a variety of assessments and interventions.
- **100% Utilization:** The wellness program is a corporate imperative rather than a safety net. When a wellness initiative is accessed only by those who are struggling, the unintended consequence is "outing" anyone who utilizes the program. On the other hand, if everyone is required to meet annually with a human resources representative to discuss satisfaction and thoughts on work conditions in addition to any wellness issues, they are provided a "safe" opportunity to express concerns and to access mental health care and other interventions. This requirement also sends the message that employee wellness is a key dimension of corporate values and a direct mediator of the success of the organization.
- **Assertive Intervention:** When employees access assistance programs early and their problems are taken seriously, their stress is managed before it becomes functionally impairing and hits the bottom line. In this scenario, health issues are diagnosed and treated early, which is the key to good treatment outcomes and long-term cost reduction. This principle fits hand-in-glove with the previous principle of "100% Utilization" and the natural increase in screening opportunities and stigma reduction it affords. Universal participation addresses concerns early on and helps reduce stigma by eliminating the misperception that participation is only for individuals who are highly dysfunctional.
- **Zero Tolerance for Discrimination:** Legislation such as the Americans With Disabilities Act of 1990 has benefited workers by aiming to prevent discrimination based on disability, including both physical and mental health conditions. Explicit discrimination, while still present, is becoming increasingly rare. What is more surreptitious, and therefore pervasive and damaging, is implicit discrimination. Firms must work to understand the subtle ways in which people with health issues are unfairly treated, whether

through implicit judgment and social ramifications, through mischaracterization of work quality, or by discouraging employees from seeking treatment. Once identified, they must be addressed directly, swiftly, and completely. This includes the complex but achievable goal of creating a safe reporting environment for any issues that arise in the workplace.
- **Training:** Managers should be trained in conflict resolution and effective communication and leadership skills to reduce workplace stress. Additionally, managers must be trained to identify job performance problems related to mental health issues and manage these issues in a respectful yet assertive way. These skills should be combined with education on cultural competency and recognizing and intervening in discrimination of all types, including that pertaining to mental health issues. Human resources personnel should be positioned as both advocates and access points for employees.

Promoting wellness and reducing stigma are powerful goals for an organization seeking to improve the health of its employees and productivity of the company. However, no matter how comprehensive and competent the effort toward supportive culture and prevention, employees will suffer from stress and mental health issues. With one in five Americans living with mental illness, this is a near certainty (Substance Abuse and Mental Health Services Administration 2014). Providing nominal health care coverage may suffice in meeting legal requirements, but as we have discussed, the cost of untreated or undertreated conditions is devastating. With this in mind, a critical corporate responsibility is ensuring access to affordable, effective treatment. The following are recommendations regarding accountability and strategies for ensuring access:

- **Health Care Education:** Employees must be empowered to recognize and understand the burden of mental health issues in themselves and their coworkers. A variety of screening tools are available through the American Psychiatric Association and other sources; these include tools for self-screening as well as resources for managers. Furthermore, employees should be educated on the various employee wellness and health care options available to them, points of access, optimal use, and sources of advocacy. Regular company-wide educational opportunities help reduce stigma, "normalize" mental health issues, and promote utilization of services. These can be in the form of meetings, educational e-mails, wellness activities, or other creative means.
- **Low Barrier to Entry:** A network of provider options must be preestablished and easily accessible. It is the employer's responsibility to ensure that options are available within the network and without excessive

wait times. The network should include primary care physicians, psychiatrists and other specialists, psychotherapists, and ancillary services such as case management and nutrition. These resources should be made available through the company's formal employee assistance program (EAP) and associated referral but should also be available to employees who wish to arrange their own care.

- **Adequate Coverage:** Any health care plan selected by the company should include robust prescription medication coverage. Medications are highly effective in treating a variety of mental health issues and, in many cases, are necessary elements of a long-term wellness plan. Health care coverage should also include robust access across a wide variety of care settings, from outpatient care to emergency services to inpatient hospitalization.
- **Metrics:** Health care plans should include the ability to track and analyze data pertaining to usage. This is critical to gauging the costs and successes of any employee wellness program.

Addressing corporate wellness is a major undertaking. Whether an organization is designing its own program or enlisting the help of a third-party consultant, the roadmap above can serve as a valuable resource from the planning phase to implementation and beyond.

Outcomes

The encouraging news is that early intervention and treatment can substantially reduce disability burden, both in terms of personal suffering and employer costs (McCulloch et al. 2001). According to the Employee Assistance Trade Association, companies average a return on investment of $3–$10 per dollar spent on EAPs (Hargrave et al. 2008). Treatment offered through EAPs has demonstrated cost savings through reduction in expenses associated with medical claims, accident benefits, mental health care and general medical costs, absenteeism, lost wages, and turnover. Perhaps more importantly, EAPs help employees. In one study, employee self-reports of impairment before and after EAP intervention were measured and assigned values in terms of lost productivity, then monetized. The bottom line is that employees improved and the firm benefited financially—on the order of a 400% return on investment (Philips 2005).

Conclusion

By this point in time, a clear case has been made for the economic benefit associated with employee wellness initiatives. Companies quite literally cannot afford to miss this opportunity to create a healthy, productive work environment. However, reasonable expectations must govern the process of cultural change. Corporate wellness is, in the grand scheme, a relatively new concept. It will take months to years for the workforce to embrace new values and begin to identify with the culture of wellness and prevention. This is particularly true for companies with long-established norms, and those that have profited in spite of a problematic culture may prove outright obstinate. Consistency and intention are the keys to progress. Even a small number of dedicated and persistent champions can drive change over time, and the effort is inherently rewarding. Advocating for wellness and mental health is not merely profitable—it is an ethical imperative and a necessity for long-lasting organizational health. Just as healthy individuals grow by working through stress, the healthy company will not crumble under difficult circumstances, but will develop even greater resilience and thrive.

Additional Resource

The American Psychiatric Association, the largest representative body for psychiatrists in the United States, is a critical source of scholarship and education for health care providers worldwide. Dedicated to evidence-based approaches to mental health treatment and advocacy, the APA has compiled resources particularly well suited to the pursuit of corporate wellness, listed and described in its own "Working Well" report, released in June 2016 (Brennan et al. 2016). For these and other resources, please visit the APA's Center for Workplace Mental Health Web site at http://workplacementalhealth.org.

References

Accreditation Council for Graduate Medical Education: ACGME Common Program Requirements. February 3, 2020. Available at: www.acgme.org/Portals/0/PFAssets/ProgramRequirements/CPRResidency2020.pdf. Accessed June 28, 2020.

Allen DG: Retaining talent: a guide to analyzing and managing employee turnover. SHRM Foundation Effective Practice Guidelines Series, 2008. Available at: www.shrm.org/hr-today/trends-and-forecasting/special-reports-and-expert-views/Documents/Retaining-Talent.pdf. Accessed March 25, 2020.

Amabile TM, Barsade SG, Mueller JS, et al: Affect and creativity at work. Administrative Science Quarterly 50:367–403, 2005

American Psychological Association: Stress in America: paying with our health. February 4, 2015. Available at: www.apa.org/news/press/releases/stress/2014/stress-report.pdf. Accessed March 25, 2020.

Arnedt JT, Owens J, Crouch M, et al: Neurobehavioral performance of residents after heavy night call vs after alcohol ingestion. JAMA 294(9):1025–1033, 2005

Attridge M, Amaral TM, Bjornson T, et al: EAP effectiveness and ROI. EASNA Research Notes 1(3):1–5, 2009

Balch CM, Oreskovich MR, Dyrbye LN, et al: Personal consequences of malpractice lawsuits on American surgeons. J Am Coll Surg 213(4):657–667, 2011

BBC: White collar, in A History of the World, 2014. Available at: www.bbc.co.uk/ahistoryoftheworld/objects/1AhY3K_mSwqaEBvZaN5eYw. Accessed July 2, 2020.

Bishop TF, Press MJ, Keyhani S, et al: Acceptance of insurance by psychiatrists and the implications for access to mental health care. JAMA Psychiatry 71(2):176–181, 2014

Boggs CJ: Workers' compensation history: the great tradeoff! Insurance Journal Online, March 16, 2015. Available at: www.insurancejournal.com/blogs/academy-journal/2015/03/19/360273.htm. Accessed March 27, 2020.

Bourne LE Jr, Yaroush RA: Stress and cognition: a cognitive psychological perspective. NASA Report, February 1, 2003. Available at: https://human-factors.arc.nasa.gov/flightcognition/download/misc/Stress%20and%20Cognition.pdf. Accessed March 25, 2020.

Brennan W, Dolan-Delvecchio K, Emmet W, et al: Working well: leading a mentally healthy business. June 2016. Available at: http://workplacementalhealth.org/getattachment/Making-The-Business-Case/Link-2-Title/working-well-toolkit.pdf?lang=en-US. Accessed March 25, 2020.

Brown SE, Ratcliffe SJ, Halpern SD: Assessing the utility of ICU readmissions as a quality metric: an analysis of changes mediated by residency work-hour reforms. Chest 147(3):626–636, 2015

Brunworth JD, Sindwani R: Impact of duty hour restrictions on otolaryngology training: divergent resident and faculty perspectives. Laryngoscope 116(7):1127–1130, 2006

Bureau of Labor Statistics: Census of fatal occupational injuries in 2018. Press Release, December 17, 2019. Available at: www.bls.gov/news.release/pdf/cfoi.pdf. Accessed March 25, 2020.

Burton WN, Conti DJ, Chen CY, et al: The role of health risk factors and disease on worker productivity. J Occup Environ Med 41(10):863–877, 1999

Colligan TW, Higgins EM: Workplace stress: etiology and consequences. J Workplace Behav Health 21(2):89–97, 2006

Compte O, Postlewaite A: Confidence-enhanced performance. American Economic Review 91(5):1536–1557, 2004

Crabtree S: Engagement keeps the doctor away. Gallup Business Journal, January 13, 2005. Available at: https://news.gallup.com/businessjournal/14500/engagement-keeps-doctor-away.aspx. Accessed March 25, 2020.

Gallup: State of the global workplace: employment engagement insights for business leaders worldwide. Gallup News, 2017. Available at: www.gallup.com/services/178517/state-global-workplace.aspx. Accessed March 25, 2020.

Glynn SJ, Boushey H: There are significant business costs to replacing employees. Center for American Progress, November 16, 2012. Available at: www.americanprogress.org/issues/economy/reports/2012/11/16/44464/there-are-significant-business-costs-to-replacing-employees. Accessed March 25, 2020.

Greenberg PE, Fournier AA, Sisitsky T, et al: The economic burden of adults with major depressive disorder in the United States (2005 and 2010). J Clin Psychiatry 76(2):155–162, 2015

Hargrave GE, Hiatt D, Alexander R, et al: EAP treatment impact on presenteeism and absenteeism: implications for return on investment. Journal of Workplace Behavioral Health 23(3):283–293, 2008

Hemp P: Presenteeism: at work-but out of it. Harv Bus Rev 82(10):49–58, 2004

Hiscox: The 2017 Hiscox guide to employee lawsuits. 2017. Available at: www.hiscox.com/documents/2017-Hiscox-Guide-to-Employee-Lawsuits.pdf. Accessed March 25, 2020.

Jena AB, Schoemaker L, Bhattacharya J: The effect of ACGME resident duty hour reforms on outcomes of physicians after completion of residency. Health Aff (Millwood) 33(10):1832–1840, 2014

Leopold RS: A Year in the Life of a Million American Workers. New York, MetLife, 2003

Liberty Mutual: Workplace Safety Index. Hopkinton, MA, Liberty Mutual Research Institute for Safety, 2016

Marlowe JF: Depression's surprising toll on worker productivity. Empl Benefits J 27(1):16–21, 2002

McCulloch J, Ozminkowski RJ, Cuffel B, et al: Analysis of a managed psychiatric disability program. J Occup Environ Med 43(2):101–109, 2001

Melek SP, Perlman D, Davenport S: Addiction and mental health vs. physical health: analyzing disparities in network use and provider reimbursement rates. Milliman Research Report, December 2017. Available at: www.milliman.com/uploadedFiles/insight/2017/NQTLDisparityAnalysis.pdf. Accessed March 25, 2020.

Morrison KW: The ROI of safety. Safety and Health Magazine, October 16, 2018. Available at: www.safetyandhealthmagazine.com/articles/10414-the-roi-of-safety. Accessed March 25, 2020.

National Institute of Mental Health: Major depression. February 2019. Available at: www.nimh.nih.gov/health/statistics/major-depression.shtml. Accessed March 25, 2020.

Occupational Safety and Health Administration: Employer responsibilities. OSHA Worker Rights and Protections, 2020. Available at: www.osha.gov/as/opa/worker/employer-responsibility.html. Accessed March 25, 2020.

Oswald AJ, Proto E, Sgroi D: Happiness and productivity. Journal of Labor Economics 33(4):789–822, 2015

Ouyang D, Chen JH, Krishnan G, et al: Patient outcomes when housestaff exceed 80 hours per week. Am J Medicine 129(9):993.e1–999.e1, 2016

Philips SB: Client satisfaction with university employee assistance programs. Employee Assistance Quarterly 19(4):59–70, 2005

Reed DA, Fletcher KE, Arora VM: Systematic review: association of shift length, protected sleep time, and night float with patient care, residents' health, and education. Ann Intern Med 153(12):829–842, 2010

Reid E: Why some men pretend to work 80-hour weeks. Harvard Business Review, April 28, 2015. Available at: https://hbr.org/2015/04/why-some-men-pretend-to-work-80-hour-weeks. Accessed March 25, 2020.

Seppala E, Cameron K: Proof that positive work cultures are more productive. Harvard Business Review Online, December 1, 2015. Available at: https://hbr.org/2015/12/proof-that-positive-work-cultures-are-more-productive. Accessed March 25, 2020.

Shanafelt TD, Balch CM, Bechamps G, et al: Burnout and medical errors among American surgeons. Ann Surg 251(6):995–1000, 2010

Shetty KD, Bhattacharya J: Changes in hospital mortality associated with residency work-hour regulations. Ann Intern Med 147(2):73–80, 2007

Stewart WF, Ricci CM, Chee E, et al: Lost productive work time costs from health conditions in the United States: results from the American Productivity Audit. J Occup Environ Med 45(12):1234–1246, 2003

Substance Abuse and Mental Health Services Administration: Results from the 2013 National Survey on Drug Use and Health: Mental Health Findings. 2014. Available at: www.samhsa.gov/data/sites/default/files/NSDUHmhfr2013/NSDUHmhfr2013.pdf. Accessed March 25, 2020.

Taylor FW: The Principles of Scientific Management. New York, Harper & Brothers, 1911

U.S. Equal Employment Opportunity Commission: ADA charge data by impairments/bases—merit factor resolutions (charges filed with EEOC) FY 1997–FY 2019. 2020. Available at: www.eeoc.gov/eeoc/statistics/enforcement/ada-merit.cfm. Accessed March 25, 2020.

Volpp KG, Rosen AK, Rosenbaum PR, et al: Mortality among hospitalized Medicare beneficiaries in the first 2 years following ACGME resident duty hour reform. JAMA 298(9):975–983, 2007

Volpp KG, Rosen AK, Rosenbaum PR, et al: Did duty hour reform lead to better outcomes among the highest risk patients? J Gen Intern Med 24(10):1149–1155, 2009

Watson Wyatt Worldwide: Staying@Work: Effective Presence at Work: Survey Report. Arlington, VA, Watson Wyatt Worldwide, 1998

Williams R: Mellon Learning Curve Research Study. New York, Mellon Corporation, 2003

21

Aging and End-of-Life Care

Alessandra Scalmati, M.D., Ph.D.
Madeleine Lipshie-Williams, M.D.
Gary J. Kennedy, M.D.

Traditional medical education created the impression that aging was an illness and that all means should be applied to extend life as long as possible, regardless of its quality. Anything less was regarded as a physician's failure. As a result, many physicians share the attitudes of society at large and are uncomfortable with old age and dying. The practice of caring for the elderly and dying in our current health care system often fails to provide comfort and a positive experience for terminally ill persons and their families.

Also, despite broad consensus on the need to integrate a psychosocial perspective into medical care for older Americans and persons at the end of life, there are not enough psychiatrists and other behavioral health providers to approach the need. Further barriers to quality care occur due to fragmentation of communication across the acute, rehabilitative, long-term, and community-based care systems. Mental health issues in older adults make needed communication and continuity of care even less likely. Poorly connected and coordinated proprietary electronic health records can make efforts to communicate between the systems frustrating, if not impossible. Patients receiving primary care at one medical center may not have their records accessible at another center or long-term care facility within the same city. Written permission for a transfer of information is required. This is a particular problem in the care of older adults when the complexity of comorbidity often requires communication between providers to avoid iatrogenic complications.

For these reasons, care for older adults and people at the end of life is approaching a moment of crisis. Psychiatrists need to have a more significant role in improving end-of-life care; however, few psychiatrists show interest in palliative and geriatric psychiatry, possibly due to fears of marginalization and lower compensation. They also may perceive a less prestigious professional identity in a medical system designed to reward those who treat disease and prolong life over those who reduce suffering (Eden et al. 2012).

Nonetheless, psychiatrists with appropriate training and support can bridge these gaps, meeting the crisis as a moment of opportunity. Psychiatrists can make major contributions to patient-centered care and systems integration. They can also influence public and policy makers' recognition of the needed shift in priorities through advocacy and education. What follows is a perspective on the delicate balance of cost and quality in psychiatric care of older adults and those at the end of their lives.

Perspectives on Advanced Age and End-of-Life Care

Within academic disability studies, the Social Disability Model (Nisker 2019) makes a distinction between *impairment* and *disability*. An impairment causes a functional limitation, whereas a disability is a disadvantage faced by those with impairments due to norms, systems, or structures in the environment. For example, a wheelchair-bound office worker is impaired, but is not disabled if the office is wheelchair accessible.

Typical medical models have conflated impairment with disability and attempt to cure the impairment rather than reduce the disability. This does not mean that medical interventions have nothing to offer, or that impairments do not cause physical limitations and psychical pain. Rather the consequences of an impairment should be accommodated if possible, to reduce the associated disability—as in the example of the wheelchair-bound office worker.

For older adults, the effects of impairment may extend beyond the patient to caretakers and the community that make up the social environment. Stakeholders must include family, caregivers, and community. For aging adults, particularly those living with chronic conditions or approaching the end of life, encounters with providers who can address both immediate and extended effects of impairments can optimize their independence by reducing their "disability." Multiple avenues of intervention exist when multiple stakeholders are involved, and collaborative approaches will often be much more satisfying for clinicians. These approaches will influence cost, quality, and accessibility of care (Nisker 2019).

Because the current model of care is based on a compensation system that rewards action-based interventions above those that are based on relationships and emotional well-being, it frequently leads to inappropriate, avoidable interventions. Stakeholders have difficulty establishing significant relationships with physicians to communicate patients' preferences and experiences. This deprives patients and their families of opportunities for important end-of-life interactions.

Even if payment models were to shift to favor the formation of these relationships, the prejudices of physicians would still need to be addressed. The notion that fulfillment and meaning cannot exist with aging, dying, and death still exists and needs to be challenged. Providers, including psychiatrists, for older adults receive minimal, if any, training in palliative care. As a result, they are often reluctant to discuss plans for death, even when doing so will ultimately provide comfort for both patients and family members. For those who are aging or at end of life, investment in home-based, person-centered care rather than disease-centered institutional care supports the well-being of individuals and communities far better than the current system. Incorporation of these models of care into medical education and residency training is a way to begin to overcome existing biases. Proposed comfort care guidelines (in place of curative care), which would facilitate this evolution in practice (Brown 2019), are discussed later in this chapter.

Determining Appropriate Care

As the aging population grows, expanding programs specifically designed to serve geriatric health needs and creating additional jobs in the field are necessary investments. An intervention studied by Foldes and colleagues (2017) is one example of such a program. It provided group support and 24-hour telephone access to coaches for family members caring for patients with Alzheimer's dementia. Compared with care as usual, the intervention significantly delayed nursing home admissions and reduced caregiver burden. Savings of approximately $40 million per year were estimated if the program were to be implemented throughout New York State. Programs such as this reduce spending in the long run, but payers are reluctant to implement them due to high up-front costs related to infrastructure and personnel. Unfortunately, long-term investments that improve public health have no immediate gain for payers who insure populations at the end of their purchasing life. This is especially so when private for-profit insurers must maximize short-term profits for shareholders.

Consequently, programs such as the one just described are not in widespread use. Commitment and planning will be required for their adoption by health care systems. Successful integration of mental health, geriatrics, and end-of-life care will need to include appropriate funding sources, easily accessible communication methods, and strategies to facilitate cultural change. Simply colocating a psychiatrist in a primary care site by providing office space, phone, and Internet access is not likely to be as effective as the process of full integration, in which the psychiatrist works directly with a team of providers including primary care, nursing, and social work. This team care facilitates screening, initiation of treatment, and treatment planning. It includes direct psychiatric consultation when mental health, substance use, or treatment resistance conditions are encountered. The integration of the psychiatric perspective is essential to the provision of "appropriate care" for older adults (Callahan et al. 2018). The demand for this innovative kind of care, involving psychiatrists with knowledge of geriatrics and palliative care, will grow as the population ages. Providing an adequate workforce to meet these needs will be challenging.

Several measures can be applied to define *appropriate care*, meaning care that is individualized but also beneficial to the population at large. Cost per quality-adjusted life years (QALY) gained and cost per disability-adjusted life years (DALY) reduced are two examples. To clarify, dialysis can restore the quality of life as well as extend the lifespan of persons with kidney failure. The expense of dialysis can be used to calculate cost per QALY gained. *Quality* is variably defined along five dimensions: mobility, self-care, usual activities, freedom from pain or discomfort, and levels of anxiety and depression (Coast et al. 2018). Similarly, dialysis can reduce the duration of disability to yield the DALY reduced measure. This calculation can be stated as a question: "For every dollar spent on dialysis, how much is the disabled time associated with chronic renal failure reduced compared with no dialysis?"

Another measure is the cost-effectiveness ratio, which represents the incremental costs divided by the incremental benefits of a treatment compared to either care as usual or another intervention. This ratio also can be exemplified with a question: "Compared with life with chronic renal failure without dialysis, how many additional years would be lived if dialysis were given?" As shown above, therapy for family members caring for a patient with dementia saved costs compared to care as usual. The caregiver intervention for persons with dementia was calculated as a net savings because nursing home admissions were delayed and the subsequent expense forestalled. Potential savings realized over 15 years in Minnesota alone would approach $1 trillion (Long et al. 2014).

These measures give some indication of what kinds of interventions provide the most quality per dollar spent, or the best value (see Chapter 1, "Defining and Measuring Value"). When outcomes are measured by metrics such as reduction in years of life lost to disability rather than cure rates or survival time, the intervention is more appropriate for both the individual and the population as a whole. This broader perspective provides a different view of what constitutes success. Considering the example of dialysis for chronic kidney disease again, treatment is palliative rather than curative, reducing disability but not eliminating the disease. Similarly, current approaches to the dementias are palliative, with quantifiable population-based benefits (Foldes et al. 2017).

Integrated Care for Older Adults

The value of integrating behavioral health personnel into primary care is well established, showing benefits in the management of comorbid diabetes, heart failure, and depression (Bruce and Sirey 2018). There are several examples of successful integrated approaches to enhancing the value of end-of-life services. One such approach is the integration of a depression care management program into Medicare home care services. This intervention conducted across seven states achieved a reduction in 30- and 60-day hospital readmission rates (Bruce et al. 2016). Nevertheless, integrating psychiatric care for Medicaid and Medicare beneficiaries was challenging in a disadvantaged community such as this.

The Montefiore Medical System's Certified Home Health Agency serves a majority of African American and Latino patients. The agency works with primary care and managed long-term care providers. It integrated a geriatric psychiatrist into the weekly team triage meeting and home visits to evaluate patients with emotional health needs. This integration has been self-sustaining in two ways: 1) by becoming incorporated as an educational component of the adult and geriatric residency training programs, and 2) by providing a fee-for-service reimbursement to the attending psychiatrist. Thus, the geriatric psychiatrist is supported as both a faculty member and a service provider. Of the patients seen, 52% received a new mental health diagnosis, with most new diagnoses being neurocognitive disorders. Of the 62% of patients who were offered psychotropic medications by the visiting psychiatrist, 90% accepted. It was suggested that this may have been due to the provision of care in a nonstigmatized home setting for older, minority adults (Ceïde et al. 2016).

In New York State, Medicare will pay for in-home mental health care if provided by a psychiatrist or psychiatric nurse practitioner. Staff of a Certified Home Health Agency, including nurses and special workers, cannot bill for mental health services. The article by Ceïde and colleagues (2016) describes one example of how a health care system can enhance value by expanding funding arrangements, which would not have supported the addition of behavioral health services in the past. The alliance of an academic medical center with a community-based agency to better train psychiatrists and provide better care for older adults is promising.

Interventions used in subacute care and rehabilitation facilities have been adapted for use with depressed patients who have advanced chronic obstructive pulmonary disease (COPD) or the sequalae of stroke (Avari and Alexopoulos 2015). A simplified psychotherapeutic approach used with depressed patients in rehabilitation for advanced COPD reduced depression as well as dyspnea, by promoting behavioral activation through physical activity and social interactions (Jackson et al. 2019). The reduction in dyspnea was unexpected, in that the initial goal was a reduction in depression. These improvements suggest a critical change in priorities for the care of older adults (Kennedy 2018). The addition of a behavioral health component to primary care may produce unexpected improvements in health overall. As argued by Applegate and colleagues (2018), the priorities for older adults with multiple comorbidities are the maintenance and optimization of the person's independence and self-direction. Rather than a disease-centered perspective, this approach is patient centered, and emotional health is a key component.

When curing a disease is no longer possible, as with a chronic illness, the goals of care should change. Moving from cure to palliation, from disease-centered to patient-centered care, is especially relevant when mental and physical illnesses are comorbid and disabling. Recent studies (e.g., Brink et al. 2019) have shown that persons with psychotic disorders have shortened lifespans relative to the general population. Although suicide is partly responsible for this phenomenon, difficulty accessing primary care and preventive services is also a significant contributor, even more so for individuals of advanced age. Experience with the integration of primary care into mental health clinics demonstrates a significant reduction of physical morbidity associated with serious and persistent mental disorders. Demonstrated benefits include reductions in obesity, improved patient self-management, and reduced risk of hospitalizations for both general medical and psychiatric issues (Bartels et al. 2018a, 2018b).

Emotional Care at Life's End

Progress in medical technology and public health has prolonged life expectancy, as well as the "active" lifespan, meaning those years of life in which the person is independent or minimally reliant on others. It has become apparent that health care providers need to focus on more than decreasing disability. A more holistic perspective takes into consideration the physical, social, cultural, and spiritual needs of older adults. This approach is necessary to promote a sense of meaning and purpose for older adults and to prevent or minimize despair and hopelessness. Respect for the patient's understanding of the aging process, in both personal and cultural contexts, is an essential aspect of patient- and community-centered care.

The use of a narrative, life-review approach in geriatric care has been a helpful way to bridge different aspects of the patient's experience (Clark 2015). This narrative technique is one of the hidden treasures of geriatric care. The patient is asked to give a brief synopsis of one or more important life events to illuminate their values and preferences. For example, one might ask older veterans to talk about their combat experience, or to describe how they felt about returning to racial segregation after fighting for one's country. More general questions, such as how they met their spouse or how they lost their parents, begin to clarify their world view and emotional life.

The integration of psychologists, social workers, psychiatrists, and spiritual counselors in palliative care and hospice teams has proven invaluable to patients and families. Terminally ill patients frequently experience depression and hopelessness, which are associated with a desire for hastened death in many cases. These desires can be mitigated by interventions to lessen depression or increase spiritual well-being (Breitbart et al. 2000; McClain et al. 2003). Meaning-centered group psychotherapy, which explores values learned and purposes achieved, was studied in a randomized controlled trial with advanced cancer patients. Results demonstrated a positive impact on patients' emotional suffering (Breitbart et al. 2010). This type of intervention may also be used for survivors of advanced cancer who live with increased disability and shortened life expectancy (van der Spek et al. 2018).

There is ample evidence to suggest that older adults suffering with depression have higher levels of physical disability, poorer overall health indicators and outcomes, and higher levels of utilization of health care services. A study conducted across Europe found an association between the loss of a sense of meaning in life and depression in older community residents, particularly older males (Volkert et al. 2017). Therefore, strategies aimed at reducing depression, hopelessness, loneliness, and social isolation will likely improve most health indicators and reduce cost of care by enhancing self-care, such as adherence to diet, exercise, and medication regimens. Some cognitive or behavioral strategies typically used to address these issues may not be as effective in older adults. Impaired cognition, particularly executive dysfunction, may require a simplified form of therapy, but age by itself is not an obstacle to most established interventions. Case reports suggest that a psychotherapeutic approach focusing on life's meaning and purpose, and the reappraisal of values and identity, is helpful for older adults facing loss and grief (Yang et al. 2018). A protocol for assessing the effectiveness of meaning-centered psychotherapy in cancer patients showed that the most successful interventions were administered in group format at the oncology clinic where patients went for follow-up. The therapy was time limited (8–12 sessions) and task focused, aiming to reengage patients with creative activities and the people who have been part of their support systems in the past (Breitbart et al. 2010). A randomized controlled trial examining a similar set of interventions for older adults would be welcome and could demonstrate a reduction in the existential despair at the end of their lives.

End-of-Life Planning and Family Counseling

It is also essential for providers to help older adults and patients at the end of life to maintain a sense of control and agency. Advanced care planning can provide the opportunity for patients and their loved ones to have a thoughtful conversation with a skilled provider about available options. A compassionate clinician can absorb the family's hopes and fears and provide realistic information without shying away from the truth or falling into euphemistic expressions. Such an encounter allows the patient and family to express preferences, mourn losses, come to terms with what is no longer possible, and attain a measure of peace. Patients and their families may approach the end of life in the context of their past experiences with health, illness, and loss, but also with love and accomplishment.

The health and well-being of older patients hinge on continuity of care and the provision of supports that allow the optimal level of independence in old age as well as comfort and security. With these in place, older adults can be a resource to their families and their communities, rather than the burden they are sometimes considered to be. Grandparents as babysitters, retired professors as tutors, and community volunteers at polling places are only some of the examples. The indirect societal costs related to the disruption of family members' roles in work and childcare are enormous and must be considered as an offset to the cost of service provision (Mittelman et al. 1996).

Family members are partners in care. They provide support for the older adults in the community. They bear witness to the history of the patient's values and preferences when the patient is no longer able to do so. Family can reinforce the message and the plan on which the team and patient have agreed. The provider's ability to engage family and caregivers in a strong collaboration can make the difference between success and failure in any plan of care. Caregivers are also subjected to high levels of stress and have an increased prevalence of anxiety and depression. Proactive interventions allowing the caregiver to maintain connections to the community include education, peer support groups, and direct care. These can have a positive impact on the health and independence of patient and caregiver alike (Mittelman et al. 1996; Teri 1999; Teri and Logsdon 2000). Envisioning caregivers as service recipients themselves is essential for good patient outcomes.

Mental health professionals possess an awareness of interpersonal and social dynamics to address families in distress, and to help other team members negotiate family conflicts that are more likely to emerge in times of crisis or loss. Successful mediation of conflicts over care choices (e.g., to undergo dialysis or not) can avoid prolonged power struggles and animosity. It can guide appropriate end-of-life care choices, avoiding expensive and inappropriate care and litigation.

The palliative care and hospice movement was born out of a concern about the excessive medicalization of patients near the end of life, which has too often left patients and family members feeling dehumanized and alone. For everyone—the patient facing the end of life, the family member facing the loss of a loved one, and even the health care provider confronted with the limit of science and technology—death represents an anxiety-provoking challenge that forces one to come to terms with one's limitations. The focus on how and where one dies often displaces the anxiety related to the confrontation of the simple reality that everyone does indeed die. Much has been written about "a good death." The fear of dying alone is often mentioned as a distressing possibility by both patients and family members, and this is even more haunting for older adults living alone in the community or living in a long-term setting (Thompson et al. 2019). Not much consensus can be found on the concept of "successful dying," according to a review published in the *American Journal of Geriatric Psychiatry* (Meier et al. 2016). Perhaps the most disturbing concern that arises is the prevalence of discordant views between patient and family as to what "success" in death might mean. This finding suggests that improvement in communication, education, and advanced planning could go a long way in facilitating the implementation of patients' wishes, and hopefully allowing for a narrowing of the gap in expectations.

Extending the Palliative Care Paradigm

The lack of geriatric mental health personnel is exacerbated by the concentration of geriatric specialists around academic medical centers, and their lack of linkage to community-based socially supportive services and home health care agencies. Transportation and physical limitations make attending those centers problematic for older adults. As the population continues to become older, the insufficient numbers and knowledge of existing providers will be even more obvious. This situation will only be ameliorated by expanding the workforce and restructuring health care systems to facilitate access to mental health care for older adults (Eden et al. 2012). A greater emphasis on palliative care will be a key element in meeting these emerging needs.

The impact of the aging population on society and the health care system is profound, and the number of older adults who will require end-of-life care is growing globally. In recent years, a shift has taken place such that more deaths are occurring in the community than in the hospital. Patients and their families are more often expressing preferences for a patient- and family-centered approach to end-of-life care and opting for the older adults to spend the last of their lives in familiar surroundings. Frequent visits to the emergency room and crisis hospitalizations deprive the patient of the opportunity to die as the patient and family desired and planned. Because communication between patients and health providers around end-of-life directives and preferences is often inadequate, potentially avoidable trips to the emergency department when older adults have difficulties continue to occur. These occurrences not only reduce the quality of the end-of-life experience but also increase expenses and burdens to the health system. Unless the deficits in communication and services are addressed, this state of affairs will only increase as the aged population grows (Bone et al. 2018a, 2018b; Jha 2019).

Hospice care has emerged in recent years as one way to avoid the overuse of hospitalization and emergency room visits, and to reduce suffering at the end of life. Part 418 of the Electronic Code of Federal Regulations (www.ecfr.gov) defines criteria for a patient to become eligible for admission to in-home hospice services: the patient must 1) be entitled to Medicare Part A and 2) have a prognosis of 6 months or less to live. Services provided include a physician assessment and certification, ongoing care by a nurse practitioner, availability of a social worker and pastoral counselor, and 4 hours daily of a hospice aide for personal care and homemaking. These services provided in the home need to be recertified after 90 days. Inpatient hospice services in long-term care facilities are also available. To facilitate the determination of when an individual may appropriately receive hospice care, online prognosis calculators (e.g., see https://eprognosis.ucsf.edu) can be used by patients, family members, and practitioners to estimate survival probabilities based on comorbidity data (Gagne et al. 2011).

Substantial evidence also supports a population-based shift from tertiary interventions to palliative primary care (Kocher and Chigurupati 2016). Although still scarce, examples of successful community-based primary and preventive mental health care are found involving urban and rural populations, different economic and racial groups, and different payers. Most of these models have benefited from public funding. Olazarán and colleagues (2010), after completing a systematic review of the literature, developed a set of recommendations related to primary care for people with Alzheimer's dementia. One of the highest rated recommendations of that review was multicomponent caregiver interventions for delay in institutionalization. Abundant nonpharmacological interventions were given the next highest rating; these included cognitive, behavioral, affective, and functional training for both the person living with dementia and the caregiver. Overall, Olazarán and colleagues (2010) found substantial evidence for beneficial outcomes and quality-of-life improvements for older adults with dementia and their caregivers, as well as potential cost savings related to the provision of primary care.

Opting to accept an impending end of life with palliative care in the home, rather than continuing to accept procedures and hospitalization, not only would improve the quality of an individual's remaining time, but also would generate enough savings to offset the costs of in-home interventions. However, the number of palliative care practitioners is low and will continue to be inadequate. As a result, more "palliative care champions" (Kamal et al. 2019) schooled in the palliative approach will need to emerge. These champions, who are not palliative care specialists, include providers from various disciplines who have additional exposure to the palliative perspective. Increased opportunities for experience with a palliative care model during training in primary care, geriatrics, or psychiatry would expand this supportive segment of the workforce.

Another model to expand the capacity for palliative care is home-based primary care, which is especially promising for frail older adults who do not meet the 6-month mortality prediction required for in-home hospice. Still, their needs are essentially palliative (Temkin-Greener et al. 2019). Brown (2019) calls for the formulation of formal guidelines with indicators of "comfort care," to clarify for physicians when to pivot from curative to palliative care and how to address the change with patients and families. Brown suggested three markers to initiate this change: 1) terminal illness which has become treatment resistant or for which treatment would be associated with high risk, 2) complications associated with the first illness or the occurrence of a second condition, and 3) frailty of a high degree. Brown's recommended guidelines would be broader than the more narrowly defined criteria for the receipt of hospice care services. These efforts to expand the availability of palliative care will provide greater comfort at the end of life and help eliminate needless expense.

The Psychiatrist's Role and Existential Angst

Facing mortality represents a unique existential challenge for both the patients and their clinicians. Working as consultants or team members, psychiatrists are able to facilitate more open communication that can assist older adults to face the existential issues that naturally arise as one faces death. These interactions between patient and psychiatrist may take place in a range of circumstances, from outpatient mental health visits to house calls for patients in palliative care. The opportunity for the patient to speak openly to a nonjudgmental third party may alleviate emotional suffering, and it enables the psychiatrist to assess the emotional status of the elder person and their natural supports.

According to Erik Erikson's psychosocial stages, the developmental task of old age is "ego integrity versus despair," or stated differently, wisdom versus dissolution (Erikson 1950). Having accomplished the more generative tasks, such as achieving financial security and building a family, a person faces a new developmental challenge. At the end of life, the task becomes acceptance of the finite quality of one's existence, the recognition of all that has been achieved and all that has not, and the realization that some hopes and dreams will remain unfulfilled. The capacity to look back at one's life with satisfaction, finding in it a sense of meaning and purpose, can help in approaching the unavoidable losses and vulnerabilities of the final years. Facing the ultimate separation from life itself is particularly salient. Confronting this task is challenging not only for the patients and their loved ones, but also for their physicians. Traditionally, physicians have drawn professional meaning by trying to avoid loss and vulnerability, through efforts to save, restore, and extend their patients' lives. This existential angst among the many stakeholders involved in late-life care is the type of question geriatric psychiatrists are trained to address (Jeste 2018). Alleviation of this type of discomfort is a quality measure that is hard to capture, but it is intuitively more valuable than extraordinary measures to prolong life, and it is significantly less costly.

Ethical Issues at End-of-Life Decisions

The U.S. health care system, focused on extending life as long as possible, has emphasized the individual rather than the family and other social supports. Ironically, these priorities increase both direct and indirect costs. Apart from the actual dollar amounts spent to prolong life, there are the emotional costs of dying painfully and being removed from familiar surroundings. Direct costs can be lowered by achievement of fewer inpatient admissions to or duration of stays in acute or long-term care facilities. Indirect costs include disruptions of family members' ability to maintain normal work schedules and to attain child care. Some of these indirect costs are reduced if patients are able to have more independence and comprehensive care. Decisions must be made regarding who bears responsibility for the costs of newer models of care, as we discuss in this section.

Health care for older adults in the United States has focused on medical treatments that are typically aggressive and cure oriented, which in too many instances only prolong suffering (Hayes et al. 2015). An example of this type of treatment is the placement of a feeding tube in a patient with advanced dementia who is losing weight despite spoon feeding. The evidence is clear that although the feeding tube may prolong life for a short time, it will not prevent other common geriatric problems such as bed ulcers or aspiration pneumonia. The gastrostomy necessary for tube insertion is an invasive procedure, and the tube can be uncomfortable once in place. Despite these considerations, some families insist on placement of the gastrostomy tube and feel that failure to do so is tantamount to killing their loved one. Choosing to continue dialysis in the context of advanced dementia is yet another example of opting for an aggressive medical treatment. These types of short-term, cure-oriented decisions have traditionally been supported by physicians and other medical staff who are biased toward keeping people alive without regard to cost or quality of life. Part of this bias involves a lack of training for how to discuss, and an inability to take time to discuss, other less aggressive and more palliative options with patients and family members.

In recent years, some attitudes about end-of-life treatments have started to change, and the medical team is much more likely to discuss options and realistic outcomes in an emotionally adept manner (Bell et al. 2019). They often advocate for alternative, more appropriate choices with regard to quality of life. These include protecting patients from burdensome or painful interventions, helping families find ways to reduce the burden of caregiving, and obtaining resources to maintain the older patient in the community. For example, instead of recommending placement of a gastrostomy tube in a patient with advanced dementia, providers should suggest continued spoon feeding, provision of comfort, and development of advanced directives about resuscitation and other interventions. Avoiding emergency department visits and putting in-home hospice care in place should also be part of the discussion. When these alternative systems are in place, families do not feel abandoned to burdensome care with a dearth of resources. Still, even with these resources available, many families insist on extraordinary measures to prolong life, and providers are often uncomfortable discussing the cost of care as a consideration for decision making.

Encouraging decisions that promote quality of life, and that direct resources to support public health, is not practical unless adequate community supports can be provided. This is especially important when mental health issues further complicate end-of-life decisions. When supports are not available, or when families choose to use hospital-based care and extraordinary measures to prolong life, who pays? Simply put, everyone bears the cost, but some people will bear more depending on their circumstances (Joynt-Maddox 2018). Insurance often influences this decision. Decisions about how and what treatment should be covered present ethical dilemmas for both public and for-profit insurers, as well as family members. Unlimited coverage will encourage families to choose more expensive options. High deductibles or arbitrary endpoints of coverage discriminate against those with few resources. Some families can afford costly interventions that have minimal benefit even if their insurance will not cover them. Other families might want these interventions but cannot afford them. When families must pay a substantial amount of the cost of prolonging the life of a loved one, how will that influence their decision? Cost-related questions are not easily answered but must be considered by those who make health care policy, as well as individuals and family members making end-of-life decisions.

When patients are covered by traditional financing arrangements, physicians and medical team members, including clergy, can help guide the most appropriate end-of-life decisions. They may agree to family members' requests for interventions that have a low probability of benefit, but this should only be the case when families are fully informed of costs and likely outcomes. Emerging models of universal coverage will need to establish parameters for end-of-life care that will influence public expenditures. The extent of coverage will in turn influence individual choices. If health care is to be considered a right, society must designate responsibility. Conflicts over where responsibilities lie are inevitable and will be part of public debate when new models for financing are considered. Health care providers, including psychiatrists, will need to assist individuals to make decisions that are best for all concerned in the context of the resources that are available to them. Training in ethics and resolution of personal conflict must be part of curricula in psychiatry and other behavioral health professions. Although the focus of this chapter is on older adults, these questions arise whenever the possibility of extending threatened life presents itself. Palliative care and family support in decision making are essential aspects of a value-oriented system of care for all ages (Kharrat et al. 2018).

There are cases in which people with a poor prognosis may wish to hasten their death to reduce their suffering. Several states have legalized procedures for physicians to assist in that process. Some European countries have even allowed euthanasia to be practiced by physicians in certain circumstances (Roest et al. 2019). These practices have generated a great deal of controversy, which are beyond the scope of this chapter. It is important to recognize, however, that these practices will generate much debate in the future and may be among the most challenging ethical issues facing end-of-life care and the pursuit of value.

Conclusion

This chapter has considered issues faced by people at the end of their lives, and the need to address them. Part of the process involves examining questions related to existence and the meaning of a life's experience, as well as being allowed to die in familiar surroundings with loved ones present. The traditional medical bias toward prolonging life regardless of cost is often inconsistent with people's wishes. Hospital-based care, trips to the emergency room, and invasive procedures are very costly and do little to extend a life of value. Quality in this arena must be defined by measures that account for the emotional well-being of individuals approaching death, rather than additional days alive alone.

Psychiatric care should be integral to services designed to facilitate a satisfying transition to death. Psychiatrists have both biomedical and psychosocial training, which allows them to be both generalists, able to integrate all aspects of treatment planning, and specialists, providing direct care for mental illnesses encountered during this period. These dual perspectives are particularly helpful when working with older adults and persons at the end of life, when multiple comorbidities and polypharmacy may be prevalent. Their training should allow them to competently prioritize interventions and maximize patient well-being, which is a critical aspect of high-value health care at the end of life. Training programs in geriatrics and palliative care emphasize this approach across systems of care from clinic, to nursing homes, to the community.

The collaborative care model for depression in primary care offers a compelling and well-established basis for integration of behavioral health care into primary care services. A growing body of evidence demonstrates both cost- and quality-related benefits of this integrated approach to dementia care. Unfortunately, deficiencies in the behavioral health care workforce, identified by the Institute of Medicine's Mental Health and Substance Use Workforce for Older Adults, may limit the availability of these arrangements (Blazer et al. 2012). The older adult health care system's transition may require better public funding (Medicaid or Medicare enhancement and expansion) to support primary and preventive mental health care for aging and dying patients. Any expansion, however, must be prioritized along with workforce expansion (Spetz and Perivakoil 2019).

The provision of palliative care and community supports will better allow older adults to bring their lives to a satisfying end. The formation of relationships with individuals at the end of their lives to make their transition more comfortable and peaceful will give providers a greater sense of accomplishment and satisfaction than that provided by the disconnected and mechanical role taken in preserving life beyond its capacity for meaning. Those relationships allow providers to continue to grow in the context of the health care team and confront their own existential issues.

The approaches described in this chapter aim to achieve the delicate balance of cost and quality in psychiatric care of older adults and those at the end of their lives; however, much remains to be done before the balance is attained.

References

Applegate WB, Ouslander JG, Kuchel GA: Implementing "patient-centered care": a revolutionary change in health care delivery. J Am Geriatr Soc 66(10):1863–1865, 2018

Avari JN, Alexopoulos GS: Models of care for late-life depression of the medically ill: examples from chronic obstructive pulmonary disease and stroke. Am J Geriatr Psychiatry 23(5):477–487, 2015

Bartels SJ, Aschbrenner KA, Pratt SI, et al: Implementation of a lifestyle intervention for people with serious mental illness in state-funded mental health centers. Psychiatr Serv 69(6):664–670, 2018a

Bartels SJ, DiMilia PR, Fortuna KL, et al: Integrated care for older adults with serious mental illness and medical comorbidity: evidence-based models and future research directions. Psychiatr Clin North Am 41(1):153–164, 2018b

Bell J, Whitney RL, Young HM: Family caregiving in serious illness in the United States: recommendations to support an invisible workforce. J Am Geriatr Soc 67(S2):S451–S456, 2019

Blazer D, Le M, Maslow K, et al (eds): The Mental Health and Substance Use Workforce for Older Adults: In Whose Hands? Washington, DC, National Academies Press, 2012

Bone AE, Evans CJ, Higginson IJ: The future of end-of-life care. Lancet 392(10151): 915–916, 2018a

Bone AE, Gomes B, Etkind SN, et al: What is the impact of population ageing on the future provision of end-of-life-care? Population-based projections of place of death. Palliat Med 32(2):329–336, 2018b

Breitbart W, Rosenfeld B, Pessin H, et al: Depression, hopelessness, and desire for hastened death in terminally ill patients with cancer. JAMA 284(22):2907–2911, 2000

Breitbart W, Rosenfeld B, Gibson C, et al: Meaning-centered group psychotherapy for patients with advanced cancer: a pilot randomized controlled trial. Psycho-Oncology 19(1):21–28, 2010

Brink M, Green A, Bojesen AB, et al: Excess medical comorbidity and mortality across the lifespan in schizophrenia: a nationwide Danish register study. Schizophr Res 206:347–354, 2019

Brown T: How to make doctors think about death. New York Times, April 27, 2019. Available at: www.nytimes.com/2019/04/27/opinion/sunday/health-death.html. Accessed March 29, 2020.

Bruce ML, Sirey JA: Integrated care for depression in older primary care patients. Can J Psychiatry 63(7):439–446, 2018

Bruce ML, Lohman MC, Greenberg RL, et al: Integrating depression care management into Medicare home health reduces risk of 30- and 60-day hospitalization: the Depression Care for PATients at Home cluster-randomized trial. J Am Geriatr Soc 64(11):2196–2203, 2016

Callahan CM, Bateman DR, Wang S, et al: State of science: bridging the science-practice gap in aging, dementia and mental health. J Am Geriatr Soc 66 (suppl 1):S28–S35, 2018

Ceïde ME, Nguyen SA, Korenblatt A, et al: Beyond primary care: integrating psychiatry into a certified home health agency to identify and treat homebound older adults with mental disorders. J Community Med Health Educ 479(6), 2016

Clark PG: Emerging themes in using narrative in geriatric care: implications for patient-centered practice and interprofessional teamwork. J Aging Stud 34:177–182, 2015

Coast J, Bailey C, Kinghorn P: Patient centered outcome measurement in health economics: beyond EQ-5D and the Quality-Adjusted Life-Year—where are we now? Ann Palliat Med 7(Suppl 3):S249–S252, 2018

Eden J, Maslow K, Le M, et al (eds): The Mental Health and Substance Use Workforce for Older Adults: In Whose Hands? Washington, DC, National Academies Press, 2012

Erikson EH: Childhood and Society. New York, WW Norton, 1950
Foldes SS, Moriarty JP, Farseth PH, et al: Medicaid savings from the New York University Caregiver intervention for families with dementia. Gerontologist 58(2):e97–e106, 2017
Gagne JJ, Glynn RJ, Avorn J, et al: A combined comorbidity score predicted mortality in elderly patients better than existing scores. J Clin Epidemiol 64(7):749–759, 2011
Hayes MM, Turnbull AE, Zaeh S, et al: Responding to requests for potentially inappropriate treatments in intensive care units. Ann Am Thorac Soc 2(11):1697–1699, 2015
Jackson DS, Banerjee S, Sirey JA, et al: Two interventions for patients with major depression and severe COPD: impact on quality of life. Am J Geriatr Psychiatry 27(5):502–511, 2019
Jeste DV: Positive psychiatry comes of age. Int Psychogeriatr 30(12):1735–1738, 2018
Jha AK: End-of-life care, not end-of-life spending. JAMA 320(7):631–632, 2019
Joynt-Maddox KE: Financial incentives and vulnerable populations—will alternative payment models help or hurt? N Engl J Med 378(11):977–979, 2018
Kamal AH, Bowman B, Ritchie CS: Identifying palliative care champions to promote high-quality care to those with serious illness. J Am Geriatr Soc 67(S2):S461–S467, 2019
Kennedy GJ: Added value of the personalized intervention for depressed patients with COPD. Am J Geriatr Psychiatry 26(2):172–173, 2018
Kharrat A, Moore GP, Beckett S, et al: Antenatal consultations at extreme prematurity: a systematic review of parent communication needs. J Pediatr 196:109.e7–115.e7, 2018
Kocher R, Chigurupati A: The coming battle over shared savings—primary care physicians versus specialists. N Engl J Med 375(2):104, 2016
Long KH, Moriarty JP, Mittelman MS, et al: Estimating the potential cost savings with the New York University caregiver intervention in Minnesota. Health Affairs (Millwood) 33(4):596–604, 2014
McClain CS, Rosenfeld B, Breitbart W: Effect of spiritual well-being on end-of-life despair in terminally ill cancer patients. Lancet 1603(9369):1603–1607, 2003
Meier EA, Gallegos JV, Thomas LPM, et al: Defining a good death (successful dying): literature review and a call for research and public dialogue. Am J Geriatr Psychiatry 24(4):261–271, 2016
Mittelman MS, Ferris SH, Shulman E, et al: A family intervention to delay nursing home placement of patients with Alzheimer disease. A randomized controlled trial. JAMA 276(21):1725–1731, 1996
Nisker J: Social model of disability must be a core competency in medical education. CMAJ 191(16):E454, 2019
Olazarán J, Reisberg B, Clare L, et al: Nonpharmacological therapies in Alzheimer's disease: a systematic review of efficacy. Dement Geriatr Cogn Disord 30(2):161–178, 2010

Roest B, Trappenburg M, Leget C: The involvement of family in the Dutch practice of euthanasia and physician assisted suicide: a systematic mixed studies review. BMC Medical Ethics 20(1):23, 2019

Spetz J, Perivakoil VS: Introduction to the special issue on the workforce for seriously ill older adults in the community. J Am Geriatr Soc 67(S2):S390, 2019

Temkin-Greener H, Szydlowski J, Intrator O, et al: Perceived effectiveness of home-based primary care teams in Veterans Health Administration. Gerontologist January 18, 2019 [Epub ahead of print]

Teri L: Training families to provide care: effects on people with dementia. Int J Geriatr Psychiatry 14(2):110–116, 1999

Teri L, Logsdon RG: Assessment and management of behavioral disturbances in Alzheimer disease. Compr Ther 26(3):169–175, 2000

Thompson G, Shindruk C, Wickson-Griffiths A, et al: "Who would want to die like that?" Perspectives on dying alone in a long-term care setting. Death Stud 43(8):509–520, 2019

van der Spek N, Jansen F, Holtmaat K, et al: Cost-utility analysis of meaning-centered group psychotherapy for cancer survivors. Psychooncology 27(7):1772–1779, 2018

Volkert J, Harter M, Dehoust M, et al: The role of meaning in life in community-dwelling older adults with depression and relationship with other risk factors. Aging Ment Health 22(10):100–106, 2017

Yang JA, Wilhelmi BL, McGlynn K: Enhancing meaning when facing later life losses. Clin Gerontol 41(5):498–507, 2018

Part V
Conclusions

22

A Value Vision for Health Care Reform

Wesley E. Sowers, M.D.

Where to Find Value in Psychiatric Care

Over the course of this book, the concept of *value* has been considered from a variety of perspectives. Various aspects of systems and services have been examined to develop some common understanding of how the current conglomerate that constitutes our system of care might be delivered from its mediocracy and transformed into a high-value system. Knowing what to do is distinct from knowing how to do it, so it has also been important to consider the "values" of various constituents, the politics and vested interests of those who have power, and the historical antecedents of the current system. This final chapter of the book is an attempt to crystallize the recommendations and strategies identified in the preceding chapters into a coherent high-value approach to health care reform and the psychiatric care that will be a critical part of it. Acknowledging that there will be no easy transition to more advantageous models for delivering high-value health care, it also summarizes some of the political forces and economic pressures that will likely be encountered in efforts to implement the models (Kodish et al. 1996; Shimm et al. 1996). Movement toward these changes will likely be an incremental, step-by-step process, so it will be necessary to establish priorities for strategic planning of advocacy efforts. Potential priorities are identified in this chapter through an analysis of the current environment and a consideration of future forces that are likely to influence the system. Likewise, potential strategies for accomplishing the identified priorities are considered, in an effort to complete a blueprint for building the system that the United States desperately needs.

Financing and Access

Probably no single issue is more significant in determining the value we obtain from the services we provide than how services are paid for, and for whom and what. The failure of fee-for-service (FFS) financing to positively contribute to the value equation has been discussed in other chapters of this book (especially in Chapters 3, "The Current System," and 6, "Innovative Financing"). FFS has created a constriction in the capacity of service providers to organize interventions optimally and has been responsible for a major part of the excessive administrative expense in our system. Allowing market forces to determine the shape of services has been another major factor contributing to the high costs of care. A variety of patches have been devised, such as value-based payments, prospective payments, and several types of bundled or capitated payments. They have been designed to circumvent the problems commonly associated with FFS, but these have not had a significant impact on the system as a whole and have added a new level of complexity to an already complicated system (Everett et al. 2012).

Simplification and unification of funding sources will be important aspects of a new vision for health care financing. Provision of coverage to the entire population would eliminate isolated, inequitable risk pools and difficulties accessing affordable insurance. In conjunction with a single source of payment, many of the unnecessary expenses associated with excessive administrative structures and delayed treatment of preventable illness would be avoided. Providing incentives for the provision of high-quality care in publicly funded systems can be challenging. Value will be realized through an emphasis on population health over individual interventions (Berwick et al. 2008). Establishing priorities for coverage will be controversial as preventive and primary care take precedence over tertiary care. In the context of a publicly financed single-source payment model providing universal coverage, private insurance and private practices could emerge to serve those who choose additional coverage, as is the case in many other countries that adhere to this model, but a universal basic health care plan will benefit everyone (see Chapter 6).

Integration

Systems that are highly fragmented, as in the United States, have difficulties with communication between service providers, coordination of care for people with complex needs, flexible responses to individual needs, and payments for interventions that cross funding streams (Substance Abuse and Mental Health Services Administration 2014; Vickers et al. 2013). Easier access to comprehensive services that are needed to address concurrent health disorders is often compromised by programs that have a monolithic focus. Integration of the various fragments currently comprising this system should create 1) efficiency of administration, 2) ease of access to a comprehensive array of services, 3) smooth transitions between levels of service intensity, 4) concurrent use of specialized services (e.g., for treating comorbid schizophrenia and heart disease), and 5) coordinated service planning and management. Reduced cost, improved outcomes, and greater consumer and provider satisfaction will be the expected result (see Chapter 7, "Integration of Services").

Psychiatric Workforce

The scope of psychiatrists' skill and practice has been markedly reduced in recent years as a result of market forces, education financing, and constriction of training curricula. The consequence of this contraction has been a focus on biological treatments in most treatment settings and limitations on the duration of contacts with clients when administering these treatments. This scenario has had a number of negative implications for psychiatrists and the Quadruple Aim on which this book has focused (as introduced in Chapter 1, "Defining and Measuring Value"). Psychiatrists have found less satisfaction in their work due to productivity pressures, documentation requirements, limits on creativity, and the resulting deterioration in the quality of their relationships with clients. This situation has too frequently led to burnout or disengagement from their work (Fava et al. 2008). Service users have likewise been dissatisfied with brief visits, the focus on medication, and their limited relationship with their doctor. This dynamic reduces the quality of care, and ultimately increases its cost (see Chapter 11, "An Expanded Role for Psychiatry").

Reversing these trends needs to begin with education. A starting place might be to create more opportunities for medical school graduates to avoid heavy debt burdens and to make concurrent adjustments in compensation expectations. Expanding the diversity of psychiatric practice will require reconfigurations of training curricula to establish a working knowledge of multiple therapeutic modalities; systems theory and dynamics; primary care, consultation, and leadership skills; and other aspects of behavioral health treatment. This training, along with opportunities to continue limited engagement with these activities after graduation, could potentially allow psychiatrists to be more effective as service planners, team members, consultants, teachers, supervisors, program planners, administrators, and clinicians (DeMello and Deshpande 2011; Falk et al. 1998). Insertion of psychiatrists into these roles will limit their availability to provide direct medication management and generation of revenue in the current FFS paradigm, but could be easily accomplished under other funding arrangements. The most efficient use of psychiatric resources will rely on the inclusion of primary care physicians, psychiatric nurse practitioners, and physician assistants (see Chapter 12, "Psychiatric Workforce Development"). Although psychiatrists may see some reduction in their monetary compensation as new systems evolve, that loss would hopefully be offset by increased job satisfaction related to a broader scope of practice (see Chapters 11 and 12).

An increasing emphasis on team management will play a significant role in developing a workforce suited to meeting the demands for psychiatric care that will inevitably grow in the future as the ecological and social environments face new challenges. Making use of a full array of professional and paraprofessional staff will allow the provision of support, coordination, and continuity of care that will be required to counteract the impact of social conditions on the health and well-being of the population. Specifically, the inclusion of allied professional prescribers, care coordinators, people with lived experience, and other prevention and recovery specialists will be essential for achieving the Quadruple Aim in the future system of care (Bell et al. 2012; Herrman et al. 2002).

Pharmacy Management and Prescribing Practices

Medication has become a significant aspect of medical treatment. The dominance of pharmacological treatment has been experienced in psychiatry as well as other medical specialties, and some of the most frequently prescribed medications are psychotropics. Much could be gained through a reformulation of the relationship between purchasers and the pharmaceutical industry and judicious governmental regulation of profit opportunities for these companies (Goldman and Cutler 2002). Single-source payers would have considerable leverage to negotiate fair pricing for the medications they would be paying for. Government funding of new drug development would increase the relevance of research to identified needs and eliminate most of the bias that has infected industry-sponsored research in the past (Barkil-Oteo et al. 2014).

This kind of transformation will not be quickly accomplished, so the burden of cost reduction and quality improvement will lie with prescribers in the short term. Evidence-informed prescribing, cost-conscious medication choices, use of less expensive diagnostic technologies, limited use of polypharmacy, and attention to opportunities for dosage reductions or discontinuation will help to diminish the cost of treatment with medication, without significant reduction in effectiveness. As the most highly trained prescribers, psychiatrists should be engaged in the management of clients with the most complex needs and as consultants to other prescribers (Moriates et al. 2015). When they are employed in this way, psychiatrists can maintain diversity in their scope of practice, as alluded to in the previous section. A more diverse set of skills will reduce the temptation of psychiatrists to rely solely on medication, rather than a more holistic array of interventions, to address client needs (see Chapter 13, "Pharmaceutical Management and Prescribing").

Technology

The explosion of technological advances in medicine over the past few decades has been phenomenal, and it has been difficult for many clinicians to keep pace with it. These advances have had obvious benefits to the system's capacity to diagnose and treat illnesses that might otherwise be missed or belatedly discovered. These advances have also brought a capacity to gather and store health information, utilize data, extend access to services, enhance communication between providers, and allow service users to be active participants in their own care. Technology will undoubtedly continue to be a significant tool in the planning and delivery of health services in the future (Farabee et al. 2016).

Despite having these benefits, technology may create some inefficiencies and dissatisfaction as well. Electronic health records (EHRs) provide a clear example of this double-edged sword. Clinicians complain that EHRs are often difficult to navigate and therefore time consuming. This is especially true for older physicians with fewer computer skills. Many find expectations of concurrent documentation difficult, distracting, impersonal, or otherwise disruptive to the clinical relationship. As a result, additional time is needed to enter clinical information, or the additional expense of hiring a scribe is incurred (Sinsky et al. 2016). To ensure that technology does not detract from the Quadruple Aim rather than enhance it, it will be important to develop improvements to confidentiality, the remote interaction experience (telehealth applications), the online and virtual interaction experience, and artificial intelligence applications that facilitate the use of EHRs. Development of greater ease of access to medical records in a unified system and creating disincentives to use unnecessary diagnostic procedures will improve the benefit/harm ratio of these technological advances (see Chapter 10, "Applications of Technology").

Diagnostics

Complexity has been characteristic of the *Diagnostic and Statistical Manual of Mental Disorders* (DSM) since its inception in 1952 (American Psychiatric Association 1952). The complexity has only grown through the development of subsequent iterations. One of the major critiques of the system is that rather than being etiologically organized, it is phenomenological, as it must be in the absence of scientifically sound evidence of causation for the majority of psychiatric illnesses. DSM-5 lists 541 diagnoses with specific criteria that must be met for assignment of each (American Psychiatric Association 2013). It is unwieldy and fraught with difficult distinctions between entries in many of the diagnostic categories (Blashfield et al. 2014).

Although DSM diagnoses have been subject to reliability and validity testing under controlled conditions, clinicians find that their application is unreliable in practice (Freedman et al. 2013). Those clinicians attempting to use the system often feel as if they must try to fit a round peg in a square hole. In many cases, clinicians opt to treat the square hole they know rather than the round peg that creates uncertainty and ineffectiveness (Wakefield 2015).

Even in the absence of an etiological classification, a diagnostic system will have value if it facilitates communication and provides a rough portrait of a particular patient's complaints. Many have suggested that a dimensional diagnostic system is better suited for this task. Simplification and consolidation should lead to greater reliability, heuristic value for treatment purposes, and capacity for patients to comprehend their condition. The use of specific diagnoses to determine eligibility for treatment should be replaced by functional assessments, because diagnosis has not proven to be as useful for understanding a person's level of incapacitation (Timimi 2014). These changes will have a relatively small impact on the cost of care, but should yield benefits in terms of quality, greater concurrence between the functional diagnosis and treatment plan, and patient and clinician satisfaction (see Chapter 14, "Diagnostic Reform").

Prevention and Health Promotion

An emphasis on curing disease (secondary and tertiary care) has characterized the U.S. health care system. Although this emphasis has enabled some remarkable results for individuals who have been very ill, it has not been successful in the development of a healthy population. Lack of access to primary care for a significant portion of the population who are uninsured or underinsured as well as the adverse social conditions that impact health contribute to the poor health indicators in this country and to disparities in the health status between various social segments (see Chapter 4, "Social Determinants of Health").

Prevention takes place on many levels, and attention to each of them will yield positive population health results. Primary prevention interventions will most often take place in public systems rather than clinical settings. Universal, selective, and indicated interventions will all have a place in reducing the incidence of illness, thereby reducing the cost of treating them and enhancing the health and well-being of the population (Gordon 1983). Primary prevention will be more easily orchestrated and funded in integrated systems with public health prioritized. The broad availability of activities designed to reduce the risk factors associated with various diseases and enhance protective elements in the environment will produce major benefits. Health promotion may be part of community-based universal interventions, but it can also be provided in the offices of psychiatrists and other clinicians. Much can be accomplished through the expansion of access to primary care and the secondary prevention interventions that can be offered in those settings (see Chapter 8, "Prevention and Health Promotion"). The participation of psychiatrists in the provision of some aspects of primary care will expand the penetration of those benefits (Kalra et al. 2012).

More ambitiously, addressing the social and environmental determinants that negatively impact health would pay significant dividends. The following will improve both the physical health and mental health of communities: reduction of poverty; expanded opportunity for education and employment; and elimination of discriminatory practices based on race, religion, gender, culture, or disability (Komro et al. 2013). Developmental supports such as access to quality prenatal care, supports for parents, and social skills or competence building, among others, will result in a lower incidence of medical and behavioral health disorders as children move into adulthood. A reduction in the prevalence of adverse childhood experiences, which so significantly impact mental health, must be part of the strategy (Felitti et al. 1998). There need to be multiple points of entry for youth to learn appropriate developmental, self-efficacy, communication, and relationship skills. Early interventions are much more likely to be successful than those implemented later in development (see Chapters 4 and 8).

There are several other issues that indirectly impact population health, many of which arise from social policy. Drug policy is one example in which social "values" have prevented rational approaches to addressing drug use and reducing the harm that results from it. Treatment rather than punishment should be predominant in policy (see Chapter 17, "Addiction Treatment and Harm Reduction"). That approach will reduce crime, community disruption, and substance use–related illnesses. Incarceration as a response to illegal substance use is another source of social disruption, in that stubborn reliance on punitive responses has been counterproductive (Steadman and Naples 2005). A transition to truly rehabilitative approaches to people who use substances and an emphasis on harm reduction will be less costly and will diminish many of the social factors that contribute to poor health outcomes.

Politics often stand in the way of necessary changes, and the lack of response to climate change is another example in which this is the case. Despite the overwhelming evidence of man's contribution to global warming and the health impacts associated with it, there have been few interventions to mitigate its deterioration (Asugeni et al. 2015). Although it may be too late to reverse damages already done, strategies are critically necessary to reduce the progression of warming, create adaptations to reduce its impact on health, and develop adequate responses to the natural disasters that will become more frequent (see Chapter 18, "Impact of Climate Change").

Finally, one area in which change may be more easily realized, and in which some significant advances have already occurred, is in the workplace. Work environments that address stress and promote health have had significant impact on the health and well-being of the employees who work within them. Mental health disorders are a leading cause of disability and low productivity. Because work is a dominant activity in the lives of most people, a major priority should be to create environments that contribute to health rather than tax it. Demonstrable improvements in productivity, profitability, and satisfaction have been realized when precious human resources are nurtured rather than exploited, as has often been the case in the past. Stress has clearly been established as a major risk factor for the development or exacerbation of both physical and emotional health disruptions (Colligan and Higgins 2006), so reduction of the workplace as a source of stress is critical, because work plays such a significant role in the lives of most of the population (see Chapter 20, "Health and the Workplace").

End of Life

Appropriately, dealing with end-of-life care was the last topic of this book, but by no means the least important. Of course, death cannot be prevented, but the care provided to those approaching the end of their lives can reduce their suffering and that of their loved ones. Extraordinary measures to prolong life are seductive to many, but they are costly and ultimately self-serving for those making decisions about their application. Ironically, facilitating peaceful transitions to death can be a major source for enhancing the value of services provided by our systems of care (Foldes et al. 2017). Emphasis on palliative care and emotional closure are important aspects of easing this transition (see Chapter 21, "Aging and End-of-Life Care").

Allocation of Resources

Significant spending would be required to implement many of the recommendations made in this book. Examples include 1) technological enhancements to extend access and facilitate communication; 2) expansion of programming and the service array for underserved areas and populations; 3) increasing the availability of medical homes and care management to all individuals in need; and 4) growth of the psychiatric workforce and the inclusion of peer specialists on treatment teams. In the areas of prevention and addressing the sociopolitical determinants of health, even greater expenditures could be anticipated related to issues such as education, housing, transportation, and safety. Where do we find the resources to support these needs?

Critics of reform often point to expenses such as these, along with threats of increased taxes related to government spending on public programs, as the main argument against implementing needed changes. Those who profit from the current system are often the most vocal and powerful critics of reform and have thus far successfully blocked efforts to realize meaningful change. In doing so, they have creatively misrepresented the value equation and obscured the opportunities for savings that would offset these expenses.

Throughout this book, authors have discussed opportunities to save money. Reducing unwarranted and unjust incarcerations, elimination of administrative waste, health and mental health promotion, implementation of prevention programs and workplace health measures, harm reduction policies, and expansion of primary care with integrated emotional health services are just a few examples. In the long term, even greater savings would be generated from effectively addressing the social and environmental ills that seriously impact population health. After considering all of these variables and recognizing the successes of other nations that have implemented such interventions, one can see the potential for cost savings. Approaches include not only the reallocation of resources and the elimination of unnecessary expenses, but also the improvement of the quality of services and health outcomes. In the following sections, structures and strategies to achieve these savings are considered.

A Vision for Health Care Reform

The passage of the Patient Protection and Affordable Care Act (ACA) in 2010 led to many improvements with regard to the reach of health care coverage and the incorporation of some prevention principles. The architecture of the ACA was constrained by the need to satisfy powerful constituencies that believed more comprehensive reforms were either too expensive or not in their interest, as well as an oppositional political climate. As a result, affordability, one of the main hopes for the ACA, was never realized and costs continued to rise. At the same time, there have been disappointingly few improvements in the outcomes obtained. To achieve a system that obtains high value, more significant reform is needed.

Several organizations and authors have proposed guidelines or principles upon which, they suggest, a new system could be built. Although some of these suggestions contain only minor tweaks to the existing system, many propose more profound alterations. The common threads contained in these formulations include affordable universal coverage; expanded primary care, prevention, and accessibility; and simplified administration (American Academy of Family Practitioners 2019; American Heart Association 2020; American Nurses Association 2010). The American Association of Community Psychiatrists (2017), in the "AACP Principles to Guide Health Care Reform," includes these elements, as well as many of the other value concepts considered in this book. Major principles derived from these documents provide a foundation for building a system that delivers value. These principles are listed in Table 22–1.

The principles listed in the table might be incorporated into the structure of a health care system in a variety of ways. Some permutations will be more attractive to some stakeholders than to others. The challenge in building a system is to address the interests of all constituents well enough to make the plan politically viable. However, a high-value system of care requires that most of the concepts in this list must be included and should not be diluted.

The universal provision of a basic plan for health care serves everyone's interest by providing a framework upon which a value-driven system can be built. The cost of inefficient, ineffective care is ultimately borne by the public, paid for by taxes. If a universal system of coverage were in place, citizens will be more likely to obtain preventive and health-promoting care through primary care providers before their ailments become severe illnesses that require expensive treatments. A single plan for everyone would also allow the simplification of administrative processes and expenses, permitting more resources to be allocated for direct care. A corollary of this principle

TABLE 22–1. Principles for health care reform

Universal coverage
Emphasis on prevention
Administrative simplicity
Accessibility
Emphasis on primary care
Workforce enhancement
Technological sophistication
Integrated holistic services
Appropriate medical education
Need-based rationing
Integrated interventions for social determinants
Limited profit opportunities
Balanced incentives for cost and quality
Pharmaceutical industry regulation
Consumer choice of providers

is the elimination of conflicts of interest inherent in the profit-driven systems that have been a hallmark of U.S. health care (Everett et al. 2012; Griffin 2020).

For a universal health care plan to be implemented, an expansion of access is essential. To accomplish this change, a more robust and relevant workforce must be developed. This is particularly important for psychiatric care, which faces growing needs and dwindling capacity as large numbers of aging psychiatrists leave the workforce. Expansion of the workforce, in which its various elements would work in concert, will be required to overcome the accessibility issues that have contributed to the poor population health outcomes in the United States. Measures that ensure a more equitable distribution of health care resources need to be part of the solution. The use of new technologies that address access issues would be difficult to exclude from a plan (Cutler 2018; Mettler 2018; Shekhar et al. 2007).

The relationship of emotional health to overall health and well-being has been considered in many of the chapters of this book. Services to protect it and treat disruptions that do occur will be an important element of any reform plan. Although an improved focus on emotional health is not articulated separately as one of the principles of reform, it is implied by several. Universal coverage and accessibility, integrated care, an emphasis on primary care and prevention, needs-based rationing, and interventions for social determinants of health status all have relevance for inclusion of emotional health interventions. Any new approach to health care must recognize that emotional health is not distinct or separate from other aspects of health. Maintaining that artificial dichotomy would constitute a first step toward dooming any new scheme (Prince et al. 2007).

Psychiatry and other emotional health professions have made significant strides in uncovering the social and psychological implications of deprivations and trauma, and in developing supportive services and evidence-based practices to address them. Much is now known about what to do; the challenge continues to be how to do it. Reforms must remove the barriers that have typically stood in the way of installation of these practices over the long term, in order to harvest their full benefits. Reimagining professional training curricula with an emphasis on health maintenance and team-based care will be necessary if the value we seek is to be realized.

Models for Reform

There are numerous examples of what reform that incorporates the principles laid out in Table 22–1 might look like, both from within our own country and from international systems. Three of those models are briefly described before practical approaches for changing the health care systems in the United States are discussed.

National Health System

A national health system is similar to the National Health Service in Great Britain (www.britannica.com/topic/National-Health-Service) or the Veterans Health Administration system in the United States (www.va.gov/health). With centralized administration, either on a regional or federal level, an all-inclusive national health system provides direct care to all citizens free of charge, eliminating billing and profit opportunities. This administrative structure allows policy to be set in accord with public health needs. Allocation of resources can reflect those needs, ensure that prevention and health promotion are prioritized, and designate appropriate workforce parameters. Organization of services, expansion of access, incorporation of new technologies, and unified, accessible documentation can all be easily incorporated within this framework, and it is conceivable that resources to address larger public health and prevention activities could be administered through a branch of such an agency.

Although this type of system appears on the surface to be an ideal format to accomplish the objectives suggested by the principles for health care reform (see Table 22–1), it also presents several challenges that need to be addressed. Rationing tertiary care according to acuity, urgency, and demand is often tricky and dependent on the availability of resources. Long waits for elective or non-life-threatening surgeries or procedures have been the source of criticism for these types of plans. Continuity of care can also be problematic unless measures are in place that support an ongoing relationship with a primary care provider. These systems are generally administered on a regional basis, with providers responsible for a defined population. This arrangement will limit choices of care recipients if they are unhappy with their providers. If carefully planned, generous funding and the reprioritization of funding allocations can reduce many of these drawbacks. Private, supplemental medical insurance coverage might also reduce some of the inconveniences of a single system for those who choose to pay for it.

Single-Payer Universal Health Insurance

A single-payer universal health insurance model is similar to the Canadian system (Martin et al. 2018) or Medicare in the United States (www.usa.gov/medicare). These systems establish a basic health insurance plan with defined coverage for predetermined services. In the United States, the plan might be administered by the states or regional health authorities with federal subsidies or might be funded and administered entirely by the federal government. Citizens and the system could incorporate a graduated copay system ranging from zero for prevention and primary care, to a high percentage for elective care, thus discouraging overuse of tertiary care or unnecessary services. Negotiated contracts with providers, based on past utilization and performance, would allow for shared risk, innovation, moderate competition, and some consumer choice. This model would eliminate many of the profit opportunities related to the insurance and pharmaceutical industries and much of the waste associated with the administration of multiple payer systems. Global funding with risk sharing and value-based payments could be used to enhance quality and economy and reduce the constrictions of FFS payments. Conceivably, unified documentation and integration of services could be mandated by central or regional authorities. Payment priorities and allocation of resources could be based primarily on need rather than wealth and direct the development of the workforce.

The advantage of a single-payer universal health insurance system is that it reorganizes the system that is already in place. It is less disruptive of the free enterprise framework, and therefore it would likely be more palatable to business and political stakeholders. It would offer greater choice to consumers and could accommodate most of the listed principles for reform. This system would also accommodate a private, supplemental insurance industry, which could conceivably use existing health care providers.

On the other hand, this system is less pliable and relies on incentives to accomplish structural priorities rather than the policy directives of the health service model described in the previous section. Depending on available resources, rationing in this system would likely create waiting times for many types of tertiary care, similar to the health service model. Although it would create greater efficiency, the single-payer universal health model does not have the same potential for administrative parsimony.

Enhanced Employer-Based Health Insurance

A third option would be to retain a predominantly employer-based health insurance system and make it work better. This is essentially what the ACA attempted to do, but it was constrained in its reforms initially and then further undercut by the shifting of political winds (eHealth 2020). The institution of mandated coverage for all would be essential in this scenario, and a public insurance option would be helpful for those who are self-employed, unemployed, or otherwise uninsured through an employer. This system would also keep overcharging by private insurers in check. Although the system would not be ideal, much of the inefficiency of the present system could potentially be eliminated through this approach and it could achieve higher-quality outcomes. These improvements can only be realized, however, by more extensive use of value-based financing, episode-of-care rates, Accountable Care Organizations, and other shared risk arrangements between payers and providers, thereby eliminating most of the weaknesses of FFS arrangements (i.e., price variability, volume incentives, administrative burden). Negotiation of pricing for pharmaceuticals across all systems would bring price lines in the United States closer to those in other developed countries, and controls on profits by insurers would eliminate much of the wasted resources in our present system.

Building this system could accomplish many of the objectives related to the principles of reform, although it would likely be more complex and challenging to do so than in the other models considered earlier. This approach represents an incremental process that could be built gradually, making it more palatable for consumers who are wary of change and who are comfortable with structures they are more familiar with. It also has the advantage of preserving consumer choice to a large extent. Despite these advantages, there are several drawbacks. Price and profit controls would still find significant resistance from businesses and economically conservative politicians, even though this model would not remove profit extraction entirely. Prevention and population health are not so easily incorporated into this type of system, and fragmentation is more difficult to erase. The low level of government administration and the preservation of multiple payers would make the blending of funding to address the social determinants of health more complex, and access issues would likely remain.

Summary of Models

These three models represent distinct approaches to enhancing the value of health care services, and each has both advantages and disadvantages. Obviously, no system is perfect, and conversions to new paradigms can be fraught with uncertainty and unintended consequences. As discussed when considering solutions to climate change (see Chapter 18, "Impact of Climate Change"), solving the value equation is a type of "wicked" problem because various stakeholders have different interests. Pleasing one stakeholder will often displease another. Although the Quadruple Aim focuses primarily on the satisfaction of consumers and providers, other stakeholders' interests will create significant barriers to its fruition. Part of the challenge, then, will be to identify methods to maximize value regardless of the system in place, as is considered in the following section.

Value Management Methodology in Psychiatric Care

All systems of health care delivery benefit from having coherent processes and practices in place to enhance clinical assessment and decision making, efficient use of resources, clear communication, and service development. Creating tools to codify these processes provides a platform for monitoring outcomes and ensuring that needs are equitably addressed according to objective criteria. When resources for care are allocated to individuals according to their needs, rather than their means or other irrelevant characteristics, population health is better served, because constituents receive the right amount of care at the right time. Having tools of this kind in place will maximize the value of services delivered by any system of financing or service organization and help prevent the overuse of unnecessary services.

Development of tools to codify coherent processes and practices should coincide with the principles of system reform discussed previously (see Table 22–1). The functional characteristics provided by instruments developed for this purpose in psychiatric care might be as follows (Sowers 2012):

- *Functional assessment:* Provide quantifiable descriptions of impairments and identify needs.
- *Simplicity and brevity:* Make it easily understood and used.

- *Decision support:* Provide guidance for service planning and service intensity decisions.
- *Data collection:* Provide a platform for outcome analysis and for individual and system performance.
- *Integration:* Allow standardization of documentation, enhanced communication, and comprehensive service array.
- *Adaptability:* Make it easily used in a variety of situations and circumstances.
- *Accessibility:* Make it intuitive for clients and providers, facilitate clinical processes and reduce redundancies, and promote person-centered care.
- *Reliability and validity:* Support consistent application from various users and provide distinct and useful results.
- *Technological compatibility:* Enable EHR integration and programming changes while ensuring ease of use.

The Level of Care Utilization System (LOCUS) is one such tool that has these characteristics. Developed by the American Association of Community Psychiatrists in 1996, it is now used widely, though not always comprehensively, in both the United States and Canada. LOCUS was considered earlier in this book as a tool to support the clinical processes associated with recovery-oriented, person-centered care (see Chapter 16, "Psychiatric Leadership"). This tool has many other uses that can further enhance value in the delivery of care. LOCUS 20, which was released in 2016 (American Association of Community Psychiatrists 2016), and CALOCUS 20 (a Child and Adolescent version), released in 2019 (American Association of Community Psychiatrists 2019) both have had three sets of minor revisions since their initial release based on feedback from users over the 20 years since these tools were introduced (Sowers et al. 2003). The durability of their basic design and content has solidified their validity beyond the psychometric properties initially established (Sowers et al. 1999). In 2019, LOCUS was recognized as a national standard for service necessity decisions for mental health in the *Witt v. United Mental Healthcare* decision by the U.S. District Court of Northern California (Wit v. United Behavioral Health 2019).

Level of Care Utilization System

Systems that allow providers to make decisions about both care and resource use, perhaps with some guidance and assumption of risk, are most efficient because they eliminate redundancies and micromanagement, which are costly. LOCUS facilitates this by defining six levels of service intensity and six dimensions for assessing which level of service intensity is most appropriate. Because Dimension IV has two subscales, there are a total of seven assessment scales. Each assessment scale is rated from 1 to 5, based on specific criteria for each increment in rating. A composite score is obtained, which ranges from 7 to 35 and weighs prominently in the determination of recommendations about level of care. The six evaluation dimensions are outlined below (see Figure 16–1 in Chapter 16 for a copy of the worksheet).

I. Risk of Harm
II. Functional Status
III. Medical, Addictive, and Psychiatric Co-Morbidity
IV. Recovery Environment, with two subscales:
   A) Level of Stress and
   B) Level of Support
V. Treatment and Recovery History
VI. Engagement and Recovery Status

The assessments may be used for initial placement recommendations, or for determination of continuing care or transition needs. The system is based on a dynamic understanding of the course of an illness, and the assessment is repeated as frequently as indicated clinically. In general, ratings are repeated most frequently during periods of greatest acuity and instability.

Levels of Care

Six "levels of care" or service intensities are defined in LOCUS. Each level is described in terms of four variables: 1) Care Environment, 2) Clinical Services, 3) Support Services, and 4) Crisis Stabilization and Prevention Services. Each level describes a flexible array of services that are available according to individual needs. On average, service utilization becomes progressively more intensive (and expensive) as one moves from the lower to the higher levels of care. A description of each level of care follows.

1. **Recovery Maintenance and Health Management:** Designed for persons who have completed treatment at a more intensive level of care and who require minimal professional support to maintain their recovery.
2. **Low Intensity Community Based Services**: Provided to persons who need ongoing treatment but who are living independently or with minimal support in the community. Access to various types of supportive services can be facilitated.
3. **High Intensity Community Based Services**: Intended for persons who require more intensive support but are able to live in the community. Multimodal treatments, supportive services, and care coordination are available.

4. **Medically Monitored Non-Residential Services:** Intended for persons who are capable of living in community settings, but only with significant support-intensive treatment and case management. Partial hospital and Assertive Community Treatment programs are available.
5. **Medically Monitored Residential Services:** Provided to persons living in an unlocked residential setting. Structured social, educational, and rehabilitative activities are available as needed.
6. **Medically Managed Residential Services:** Provided to individuals living in a locked setting capable of providing close monitoring, attention, and safety. Multimodal treatment will be available, along with support of activities of daily living.

Placement Decisions

Placement criteria are provided in LOCUS for each level of care, listed above. A decision about an individual's placement is based on the most appropriate dimensional ratings for the particular level of care and the composite score from the assessment scale. In some cases, independent criteria (e.g., suicidal intentions) would supersede other requirements for level of care determinations. LOCUS has a simple and rapid methodology for arriving at placement recommendations.

Child and Adolescent Level of Care Utilization System

CALOCUS was developed in 1998 and follows the general format of the LOCUS for adults. It is modified to incorporate principles of child and adolescent development, a family and youth empowerment focus, and an emphasis on community-based systems of care (Fallon et al. 2006; Sowers et al. 2003). Similarly, the levels of care in CALOCUS are modified to reflect wrap-around approaches and the broader community service collaboration required to meet children's needs. The similarities between the two instruments make transitions between child and adult service systems go more smoothly and help bridge the gap between the two treatment communities. They both encourage a consistent and intuitive clinical thinking process, which is useful regardless of what service system is involved.

Scope of Use

As noted, the use of LOCUS has the potential to advance value in many ways, regardless of the system in which it is employed. (Note that for the sake of simplicity, in the remainder of this discussion, "LOCUS" and "the instrument" refer to both LOCUS and CALOCUS.) The primary intent of the instrument at its inception was to provide a simple yet comprehensive assessment of service needs and to match them to one of the six levels of service intensity defined by the instrument. In doing so, it promotes needs-based rationing (clients get exactly what they need, not more nor less, when a comprehensive continuum is in place) and individualized service planning. The simplicity and intuitiveness of its content facilitates the establishment of person-centered care and collaboration, enhancing client choice over what services they receive. By employing assessment components that include severity of mental illness, addiction, physical illness, stressors, and supports, as well as engagement and past experience in treatment, LOCUS allows a holistic approach to service planning. Broad use of this instrument would provide a clear language for communication between clinical entities and a framework to facilitate documentation and integration of services (Sowers 2012).

At the provider system level, LOCUS can help reduce administrative burden and waste, even in current FFS systems. When both payers and providers can embrace the same standard, micromanagement by payers can be reduced or eliminated, and providers can manage service intensity without interference, apart from occasional auditing to ensure proper use. Use of such a system therefore enhances the percentage of available resources devoted to services and reduces potential clinician burnout related to onerous utilization reviews. Identification of the social-environmental factors affecting emotional health helps in establishing a prevention incentive and highlights their contribution to the cost of care. Because of its ease of administration, LOCUS can be completed with minimal training by individuals from a variety of backgrounds, making it useful for screening in primary care settings, schools, and workplaces to identify difficulties before they become severe.

From a quality perspective, when LOCUS is used in a digital format, data can be easily harvested to chart the course of impairments, collective outcomes, and utilization analysis. This capacity is especially important for the management of larger systems of care (regional or state health administrations). Collecting data related to average service needs of the assessed population at a given time relative to the availability of services at a particular level of care can identify which types of services need to be created or which existing services need to be expanded. This function contributes to the establishment of a comprehensive continuum of service elements that can most efficiently meet the needs of a population.

LOCUS might also be used to develop case-related reimbursement rates (similar to diagnosis-related groups or capitation payment systems). These case-related rates would facilitate risk sharing by balancing incentives for payers and providers. With information related to the average cost of care at one of the six levels of service intensity, along with average length of service for people assigned to that service intensity, a fixed payment rate could be established for persons assigned to that level. For example, if the all-inclusive average cost of caring for people assigned to the most intense level of service (i.e., inpatient hospitalization) is $900 daily, and the average level of service for people assigned to that level is 5 days, then a rate of $4,500 could be established for each person admitted to that level of care. Prospective payments to providers based on past utilization records derived from LOCUS could also be developed. In either case, providers would have incentives to work within their means. Stratified case rates could also be developed using LOCUS ratings; these would account for chronicity and severity of illness in order to avoid inaccuracy of payments related to an uneven case mix (e.g., people with more chronic, severe mental illness would have longer stays and higher average costs).

Although an instrument such as LOCUS cannot provide all the elements required for high-value care, it does help to enhance the value equation. Implementation of this type of system will contribute to an incremental approach to higher value obtained from emotional health services. Even as systems evolve toward greater efficiency and population health, a framework of this type will continue to provide many useful advantages for managing services and resources effectively and guiding the pursuit of quality.

Confronting Barriers and Establishing Priorities

As described throughout this book, there are a variety of obstacles to the reform of the U.S. health care system, and the tenacity of this dysfunctional system, which delivers a low level of value, is a testament to the strength of these barriers. Although there have been some partial improvements in coverage and payment arrangements over the years (e.g., Medicare, Medicaid, Children's Health Insurance Program, Affordable Care Act), the more significant reforms needed to achieve a high-value system overall have met stiff resistance (Birn et al. 2003).

Businesses have exerted tremendous influence in protecting their ability to profit from the health care system and have spent an enormous amount of money in doing so. Pharmaceutical, insurance, and device manufacturing industries have vigorously promoted their products and organized campaigns to defeat any proposal that would limit the profits they extract from the system. Although many of these companies profess to be concerned about quality and the health of individuals, their first priority is making money, so any plan that impedes that objective will not be greeted gladly (Shimm et al. 1996). These industries are unlikely to be swayed by arguments that change would be for the greater good of the population. They typically create fears that government involvement will limit people's choices, limit their access to desired services, create job losses, and raise taxes. Information campaigns have so far been successful in convincing the public to stay the course and to support politicians who will vote to do so (Edmonds 2016).

Politics and politicians present another significant obstacle to change, particularly in the acrimonious partisan atmosphere of recent years. Even those legislators who understand the best interests of the public's health are often intimidated by party politics opposing change, or by the fear of alienating constituents who have a limited understanding of the issues and who are easily influenced by oppositional propaganda. Elected officials may feel the need to favor business interests that support their campaigns. Running for office has become increasingly expensive, and the outcome is heavily dependent on spending. Because power resides with those who have seniority in legislative bodies, it is very important to them to get reelected, and without assurances that other sources of support will be available, many politicians will be reluctant to support policies that threaten their donors, even when they know the worth of those policies.

Another barrier to change that must be confronted is the medical profession itself. The American Medical Association and other medical organizations have traditionally been quite resistant to change (Edmonds 2016; Zwier 2017). This attitude has begun to shift in recent years as more physicians migrated to public sector employment or large group practices—a change that occurred as the autonomy of solo private practices became more difficult to maintain in the evolving economic climate. There are still conservative elements of the medical community that do not trust imposition of controls that are not generated by the profession. Unfortunately, the profession has not done a very good job over the years of governing itself and creating standards and practices that promote value, or of advocating for policies that support population health and primary care. The supply of physicians has been unequal to the need for care, and with the skew of career selection leaning heavily toward the specialties, resources are often spent treating advanced illness and providing tertiary care. The issue of professional burnout and dissatisfaction has been raised in many chapters of this book; although the systems of care bear a large part of the responsibility for this situation, the medical profession has grossly misjudged its best interests and has contributed to its own detriment by acquiescing to market forces and eschewing practices to protect the quality of care and lower costs (Birn et al. 2003).

Taking these barriers into consideration, how does the psychiatric profession set priorities for change? Part II of this book identified several ways that systems must change to improve value, and Part III looked at value interventions on the level of service delivery. Many of these latter interventions could be carried out even in the absence of significant systems change. Incremental change is usually more digestible than radical or sudden changes, so it may be advantageous to focus first on those changes that can be made in the clinical work provided by psychiatrists and other behavioral health clinicians; this is the "low-hanging fruit." At the same time, advocacy for systemwide change, which will have the greatest impact once accomplished, must be pursued vigorously.

One way to think about priorities, as well as the strategies needed to implement them, is to categorize them according to complexity and the difficulty of achieving them. Although some of these interventions are related specifically to psychiatric care, many are universal and apply to the health care system as a whole. Table 22–2 divides the various interventions that have been considered in this book into three tiers of complexity. *Complexity* takes into account *constituency* (the level of diversity of stakeholders and their interests) and *resistance* to the barriers that are likely to be encountered.

Tier 1 interventions are those that can be changed most easily because constituents are relatively homogeneous in terms of their interests (health care providers, professionals, educators) and are fairly sophisticated in their ability to understand value concepts. These interventions face relatively few obstacles to their implementation. The major barriers to change for this group of interventions are ignorance and the challenge of educating constituents regarding the advantages of change and creating consensus. Several of these interventions have already found some traction and have demonstrated effectiveness in a piecemeal fashion. Their use will be more easily expanded with other systematic reforms, but most are possible even within the health care structures currently in place.

Tier 2 interventions have a more diverse constituency and the potential for greater conflicts of interest. These interventions also face greater obstacles to implementation, because they may cause dissatisfaction and resistance from some stakeholders. For example, pharmaceutical companies will likely resist regulation and pricing limitations, and groups with privacy concerns may oppose expanded access to health records. Partisan politics will come into play as many of these interventions are proposed, as has been the case in the past. A great deal more effort and advocacy will be needed to overcome the opposition put forth by those who wish to preserve their interests (e.g., profit), and in some cases, additional resources will be required (e.g., technological advances).

TABLE 22–2. Tiers of complexity for value interventions in psychiatric care

Tier 1 interventions: simple constituency—low resistance

- Training—residency training and continuing medical education
  - Secondary prevention and health promotion
  - Primary care interface—simple integration
  - Diversified curricula—expanded scope of practice
  - Cost consciousness in prescribing and diagnostic testing
- Implementation of value management tools (e.g., Level of Care Utilization System, American Society of Addiction Medicine Criteria)
- Expansion of alternative value-based funding options (e.g., Accountable Care Organizations, value-based funding)
- Revised/expanded practice guidelines and quality indicators
- Expansion of healthy workplace practices
- Expansion of peer specialist workforce
- Large-scale implementation of evidence-based practices

Tier 2 interventions: diverse constituency—moderate resistance

- Expanded workforce—nurse practitioner and physician assistant complementation
- User-friendly technology—simplified workflow
- Pharmaceutical regulation and negotiated pricing
- Universal "Cloud-based" medical records—enhanced access
- Universal coverage and parity—public insurance options
- Simplified diagnostic systems—functional assessment practices
- Delegation of risk and resource management to providers

Tier 3 interventions: complex constituency—high resistance

- Primary prevention—public health and integration of social determinants
  - Corrections reform—rehabilitation and reintegration
  - Drug policy reform—treatment and harm reduction strategies
  - Climate change preparation and mitigation
  - Elimination of poverty and expansion of opportunity for all
- Universal basic health plan
- Single-source financing—elimination of profit extractions

Tier 3 interventions present the greatest challenge for implementation, but also offer the greatest benefit for value and population health once they are accomplished. The constituency for these interventions is society at large with all its variation and complex and divergent interests. These interventions face mighty opposition from those entities that currently profit from the system that is in place, and business concerns will likely bring the force of their influence to the politicians who must ultimately agree to make these changes. Many of these changes would require a degree of government investment, regulation, and administration that would be unpalatable to many libertarian and conservative groups who are suspicious of government control. It would also be necessary to overcome the fractious state of society with a recognition that everyone benefits in some way from measures that protect the health of all members of society.

Conclusion: Finding Value

We began our search for value in psychiatric care from a place that demonstrated very little value. As the journey progressed, we discovered many opportunities to enhance value. In most respects, we know the things we must do, but the challenge lies in how to do them. Many forces have aligned to obstruct progress toward the installation of the various interventions that can improve the value of the services provided by the U.S. health care systems, and strategies are necessary that recognize that incremental change is needed and is most likely to be successful. Various interventions can be implemented without significant change in the infrastructure currently in place, and these changes should be made without delay. Many of the other measures that are anticipated to enhance value will require greater patience and tenacity in their pursuit.

Although we have emphasized value in psychiatric care, it has been noted repeatedly through this book that physical health and emotional health are inextricably intertwined. Many aspects of the improved value interventions that have been outlined cannot be realized by implementation in only one part of the system. One important principle that emerges from our investigations is that reform must incorporate the integration of all aspects of health care, and that emotional health must be a prominent part of that design. A corollary of this is the necessity of collaboration with the full array of stakeholders: allied professionals, administrators, payers, service users, government representatives, educators, law enforcement and correction officials, climatologists, journalists, and the public at large. It is only through these connections and a search for common ground that we can reach the lofty goal of high-value health care and well-being for all members of our society.

References

American Academy of Family Practitioners: Health care for all: a framework for moving to a primary care-based health care system in the United States. December 10, 2019. Available at: www.aafp.org/about/policies/all/health-care-for-all.html. Accessed March 31, 2020.

American Association of Community Psychiatrists: LOCUS: Level of Care Utilization System for Psychiatric and Addiction Services, Adult Version 20. 2016. Available at: www.communitypsychiatry.org/resources/locus. Accessed April 8, 2020.

American Association of Community Psychiatrists: AACP principles to guide health care reform. 2017. Available at: https://drive.google.com/file/d/0Bx-GKNvcx-xl-a09hTE12b1hsOWs/view. Accessed March 31, 2020.

American Association of Community Psychiatrists: CALOCUS: Child and Adolescent Level of Care Utilization System—Child and Adolescent Version 20. July 2019. Available at: www.communitypsychiatry.org/resources/locus. Accessed March 12, 2020.

American Heart Association: Principles on health care reform. 2020. Available at: www.heart.org/idc/groups/heart-public/@wcm/@adv/documents/downloadable/ucm_306161.pdf. Accessed March 31, 2020.

American Nurses Association: Health system reform: nursing's goal of high quality, affordable care for all. 2010. Available at: www.nursingworld.org/~4ae32b/globalassets/docs/ana/health-system-reform---final--haney---6-10-10.pdf. Accessed March 31, 2020.

American Psychiatric Association: Diagnostic and Statistical Manual of Mental Disorders. Washington, DC, American Psychiatric Association, 1952

American Psychiatric Association: Diagnostic and Statistical Manual of Mental Disorders, 5th Edition. Washington, DC, American Psychiatric Association, 2013

Asugeni J, MacLaren D, Massey PD: Mental health issues from rising sea level in a remote coastal region of the Solomon Islands: current and future. Australas Psychiatry 23(6 Suppl):22–25, 2015

Barkil-Oteo A, Stern DA, Arbuckle MR: Addressing the cost of health care from the front lines of psychiatry. JAMA Psychiatry 71(6):619–620, 2014

Bell C, McBride D, Redd J, et al: Team-based treatment, in Handbook of Community Psychiatry. Edited by McQuistion H, Sowers W, Ranz J, et al. New York, Springer Science+Business Media, 2012, pp 211–221

Berwick DM, Nolan TW, Whittington J: The Triple Aim: care, health, and cost. Health Aff (Millwood) 27(3):759–769, 2008

Birn A, Brown T, Fee E, et al: Struggles for national health reform in the United States. Am J Public Health 93(1):86–91, 2003

Blashfield RK, Keeley JW, Flanagan EH, et al: The cycle of classification: DSM-I through DSM-5. Annu Rev Clin Psychol 10:25–51, 2014

Colligan TW, Higgins EM: Workplace stress: etiology and consequences. J Workplace Behav Health 21(2):89–97, 2006

Cutler D: What is the U.S. health spending problem? Health Aff (Millwood) 37(3):493–497, 2018

DeMello JP, Deshpande SP: Career satisfaction of psychiatrists. Psychiatr Serv 62(9):1013–1018, 2011

Edmonds SA: Where is the resistance to health care reform? Healio: Primary Care Optometry News, February 5, 2016. Available at: www.healio.com/optometry/regulatory-legislative/news/blogs/%7B3baabe84-ac07-4587-9890-e438b5f15b05%7D/scott-a-edmonds-od-faao/blog-where-is-the-resistance-to-health-care-reform. Accessed March 31, 2020.

eHealth: History and timeline of the Affordable Care Act. March 2, 2020. Available at: www.ehealthinsurance.com/resources/affordable-care-act/history-timeline-affordable-care-act-aca. Accessed March 31, 2020.

Everett A, Sowers W, McQistion H: Financing of community behavioral health services, in Handbook of Community Psychiatry. Edited by McQuistion H, Sowers W, Ranz J, et al. New York, Springer Science+Business Media, 2012, pp 45–59

Falk N, Cutler D, Birecree E, et al: The community psychiatrist: King Lear, Hamlet, or Fishmonger? Traditional vs. nontraditional roles and settings. Journal of Practical Psychiatry and Behavioral Health 4(6):346–355, 1998

Fallon T, Pumariega A, Sowers W, et al: A level of care instrument for children's systems of care: construction, reliability, and validity. J Child Fam Stud 15(2):143–155, 2006

Farabee D, Calhoun S, Veliz R: An experimental comparison of telepsychiatry and conventional psychiatry for parolees. Psychiatr Serv 67(5):562–565, 2016

Fava GA, Park SK, Dubovsky S: The mental health clinic: a new model. World Psychiatry 7(3):177–181, 2008

Felitti VJ, Anda RF, Nordenberg D, et al: Relationship of childhood abuse and household dysfunction to many of the leading causes of death in adults. American Journal of Preventive Medicine 14(4):245–258, 1998

Foldes SS, Moriarty JP, Farseth PH, et al: Medicaid savings from the New York University Caregiver Intervention for families with dementia. Gerontologist 58(2):e97–e106, 2017

Freedman R, Lewis D, Michels R, et al: The initial field trials of DSM-5: new blooms and old thorns. Am J Psychiatry 170(1):1–5, 2013

Goldman C, Cutler DL: Pharmaceutical industry support of psychiatric research and education: ethical issues and remedies, in Ethics in Community Mental Health Care: Commonplace Concerns. Edited by Backlar PB, Cutler DL. New York, Kluwer Academic, 2002, pp 209–233

Gordon R: An operational classification of disease prevention. Public Health Rep 98(2):107–109, 1983

Griffin J: The history of healthcare and organized medicine in America. JP Griffin Group, March 27, 2020. Available at: www.griffinbenefits.com/employeebenefitsblog/history_of_healthcare. Accessed April 1, 2020.

Herrman H, Trauer T, Warnock J: Professional Liaison Committee (Australia) project team: the roles and relationships of psychiatrists and other service providers in mental health services. Aust NZJ Psychiatry 36(1):75–80, 2002

Kalra G, Christodoulou G, Tsipas N, et al: Mental health promotion: guidance and strategies. Eur Psychiatry 27(2):81–86, 2012

Kodish E, Murray T, Whitehouse P: Conflict of interest in university-industry research relationships: realities, politics, and values. Acad Med 71(12):1287–1290, 1996

Komro KA, Tobler AL, Detiole AL, et al: Beyond the clinic: improving child health through evidence-based community development. BMC Pediatr 13:172, 2013

Martin D, Miller A, Quesnel-Vallee A, et al: Canada's universal health-care system: achieving its potential. Lancet 381(10131):1718–1735, 2018

Mettler S: The Government-Citizen Disconnect. New York, Russell Sage Foundation, 2018

Moriates C, Arora V, Shah N: High-value medication prescribing, in Understanding Value-Based Health Care. New York, McGraw-Hill Education, 2015, pp 253–278

Prince M, Patel V, Saxena S, et al: No health without mental health. Lancet 370(9590):859–877, 2007

Shekhar S, Thornicroft G, Knapp M, et al: Resources for mental health: scarcity, inequity, and inefficiency. Lancet 370(95):878–889, 2007

Shimm D, Spece R, DiGregorio M: Conflicts of interest in relationships between physicians and the pharmaceutical industry, in Conflicts of Interest in Clinical Practice and Research. Edited by Spece R, Shimm D, Buchanan A. New York, Oxford University Press, 1996, pp 321–357

Sinsky C, Colligan L, Li L, et al: Allocation of physician time in ambulatory practice: a time and motion study in 4 specialties. Ann Intern Med 165(11):753–760, 2016

Sowers W: Service and resource management, in Handbook of Community Psychiatry. Edited by McQuistion H, Sowers W, Ranz J, et al. New York, Springer Science+Business Media, 2012, pp 533–542

Sowers W, George C, Thompson K: Level of care utilization system for psychiatric and addiction services: preliminary reliability and validity testing. Community Ment Health J 35(6):545–563, 1999

Sowers W, Pumariega A, Huffine C, et al: Level-of-care decision making in behavioral health services: the LOCUS and CALOCUS. Psychiatr Serv 54(11):1461–1463, 2003

Steadman HJ, Naples M: Assessing the effectiveness of jail diversion programs for persons with serious mental illness and co-occurring substance use disorders. Behav Sci Law 23(2):163–170, 2005

Substance Abuse and Mental Health Services Administration: Center for Integrated Health Solutions: essential elements of effective integrated primary behavioral health terms. 2014. Available at www.integration.samhsa.gov/workforce/team-members/Essential_Elements_of_an_Integrated_Team.pdf. Accessed August 26, 2019.

Timimi S: No more psychiatric labels: why formal psychiatric diagnostic systems should be abolished. Int J Clin Health Psychol 14(3):208–215, 2014

Vickers KS, Ridgeway JL, Hathaway JC, et al: Integration of mental health resources in a primary care setting leads to increased provider satisfaction and patient access. Gen Hosp Psychiatry 35(5):461–467, 2013

Wakefield J: DSM-5, psychiatric epidemiology and the false positives problem. Epidemiol Psychiatr Sci 24(3):188–196, 2015

Wit v United Behavioral Health, Case No. 14-cv-02346-JCS, February 28, 2019. Available at: www.courtlistener.com/recap/gov.uscourts.cand.277588/gov.uscourts.cand.277588.418.0.pdf. Accessed March 31, 2020.

Zwier P: Challenges of health care reform in 2017. 2017. Available at: http://law.emory.edu/ecgar/content/volume-4/issue-special/essays-interviews/challenges-health-care-reform-2017.html. Accessed March 31, 2020.

Index

Page numbers printed in **boldface** *type refer to tables or figures.*